AF352361

CLINICAL APPLICATIONS OF CYTOKINES AND GROWTH FACTORS

CLINICAL APPLICATIONS OF CYTOKINES AND GROWTH FACTORS

edited by

JOHN R. WINGARD
University of Florida College of Medicine, USA

and

GEORGE D. DEMETRI
Dana Farber Cancer Institute, Harvard Medical School, USA

Distributors for North, Central and South America:
Kluwer Academic Publishers
101 Philip Drive
Assinippi Park
Norwell, Massachusetts 02061 USA

Distributors for all other countries:
Kluwer Academic Publishers Group
Distribution Centre
Post Office Box 322
3300 AH Dordrecht, THE NETHERLANDS

Library of Congress Cataloging-in-Publication Data

Clinical applications of cytokines and growth factors / edited by John
   R. Wingard and George D. Demetri.
        p.   cm. -- (Developments in oncology ; 80)
     Includes index.
     ISBN 0-7923-8486-5
     1. Blood--Diseases--Immunotherapy. 2. Hematopoietic growth
factors--Therapeutic use.   3. Growth factors--Therapeutic use.
     I. Wingard, John R., 1947-   . II. Demetri, George D., 1956-
III.   Series.
     [DNLM: 1. Cytokines--pharmacology. 2. Cytokines--therapeutic use.
3. Growth Substances--pharmacology. 4. Growth Substances-
-therapeutic use.   W1 DE998N v.80 1999]
     RC636.C54   1999
     616.07'9--dc21
     DNLM/DLC
     for Library of Congress   99-22740
                                                                    CIP

Printed on acid-free paper.

Printed in the United States of America

TABLE OF CONTENTS

List of Contributors viii

Introduction xi

I. **Biology of Hematopoietic and Lymphopoietic Cytokines**

1. Cytokines, Growth Factors, and Hematopoiesis
   G. BAGBY and M. HEINRICH 2

2. The Interaction of Cytokines with Stem Cell and Stromal Cell
   Physiology
   P. SIMMONS, D.N. HAYLOCK, J-P LEVESQUE, and
   A.C.W. ZANNETTINO 56

3. The Interaction of Cytokines with T-cell and Natural Killer Cell
   Physiology
   R.A. CARTER and E.K. WALLER 74

4. Improving on Nature by Re-Engineering Hematopoietic Growth
   Factors
   Y.FENG and J. MCKEARN 90

II. **Management of Neutropenia and Neutropenic Fever**

5. The Influence of Colony Stimulating Factors on Neutrophil
   Production, Distribution, and Function
   J.M. GAVIRIA, W.C. LILES, and D.C. DALE 118

6. Evidence-Based Use of Hematopoietic Cytokines in Clinical
   Oncology
   G.D. DEMETRI 137

7. Economic, Public Health, and Policy Implications of Hematopoietic
   Growth Factors, High-Dose Chemotherapy, and Stem Cell Rescue
   C.L. BENNETT and T.J. STINSON 150

8. Outpatient Management of Neutropenic Fever: Antibiotics, Growth
   Factors or Both?
   E.B. RUBINSTEIN, L.S. ELTING, C.C. SUN, and
   K.V.I. ROLSTON 159

9. The Use of Hematopoietic Growth Factors for Recruitment of
   Leukocytes for Transfusion
   D.B. JENDIROBA, B. LICHTIGER, and E. J FREIREICH 178

III.   Management of Anemia

10. Pathophysiology of the Anemia of Malignancy
J.W. ADAMSON 187

11. The Use of Recombinant Erythropoietin in the Treatment and
Prevention of Cancer and Chemotherapy Related Anemia
J. L. SPIVAK 198

IV Management of Thrombocytopenia

12. Regulation of Human Megakaryocytopoiesis
R. HOFFMAN and M.W. LONG 218

13. The Effects of Multilineage Cytokines on Platelet Recovery
R. VIJ and J. DIPERSIO 237

14. Clinical Studies of Thrombopoietin
R. BASSER 269

V. The Role of Cytokines to Enhance Cancer Chemotherapy

15. Dose Intensification in Solid Tumor Chemotherapy
H. VAN DEVENTER and T. SHEA 279

16. Conventional and High Dose Chemotherapy for Lymphomas
K.W. VAN BESIEN 300

17. Hematopoietic Growth Factors in Acute Leukemia
R. STONE 313

VI. Management of Marrow Failure States

18. Cytokines for the Treatment of Myelodysplastic Syndromes
and Other Bone Marrow Failure States
R. S. NEGRIN 326

VII   The Use of Cytokines in Blood and Marrow Transplantation

19. Stem Cell Collection for Hematopoietic Transplantation: Stem
Cell Sources, Mobilization Strategies, and Factors that Influence
Yield
J.R. WINGARD and F.M. WEEKS 341

20. Mechanisms of Growth Factor Mobilization of Hematopoietic
Progenitors
D. LINK 357

21. The Use of Cytokines to Enhance Collection of Stem Cells for
     Marrow and Blood Transplantation
     S. ROMAN-UNFER and E.J. SHPALL 369

22. The Use of Cytokines During Blood and Marrow Transplantation
     J. NEMUNAITIS 381

Index 403

List of Contributors

JOHN W. ADAMSON, M.D., Director of Research, Lindsley F. Kimball Research Institute, New York Blood Center, New York, NY 10021

GROVER BAGBY, M.D., Professor of Medicine and Molecular Medical Genetics, Director, Oregon Cancer Center, Oregon Health Sciences University, Portland, OR 97201

RUSSELL BASSER, MBBS., Centre for Developmental Cancer Therapeutics, Royal Melbourne Hospital, Victoria, Australia, 3050

CHARLES L. BENNETT, M.D., Ph.D., Associate Professor, Northwestern University, VA Chicago Health Care Systems, Lakeside Division, Medical Science Building, Chicago, IL 60611

RICHARD A. CARTER, M.D., Assistant Professor of Medicine, Emory University School of Medicine, Atlanta, GA 30322

DAVID C. DALE, M.D., Professor of Medicine, Department of Medicine, University of Washington, Seattle, WA 98195

GEORGE D. DEMETRI, M.D., Assistant Professor of Medicine, Department of Adult Oncology, Dana-Farber Cancer Institute and Harvard Medical School, Boston, MA 02115

JOHN DIPERSIO, M.D., Professor of Medicine, Pathology, and Pediatrics, Chief, Division of BMT and Stem Cell Biology, Washington University School of Medicine, St. Louis, MO 63110

LINDA S. ELTING, Dr.P.H., Associate Professor of Epidemiology, MD Anderson Cancer Center, Houston, TX 77030

YIQING FEN, Ph.D., Senior Research Investigator, SEARLE/A Monsanto Company, St. Louis, MO 63198

EMIL J FREIREICH, M.D., D.Sc. (Hon), Professor of Medicine, University of Texas MD Anderson Cancer Center, Houston, TX 77030

J. MILTON GAVIRIA, M.D., Senior Fellow, Division of Infectious Disease, Department of Medicine, University of Washington, Seattle, WA 98195

DAVID N. HAYLOCK, B.App.Sci.,Hanson Centre for Cancer Research, Division of Haematology, Institute of Medical and Veterinary Science, Adelaide, Australia, SA5000

MICHAEL HEINRICH, M.D., Associate Professor of Medicine, Oregon Health Sciences University, Portland, OR 97201

RONALD HOFFMAN, M.D., Eileen Heidrick Professor of Oncology, Chief, Hematology/Oncology Section, Molecular Biology Research Laboratory, University of Illinois College of Medicine, Chicago, IL 60607

DAVID B. JENDIROBA, M.D., Graduate Research Assistant, University of Texas MD Anderson Cancer Center, Houston, TX 77030

JEAN-PIERRE LEVESQUE, PH.D, Hanson Centre for Cancer Research, Division of Haematology, Institute of Medical and Veterinary Science, Adelaide, Australia, SA5000

BENJAMIN LICHTIGER, M.D., Ph.D., Professor of Medicine, University of Texas MD Anderson Cancer Center, Houston, TX 77030

W. CONRAD LILES, M.D., Ph.D., Assistant Professor, Division of Infectious Diseases, Department of Medicine, University of Washington, Seattle, WA 98195

DANIEL LINK, M.D., Assistant Professor, Washington University School of Medicine, St. Louis, MO 53110

MICHAEL W. LONG, M.D., Associate Professor, Pediatric Hematology/Oncology Section, University of Michigan School of Medicine, Ann Arbor, MI

JOHN MCKEARN, Ph.D., Executive Director of Discovery Research, SEARLE/A Monsanto Company, St. Louis, MO 63198

ROBERT S. NEGRIN, M.D., Associate Professor of Medicine, Stanford University Hospital, Stanford, CA 94305

JOHN NEMUNAITIS, M.D., Regional Director, PRN Research, Inc.; Director, TOPA Research, Physician Reliance Network, Dallas, TX 75246

KENNETH V.I. ROLSTON, M.D., Professor of Medicine, MD Anderson Cancer Center, Houston, TX 77030

SUSAN ROMAN-UNFER, M.D., Bone Marrow Transplant Fellow, University of Colorado Health Science Center, Bone Marrow Transplant Program, Denver, CO 80262

EDWARD B. RUBENSTEIN, M.D., Associate Professor, University of Texas MD Anderson Cancer Center, Houston, TX 77030

THOMAS SHEA, M.D., Professor of Medicine, Department of Medicine, Division of Hematology/Oncology, University of North Carolina, Chapel Hill, NC 27599

ELIZABETH J. SHPALL, M.D., Professor of Medicine, University of Colorado Health Science Center Bone Marrow Transplant Program, Denver, CO 80262

PAUL SIMMONS, M.D., Matthew Roberts Laboratory, Division of Hematology, Hanson Centre for Cancer Research, Adelaide, Australia, SA5000.

JERRY L. SPIVAK, M.D., Professor of Medicine and Oncology, Johns Hopkins University School of Medicine, Baltimore, MD 21205

TAMMY J. STINSON, M.S., Research Analyst, VA Chicago Health Care Systems, Lakeside Division, Medical Science Building, Chicago, IL 60611

RICHARD STONE, M.D., Associate Professor of Medicine, Harvard University, Dana Farber Cancer Institute, Boston, MA 02114

CHARLOTTE C. SUN, M.P.H., Graduate Research Assistant, University of Texas MD Anderson Cancer Center, Houston, TX 77030

KOEN B. VAN BESIEN, M.D., Associate Professor of Medicine, Director, Stem Cell Transplantation, University of Illinois-Chicago, Chicago, IL 60612

HENRIK VAN DEVENTER, M.D., Research Fellow, Department of Medicine, Division of Hematology/Oncology, University of North Carolina, Chapel Hill, NC 27599

RAVI VIJ, M.D., Fellow, Division of Bone Marrow Transplantation and Stem Cell Biology, Washington University School of Medicine, St. Louis, MO 63110

EDMUND K. WALLER, M.D., Ph.D., Assistant Professor of Medicine, Emory University School of Medicine, Atlanta, GA 30322

FREDERICK M. WEEKS, M.D., Assistant Professor of Medicine, Division of Hematology/Oncology, University of Florida College of Medicine, Shands Hospital, Gainesville, FL 32610

JOHN R. WINGARD, M.D., Professor of Medicine, Director, Bone Marrow Transplant Program, Division of Hematology/Oncology, University of Florida College of Medicine, Shands Hospital, Gainesville, FL 32610

ANDREW C.W. ZANETTINO, Ph.D., Hanson Centre for Cancer Research, Division of Haematology, Institute of Medical and Veterinary Science, Adelaide, Australia, SA5000

Introduction

The hematopoietic system plays roles that are crucial for survival of the host: delivery of oxygen to tissues, arrest of accidental blood leaking from blood vessels, and fending off of invading microbes by humoral, cell-mediated, and phagocytic immunity.

The activity of the hematopoietic system is staggering: daily, a normal adult produces approximately 2.5 billion erythrocytes, 2.5 billion platelets, and 1 billion granulocytes per kilogram of body weight. This production is adjusted in a timely fashion to changes in actual needs and can vary from nearly none to many times the normal rate depending on needs which vary from day to day, or even minute to minute. In response to a variety of stimuli, the cellular components of the blood are promptly increased or decreased in production to maintain appropriate numbers to optimally protect the host from hypoxia, infection, and hemorrhage.

How does this all happen and happen without over or under responding? There has been extraordinary growth in our understanding of hematopoiesis over the last two decades. Occupying center stage is the pluripotent stem cell and its progeny. Hematopoietic stem cells have been characterized by their capacity for self renewal and their ability to proliferate and differentiate along multiple lineages. Few in number, the stem cell gives rise to all circulating neutrophils, erythrocytes, lymphoid cells, and platelets. In hematopoietic transplantation, the stem cell is capable of restoring long-term hematopoiesis in a lethally irradiated host.

Expansion of the numbers of progeny of stem cells provides the host with an enormous capacity for hematopoietic homeostasis. As important as stem cells are, however, it is now recognized that it is only through very complex interactions with other cells in the stromal microenvironment, physical contact with matrix proteins in the bone marrow, and exposure to soluble proteins which have growth stimulatory and growth inhibitory properties, such as hematopoietic growth factors and various adhesion molecules, that stem cells can do their jobs. Thus, these "supporting actors" are every bit as important as stem cells in the regulation of hematopoiesis. The growth factors, their actions, and their clinical roles, are the subject of this volume.

Hematopoietic growth factors are a family of glycoproteins that regulate proliferation, differentiation, and function of hematopoietic cells. The specific function of these molecules are complex and redundant. Their activity may be lineage-specific or affect cells of multiple lineages. These molecules are synthesized by lymphocytes, monocytes, stromal cells, and a host of other cell types as well.

The identification and isolation of their genes has led to mass production of recombinant hematopoietic growth factor molecules. The availability of these molecules, in turn, have made possible in vitro studies on progenitor cell proliferation and function to achieve better understanding of hematopoiesis and, subsequently, clinical trials.

Today, several growth factors are available to the clinician as treatments for various pathologic pertubations of hematopoiesis. Their use has also advanced our capacity to safely deliver cancer chemotherapy. Hematopoietic growth factors have become an everyday tool for the practicing oncologist.

In this volume, recognized experts review the biological interactions between hematopoietic progenitors, growth factors and cytokines, and the stromal microenvironment that have provided the scientific basis for our current understanding of the hematopoiesis. In subsequent sections, the pathophysiology of neutropenia, anemia, and thrombocytopenia are presented, along with discussions of the clinical challenges these pose for the practicing oncologist and hematologist and the roles of various hematopoietic growth factors in therapeutic strategies for these entities.

The roles of chemotherapy dose intensity and dose density are of crucial importance as theoretical and practical frameworks to plan strategies to optimize treatment protocols for solid tumors, lymphomas, and leukemia. These issues are discussed to provide the oncologist with an up to date assessment of the contribution (or lack thereof in some cases) of hematopoietic growth factors in establishing data to confirm or refute various theoretical premises of cancer chemotherapy.

In the final section, the role of hematopoietic growth factors in the field of hematopoietic cell transplantation is discussed. Certainly transplantation, as a vehicle to achieve the ultimate in dose intensity, has now established a role for itself in clinical oncology as an established treatment with superior outcomes for a number of disease scenarios when compared to less aggressive treatment options. However, its role remains investigational in other situations. Because of high rates of morbidity and mortality, this treatment strategy was limited in its applications throughout much of the 1980's. With the advent of hematopoietic growth factors, mortality, morbidity, length of hospitalization, and treatment costs have dramatically fallen. The use of hematopoietic growth factors to mobilize hematopoietic progenitors has led most transplant centers to abandon the use of bone marrow as a source of stem cells in favor of "mobilized" peripheral blood progenitor cells. This shift has furthered patient acceptance and led to even greater degrees of safety and decreases in costs.

The authors of the chapters were asked to provide thorough and up to date, yet succinct, reviews of our current knowledge to provide a resource for clinical oncologists and hematologists. It is hoped that this volume will not only provide an up to date resource of what is known, but also provide insights into the gaps in our current state of knowledge and point to the challenges for future clinical studies.

Acknowledgement

The editors wish to thank Connie Cohoon for her hard work in editing, compiling, and formatting this volume.

I

Biology of Hematopoietic and Lymphopoietic Cytokines

1. Cytokines, Growth Factors and Hematopoiesis

Grover C. Bagby, Jr., Michael C. Heinrich

Introduction

The bone marrow responds to environmental stimuli in predictable and sensible ways effectively protecting the host from the vicissitudes of life on earth. A specific stimulus of hypoxia, for example, will result in the expansion of the erythroid bone marrow and subsequent erythrocytosis, but the bone marrow will not increase production of B-lymphocytes or neutrophils. This response evolves from hypoxia-induced increases in circulating levels of erythropoietin (EPO), a glycoprotein hormone that specifically stimulates the proliferation and differentiation of cells of the erythroid lineage[1]. EPO is but one of about thirty well-characterized hematopoietic growth factors that regulate the production and activity of blood cells. Additional ones will surely be characterized each year at an increasing pace.

Recombinant hematopoietic growth factors have recently become available, enabling hundreds of laboratories to test specific control points for blood cell production. *In vitro* experiments in many laboratories using genomic and cDNA clones, *in vitro* transcripts, and recombinant proteins have uncovered new levels of complexity and provided new explanations of how biologic organisms work. Studies using mice carrying germline disruptions of such genes have been even more informative, even surprising. Today, there is an excitingly clear picture of a complex and highly efficient intercellular molecular communication system. That system is the subject matter of this chapter.

We present here a brief compilation of the hematopoietic growth factors organized into three functional groups: (a) proteins that function largely in support of a specific lineage; (b) proteins with an effect on multipotential hematopoietic cells - so called "early acting" factors, and (c) proteins that regulate hematopoiesis indirectly by inducing expression of direct acting growth factor genes in auxiliary cells. This organizational framework is, in some cases, arbitrary. GM-CSF for example, is assigned to the granulopoietic lineage notwithstanding it's capacity to influence non granulopoietic cells, because the *biologically dominant effect* of the factor when administered to humans, is on production and activation state of phagocytic leukocytes. Knockout mice have helped solidify some assignments. M-CSF is assigned to the granulopoietic lineage because a major manifestation of M-CSF deficiency is monocytopenia[2]. This organizational framework is important only conversationally, not biologically. Most of the hematopoietic growth factors do more than one thing and can act on more than one cell type. Consequently, because the lineage assignments we have made are sometimes arbitrary (e.g. IL-5 is in the granulopoiesis section, but has clear effects on lymphoid cells too), we have listed many of the biological activities of these proteins in Table 1. These are complexities that must dissuade the reader from locking each factor into an arbitrary box.

Table 1. Heterogeneous biological activities of the hematopoietic growth factors and interleukins.

Erythropoietic Factors

EPO
Stimulates clonal growth of CFU-E and a subset of BFU-E
Suppresses apoptosis in erythroid progenitor cells
Induces release of reticulocytes from marrow
Induces globin synthesis in erythroid precursor cells
Stimulates murine megakaryocyte colony growth and terminal maturation *in vitro* but has no apparent thrombopoietic activity *in vivo*
Mitogen for neonatal rat cardiac myocytes

SF
Promotes the proliferation and differentiation of pre-CFCs
Acts synergistically with IL-3, GM-CSF, and EPO to support clonal growth of CFU-GEMM, BFU-E, and CFU-Mk
Enhances hematopoietic colony growth in cultures of marrow cells from   patients with congenital marrow failure states
Stimulates the proliferation and differentiation of mast cell precursors
Chemotactic for mast cells
Independently stimulates mast cell degranulation and enhances IgE-dependent mediator release from mast cells
Stimulates expansion of committed progenitor cell compartment *in vivo*
Stimulates mast cell hyperplasia *in vivo*
Supports melanocyte development and migration
Supports gametogenesis

IGF-I (hematopoietic effects of)
Induces erythroid colony formation at high doses in absence of EPO
Induces DNA synthesis in erythroid progenitor cells
Anti-apoptotic effects in erythroid progenitor cells and IL-3 dependent cells

Granulopoietic Factors

GM-CSF
Stimulation of multilineage hematopoietic progenitor cells
Stimulation of BFU-E growth
Stimulation of granulocyte, macrophage, and eosinophil colony growth
Stimulates functional activity of eosinophils, neutrophils, monocytes and macrophages
Induces IL-1 gene expression in neutrophils and peripheral blood mononuclear leukocytes
Co-stimulates T-cell proliferation with IL-2 Induces or co-induces TNFα gene expression with IFN-γ in monocytes
Stimulates proliferation of myeloid leukemic cells
Stimulates growth of certain non-hematopoietic cancer cells *in vitro*
Induces migration and proliferation of vascular endothelial cells *in vitro*

G-CSF
Stimulates growth of progenitor cells committed to the neutrophil lineage
Stimulates neutrophil maturation of certain leukemic cells
Activates phagocytic function of mature neutrophils
Stimulates quiescent pluripotent hematopoietic progenitor cells to enter G1-S

Stimulates mobilization of stem cells and progenitors from hematopoietic niches
  into peripheral blood
Maintenance of steady-state neutrophil numbers

M-CSF   Induction of monocyte/macrophage growth and differentiation
Activation of macrophage phagocytic function
Activation of macrophage secretory function
Maintenance of steady state monocyte levels
Maintenance of steady state osteoclast numbers

IL-5   Stimulates eosinophil production and activation
Activates cytotoxic T-cells
Induces or co-induces immunoglobulin secretion

<u>Megakaryocytopoietic Factors</u>

TPO: Stimulates *in vitro* growth of CFU-MK, megakaryocytes, and platelets
Stimulates clonal growth of individual $CD34^+CD38^-$ cells.
Synergizes with Steel factor, IL-3 and FL
In single CD34+CD38+ cells, TPO synergized with SF and IL-3 but not Flt3
  ligand. No increase in colony growth nor colony size is seen when TPO is added
  to multi-cytokine combinations
Increases megakaryocyte ploidy *in vitro* and in vivo
Enhances the proliferation and differentiation of yolk-sac erythroid lineage
  precursors
Stimulates production of PDGF, platelet factor 4 and b-thromboglobulin from
  megakaryocytes
Supports continuous growth of cytokine-dependent human leukemic cell lines
Stimulates adhesion of hematopoietic progenitor cells to fibronectin by activation
  of VLA-4 and VLA-5
No direct effect on platelet aggregation but primes the response to ADP,
epinephrine and thrombin. Also increases platelet release of ATP and
thromboxane B2 production and platelet expression of CD62 (P-selectin).
Stimulates proliferation of c-mpl positive AML blasts

IL-11   Stimulates proliferation of murine plasmacytoma and hybridoma cell lines
Stimulates CD4+ T-cell-dependent proliferation of antigen-specific plaque-
  forming B-cells
Shortens the duration of G_o of primitive hematopoietic progenitor cells
Acts synergistically with IL-3 or SF to stimulate the clonal growth of erythroid
  (BFU-E and CFU-E) and primitive megakaryocytic (BFU-Mk) progenitors
Increases the ploidy of cultured megakaryocytes
Increases peripheral platelet and neutrophil counts
Increases the numbers and cycling activity of committed progenitor cells
Hastens hematopoietic recovery following cytotoxic chemotherapy, ionizing
  radiation, and bone marrow transplantation
Acts as an autocrine growth factor for certain megakaryoblastic cell lines
Stimulates hepatic acute phase reactant production
Suppresses adipogenesis in pre-adipocytes

<u>**Lymphopoietic Factors**</u>

IL-7 Induces clonal growth of pre-B cells
Stimulates growth of pre-T cells
Stimulates growth of CLL, acute leukemia, and   Sezary cells.
Enhances IL-3 and GM-CSF production by activated T cells.
Induces expression of IL-6, IL-1, TNFα, and IL-8 in peripheral blood monocytes.

IL-2 Induces proliferation and activation of T-lymphocytes
Induces proliferation and activation of B-lymphocytes
Induces proliferation and activation of natural killer (NK) cells
Induces expression of IL-1 in monocytes and macrophages
Co-induces (with IL-1) expression of interferon-g in T-cells

IL-15 Induces proliferation and activation of T cells
Synergizes with IL-12 to induce proliferation and activation of T cells
Induces proliferation and activation of B cells
Induces proliferation and activation of NK cells
IL-15 (as a single factor) induces differentiation of $CD3^-CD56^+$ NK cells from $CD34^+$ HPC.
SF synergizes with IL-15 to increase expansion without altering differentiation state of expanded NK cells
Induces antitumor responses in animal models in which the tumor is also responsive to IL-2 treatment
Induces angiogenesis *in vivo*
Stimulates accumulation of contractile proteins in muscle fibers of differentiated myocytes
Stimulates the expansion of PBMC anti-HIV specific CTL
Stimulates mast cell proliferation

IL-4 Induces proliferation of activated B-cells
Inhibits IL-2-stimulated proliferation of B-cells
Co-induces immunoglobulin secretion and isotype switching
Induces proliferation of T-cells
Induces proliferation of fibroblasts
Co-induces (with PMA) IL-2 receptor expression in T-cells
Inhibits induction and function of lymphokine activated killer (LAK) cells
Inhibits IL-1 release
Induces expression of M-CSF and G-CSF genes in monocytes

IL-10 Inhibits monocyte/macrophage-dependent synthesis of T_h1-derived cytokines (IL-2, IFNγ, lymphotoxin) in man and mouse
Inhibits monocyte/macrophage-dependent synthesis of "T_h2-type" (IL-3, IL-4, IL-5) and NK-derived cytokines (IFNγ and TNFα)
Inhibits monocyte/macrophage-dependent T-cell proliferation
Inhibits proliferation of and IL-2 production by purified T-cells
Acts as co-stimulator of B-cell proliferation
Represses constitutive and IFNγ -induced MHC class II antigen expression on mononuclear phagocytes
Inhibits the production of IL-1, TNFα, IL-6, IL-8, G-CSF, GM-CSF, and IL-10 by mononuclear phagocytes

Inhibits the production of reactive oxygen species and NO by mononuclear phagocytes

IL-12   Induces the differentiation of naive T helper cells into T_h1 cells
Augments functional activity of NK cells
Acts synergistically with TNFα to stimulate IFNγ production by NK cells
Induces LAK activity in NK cells

IL-13   Shares many biological activities with IL-4 but is not known to influence T-lymphocytes
Enhances expression of lymphocyte antigens in B cells
Enhances B-cell proliferation
Promotes isotype switching to permit IgE expression
Enhances production of IgG_4 and IgM
Inhibits IFNγ production by NK cells exposed to IL-2
Induces VCAM-1 in endothelial cells but not E-selectin or ICAM-1

IL-14   Stimulates the proliferation of anti-m or
Staphylococcus Aureus Cowan treated B cells
Synergizes with IL-2 to stimulate proliferation of anti-m B cells
Stimulates proliferation of pre-B cell All, hairy cell leukemia cells, prolymphocytic leukemia and chronic lymphocytic leukemia cells
Inhibits secretion of immunoglobulin by activated B cells.
Autocrine growth factor for some B cell lymphoma cell lines.

IL-16   Chemotactic for CD4+ T cells, monocytes, eosinophils at nanomolar concentrations
Growth factor for CD4+ T cells
Induces functional IL-2 receptors on CD4+ T cells
Inhibits HIV-1 replication *in vitro*
Inhibits proliferation in mixed lymphocyte reactions

Multipotential Factors ("early acting factors")

IL-3   Stimulates multilineage colony growth
Stimulates growth of primitive hematopoietic cell lines with multilineage potential
Stimulates BFU-E proliferation *in vitro*
Stimulates proliferation of murine CFU-S
Induces B-lymphocyte differentiation
Co-stimulates T-cell proliferation with IL-2
Induces macrophages to express M-CSF (this may explain reports that IL-3 induces clonal growth of pulmonary alveolar macrophages)
Stimulates growth of myeloid leukemic cells *in vitro*
Primes hapten-specific contact hypersensitivity responses

FL   Stimulates proliferation of some AML and ALL blasts
Stimulates proliferation and differentiation of dendritic cells *in vitro* and *in vivo*
Addition of FL to multi-cytokine combinations augments retroviral transduction of HPC
Stimulates anti-tumor responses in murine models of syngeneic cancer
Mobilizes peripheral blood stem cells weakly as a single agent but markedly

synergizes with G-CSF
Weak colony stimulating activity as single agent but synergizes with IL-3, GM-CSF, SF, IL-11, IL-6, G-CSF, IL-7, and multi-cytokine combinations

IL-9

Stimulates the clonal growth of BFU-E in combination with Epo
Stimulates the clonal growth of fetal CFU-Mix and CFU-GM
Augments IL-3-induced growth of murine bone marrow-derived mast cells
Stimulates the proliferation of preactivated PBMC-derived T-cell lines

IL-6

Synergistic with IL-3 in CFU-GEMM colony growth
Synergistic with M-CSF in macrophage colony growth and with GM-CSF in granulocyte colony growth
Synergistic with IL-4 in inducing T-cell proliferation, immunoglobulin secretion, and hematopoietic colony formation
Synergistic with IL-2 and IL-1 in inducing T-cell proliferation
Co-induces differentiation of B-cells
Induces terminal differentiation of myeloid leukemic cell lines
Induces neuronal differentiation in certain pheochromocytoma cell lines
Co-induces cytotoxic T-cells *in vitro*
Stimulates plasmacytoma growth
Induces acute phase responses *in vivo*
Induces acute phase protein synthesis in hepatocytes
Stimulates megakaryocytopoiesis *in vitro* and *in vivo*

Indirect Acting Factors

IL-1

Induces expression of GM-CSF, G-CSF, IL-6 and IL-1 in fibroblasts, endothelial cells, keratinocytes, and thymic epithelial cells
Induces proliferation of pre-activated T-cells
Induces acute phase protein synthesis
Induces fever and sleep *in vivo*
Stimulates release of ACTH
Promotes transendothelial passage of neutrophils
Synergizes with IL-3 in stimulating proliferation in primitive hematopoietic progenitor cells *in vitro*
Stimulates prostaglandin E production in fibroblasts, monocytes, and neutrophils
Modulates EGF receptor expression

TNFα

Induces expression of GM-CSF, G-CSF, IL-6, and IL-1 in fibroblasts and endothelial cells
Enhances mitogen induced GM-CSF expression in T-cells
Induces release of GM-CSF and M-CSF *in vivo*
Inhibits virus replication synergistically with interferons
Stimulates prostaglandin E production in fibroblasts and neutrophils
Enhances parasite and tumor cell cytotoxicity of eosinophils and macrophages
Inhibits proliferation of hematopoietic progenitor cells lymphocytes and certain leukemia cell lines *in vitro*
Mediates the hemodynamic and toxic effects of endotoxin
Induces expression of IL-6 in fibroblasts
Induces expression of adhesion molecules in myeloid cells
Activates phagocytic function of neutrophils

Induces expression of IL-8

Increases production of plasminogen-activator inhibitor in vascular endothelial cells

Suppresses transcription of the thrombomodulin gene in endothelial cells

Modulates EGF receptor expression

Promotes transendothelial passage of neutrophils

Activates NF-k B trans-activating protein in lymphoid cells

IL-17   Induces secretion of IL-6, IL-8, PGE2 and G-CSF from stromal cells.

Synergizes with TNF-α and IFN-g to induce stromal cell production of GM-CSF and IL-1

Upregulates ICAM-1 expression by fibroblasts.

IL-18   Induces IFN-g production from T cells, B cells, NK cells, peripheral blood mononuclear cells.

Synergizes with IL-12 to enhance production of IFN-g by activated T cells.

Induces GM-CSF production from T cells.

Inhibits production of osteoclast-like multinucleated giant cells in co- cultures of osteoblasts and hematopoietic cells.

Augments NK activity in human and mouse PBMC.

Inhibits IL-10 production by T cells.

Enhances *fas*-mediated cytotoxicity of murineTh1 but not Th0 or Th2 cells.

The Chemokine, IL-8

IL-8   Modulates neutrophil production in the steady state (potential feedback inhibitor of that lineage)

Stimulates neutrophil chemotaxis, exocytosis, respiratory burst, shape change, adhesion molecule expression, and complement receptor type 1 expression

Stimulates T-lymphocyte chemotaxis

Stimulates basophil chemotaxis, histamine release, and leukotriene release

Stimulates endothelial cell chemotaxis and proliferation

Stimulates angiogenesis

This is not, however, molecular anarchy. Certain rules of order are very consistent in cytokine biology (Table 2). Some factors influence production of blood cells directly by binding to receptors on progenitor cells, others influence the process indirectly by binding to receptors pm auxiliary cells which then respond by releasing growth factors, some do both. Some factors can induce cell division, others only serve to permit the survival of progenitors of a given lineage. "Lineage specific" factors influence the replication or survival of primitive cells and also activate the function of the terminally differentiated cells of that lineage. Some factors act synergistically with other cytokines. Auxiliary cells and progenitor cells can "cross-talk" and exhibit signal amplification circuits.

Hematopoietic Growth Factor Receptors

There are at least six receptor superfamilies involved in controlling the behavior of hematopoietic cells. Most receptors for hematopoietic growth factors are members of the Type I cytokine receptor family.

The Hematopoietic Growth Factor Receptor Superfamily (Type I cytokine receptors). These receptors do not possess intrinsic kinase activity. They lead to phosphorylation of cellular substrates by serving as docking sites for adaptor molecules that do have kinase activity. The characterization of receptors for many of the growth factors has permitted the identification of a group that includes receptors for LIF, IL-1, IL-2, IL-3, IL-4, IL-5, IL-6, IL-7, IL-9, IL-13, IL-18, GM-CSF, G-CSF, EPO, prolactin, growth hormone, ciliary neurotrophic factor, and c-*mpl*[3;4]. There are a number of repetitive structural and functional themes in this superfamily (Fig. 1) including: (1) four cysteine residues in the extracellular domain, (2) the sequence W-S-X-W-S in the ligand binding extracellular domain that may optimize the tertiary structure of the receptors[5], (3) a capacity for enhanced binding and or signal transduction when expressed as a heterodimer or homodimer, (4) lack of a known catalytic domain in the cytoplasmic portion of the molecule, and (5) the presence of fibronectin type III domains [6] in the extracellular regions.

Apart from these shared homologous domains, there is minimal sequence homology among these receptors and the size of their cytoplasmic domains are quite variable. Another shared feature of many hematopoietic growth factor receptors is their ability to transduce signals that prevent programmed cell death (apoptosis), in some cases without inducing mitogenic signals. This is particularly true of the lineage specific factors, EPO, M-CSF, IL-5 and IL-7, each of which is reviewed below[7-12].

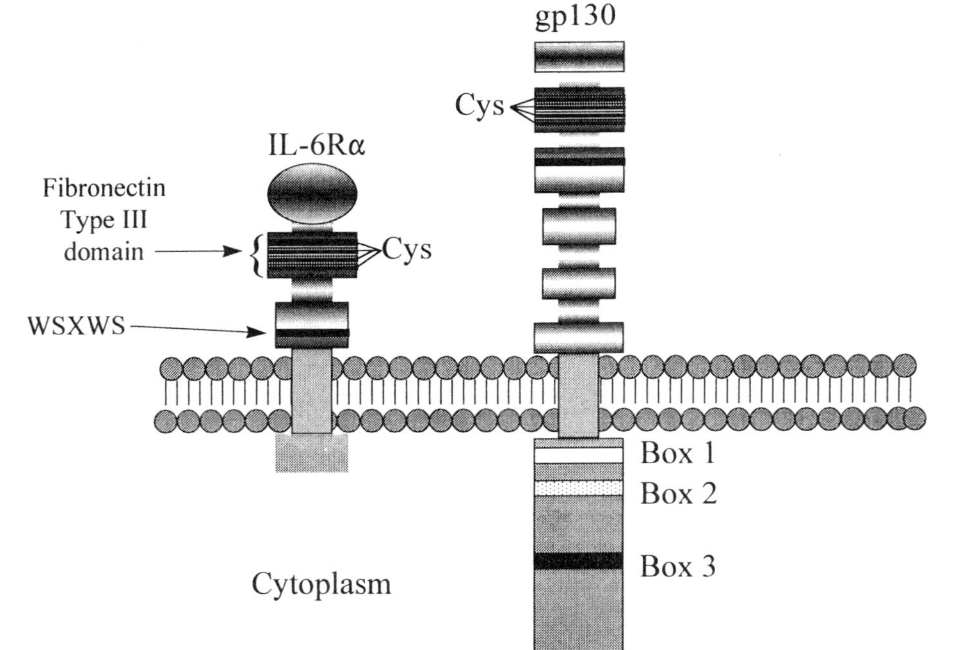

Figure 1. Class I cytokine receptors. This family includes receptors for EPO, TPO, GM-CSF, G-CSF, LIF, prolactin, growth hormone, and interleukins 2,3,4,5,6,7,9,11,12, and 15. Shown here are the two components of the high affinity IL-6 receptor, IL-6α and gp130. Regions of homology are found both in the extracellular and cytoplasmic regions. The conserved extracellular regions of class I receptors contains fibronectin type III regions which contain the ligand binding pockets, four conserved cysteine residues, and a Trp-Ser-any-Trp-Ser (WSXWS) box, each of which is essential for receptor function, although in the unique case of the erythropoietin receptor, recent saturation mutagenesis of the WSXWS box revealed no mutation that interdicted signaling. Cytoplasmic domains contain conserved residues as well in regions termed box-1 and box-2 located close to the membrane.

With some receptor complexes, the capacity to transduce a set of biological signals depends upon discrete functional domains in one or more of the receptor chains. For example, specific sets of signalling pathways can be disrupted by mutagenesis without interdicting all functions of the receptor[13].

The receptors for many hematopoietic growth and differentiation factors share peptide subunits with other receptors. This kind of swapping is seen in granulopoiesis and lymphopoiesis. For example, IL-5, GM-CSF, and IL-3 have unique low affinity (α-chain) receptors, but they share the same β-chain[14; 15] and association of the two chains results in the formation of a specific high-affinity subunit capable of effective signal transduction (Figure 2).

Other chain swapping systems are cartooned in Figure 3. The most highly shared receptor system occurs in lymphopoiesis in which six different cytokines, IL-2, 4, 7, 9, 13 and 15 share certain subunits in common and in which IL-2 and IL-15 share two common subunits (Fig. 3).

In many instances, soluble forms of the receptor are released, sometimes resulting from translation of differentially spliced mRNA. Soluble forms have been described for IL-4, IL-5, Il-7, G-CSF, SF, EPO, and GM-CSF receptors[16-20]. Although the biological meaning of this phenomenon is not yet fully understood, the soluble forms may act as cmpetitive binding proteins for the ligand and, as is clarly the case for the soluble IL-4 receptor [20] , serve as natural in vovo antagonists for specific cytokines.

<u>Receptors with cytoplasmic tyrosine kinase domains</u>. Amino acid sequence analysis has permitted the categorization of three subclasses of a tyrosine receptor family. Subclass 1 includes the neu/HER2 proto-oncogene and epidermal growth factor, subclass 2 includes the insulin and IGF-1 receptors, and type 3, the receptors for M-CSF, SF, Flt3/flk-2 lingand (FL) and plagelet derived growth factor (PDGF). *C-kit*, the *flt3* gene and c-*fms* are genes that encode three related hematopoietic growth factor receptors, the ligands for which are SF, FL, and M-CSF respectively. All receptors with tyrosine kinase activity possess large glycosylated extracellular domains, a single transmembrane spinning region, and a cytoplasmic domain that contains one or more tyorsine kinases catalytic (Figure 4).

<u>Type II cytokine receptors</u>. The class II subgroup of cytokine receptors include the interferon receptors, and the receptors for tissue factor and IL-10. Each has an extracellular domain containing a region resembling the fibronectin III domain found in the type I receptors[21], which may serve as the ligand binding site. While the signaling pathways for IL-10 are not fully elucidated, the interferon signaling pathways have been widely studied and are outlined in Figure 5.

<u>Chemokine receptors</u>. The chemokine receptor family includes receptors for a few factors relevant to blood cell production; IL-8 and mip-1α, for example, both serve, at least in part, as braking factors, slowing progenitor cell proliferation. The chemokine receptors are seven transmembrane spanning G protein linked receptors[22] that are divided into three families based on their variability in cysteine residues; α or CXC, β or CC, and γ or C[23]. It is clear that some of these chemotactic factors (e.g. IL-8 and mip) may also serve as feedback inhibitors of hematopoiesis[24,25].

<u>Tumor necrosis factor receptor (TNFR) family</u>. The TNF-R family includes TNFRI, TNFR2, *fas*, CD40, NGF receptor, CD27, CD30, and OX40. Each has one or more distinct biological effects. Both TNFα and *fas* have the capacity to profoundly

11

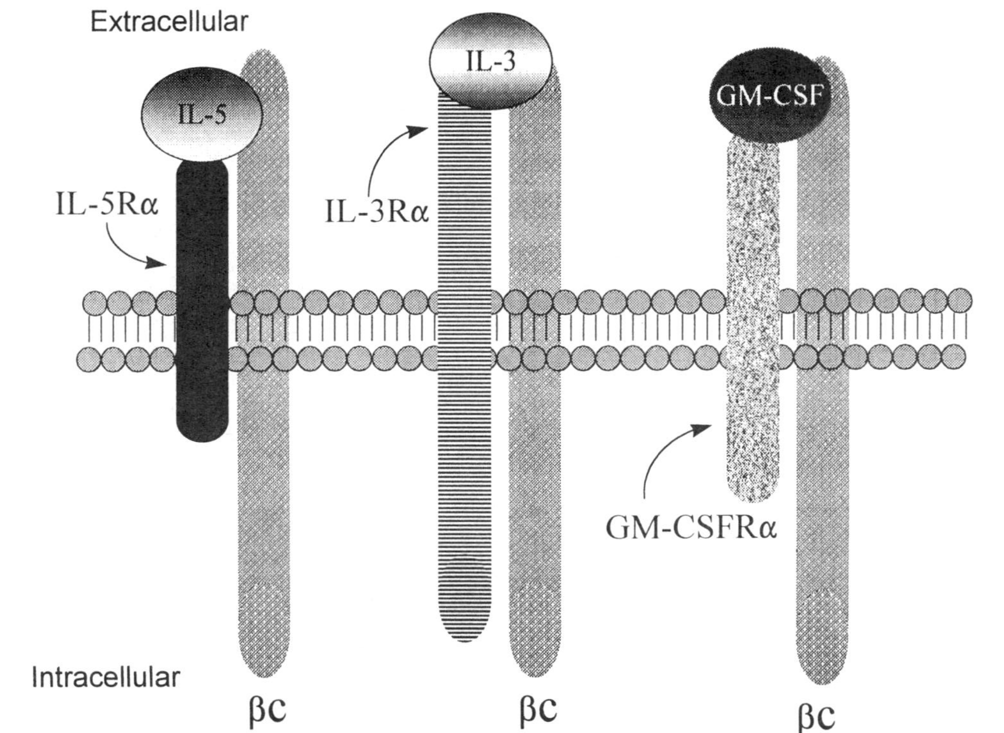

Figure 2. Receptor chain swapping. Three sets of hematopoietic growth factor receptors share some of their heteromeric receptor chains. Shown here are the heterodimeric IL-3, IL-5, and GM-CSF receptors each of which have unique alpha chains and each of which associate with a common beta chain (βc) that increases the binding affinity of the complex when compared to the alpha chains alone. Not shown here is the IL-6 set in which alpha chains interact with a second 130 kDa chain (gp130) that is also shared as the second partner with LIFR, OSMR, CNTFR (not shown) and the IL-11Rα chains.

suppress hematopoiesis by triggering programmed cell death in progenitor cells[26-29].

Fas mediated apoptosis of stem cells and progenitors may represent a major pathophysiological mechanism of bone marrow failure in acquired[30] and hereditary bone marrow failure states[31]. TNF receptors transduce complex signals via multiple pathways that induce programmed cell death in some cells and induce secretion of hematopoietic growth factors in others. The majority of these receptors contain Cysteine-rich repeats in the extracellular domains and have cytoplasmic portions containing 80 amino acid "death domains" required for transducing apoptotic signals and for NF-κB activation. The *fas* activation pathway, shown as a paradigm of this superfamily, is shown in Figure 6.

Hematopoietic Control

Erythropoiesis (Figure 7). Factors involved in *effective* production of red cells include IL-3[32-34], IL-9[35; 36], IL-11[37], SF, insulin-like growth factor-1 (IGF-1)[38], thrombopoietin (TPO)[39], and GM-CSF[39,40;41], which induce proliferation of primitive erythroid progenitors. Other factors might play a role as well, including angiotensin II[42]. Few of these factors will induce erythroid cellular proliferation in the absence of the lineage-specific factor EPO, which is the pivotal humoral factor that functions to prevent programmed cell death of the most committed erythroid progenitor cells and their progeny[12]. However, SF and IGF-1 have also emerged as unique regulators of erythropoiesis as well[43]. These three factors will be reviewed here.

Erythropoietin (EPO). Erythropoietin (EPO), an 18 kDa protein[44] (34-39 kDa when fully glycosylated[45]) encoded by a gene stationed on the long arm of chromosome 7 [46], is expressed largely by cells in the liver in embryonic life [47; 48], cells of the kidney [49] and, to a lesser extent, liver [47] in adult life, and by certain hepatoma cell lines[50]. The production of erythropoietin is induced by hypoxia, a mechanism which may involve the initial activation[50], of heme proteins that stimulate EPO gene expression[51]. The EPO receptor (EPO-R) genes, located on human chromosome 19, encodes a classic type I cytokine receptor (Fig. 1) that utilizes the jak/stat pathway for signal transduction[52]. Specifically, tyrosine phosphorylation of the EPO-R creates docking sites for SH2 domain(s) in signaling molecules that include STAT2, STAT5, protein tyrosine phosphatases SH- PTP1 and SH-PTP2, and phosphoinositide 3-kinase (PI3 kinase)[53,54]. Subsequent association of EPO-R with SHP-1 terminates signaling[55]. Other signaling pathways, including those involving protein kinase C family members, may also be involved and the linkage of these pathways with the JAK-STAT pathway is unclear[56].

The effects of EPO on progenitor cell proliferation are optimal in the presence of SF and its effects on terminal erythroid differentiation are optimized by IGF-1[12]. EPO has been reported to stimulate various levels of megakaryocytopoiesis *in vitro* and platelet production in experimental animals [57] and high affinity EPO receptors have been reported in rodent megakaryocytes[58]. However, the physiologic relevance of these observations is unclear because (a) the effect is not seen in serum free cultures [59] or in cultures of cells enriched for progenitors[60] (and relatively free, therefore, of accessory cells) and, (b) therapy with recombinant human EPO has shown no consistent effects on platelet counts.

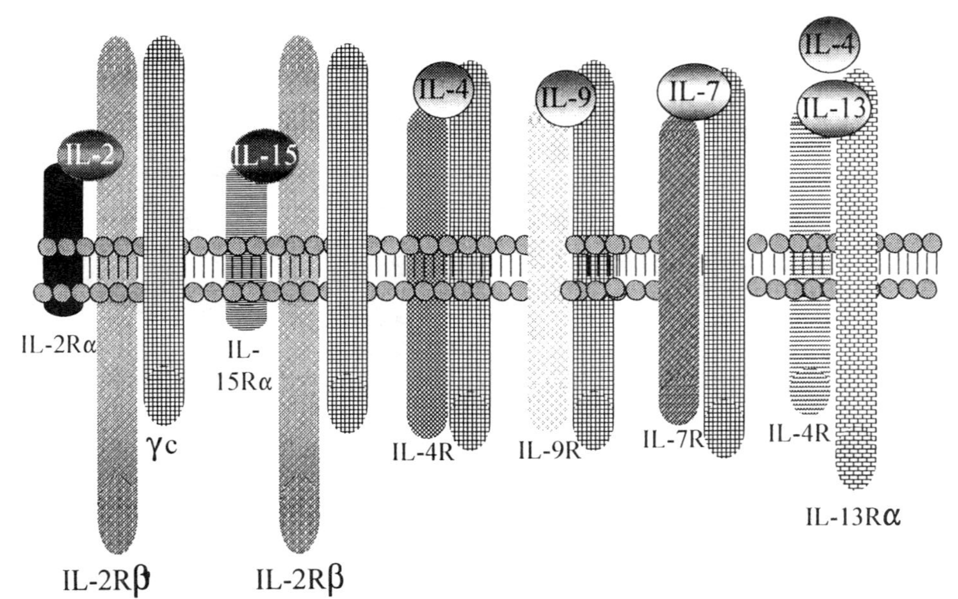

Figure 3. Receptor chain swapping; the Il-2/IL-15 paradigm. Six receptors are involved in chain swapping. IL-2, IL-15, IL-4, IL-7, IL-9, and IL-13. Of note are the heterotrimeric IL-2 and IL-15 receptors which share not one, but two chains.

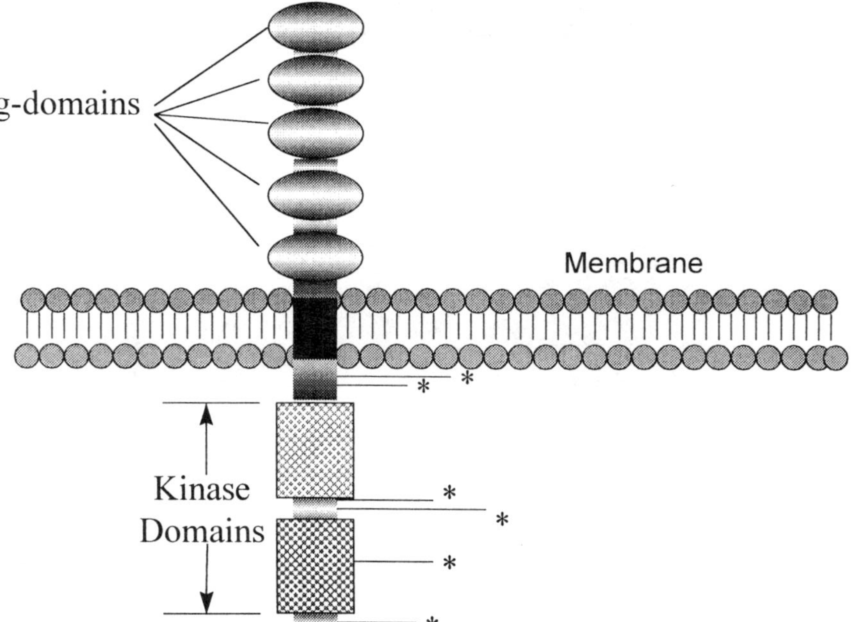

Figure 4. Cytoplasmic tyrosine kinase (TK) receptors. A prototype TK receptor, c-*kit*, is shown here. The extracellular domain contains no fibronectin like modules or WSXWS motifs, but has five immunoglobulin like domains (oval shaped). There are at least 6 potential sites for tyrosine phosphorylation (asterisks) in the cytoplasmic region, each of which may serve as docking sites for adaptor proteins containing SH2 domains. When growth factors bind to this class of receptors, receptor chains dimerize, auto-transphosphorylate, and then serve as docking sites for a variety of adaptor proteins that serve as signal transducers. These adaptor proteins contain SH2 domains which specifically associate with proteins on phosphotyrosines and adjacent carboxyterminal residues.

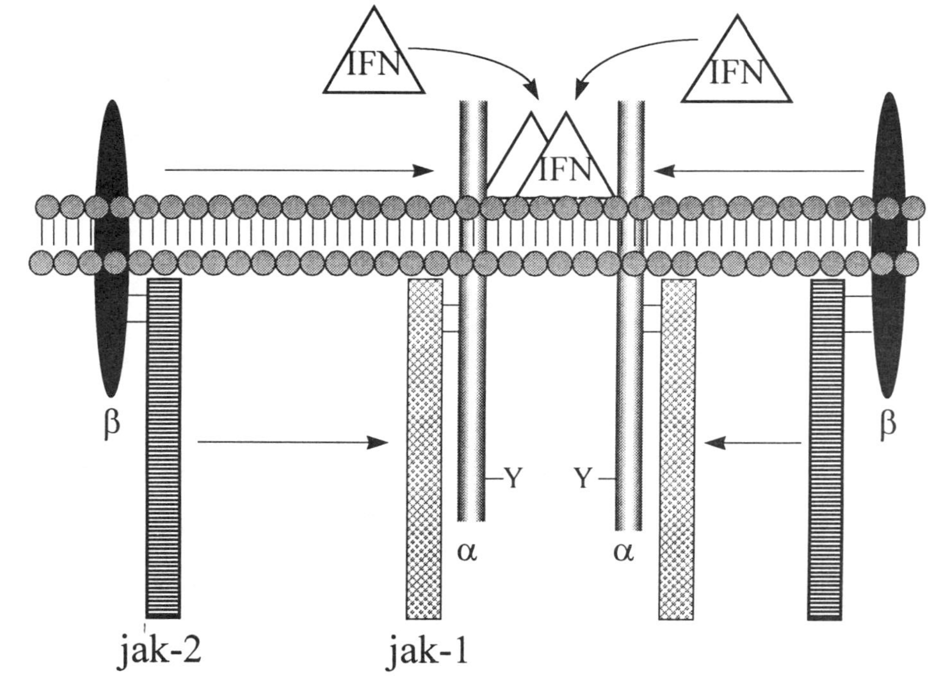

Figure 5. Class II subgroup of cytokine receptors. Shown here is the ligand-binding induced assembly of the IFNγ receptor. Binding of the IFN molecules to the IFNγRα chains, with which jak-1 (Janus kinase 1) is associated, causes the association of alpha with beta chains of the receptor (the beta chain is associated with jak-2). The Jak-1/Jak-2 complex phosphorylates tyrosines on the alpha chain at least one of which become a docking site for stat1 (not shown). When stat1 docks, it too is phosphorylated on tyrosines, dissociates from the alpha chain and forms a homodimer which is then transported to the nucleus to bind to gamma activating sequences (GAS elements). A variety of hematopoietic growth factor complexes utilize stat molecules for signal transduction.

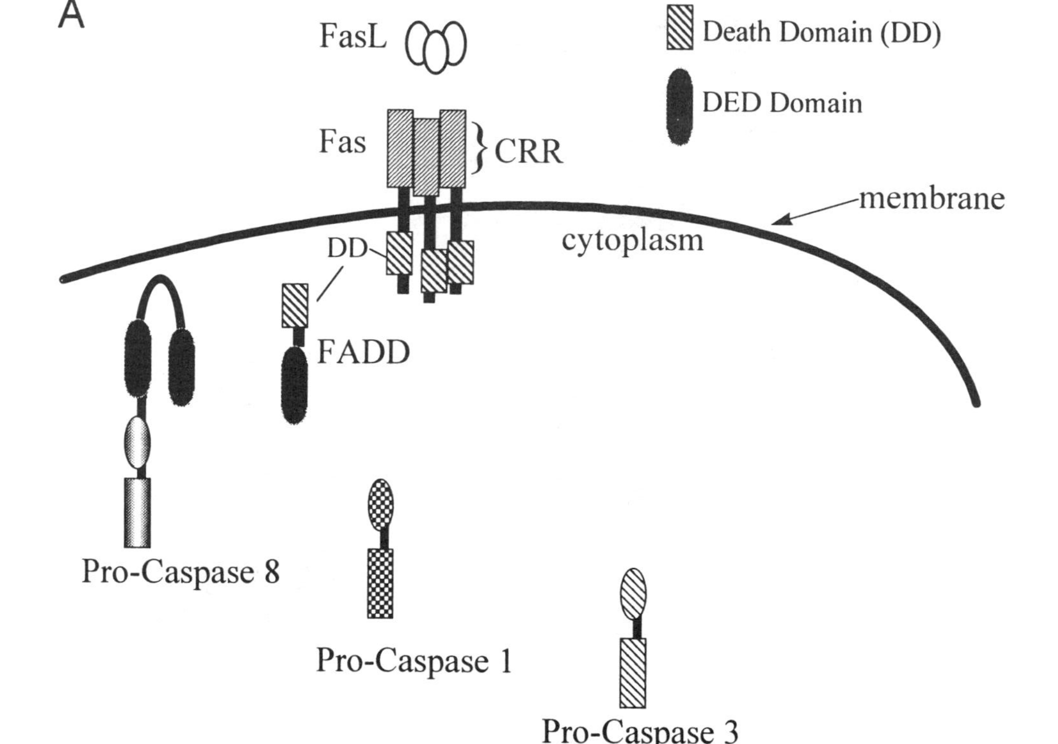

Figure 6A.   The Fas activation pathway: The TNF-R family includes TNFRI, TNFR2, *fas*, CD40, NGF receptor, CD27, CD30, and OX40. Both TNFα and *fas* have the capacity to profoundly suppress hematopoiesis by triggering programmed cell death in progenitor cells. *Fas* mediated apoptosis involves the trimeric fas complex (containing a cysteine rich region [CRR] in the extracellular domain and a death domain in the cytoplasmic region) and a set of signaling molecules, many of which are proenzymes.

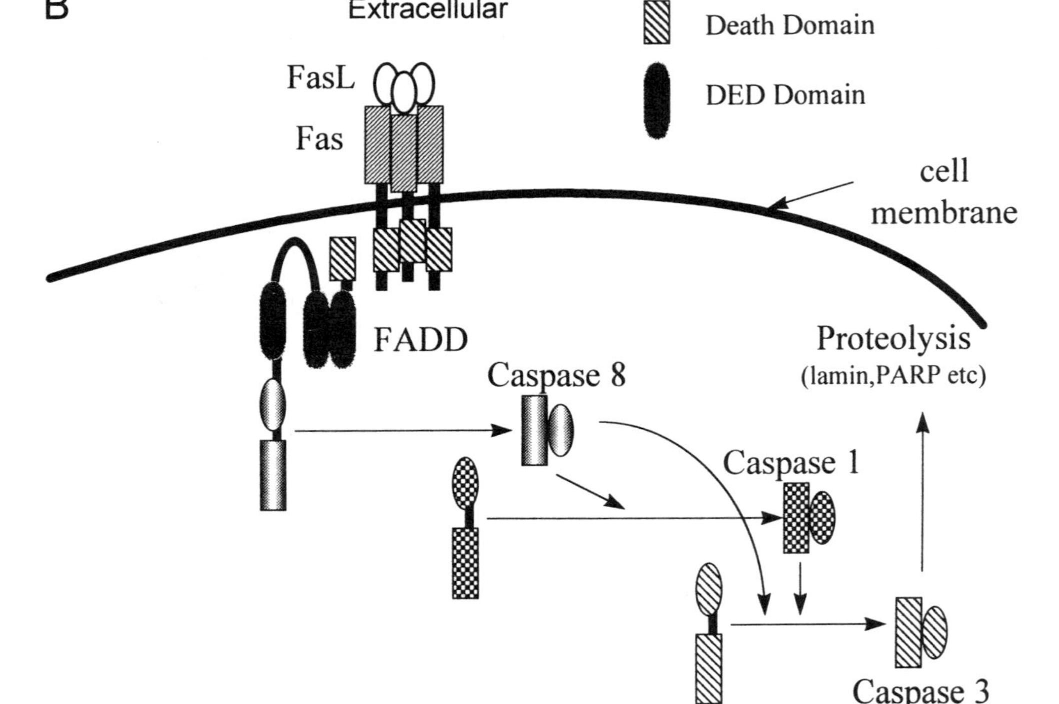

Figure 6B. After binding FasL, the death domains of fas and FADD associate, prompting the association of the DED domains of pro-caspase 8 (FLICE) and FADD. Association with FADD induces autocatalytic cleavage of pro-caspase 8 to produce Caspase . Caspase 8 cleaves pro-caspase 1 to caspase 1 (IL-1 converting enzyme, ICE) which in turn cleaves pro-caspase 3 to caspase 3 (CPP32). Caspase 8 can cleave pro-caspase 3 directly as well. Caspase 3 is responsible for proteolysis of a wide variety of structural cellular proteins including lamin and poly-ADP ribose polymerase (PARP).

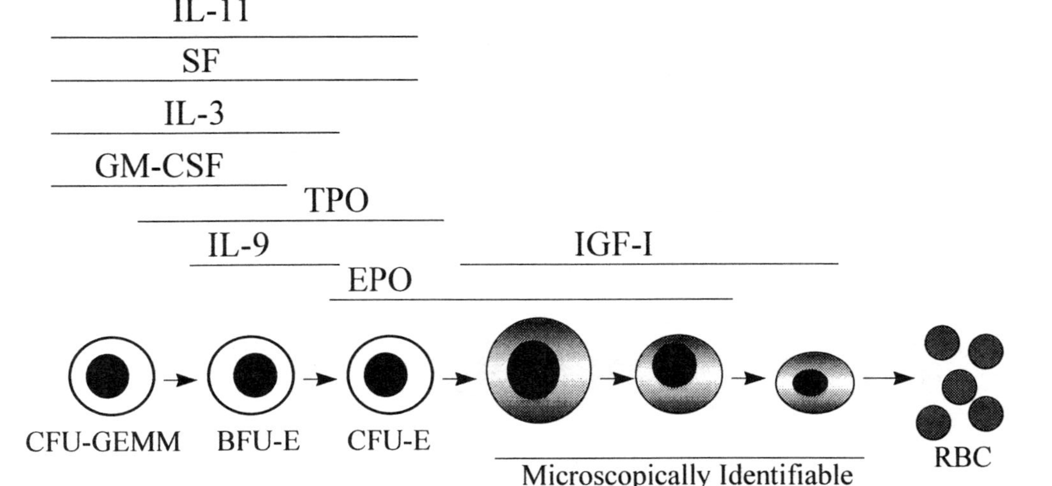

Figure 7. Humoral control of erythropoiesis. A number of growth factors control multipotential progenitor cell replication and primitive erythroid progenitor cell growth (BFU-E), but the two most lineage specific differentiation and survival factors known are erythropoietin and IGF-1. While these two factors are sufficient for erythroid differentiation, the necessary factors seem to be Steel factor and EPO because deficiencies of either of these factors results in anemia.

EPO was the first hematopoietic growth factor to be identified experimentally and the use of the recombinant protein has been shown to be effective in the management of anemia associated with renal failure[61]. Other clinical uses of EPO have also emerged. Patients with myelodysplasia [62], those with progressive anemia in the setting of cancer therapy [63], and patients who refuse blood transfusions[64], are candidates for erythropoietin therapy, generally given subcutaneously, three times weekly, at 100 units/kg/dose. AIDS patients with endogenous erythropoietin levels of less than 500 IU/L, need fewer red cell transfusions, have higher hemoglobin levels and report an improvement in quality of life when treated with EPO[65].

EPO

<u>Chromosome:</u> **7q21**
<u>Gene product:</u> **34-39 kDa**
<u>Produced by:</u> **kidney in adult, liver during development, hepatoma lines**
<u>Induced by:</u> **hypoxia**
<u>Receptor:</u> **class I cytokine receptor encoded by a single gene on human chromosome 19p13.3-p13.2 utilizing jak2 and stat5 for signaling**
<u>Consequences of EPO deficiency:</u> **anemia in man, homozygous deletion of EPO or EPO-R in mice is lethal, resulting in embryonic anemia and death**

<u>Steel Factor (SF).</u> SF is a highly glycosylated 28-36 kDa protein encoded by a gene on human chromosome 12q22[66]. The widely expressed gene gives rise, via alternate splicing, to two mRNA species, one containing exon 6 (exon 6$^+$) and a second in which exon 6 has been spliced out (exon 6$^-$)[67, 68]. The ratio of exon 6$^+$ to exon 6$^-$ transcripts is approximately 3:1[69]. SF expression has been demonstrated in fibroblasts, bone marrow stromal ("fibroblast-like") cells, vascular endothelial cells, and Sertoli cells, as well as in various embryonic tissues[69],[70]. No inductive cytokines for SF expression have yet been convincingly documented[69], although TGFβ represses SF expression[71]. SF is elaborated in both membrane-bound and soluble forms, the latter resulting from protease cleavage of the exon 6$^+$ transcript-encoded protein at an exon 6-encoded consensus cleavage site[68]. The membrane-bound and soluble forms of SF display equivalent bioactivity in clonogenic assays *in vitro*[67]. However, the particular relevance of the membrane-bound form to normal hematopoiesis, gametogenesis, and pigmentation is clearly illustrated by mice homozygous for the *Sl^d* allele in which a genomic deletion gives rise to a soluble protein lacking the anchoring transmembrane and cytoplasmic domains[68]. Although the soluble protein retains full biologic activity *in vitro*, these animal are anemic, sterile, and nonpigmented[68;72].

SF promotes the proliferation and differentiation of the most primitive hematopoietic progenitor cells ("pre-CFCs") into committed progenitor cells (CFU-GEMM, BFU-E, CFU-GM, and CFU-Mk)[73, 74]. While SF has no independent colony-stimulating activity, it acts synergistically with IL-3, GM-CSF, and erythropoietin to promote CFU-GEMM-, BFU-E-, and CFU-Mk-derived colony growth[75,76]. SF administration *in vivo* induces a marked expansion in the compartment of committed hematopoietic progenitor cells and striking mast cell hyperplasia[77,78]. Outside the hematopoietic system, appropriate developmentally regulated SF expression is necessary for normal melanocyte development and migration and gametogenesis[79].

Because SF has an influence on primitive hematopoietic cells of other lineages and on multipotential cells [80], some categorize this factor as an "early acting" hematopoietic growth factor. However, persuasive evidence that SF plays an essential role in erythropoiesis derives from; (a) the anemia that attends SF deficiency in mice and (b) the capacity of SF to enhance DNA synthesis in isolated erythroid progenitor cells[12], and (c) findings that EPO-R and c-kit, the SF receptor, are co-expressed in erythroid progenitor cells[81] and that these receptors interact in erythroid cells [82].

SF

Chromosome: 12q22-24
Gene product: approximately 40 kDa
Produced by: fibroblasts, endothelial cells, bone marrow stromal cells, Sertoli cells, hepatocytes, various embryonic tissues
Expression: constitutive
Receptor: c-kit protein (CD117), a receptor tyrosine kinase encoded by a gene on human chromosome 4q11-q13 (the piebald locus) and murine chromosome 5 (the white spotting locus), certain mutations of which are oncogenic
Consequences of SF Deficiency (mice): anemia, mast cell deficiency, reduced stem cell numbers

---

Insulin-like growth factor-1, IGF-1. IGF1 and IGF2 (reviewed in [83])(located on chromosomes 12q22-q24.1 and 11p15, respectively [84]) are small peptide (70 and 67 residues respectively) homologues of proinsulin[85]. The role of IGF-2 in hematopoietic cells is unclear. The major site of IGF-1 synthesis is the liver. IGF-1 has multiple effects on a wide variety of cells and its receptor (IGF1R) is expressed ubiquitously. The bioactivity of IGF-1 is largely mitogenic and is known to regulate growth of both normal and malignant cells [86; 87]. IGF-I knockout mice exhibit extreme embryonic and postnatal growth retardation, neurological defects and prenatal mortality (reviewed in[88]). Growth failure and neurological deficits have also been described in humans with IGF-1 deficiency[89]. IGFI-R is a receptor protein kinase encoded by a 100 kb gene on human chromosome 15q26. [90] It is synthesized as a single precursor that dimerizes and processed into alpha and beta subunits which form a heterotetrameric receptor complex[91]. The activated receptor phosphorylates the Crk adaptor protein which associates with the guanine releasing proteins Sos and C3G in the ras signaling pathway[92].

First noted by Sawada et al[93], the erythropoietic activity of IGF-1 was confirmed by Axelrad's group, using serum free cultures of erythroid progenitor cells from adult human peripheral blood. They discovered that erythroid progenitor cells formed erythroid colonies in the presence of IGF-1 even in the absence of EPO[94]. Moreover, the activities of EPO and IGF-1 overlapped because combinations of these factors resulted in clonal growth that was less than the sum of colony formation with each factor alone[94]. The same group also demonstrated that progenitors from polycythemia vera patients were two orders of magnitude more sensitive to IGF-1 than were normal cells[95], and that the effect was transduced through the IGF1R[96]. The effects of IGF-1 are both mitogenic and anti-apoptotic in erythroid progenitor cells[38], and in IL-3 responsive cell lines as well [97]. For these reasons, and notwithstanding the myriad effects of IGF-I and II on many types of cells, we include IGF-1 as an important erythropoietic factor that shares biological activities with both SF and EPO.

Insulin Like Growth Factor 1 (IGF-1)
<u>Chromosomal location:</u> human chromosomes 12q22-q24.1
<u>Gene product:</u>   70 amino acids
<u>Produced by:</u> liver
<u>Induced by:</u> growth hormone
<u>Receptor:</u> receptor protein kinase family member, synthesized as single precursor (151 kDa, encoded by a gene on human chromosome 15q25-q26[83]) and processed into alpha (80 kDa) and beta (70 kDa) subunits that form heterotetramers.
<u>Consequences of IGF-1 Deficiency:</u> embryonic and post natal growth retardation, neurological deficits[88; 89] homozygous inactivating IGF-I lesions are lethal

---

Granulopoiesis (Figure 8)

<u>Neutrophils</u>. As shown in Fig. 3, the production of neutrophilic leukocytes involves a variety of different factors including GM-CSF, IL-3, M-CSF, and G-CSF. Other factors including IL-11, SF, and FL stimulate or enhance neutrophil clonal growth *in vitro*. Recent studies on G-CSF knockout mice indicate that the most significant lineage specific factor for neutrophils is G-CSF [98].

 <u>GM-CSF</u>. GM-CSF, is a glycoprotein of 14-35 kDa [99] (the molecular weight varies with the degree of glycosylation) reflects variable degrees of glycosylation) encoded by a gene located on the long arm of chromosome 5 [100]. The biological activities of GM-CSF are reviewed in Table 1. GM-CSF activates the functional activity of most phagocytes including neutrophils[101], macrophages[102,103], and eosinophils[104,105] demonstrating a recurrent theme in hematopoietic control; namely, that lineage specific growth factors frequently activate the functional activity of the terminally differentiated progeny (Figure 9). In fact, in GM-CSF deficient mice, the major morbidity results from the absence of normal phagocytic function rather than a failure to produce phagocytes.

 The GM-CSF receptor is a type I cytokine receptor with a 44 kDa alpha (CD116) and 96 kDa beta (CDw131) chain. The receptor is expressed by mononuclear phagocytes, neutrophils, endothelial cells, eosinophils, and fibroblasts. The beta chain is shared with the alpha chains for IL-3 and IL-5 (Figure 2).

 GM-CSF therapy enhances the production of neutrophils, monocytes, and eosinophils[106]. *In vitro* GM-CSF induces neutrophil, macrophage and eosinophil colony growth, but there is no compelling evidence that GM-CSF alone induces neutrophil differentiation in the absence of G-CSF[107-109]. Thus, it is likely that neutrophilic leukocytosis in recipients of GM-CSF reflects the capacity of GM-CSF to induce expression of other factors, especially IL-1 [110], which induces expression of G-CSF [111] by a variety of cell types.

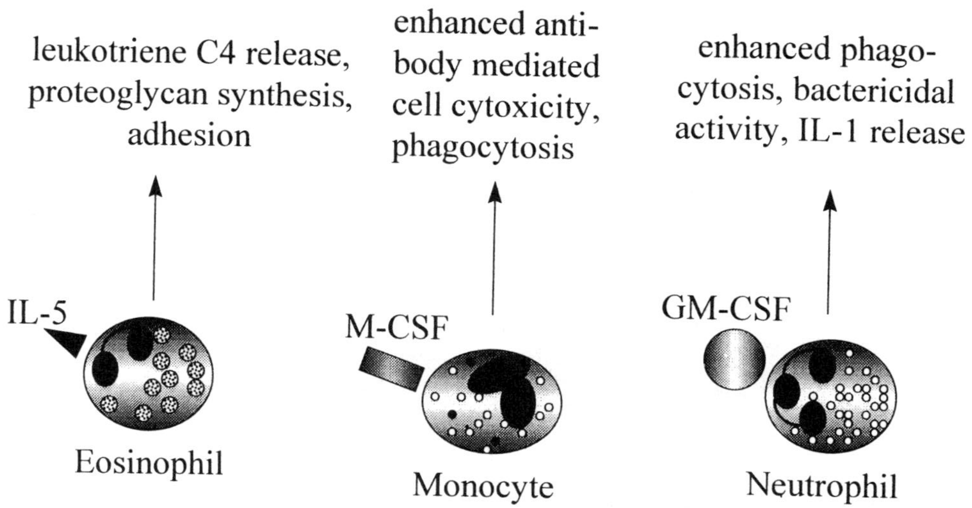

Figure 8. Humoral control of granulopoiesis. A number of growth factors control multipotential progenitor cell replication, but production of specific phagocytic lineages depends upon specific factors. G-CSF is necessary for neutrophils production. M-CSF is necessary for monocyte production. IL-5 is a strong growth and survival factor for eosinophils. The production of basophils and mast cells is less well understood but the mast cell deficiency found in Steel factor deficient mice suggests that SF is a necessary factor for this process which is also influenced by IL-3 and TGFβ.

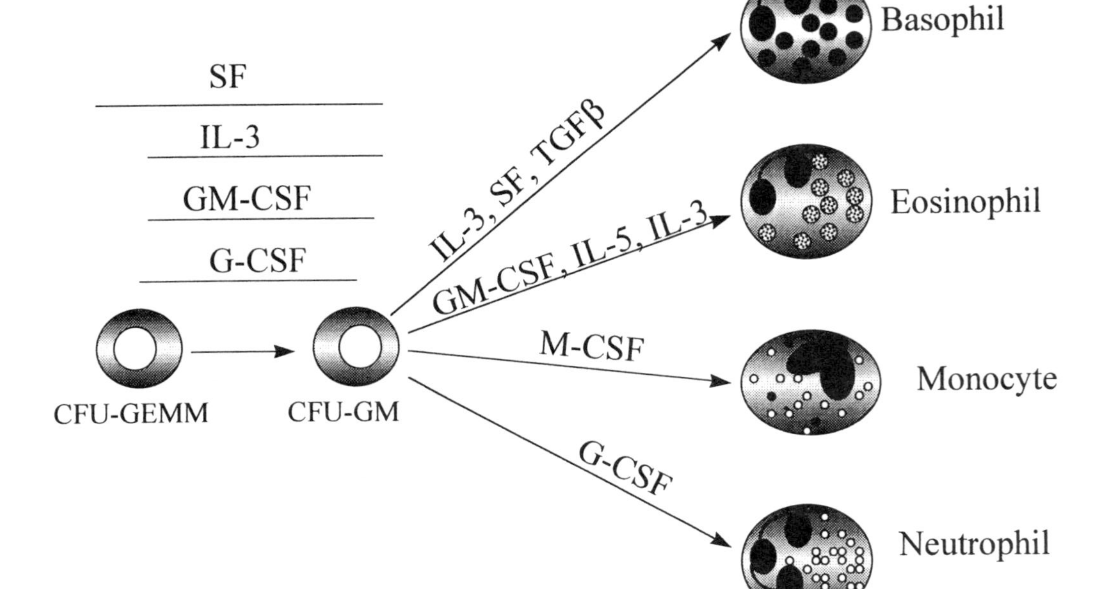

Figure 9. Activation of phagocyte function by growth and survival factors. Lineage specific growth and survival factors influence the functional activity of terminally differentiated cells of the same lineage. GM-CSF activates the functional activity of most phagocytes including neutrophils. In fact, in GM-CSF deficient mice, the major morbidity results from the absence of normal phagocytic function rather than a failure to produce phagocytes. M-CSF and IL-5 activate function of monocytes and macrophages and eosinophils respectively.

Chromosome: 5q31.1
Gene product: 18-28 kDa
Produced by: mast cells, T lymphocytes, endothelial cells, fibroblasts, and thymic epithelial cells
Induced by: TNF-α, IL-1, LPS, phorbol esters, calcium ionophore A23187
Receptor: Heterodimer composed of GM-CSF-specific α subunit (CD116, on chromosomes Xp22.32, Yp11.3 in the pseudo-autosomal regions) and a β subunit (CDw131 on chromosome 22q12.2-13.1) shared with high-affinity IL-3 and IL-5 receptors
Knockout mouse: Susceptibility to infections by obligate intracellular organisms, pulmonary lesions resembling pulmonary alveolar proteinosis

G-CSF. G-CSF, an 18 kDa protein encoded by a gene on the long arm of chromosome 17 [112] stimulates proliferation of granulocyte progenitor cells [113-115] and activates neutrophil function[116,117]. G-CSF is produced by a wide variety of mesenchymal cells under the influence of inductive factors such as IL-1,[111], endotoxin [118], and TNFα[119]. The 115 kDa G-CSF receptor is a member of the type I cytokine receptor family with one N-terminal immunoglobulin domain[120], four fibronectin domains in the extracellular region, and a WSXWS motif necessary for signal transduction[19]. Although some argue that G-CSF has a proliferative influence on pluripotent stem cells [121,122]. G-CSF deficient mice show selective chronic neutropenia and have neutrophil counts only 20% of control animals[108], G-CSF receptor mutations may cause certain severe congenital neutropenic syndromes [123], dogs that develop neutralizing antibodies to G-CSF develop neutropenia [124], and the use of G-CSF in clinical situations has one dominant effect, the induction of neutrophil production and release. Recombinant human G-CSF is widely used in clinical practice and the indications for its use will be reviewed in subsequent chapters in Section II.

G-CSF

Chromosome: 17q11.2-q12
Gene product: 18 kDa
Produced by: monocytes, macrophages, endothelial cells, fibroblasts
Induced by: IL-1, TNF-α, endotoxin
Receptor: G-CSFR (CD114, on chromosome 1p35-34.3), 89.5 kDa polypeptides, 4 forms each differing only at the C-terminus, probably generated by alternative splicing.
Knockout Mouse: Neutropenia and failure to develop a neutrophilic leukocytosis response to infections.

Monocytes/macrophages. Mononuclear phagocytes are phylogenetically the most primitive elements of the blood being closely related functionally to the phagocytic coloemocytes of invertebrates [125, 126]. *In vitro*, both GM-CSF and macrophage-CSF (M-CSF) both regulate survival and function of monocytes, but only M-CSF deficient mice have monocytopenia and macrophage deficiency [2, 127] A complete deficiency of mononuclear phagocytes is probably incompatible with life.

M-CSF. M-CSF, is encoded by a gene on the short arm of chromosome 1[128]. M-CSF which gives rise to two glycoprotein species (70-90kDa and 40-50kDa) as a result of alternative splicing [100, 129] and stimulates monocyte/macrophage proliferation[113]. M-

CSF also activates secretory[130] and phagocytic[131,132] function. The mononuclear phagocyte is an essential regulatory cell for hematopoietic cells of many lineages [133]. It is, therefore, no surprise that osteopetrotic (*op/op*) mice with a naturally occurring M-CSF deficiency [2, 127], routinely exhibit bone marrow failure[127]. As is the case with G-CSF for neutrophils and EPO for erythroid cells, M-CSF serves as the major survival factor for mononuclear phagocytes [134]. Specifically, marrow failure and osteopetrosis in M-CSF deficient mice can be restored by enforcing expression of the anti-apoptotic protein, Bcl-2 in mononuclear phagocytes of *op/op* mice[134]. Thus, M-CSF augments monocyte survival permitting them to respond to internal and external cues for their differentiation. The M-CSF receptor, the c-fms proto-oncogene product encoded by a gene on human chromosome 5q32-33, is a type III tyrosine kinase family member.

M-CSF

<u>Chromosome:</u> **1p21-p13**
<u>Gene product:</u> **40-90 kDa**
<u>Produced by:</u> **monocytes, macrophages, fibroblasts, epithelial cells, vascular endothelial cells, osteoblasts**
<u>Induced by:</u> **IL-3, IL-4, TNF-α, endotoxin**
<u>Receptor:</u> **a 165 kDa cell-surface receptor tyrosine kinase, encoded by c-fms, a cellular proto-oncogene located on human chromosome 5q33-34, is the cellular homologue of the v-fms oncogene of the McDonough strain of feline sarcoma virus.**
<u>M-CSF deficient mice:</u> **severe deficiency of macrophages and osteoclasts, hematopoietic failure, osteopetrosis**

<u>Eosinophils</u>. Eosinophil production depends on GM-CSF, IL-3 and IL-5 [135], the latter being the more cell-type-specific of the three, at least in granulopoiesis (IL-5 exerts effects in lymphoid cells too). Again, just as G-CSF and EPO are survival factors for their respective lineages, IL-5 prolongs the survival of eosinophils [10] and incubation of human bone marrow cells in suspension culture with IL-5 induces production of a greater fraction of eosinophils[136, 137].

<u>IL-5</u>. Interleukin 5 [136,138], the gene for which is also located on the long arm of chromosome 5 [139], stimulates both proliferation of progenitors and function of the progeny (Figure 8). IL-5 is produced by T-lymphocytes induced by antigen, mitogens, and phorbol esters [136,138]. The high-affinity IL-5 receptor is a dimer composed of an IL-5 specific ligand-binding a-chain and a b-chain also common to the GM-CSF and IL-3 receptors [14,15].

IL-5

<u>Chromosome:</u> **5q31.1**
<u>Gene product:</u> **50-60 kDa**
<u>Produced by:</u> **T lymphocytes**
<u>Induced by:</u> **antigen, mitogen, phorbol esters**
<u>Receptor:</u> **heterodimer composed of IL-5-specific α-subunit (CDw125, human chromosome 3p26-p24) and β-subunit (CDw131, human chromosome 22q12.2-q13.1, shared with the high-affinity GM-CSF and IL-3 receptors)**
<u>IL-5 deficiency:</u> **failure to mount an appropriate eosinophilic response**

The lymphopoietic functions of IL-5 are reviewed in Table 1. The role of IL-5 in production and migration of eosinophils is clearly demonstrated by experiments in which anti-IL-5 antibodies inhibit parasite induced eosinophilia in mice[140], and in which mice with IL-5Rβ chain deficiency also failed to mount an eosinophilic response to N. brasiliensis [141].

Basophils. The production of basophils and mast cells is induced by IL-3 (reviewed below) and SF (reviewed above), which seem to be sufficient *in vitro* to stimulate production and viability of this cell type, although the relationship between these factors and IL-4 has not been clarified[142].

Megakaryocytopoiesis (Figure 10)

IL-3[143,144], IL-6[145,146], IL-11[147,148], LIF [149], SF [150], and EPO [57; 151] have been reported to influence production and/or maturation of megakaryocytes. However, the most profound effects on platelet counts have been seen using TPO and IL-11.

Thrombopoietin (TPO). TPO, an 36-kd protein (65-85 kD when full glycosylated)[152] encoded by a gene on the long arm of chromosome 3 [152,153], is constitutively produced by a variety of organs/cell types including hepatocytes, proximal convoluted tubule cells of the kidney, bone marrow stromal cells, muscle, brain and spleen cells[154-156]. The TPO receptor is the gene product of c-mpl, the human homologue of the murine myeloproliferative leukemia virus, encoded by a gene on human chromosome 1 (1p34) and the D band of murine chromosome 4 [157]. The extracellular domain of c-mpl resembles the hematopoietic growth factor superfamily[158].

Hepatocytes are the primary source of serum thrombopoietin in humans. Indeed, serum thrombopoietin levels are low to undetectable in patients with cirrhosis and thrombocytopenia and increase within two days after orthotopic liver transplantation[159,160]. Circulating thrombopoietin binds via the c-mpl protein to platelets and to a lesser extent megakaryocytes, is internalized and then degraded[161]. Thrombopoietin levels are inversely related to the platelet count in patients with thrombocytopenia and can be decreased by platelet transfusion[162-164]. Serum thrombopoietin is also inversely related to megakaryocyte mass [155, 165]. The increase in TPO levels seen in thrombocytopenia do not appear to be due to any increase in TPO production but instead results from a decrease in TPO binding to platelets and/or megakaryocytes[155, 161, 163].

The *in vivo* role of TPO in regulating hematopoiesis has been demonstrated in mice nullizygous for TPO or its receptor. Such mice have marked thrombocytopenia (platelet counts 5-10% of normal) but have normal hematocrits, white blood cell counts and peripheral numbers of neutrophils, lymphocytes, monocytes and eosinophils[166,167,168]. The platelets in such knockout mice seem to function normally, demonstrating that TPO/c-mpl is not absolutely required for production of normal platelets but that TPO is the primary regulator of platelet mass *in vivo*. It also has additional, multilineage effects. In c-mpl -/- mice, bone marrow, spleen and peripheral blood contain significant reductions of CFU-GM, BFU-E, and CFU-GEMM [166,167]. Day-12 CFU-S and long-term repopulating cells are reduced by an order of magnitude in c-mpl -/- mice [169,170]. The magnitude of the stem cell deficiency in these mice is equivalent to that seen in flk2/flt3 -/- mice indicating that TPO, like flt3 ligand and SF are necessary for optimal stem cell maintenance *in vivo*.

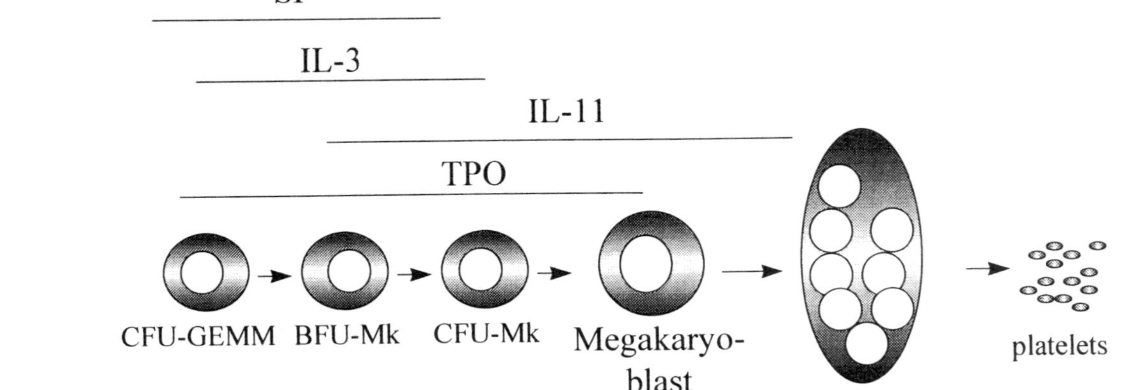

Figure 10. Humoral control of megakaryocyte and platelet production. The two humoral factors that influence this process directly include IL-11 (currently approved for clinical use) and thrombopoietin (TPO), both of which induce more rapid recovery of platelets after bone marrow injury. BFU-Mk = burst forming unit of megakaryocytopoiesis, CFU-Mk = colony forming unit of megakaryocytopoiesis.

TPO has been used to date in a limited number of human clinical trials. Treatment with a single dose or with daily doses of TPO result in a dose dependent but late increase in platelet count associated with an increase in bone marrow megakaryocytes[171-173]. There is conflicting data on the effect of TPO on bone marrow progenitors but it is clear that TPO treatment causes mobilization of hematopoietic progenitors [171-173].

TPO

<u>Chromosome:</u> **human 3q27-28, mouse chromosome 16**
<u>Gene product:</u> **65-85 kDa**
<u>Produced by:</u> **wide variety of somatic cells including bone those of marrow stroma, spleen, renal tubule, liver, muscle, brain**
<u>Receptor:</u> **c-mpl, chromosome 1p34,**
<u>TPO deficiency (or c-mpl deficiency):</u> **marked thrombocytopenia but no anemia or leukopenia.**

IL-11. The IL-11 cDNA was isolated from the primate bone marrow stromal cell line PU-34[147]. The 19 kDa protein is encoded by a gene located on human chromosome 19[174]. IL-11 is produced by fibroblasts and bone marrow stromal cells, and its production is markedly increased by IL-1[147, 175;,176]. The IL-11 receptor is a type I cytokine receptor heterodimer consisting of IL-11Rα, structurally related to CD126 (IL-6Rα) and gp130 [177, 178]. the latter being shared with the alpha chains of LIF, OSM, CNTF, and IL-6 (Figure 2).

IL-11 is a pleiotropic cytokine with growth stimulatory effects, which overlap those of IL-6, on multiple classes of lymphoid and myeloid cells[176,179]. These bioactivities are reviewed in Table 1. Of relevance to our categorization of IL-11 as a megakaryocytic growth factor, in combination with IL-3, IL-11 induces an upward shift in the ploidy values of cultured megakaryocytes.[180] *In vivo*, IL-11 administration stimulates megakaryocytopoiesis, increases peripheral platelet and neutrophil counts, and increases the numbers and cycling activity of all classes of committed hematopoietic progenitor cells[181, 182]. Taking these important bioactivities into account, it is rather surprising that IL-11Rα knockout mice have no hematological defect, indicating that IL-11 is completely dispensable for hematopoiesis, at least in mice [183].

IL-11

<u>Chromosome:</u> **19q13.3-13.4**
<u>Gene product:</u> **19-24 kDa**
<u>Produced by:</u> **fibroblasts, bone marrow stromal cells**
<u>Induced by:</u> **IL-1, PMA, calcium ionophore A23187**
<u>Receptor:</u> **Heterodimer consisting of the 43 kDa IL-11Rα chain encoded by a gene located on human chromosome 9p13 and the CD130 (gp130) molecule (Figure 2B) encoded by a gene on chromosome 5q11.**
<u>Knockout mouse:</u> **no hematological defect detected**

Notwithstanding its dispensability, the clear influence of IL-11 on megakaryocytes underscores the potential therapeutic value of this cytokine in the management of thrombocytopenia and chemotherapy- or radiation-induced myelosuppression. Indeed,

IL-11 has been approved for prevention of severe thrombocytopenia and to reduce platelet transfusion requirements for patients receiving cytotoxic chemotherapy for non-myeloid malignancies.

Lymphopoiesis (Figure 11)

The growth and development of lymphoid cells from the common lymphoid progenitor [184] occurs in multiple anatomical locations where different factors may influence these processes. Many of the hematopoietic growth factors and interleukins have been shown to play a role in the growth and development of B-cells (Fig. 4A), and T-lymphocytes (Fig. 4B). Natural killer cell control is less well understood, although the role of IL-12 and IL-15 in this process seems quite clear. (Fig. 4C)

IL-7. IL-7 is a true lymphopoietic factor. A 17 kDa protein encoded by a gene on human chromosome 8q12-13[185]. IL-7 is produced by bone marrow stromal cells [186] and intestinal epithelial cells[187], and binds to a heteromeric receptor which shares a common gamma chain with the receptors for IL-2, 4, 7, 9, and 15 (Figure 2C). The IL-7Rα chain (CD127) is a type I cytokine receptor expressed on bone marrow lymphoid progenitor cells, thymocytes, mature T-cells and mononuclear phagocytes. As shown in Table 1, the biological activity of IL-7 is heavily weighted toward the lymphoid lineage, inducing the clonal growth of normal pre-B cells[186,188], pre-T cells,[189] and various types of neoplastic lymphoid cells[190]. It acts synergistically with flt3-ligand and IL-10 to augment growth of primitive B lymphocytes[191]. Like other hematopoietic growth factors, it can act indirectly as well by enhancing production of other growth factors, IL-3 and GM-CSF production by activated T-cells[192] and IL-6, IL-1, TNF-α, and IL-8 production by peripheral blood monocytes[193; 194] for example. The clear lymphopoietic function of this cytokine is best clarified by findings of lymphopenia and severe combined immunodeficiency in IL-7 [195] or IL-7Rα[196] knockout mice. Mutant mice have lymphocytopenia and have reduced B-cell and T-cell numbers in lymphoid organs including spleen and thymus.

IL-7

Chromosome: 8q12-13
Gene product: 17 kDa
Produced by: marrow stromal cells, spleen, and thymus tissue
Receptor: Class I cytokine heterodimeric receptor, unique 49 kDa alpha chain (CD127, chromosome 5p13) and a 40 kDa common gamma chain, γ_c (CD132, chromosome Xq13) which the alpha chain shares with those of IL-2, IL-4, IL-9, IL-13, and IL-15.
Knockout mice: lymphopenia and severe reductions in B-cell and T-cell cellularity of all lymphoid organs including nodes, spleen, marrow and thymus

---

IL-2. IL-2 is encoded by a gene located on chromosome 4[197]. The 23-kd gene product is produced by T lymphocytes induced by mitogens, antigens, certain antibodies, phorbol esters, and lectins [198-200]. The IL-2 receptor (IL-2R), a heterotrimer of 55 (α)-, 75 (β)-, and 64 (γ)-kDa subunit, [199, 201,202], is expressed by T cells [203], B cells [204-206], and natural killer (NK) cells [207]. The biologic activities of IL-2 are broad and are reviewed in Table 1. It is clear that this cytokine is *not required for lymphopoiesis* per se because IL-2 knockout mice do not suffer from lymphopenia or immune deficiency[208], in fact, the mice develop a syndrome of generalized inflammatory disease that involves multiple organs[209,210], often with severe fatal colitis.

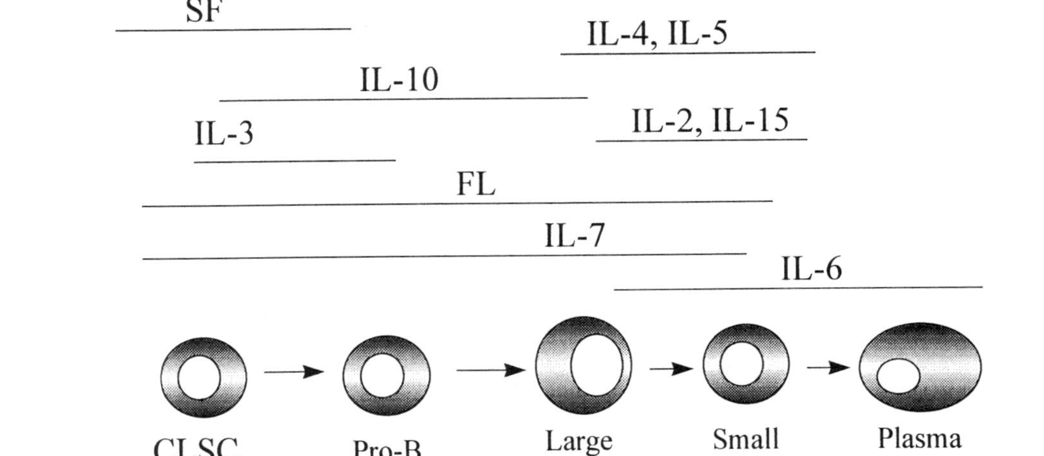

Figure 11. Humoral control of B-lymphopoiesis. Some of the many factors involved in regulating growth and differentiation of lymphoid cells are sufficient to induce growth or differentiation or both. However, most of the factors act synergistically, some always need "help" (IL-6 induces B-cell differentiation only in the presence of IL-2 and IL-10 enhances pro-B cell differentiation only in the presence of flt3 ligand (FL) and IL-7). CLSC = committed lymphoid stem cell.

These surprising results indicate that IL-2 functions most prominently as a modulator, or negative regulator of the immune response and its absence, marked by uncontrolled activation and expansion of CD4+ T cells[209], disrupts the management of self tolerance[209,210].

IL-2

<u>Chromosome:</u> **4q**
<u>Gene product:</u> **23 kDa**
<u>Produced by:</u> **T lymphocytes**
<u>Induced by:</u> **mitogens, antigens, some antibodies, phorbol esters, lectins, and IL-1**
<u>Receptor and subunits:</u> **α/β/γ heterotrimer on T lymphocytes, B lymphocytes, and NK cells. α, (CD25, chromosome 10p14-p15); β, (CD122, chromosome 22q11.2-q13); γ, (CD132, Chromosome Xq13)**
<u>Knockout mice:</u> **generalized fatal immunoproliferative disorder involving multiple organs; loss of self-tolerance**

<u>IL-15</u>. IL-15 is a 14 kD polypeptide produced by a variety of cells including monocytes, macrophages, epithelial cells, muscle cells, fibroblasts, keratinocytes and hematopoietic stromal cells [211, 212]. The gene for human IL-15 maps to chromosome 4q31 in close proximity to the IL-2 gene (4q26-27)[213]. IL-15 and IL-2 exert overlapping effects in lymphopoiesis, despite a lack of significant homologies between the IL-2 and IL-15 coding sequences [212, 213]. The receptors for IL-15 and IL-2 share two subunits (the IL-2Rβ and common gamma chain) IL-15, like IL-2, is a potent modulator of NK cell activity. IL-15, used as a single agent, induces differentiation of CD3⁻CD56⁺ NK cells from CD34⁺ hematopoietic progenitor cells. SF synergizes with IL-15 to increase this expansion without altering differentiation state of expanded NK cells [214]. IL-15 may be required for the generation of functional murine NK cells[215]. Definitive testing of this hypothesis will require the generation of IL-15 -/- mice or the use of blocking antibodies to IL-15 specific subunit of the IL-15 receptor complex.

Like IL-2, IL-15 supports the proliferation and maturation of B cells and is co-stimulatory with anti-m antibody, phorbol ester or CD40-ligand.

IL-15

<u>Gene:</u> **human chromosome 4q31 (in close proximity to IL-2 [4q26-27])**
<u>Gene Product:</u> **14 kD**
<u>Produced by:</u> **Monocytes, macrophages, epithelial cells, skeletal muscle cells, bone marrow and thymic stromal cells[212]**
<u>Induced by:</u> **UV light, BCG, LPS, IL-10**
<u>Receptor:</u> **Heterotrimeric complex consisting of: IL-15 specific a-subunit (chromosome 10p14-p15), IL- 2Rb (CD122, 70 kDa, chromosome 22q11.2-q13), and IL-2Rg (CD132, 64 kDa, chromosome Xq13) subunits**

While the bioactivities of IL-2 and IL-15 are quite similar, there are several some important differences. First, IL-2 is exclusively produced by activated T cells whereas IL-15 is secreted by a much broader range of cell types but not by T cells. The widespread production of constitutive and inducible IL-15 protein may serve to target immune effector cells to sites of peripheral inflammation-infection [216, 217]. Second, only T cells, monocytes and B cells express mRNA for the IL-2Ra subunit whereas expression of mRNA for the IL-15Ra subunit is fairly ubiquitous. Third, the effects of IL-2 are restricted to hematopoietic cells whereas there is evidence that IL-15 can directly modulate some types of non-hematopoietic cells [218]. For example, IL-15 induces tryosine phosphorylation of endothelial cell proteins *in vitro* and stimulates angiogenesis *in vivo*[219].

IL-4. The IL-4 gene resides on the long arm of chromosome 5 [220-222] and encodes an 18 kDa protein [223; 224] produced by T-lymphocytes induced by phorbol esters, lectins, and certain antigens [225]. While it largely affects lymphoid cells, it can influence non-lymphoid lineages [226,227]. IL-4 deficient mice are viable and have defective Th2 cytokine production after nematode infections.

IL-4

Chromosome: 5q23-q21
Gene product: 18 kDa
Produced by: T lymphocytes (both CD4$^+$ and CD8$^+$)
Induced by: phorbol esters, calcium ionophore A23187
Receptor: heterodimeric member of the cytokine receptor superfamily; ~87 kDa α-chain (CD124, chromosome 16p11.2-p12.1) and the ~40 kDa γ_c chain (CD132, chromosome Xq13) which is shared with the complex receptors for IL-2, IL-7, IL-9, and IL-15.
Knockout mice: defective Th2 cytokine responses, resistance to murine retroviral immunodeficiency syndrome

---

IL-10. Human IL-10 is an 18 kDa protein [228] which is expressed as a noncovalent homodimer[229] and is encoded by a gene on chromosome 1[230]. The IL-10 receptor is a 90-110 kDa class II cytokine receptor family member (Fig 5), consisting of two extracellular fibronectin type III domains but no WSXWS motif and a 318 amino acid cytoplasmic region. IL-10 is truly pleiotropic (Table 1). IL-10 knockout mice challenged with Aspergillus fumigatus have an exaggerated immune response including increased release of IL-4, IL-5, and IFNγ and a higher than normal mortality rate. Similar results are found in the same murine model challenged with Toxoplasma[231]. Some strains of IL-10 deficient mice also develop chronic enterocolitis followed by carcinoma of the colon [232]. These findings confirmed earlier studies that first characterized IL-10 as "cytokine synthesis inhibitory factor (CSIF)" because of its capacity to inhibit the production of cytokines by T-lymphocytes[233].

IL-10

Chromosome: 1q31-q32
Gene product: 18 kDa
Produced by: T cells, activated B cells and B-cell lymphomas, mononuclear phagocytes, keratinocytes
Induced by: LPS, anti-CD3, PMA
Receptor: class II receptor family, 90-110 kDa, human chromosome 11
Knockout mice: exaggerated immune responses to obligate intracellular parasites, inflammatory bowel disease

---

IL-12. IL-12 is a 75 kDa heterodimer composed of disulfide-linked 35 and 40 kDa (p35 and p40, respectively) subunits[234,235].   Isolation of their respective cDNAs demonstrated that p35 and p40 are encoded by distinct genes and that expression of both is necessary for production of the biologically active molecule[236,237]. The two subunits of the IL-12 receptor consist of IL12RB2 (human chromosome 1p31.2) and IL12B1 (human chromosome 19p13.1)[238]. The IL12RB1 chain contains 5 fibronectin III domains and has a high degree of homology to CD130[239]. Interleukin-12 knockout mice, viable and fertile, are immunologically compromised. Although they display no gross developmental abnormalities, the capacity of these mice to mount a Th1 response and to release IFNγ in response to endotoxin is impaired and murine strains ordinarily resistant to Leishmania major become sensitive to this organism when IL-12 deficient[240,241].

IL-12

Gene product: 75-kd heterodimer of 35- and 40-kd subunits
Produced by: mononuclear phagocytes, EBV-transformed B-cell lines
Induced by: LPS, various pathogens
Receptor: single class of high-affinity receptors approximately 110 kDa in size
Knockout mice: unable to mount a Th1 response, can't release IFNγ in response to endotoxin, can't resist Leishmanial infection

---

IL-13. IL-13, a 10 kDa Th2 cytokine encoded by a gene located on human chromosome 5q31 (in the cluster that also contains IL-3, IL-5, IL-4, and GM-CSF)[242], shares many biological activities with IL-4. The similarity in biological activity of IL-4 and IL-13 is probably due to shared signal transduction pathways and receptor structure[243]. Consistent with the current model of the IL-13 receptor, a mutant IL-4 protein has been described that competitively antagonizes the activity of both IL-4 and IL-13[244]. The bioactivities of IL-13 are reviewed in Table 1. Of particular interest is the capacity of IL-13 to repress HIV-1 replication in alveolar- and peripheral blood derived-macrophages[245,246].

IL-13

Chromosome: 5q23-q21 (Note that IL-4 and IL-13 are located within 12 kb in a "head to tail" orientation[251]
Gene Product: Isoforms of 9 and 17 kD. 17 kD probably represents a N-glycosylated isoform.[252]
Produced by: Th2 T cells, basophils, stromal cells
Induced by: CD28 ligation,[252] Ionomycin, PMA,[253], anti-IgE[254]
Receptor: Heterodimer consisting of IL-13-specific "-subunit, IL-4-specific "-subunit and possibly a third subunit; g-c subunit shared by IL-2, -4, -7 , -9 and −15 is not required for IL-13 signal transduction

---

Although the actions of IL-4 and IL-13 are largely redundant several distinctions can be made: first, IL-13, unlike IL-4, has no significant effect on T cells[247], second, the kinetics of IL-13 secretion following T cell activation differ from those of IL-4[248]. Finally, IL-13 does not regulate pre-B cell differentiation. IL-13 may have a future role in the treatment of macrophage-mediated inflammatory conditions such as septic shock and some autoimmune diseases. In mice, treatment with IL-13 protects against

LPS-induced lethal endotoxemia [249]. Another clinical use for IL-13 may be in the treatment of HIV infection possibly in combination with other immune modulators such as IL-16 [245,250].

IL-14. IL-14 a 60 kDa polypeptide produced by normal T cells, T cell clones, and cell lines generated from patients with T or B cell lymphomas [255]. IL-14 secretion is induced by PHA stimulation but not by treatment with LPS, phorbol ester or concanavalin A [256,257]. IL-14 binds to a 90 kD receptor that is only expressed by cells of B cell lineage [255,258]. As predicted by the cellular distribution of IL-14R expression, only cells of B cell lineage respond to IL-14.

In contrast to the results with normal B cells, neoplastic B cells are often responsive to IL-14 without requirement for a co-mitogenic stimulus. In the majority of cases of pre-B ALL, hairy cell leukemia, prolymphocytic leukemia or B-cell CLL the malignant cells will be stimulated to proliferate *in vitro* by addition of IL-14 [258,259]. In some patients, autocrine or paracrine production of IL-14 by malignant B cells may play a pathologic role [260]. Abnormalities of IL-14 receptor signal transduction may also be involved in certain non-malignant disease states including systemic lupus erythematosus [261].

IL-14

Chromosome: Not assigned
Gene Product: 60 kDa
Produced by: T cells, T and B lineage lymphoma cells
Induced by: PHA
Receptor: 90 kDa

IL-16. IL-16, formerly known as lymphocyte chemoattractant factor, is unique among the interleukins in that its cognate receptor (CD4) is an immune costimulatory molecule rather than a typical growth factor receptor [262]. IL-16 is a 16-18 kD protein that is formed by caspase 3 proteolytic cleavage of the pro-IL-16 polypeptide [263]. The main cellular source of IL-16 appears to be CD8+ T cells, although eosinophils and mast cells also produce IL-16 protein [264-266]. The bioactivities of IL-16 are reviewed in Table 1. IL-16 receptor deficient mice (CD4 -/-) have been described, but the phenotype in these mice is more likely due to a loss of the co-stimulatory actions of CD4 in T cell development than from a loss of IL-16 ligand binding activity [267].

IL-16 represses HIV-1 promoter activity (quantified using an HIV-1 LTR-reporter sequence)[268], and although IL-16 does not suppress HIV-1 replication in naturally infected peripheral blood mononuclear cells[269], when expressed in CD4+ human cells, IL-16 renders these cells resistant to HIV-1 infection [270].

IL-16

Chromosome: unknown
Gene Product: 16-18 kD, production of functional IL-16 requires cleavage of pro-IL-6 polypeptide by caspase 3[263]
Produced by: CD8+ T cells, mas56t cells
Induced by: serotonin, antigen challenge, C5a, PMA, histamine
Bioactivity: see Table 2

Factors with Multilineage Activity ("Early Acting" Factors)

At least 6 growth factors, IL-3 [271,272], GM-CSF [273,274], SF [275], FL [276], IL-9, IL-6, IL-10[229], and TPO [277,278], have obvious direct effects on multilineage progenitor cells and are thus capable of stimulating hematopoietic precursors before they have become fully committed to one lineage or another. Because of the heavily tilted lineage specific effects of most of these factors, only IL-3, FL, IL-9 and IL-6 are reviewed below in the category of early acting factors.

IL-3. IL-3 was one of the earliest recognized multipotential hematopoietic growth factors[113,114,279]. The human IL-3 gene (5q31.1, only 9kb upstream of the gene for GM-CSF) encodes a 14-28 kDa protein that influences the growth of multiple lineages. To date, only T-lymphocytes (induced by mitogens, phorbol esters, and certain antigens) [280], mast cells [281], and certain cell types in mouse brain tissue[282] have been found to express the IL-3 gene. Although T-lymphocytes can be induced to produce both IL-3 [283; 284] and GM-CSF [284], there is clear cut evidence that each is regulated independently of the other[285].

The direct growth-stimulatory effects of IL-3 seem to be largely limited to very primitive committed progenitors like the BFU-E [286-288] and hematopoietic progenitor cells with multilineage potential [287,289] possibly even CFU-S[290]. When expressed by human stromal cells engineered to produce human IL-3, SF, FL, or IL-7, only IL-3 expressing cells were capable of supporting sustained human hematopoiesis in a murine xenograft model[291]. Interestingly, notwithstanding all of its direct and indirect hematopoietic effects, IL-3 is completely dispensable for normal steady state hematopoiesis because no hematopoietic defects have been found in IL-3 knockout mice [292].

IL-3

Chromosome: 5q31.1
Gene product: 14-28 kDa
Produced by: T lymphocytes, mast cells
Induced by: mitogens, phorbol esters, calcium ionophore A23187, IgE receptor activation (mast cells)
Receptor: heterodimer of IL-3-specific α subunit (CDw123, chromosome Xp22.3, Yp13.3) and a β subunit (CDw131, chromosome 22q12.2-q13.1) shared in common with IL-5 and GM-CSF receptors
Knockout Mice: No hematopoietic defect in steady state; deficient delayed type hypersensitivity[292]

FL. FL is the cognate ligand for the flt3/flk2 receptor tyrosine kinase [293]. Flt3/flk2 is a member of the type III receptor tyrosine kinase family (reviewed in [294]) Indeed, the flt3/flk2 gene shares a common genomic structural organization with c-kit and c-fms [295]. Human flt3/flk2 is a 993 amino acid protein with a predicted molecular mass of 110 kD and contains ten potential sites for N-linked glycosylation. Cell-associated flt3/flk2 has a molecular mass of 155-160 kD, the difference in apparent versus predicted molecular mass is attributed to glycosylation [296,297].

As is the case for M-CSF and SF, both soluble and membrane-bound FL protein isoforms have biologic activity [298,299]. The relative biologic significance of membrane-bound and soluble isoforms of FL have not been determined.

Normal serum levels of FL in humans are less than 100 pg/ml. Levels of FL are not increased in patients with anemia only, but increase dramatically in patients with pancytopenia such as seen with aplastic anemia, Fanconi anemia or chemotherapy and/or radiation induced myelosuppression [294,300].

The biological activity of FL is substantial (Table 1). In general, FL has little *in vitro* colony stimulating activity as a single agent but has potent synergism with a variety of other hemopoietins including SF [293,301], IL-3 [293,301], IL-7 [301], GM-CSF [302], G-CSF [302,303], IL-6 [293], M-CSF [302], IL-11 [304,305], as well as with multi-cytokine combinations [306,307].

FL responsive hematopoietic cells appear to be more primitive and have greater lineage restriction than SF responsive cells. FL supports the *in vitro* proliferation of LTCIC, CFU-S and long-term repopulating cells [308-311]. FL increases recruitment of primitive HPC into the cell cycle and inhibits apoptosis [310,312].

Considering the heterogeneous "early acting" effects of this cytokine on hematopoiesis, it is surprising, just as it was with IL-11Rα knockout mice, that no marrow failure state is found in mice with targeted disruptions of the flk2/flt3 gene [313]. These mice, unlike mice nullizygous for SF or c-kit, are viable and had no gross abnormalities of bone marrow or spleen cellularity, peripheral blood counts or morphology. There are, however, subclinical deficiencies in B-lymphopoiesis and a clear stem cell defect in transplant experiments; Flt3/flk2 nullizygous marrow was 4.5-fold less efficient in repopulating peripheral blood, 2.5-fold less efficient in repopulating marrow and spleen, and 8- fold less efficient in thymic repopulation. Thus, the flt3/flk2 gene appears to be crucial for stem cell transplantation especially for lymphoid reconstitution.

FL

Chromosome: 19q13.3
Gene Product: Various isoforms are produced by alternative splicing. Membrane and soluble isoforms exist
Produced by: mRNA expressed by most tissues examined including spleen, lung, stromal cells, peripheral blood mononuclear cells, T cell clones
Induced by: IL-1α, pancytopenia
Receptor: Flt3/flk2, a type III receptor tyrosine kinase, human chromosome 13q12-13
Knockout Mice: 50% reduction in pro-B cells, 25% reduction in pre-B cells, 6-fold reduction in B-cell colony forming potential, reduced repopulating capacity of stem cells

---

IL-9. The IL-9 [314; 315] gene is on the portion of the long arm of chromosome 5 [316,317] that also carries the genes that encode GM-CSF, IL-3, IL-4, IL-5, the M-CSF receptor (c-fms), and a number of other cytokines and growth factor receptors. IL-9 is produced by activated T-lymphocytes, primarily CD4+ lymphocytes[318,319], and both IL-4 and IL-10 can induce IL-9 gene expression, but *in vivo*, IL-10 is the most critical because IL-9 expression is low in IL-10 knockout mice, but is not low in IL-4 knockout mice[320]. The IL-9 receptor is a member of the hematopoietic growth factor superfamily (Figure 2) and is expressed in membrane-bound and soluble forms[321]. The receptor is expressed on erythroid, myeloid, and lymphoid precursor cells as well as activated T-cells and T-cell lines. In combination with erythropoietin, IL-9 supports BFU-E-derived colony growth [322,323], supports the clonal growth of fetal erythroid, multipotential, and granulocyte-macrophage progenitors[323], but does not exhibit megakaryocytopoietic activity.

IL-9

<u>Chromosome:</u> 5q31.2-31.3
<u>Gene product:</u> 20-30 kDa
<u>Produced by:</u> **T lymphocytes**
<u>Induced by:</u> **PHA, PMA, calcium ionophore A23187, anti-CD3, IL-1, IL-2, HTLV-I or -II**
<u>Receptor:</u> **522-amino acid member of hematopoietic growth factor receptor superfamily**

<u>IL-6</u>. The IL-6 gene resides on the short arm of chromosome 7 [221; 324] and encodes a 21-26 kDa protein [325]. The expression of the gene is seen in heterogeneous cell types including fibroblasts[326], endothelial cells[327], monocyte/macrophages[326], and T-lymphocytes [328]. IL-6 is induced by IL-1[111], TNF-α [329], mitogens [328], and endotoxin[330].

Largely a synergistic factor, recombinant human IL-6 has no clearly demonstrable direct effect on the proliferation of any human hematopoietic progenitor cell on its own although it stimulates murine granulocyte/macrophage colony formation [331; 332] and is unambiguously an autocrine and paracrine growth factor for malignant lymphoid and myeloma cell lines [333-336].

IL-6 deficiency adversely affects survival of hematopoietic stem cells and early progenitor cells of multiple lineages [337]. A recent study on IL-6 deficient mice, suggests strongly that IL-6 also functions as an essential antiinflammatory cytokine that, like IL-10, modulates the intensity of the inflammatory response[338],

---

IL-6

<u>Chromosome:</u> 7p
<u>Gene product:</u> 21-26 kDa
<u>Produced by:</u> **macrophages, endothelial cells, fibroblasts, T lymphocytes**
<u>Induced by:</u> **IL-1, mitogens, endotoxin**
<u>Receptor:</u> **Heterodimer consisting of; the ligand binding protein IL-6Rα (CD126), a 450-amino acid low affinity binding protein encoded by a gene on 1q21 and the protein gp130 (CD130) encoded by a gene located on 5q11 which also serves as a beta chain for CNTF, IL-11, oncostatin M, and LIF.**
<u>Knockout mouse:</u> **reduced survival of hematopoietic stem cells and multilineage progenitors, reduced T cell numbers, reduced proliferation and maturation of erythroid and myeloid cells**

Factors That Function as Inducers of Growth Factor Gene Expression

Some proteins which regulate hematopoiesis *in vivo* and *in vitro* do so indirectly (Table 2). That is, in some cases they incite bystander cells, also known as "accessory" or "auxiliary" cells, to release direct-acting factors.

<u>IL-1</u>. IL-1 was formerly known as endogenous pyrogen, lymphocyte activating factor, and many other names. IL-1 exists in two molecular forms (IL-1a and IL-1b) which are encoded by two genes on chromosome 2. Each of these genes encodes 31

kDa precursor molecules which are cleaved by IL-1 converting enzyme[339] to 17 kDa peptides. IL-1, originally thought to be produced only by monocytes and macrophages, is produced by almost all cells. Gene expression is induced by endotoxin, IL-1, GM-CSF, TNF-α and IL-2. The bioactivity of IL-1 is tremendously broad and there is good evidence that it regulates expression of most genes encoding mediators of inflammation. IL-1 has no colony-stimulating activity itself. However, when administered *in vivo*, IL-1 universally induces neutrophilic leukocytosis, which results from the induction of G-CSF and GM-CSF expression by other cells, including fibroblasts, endothelial cells [111], thymic epithelial cells [340] and T-lymphocytes.

IL-1α and β

Chromosome: 2q
Gene product: 31-kd precursor, mature 17-kd cleavage product
Produced by: most cells
Induced by: endotoxin, IL-1, GM-CSF, TNF-α, IL-2
Receptors: CDw121b, a 68 kDa protein encoded by a gene on 2q12-q22, and CD121a, an 80-kDa protein encoded by a gene on the same chromosome (2q12). Both are members of immunoglobulin superfamily
Knockout mice: IL-1β: minor defects. IL-1RI: no dramatic effects on immune system or hematopoiesis.

TNF-α. TNF-α, a 17 kDa protein (a cleavage product of a 29 kDa membrane associated protein) encoded by a gene stationed on chromosome 6 [341] near the major histocompatibility complex [342], shares with IL-1 a large number of heterogeneous biological activities (Table 2) and, like IL-1, functions largely to induce the expression of other subordinate genes which, in turn, function as more specific regulators of hematopoietic responses to inflammation. That EPO gene expression is not induced by TNF-α may account for the vulnerability of erythroid cells in anemic patients with chronic inflammatory diseases in which the organism induces TNFα gene expression[343, 344]. When factors like TNF-α have confusing double-edged biological functions (e.g. suppress colony growth and induce growth factor gene expression), it takes an *in vivo* model to assign weight to the *in vitro* responses reported. This has been done recently and it is clear that the stimulatory effect of TNF-α dominates in granulopoiesis [345,346] but inhibitory effects dominate erythropoiesis [343,347].

TNF-α

Chromosome: 6p
Gene product: 17 kDa (cleaved by TNF converting enzyme from a 26 kDa precursor)
Produced by: macrophages, B lymphocytes, NK cells
Induced by: endotoxin, GM-CSF, IL-3, poly(I):poly(C), phorbol esters, calcium ionophore A23187
Receptor: 55 kDa protein homologous to nerve growth factor receptor
Bioactivity: see Table 2
Knockout mice: TNF-RI deficient mice: hypersensitive to bacterial infections, failure of endotoxin to induce iNOS, failure of TNF to induce IL-6, GM-CSF, ICAM-1, and VCAM-1

IL-17. IL-17 is a 22 kDa cytokine homologous to the predicted amino acid sequence of open reading frame 13 (ORF13) of Herpesvirus samiri. This homology is analogous to the presence of an IL-10 homologue in the genome of the Epstein-Barr virus [348]. The gene encoding the receptor for the human IL-17R has recently been cloned and resides on chromosome 22q11.22-23. IL-17R is ubiquitously expressed and protein is expressed by all hematopoietic and epithelial cell lines that have been tested [349,350]. IL-17 is produced by activated memory T cells and induces stromal cells to secrete inflammatory and hematopoietic cytokines including IL-6, IL-8, PGE2, G-CSF and GM-CSF[351], and ICAM-1[350].

IL-17

Chromosome: unknown
Gene Product: 15 and 22 kD isoforms. The 22 kD protein is produced by glycosylation of the 15 kD isoform.
Produced by: activated T cells; in mice, IL-17 is only produced by TCR ab+/CD4-/CD8- cells.
Induced by: PMA, ionomycin, CD3 ligation, PHA
Receptor: Predominant species 128-132 kDa, minor species of 105-107 kD (non-glycosylated form); human chromosome 22q11.22-23

IL-18. IL-18, an 18 kD protein produced by macrophages and keratinocytes[352], induces IFN-γ production from lymphoid cells including unfractionated peripheral blood mononuclear cells. Pro-IL-18 is cleaved by the IL-1- converting enzyme (ICE, caspase-1) to yield the active protein [353,354]. The receptor for IL-18 is a member of the IL-1 receptor family, also known as IL-1-receptor related protein (IL-1RRP) [355].

IL-18

Also known as: Interferon-γ-inducing factor, IL-1γ
Chromosome: unknown
Gene Product: 18 kD
Produced by: keratinocytes, Kupffer cells, activated macrophages, osteoblastic stromal cells
Induced by: LPS
Receptor: 60-100 kD protein (previously known as IL-1R related protein)
Bioactivity: see Table 2

Summary

Our current knowledge of hematopoietic control derives, in large part, from five pathways of laboratory and clinical investigation each of which inform and sometimes surprise us. These include: (1) hematopoietic cell culture methods, (2) characterization of cytokine and growth factor genes and the proteins they encode, (3) the identification of lineage- and stage-specific cytokine receptor molecules, (4) the development of cytokine and cytokine receptor knockout mice and (5) clinical trials of recombinant hematopoietic growth factors. Despite the complexities of hematopoietic control, cause-and-effect relationships are clearly testable using a combination of the five approaches. Because many of these cells and hematopoietic factors have homologues in primitive organisms, and because disruptions of selected components of the control system can result in a wide variety of clinical disorders from leukemia to aplastic anemia, this extraordinarily efficient molecular network is a paradigm with profound implications for not only clinicians but for developmental biologists, cell biologists, and molecular biologists as well.

References

1.   Nijhof W, Wierenga PK, Sahr K, ct al.: Induction of globin mRNA transcription by erythropoietin in differentiating erythroid precursor cells. Exp.Hematol. 15:779, 1987
2.   Wiktor-Jedrzejczak W, Bartocci A, Ferrante AW, Jr., et al: Total absence of colony-stimulating factor 1 in the macrophage- deficient osteopetrotic (op/op) mouse [published erratum appears in Proc Natl Acad Sci U S A 1991 Jul 1;88(13):5937]. Proc.Natl.Acad.Sci.U.S.A. 87 :4828, 1990
3.   Nicola NA, Metcalf D: Subunit promiscuity among hemopoietic growth factor receptors. Cell 67:1, 1991
4.   Bazan JF: Structural design and molecular evolution of a cytokine receptor superfamily. Proc.Natl.Acad.Sci.USA 87:6934, 1990
5.   Hilton DJ, Watowich SS, Katz L, et al: Saturation mutagenesis of the WSXWS motif of the erythropoietin receptor. J.Biol.Chem. 271:4699, 1996
6.   Patthy L: Homology of a domain of the growth hormone/prolactin receptor family with type III modules of fibronectin [letter]. Cell 61:13, 1990
7.   Baffy G, Miyashita T, Williamson JR, et al: Apoptosis induced by withdrawal of interleukin-3 (IL-3) from an IL-3-dependent hematopoietic cell line is associated with repartitioning of intracellular calcium and is blocked by enforced Bcl-2 oncoprotein production. J.Biol.Chem. 268:6511, 1993
8.   Magnelli L, Cinelli M, Turchetti A, et al: Apoptosis induction in 32D cells by IL-3 withdrawal is preceded by a drop in the intracellular calcium level. Biochem.Biophys.Res.Commun. 194:1394, 1993
9.   Collins MK, Marvel J, Malde P, et al: Interleukin 3 protects murine bone marrow cells from apoptosis induced by DNA damaging agents. J.Exp.Med. 176:1043, 1992
10.   Yamaguchi Y, Suda T, Ohta S, et al: Analysis of the survival of mature human eosinophils: Interleukin- 5 prevents apoptosis in mature human eosinophils. Blood 78:2542, 1991
11.   Brach MA, deVos S, Gruss HJ, et al: Prolongation of survival of human polymorphonuclear neutrophils by granulocyte-macrophage colony-stimulating factor is caused by inhibition of programmed cell death. Blood 80:2920, 1992
12.   Muta K, Krantz SB, Bondurant MC, et al: Distinct roles of erythropoietin, insulin-like growth factor I, and stem cell factor in the development of erythroid progenitor cells. J.Clin.Invest. 94:34, 1994
13.   Dorsch M, Fan PD, Danial NN et al: The thrombopoietin receptor can mediate proliferation without activation of the Jak-STAT pathway. J.Exp.Med. 186:1947, 1997
14.   Tavernier J, Devos R, Cornelis S, et al: A human high affinity interleukin-5 receptor (IL5R) is composed of an IL-5-specific a chain and a b chain shared with the receptor for GM-CSF. Cell 66:1175, 1991
15.   Kitamura T, Sato N, Arai K, et al : Expression cloning of the human IL-3 receptor cDNA reveals a shared b subunit for the human IL-3 and GM-CSF receptors. Cell 66:1165, 1991
16.   Kuramochi S, Ikawa Y, Todokoro K: Characterization of murine erythropoietin receptor genes. J.Mol.Biol. 216:567, 1990
17.   Goodwin RG, Friend D, Ziegler SF, et al: Cloning of the human and murine interleukin-7 receptors: Demonstration of a soluble form and homology to a new receptor superfamily. Cell 60:941, 1990
18.   Honda M, Yamamoto S, Cheng M, et al: Human soluble IL-6 receptor: Its detection and enhanced release by HIV infection. J.Immunol. 148:2175, 1992
19.   Fukunaga R, Seto Y, Mizushima S, et al: Three different mRNAs encoding human granulocyte colony- stimulating factor receptor. Proc.Natl.Acad.Sci.USA 87:8702, 1990
20.   Fanslow WC, Clifford KN, Park LS, et al: Regulation of alloreactivity in vivo by IL-4 and the soluble IL- 4 receptor. J.Immunol. 147:535, 1991
21.   Bazan JF: Haemopoietic receptors and helical cytokines. Immunol.Today 11:350, 1990
22.   Premack BA, Schall TJ: Chemokine receptors: Gateways to inflammation and infection. Nature Med. 2:1174, 1996
23.   Mackay CR: Chemokines: What chemokine is that. Curr.Biol. 7:R384, 1997

24. Aronica SM, Mantel C, Gonin R, et al: Interferon-inducible protein 10 and macrophage inflammatory protein-1a inhibit growth factor stimulation of Raf-1 kinase activity and protein synthesis in a human growth factor- dependent hematopoietic cell line. J.Biol.Chem. 270:21998, 1995

25. Shuster DE, Kehrli ME, Jr., Ackermann MR: Neutrophilia in mice that lack the murine IL-8 receptor homolog. Science 269:1590, 1995

26. Barcena A, Park SW, Banapour B, et al: Expression of Fas/CD95 and Bcl-2 by primitive hematopoietic progenitors freshly isolated from human fetal liver. Blood 88:2013, 1996

27. Nagafuji K, Shibuya T, Harada M, et al: Functional expression of Fas antigen (CD95) on hematopoietic progenitor cells. Blood 86:883, 1995

28. Maciejewski JP, Selleri C, Sato T, et al: Nitric oxide suppression of human hematopoiesis in vitro. Contribution to inhibitory action of interferon-gamma and tumor necrosis factor-alpha. J.Clin.Invest. 96:1085, 1995

29. Maciejewski J, Selleri C, Anderson S, et al: Fas antigen expression on CD34+ human marrow cells is induced by interferon gamma and tumor necrosis factor alpha and potentiates cytokine-mediated hematopoietic suppression in vitro. Blood 85:3183, 1995

30. Maciejewski JP, Selleri C, Sato T, et al: Increased expression of Fas antigen on bone marrow CD34$^+$ cells of patients with aplastic anaemia. Br.J.Haematol. 91 :245, 1995

31. Rathbun RK, Faulkner GR, Ostroski MH, et al: Inactivation of the Fanconi anemia group C (FAC) gene augments interferon-gamma-induced apoptotic responses in hematopoietic cells. Blood 90:974, 1997

32. Yang Y-C, Ciarietta AB, Temple PA, et al: Human IL-3 (multi-CSF): identification by expression cloning of a novel hematopoietic growth factor related to murine IL-3. Cell 47:3, 1986

33. Ponting IL, Heyworth CM, Cormier F, et al: Serum-free culture of enriched murine haemopoietic stem cells. II: Effects of growth factors and haemin on development. Growth.Factors. 4:165, 1991

34. Monette FC: The role of interleukin-3 and heme in the induction of erythropoiesis. Ann.NY Acad.Sci. 554:49, 1989

35. Bourette RP, Royet J, Mouchiroud G, et al: Murine interleukin 9 stimulates the proliferation of mouse erythroid progenitor cells and favors the erythroid differentiation of multipotent FDCP-mix cells. Exp.Hematol. 20:868, 1992

36. Schaafsma MR, Falkenburg JHF, Duinkerken N, et al: Interleukin-9 stimulates the proliferation of enriched human erythroid progenitor cells: Additive effect with GM-CSF. Ann.Hematol. 66:45, 1993

37. Quesniaux VFJ, Clark SC, Turner K, et al: Interleukin-11 stimulates multiple phases of erythropoiesis in vitro. Blood 80:1218, 1992

38. Muta K, Krantz SB: Apoptosis of human erythroid colony-forming cells is decreased by stem cell factor and insulin-like growth factor I as well as erythropoietin. J.Cell Physiol. 156:264, 1993

39. Kaushansky K, Broudy VC, Grossmann A, et al: Thrombopoietin expands erythroid progenitors, increases red cell production, and enhances erythroid recovery after myelosuppressive therapy. J.Clin.Invest. 96:1683, 1995

40. Broxmeyer HE, Cooper S, Vadhan-Raj S: Cell cycle status of erythroid (BFU-E) progenitor cells from the bone marrows of patients on a clinical trial with purified recombinant human granulocyte-macrophage colony- stimulating factor. Exp.Hematol. 17:455, 1989

41. Valtieri M, Gabbianelli M, Pelosi E, et al: Erythropoietin alone induces erythroid burst formation by human embryonic but not adult BFU-E in unicellular serum-free culture. Blood 74:460, 1989

42. Mrug M, Stopka T, Julian BA, et al: Angiotensin II stimulates proliferation of normal early erythroid progenitors. J.Clin.Invest. 100:2310, 1997

43. McKenna HJ, De Vries P, Brasel K, et al: Effect of flt3 ligand on the ex vivo expansion of human CD34+ hematopoietic progenitor cells. Blood 86:3413, 1995

44. Lin F-K, Suggs S, Lin C-H, et al: Cloning and expression of the human erythropoietin gene. Proc.Natl.Acad.Sci.USA 82:7580, 1985

45. Browne JK, Cohen AM, Egrie JC, et al: Erythropoietin: gene cloning, protein structure and biological properties. Cold Spring Harbor Symp.Quant.Biol. 51:693, 1986

46. Powell JS, Berkner KL, Lebo RV, et al: Human erythropoietin gene: high level expression in stably transfected mammalian cells and chromosome localization. Proc.Natl.Acad.Sci.USA 83:6465, 1986

47. Fried W: The liver as a source of extrarenal erythropoietin. Blood 40:671, 1972

48. Zanjani ED, Ascensao JL, McGlave PB, et al: Studies on the liver to kidney switch of

erythropoietin production. J.Clin.Invest. 67:1183, 1981

49. Jacobson LO, Goldwasser E, Fried W, et al: Studies on erythropoiesis. VII. The role of the kidney in the production of erythropoietin. Trans.Assoc.Am.Physicians 70:305, 1957

50. Goldberg MA, Glass GA, Cunningham JM, et al: The regulated expression of erythropoietin by two human hepatoma cell lines. Proc.Natl.Acad.Sci.USA 84:7972, 1987

51. Goldberg MA, Dunning SP, Bunn HF: Regulation of the erythropoietin gene: Evidence that the oxygen sensor is a heme protein. Science 242:1412, 1988

52. Witthuhn BA, Quelle FW, Silvennoinen O, et al: JAK2 associates with the erythropoietin receptor and is tyrosine phosphorylated and activated following stimulation with erythropoietin. Cell 74:227, 1993

53. Klingmuller U, Wu H, Hsiao JG, et al: Identification of a novel pathway important for proliferation and differentiation of primary erythroid progenitors. Proc.Natl.Acad.Sci.U.S.A. 94:3016, 1997

54. Lodish HF, Hilton DJ, Klingmuller U, et al: The erythropoietin receptor: biogenesis, dimerization, and intracellular signal transduction. Cold Spring Harb.Symp.Quant.Biol. 60:93, 1995

55. Klingmuller U: The role of tyrosine phosphorylation in proliferation and maturation of erythroid progenitor cells--signals emanating from the erythropoietin receptor. Eur.J.Biochem. 249:637, 1997

56. Tsushima H, Urata Y, Miyazaki Y, et al: Human erythropoietin receptor increases GATA-2 and Bcl-x$_L$ by a protein kinase C dependent pathway in human erythropoietin- dependent cell line AS-E2. Cell Growth Differ. 8:1317, 1997

57. McDonald TP, Cottrell MB, Clift RE, et al: High doses of recombinant erythropoietin stimulate platelet production in mice. Exp.Hematol. 15:719, 1987

58. Fraser JC, Tan AS, Lin FK, et al: Expression of specific high-affinity binding sites for erythropoietin on rat and mouse megakaryocytes. Exp.Hematol. 17:10, 1989

59. Clark DA, Dessypris EN: Effects of recombinant erythropoietin on murine megakaryocytic colony formation in vitro. J Lab.Clin.Med. 108:423, 1986

60. Lu L, Bruno E , Briddell RA, et al: Effects of hematopoietic growth factors on in vitro colony formation by human megakaryocyte progenitor cells. Behring.Inst.Mitt. 181, 1988

61. Winearls CG, Oliver DO, Pippard MJ, et al: Effect of human erythropoietin derived from recombinant DNA on the anaemia of patients maintained by chronic haemodialysis. Lancet 2:1175, 1986

62. Hellström-Lindberg E, Negrin R, Stein R, et al: Erythroid response to treatment with G-CSF plus erythropoietin for the anaemia of patients with myelodysplastic syndromes: proposal for a predictive model. Br.J.Haematol. 99:344, 1997

63. Henry DH: Recombinant human erythropoietin treatment of anemic cancer patients. Cancer Pract. 4:180, 1996

64. Bennett DR, Shulman IA: Practical issues when confronting the patient who refuses blood transfusion therapy. Am.J.Clin.Pathol. 107:S23, 1997

65. Henry DH, Beall GN, Benson CA, et al: Recombinant human erythropoietin in the treatment of anemia associated with human immunodeficiency virus (HIV) infection and zidovudine therapy. Overview of four clinical trials [see comments]. Ann.Intern.Med. 117:739, 1992

66. Anderson DM, Williams DE, Tushinski R et al: Alternate splicing of the mRNAs encoding human mast cell growth factor and localization of the gene to chromosome 12q22-q24. Cell Growth Differ. 2:373, 1991

67. Anderson DM, Lyman SD, Baird A, et al: Molecular cloning of mast cell growth factor, a hematopoietin that is active in both membrane bound and soluble forms. Cell 63:235, 1990

68. Flanagan JG, Chan DC, Leder P: Transmembrane form of the *kit* ligand growth factor is determined by alternative splicing and is missing in the *Sl^d* mutant. Cell 64:1025, 1991

69. Heinrich, MC, Dooley DC, Freed AC, et al: Constitutive expression of steel factor gene by human stromal cells. Blood 82:771, 1993

70. Keshet E, Lyman SD, Williams DE, et al: Embryonic RNA expression patterns of the c-*kit* receptor and its cognate ligand suggest multiple functional roles in mouse development. EMBO J. 10:2425, 1991

71. Heinrich MC, Dooley DC, Keeble WW: Transforming growth factor beta 1 inhibits expression of the gene products for steel factor and its receptor (c-kit). Blood 85:1769, 1995

72. Huang EJ, Nocka KH, Buck J, et al: Differential expression and processing of two cell associated forms of the Kit-ligand: KL-1 and KL-2. Mol.Biol.Cell 3:349, 1992

73. Brandt J, Briddell RA, Srour EF, et al R: Role of c-kit ligand in the expansion of human

hematopoietic progenitor cells. Blood 79:634, 1992
74. Bernstein ID, Andrews RG, Zsebo KM: Recombinant human stem cell factor enhances the formation of colonies by CD34$^+$ and CD34$^+$lin$^-$ cells, and the generation of colony-forming cell progeny from CD34$^+$lin$^-$ cells cultured with interleukin-3, granulocyte colony- stimulating factor, or granulocyte-macrophage colony-stimulating factor. Blood 77:2316, 1991
75. Tsuji K, Lyman SD, Sudo T, et al: Enhancement of murine hematopoiesis by synergistic interactions between Steel factor (ligand for c-kit), interleukin-11, and other early acting factors in culture. Blood 79:2855, 1992
76. Broxmeyer HE, Cooper S, Lu L et al: Effect of murine mast cell growth factor (c-kit proto-oncogene ligand) on colony formation by human marrow hematopoietic progenitor cells. Blood 77:2142, 1991
77. Andrews RG, Knitter GH, Bartelmez SH, et al: Recombinant human stem cell factor, a c-*kit* ligand, stimulates hematopoiesis in primates. Blood 78:1975, 1991
78. Tsai M, Shih L, Newlands GFJ et al: The rat c-kit ligand, stem cell factor, induces the development of connective tissue-type and mucosal mast cells in vivo. Analysis by anatomical distribution, histochemistry and protease phenotype. J.Exp.Med. 174:125, 1991
79. Murphy M, Reid K, Williams DE, et al: Steel factor is required for maintenance, but not differentiation, of melanocyte precursors in the neural crest. Dev.Biol. 153:396, 1992
80. Bodine DM, Orlic D, Birkett NC, et al: Stem cell factor increases colony-forming unit-spleen number in vitro in synergy with interleukin-6, and in vivo in *Sl/Sl^d* mice as a single factor. Blood 79:913, 1992
81. De Jong MO, Westerman Y, Wagemaker G, et al: Coexpression of Kit and the receptors for erythropoietin, interleukin 6 and GM-CSF on hemopoietic cells. Stem.Cells 15:275, 1997
82. Wu H, Klingmuller U, Acurio A, et al: Functional interaction of erythropoietin and stem cell factor receptors is essential for erythroid colony formation. Proc.Natl.Acad.Sci.U.S.A. 94 :1806, 1997
83. Stewart CEH, Rotwein P: Growth, differentiation, and survival: multiple physiological functions for insulin-like growth factors. Physiol.Rev. 76:1005, 1998
84. Morton CC, Byers MG, Nakai H, et al: Human genes for insulin-like growth factors I and II and epidermal growth factor are located on 12q22----q24.1, 11p15, and 4q25----q27, respectively. Cytogenet.Cell Genet. 41:245, 1986
85. Adamo ML, Neuenschwander S, LeRoith D, et al: Structure, expression, and regulation of the IGF-I gene. Adv.Exp.Med.Biol. 343:1, 1993
86. Osborne CK, Clemmons DR, Arteaga CL: Regulation of breast cancer growth by insulin-like growth factors. J.Steroid.Biochem.Mol.Biol. 37:805, 1990
87. Kaicer EK, Blat C, Harel L: IGF-I and IGF-binding proteins: stimulatory and inhibitory factors secreted by human prostatic adenocarcinoma cells. Growth.Factors. 4:231, 1991
88. Warburton C, Powell-Braxton L: Mouse models of IGF-I deficiency generated by gene targeting. Receptor. 5:35, 1995
89. Woods KA, Camacho-Hubner C, Savage MO, et al: Intrauterine growth retardation and postnatal growth failure associated with deletion of the insulin-like growth factor I gene [see comments]. N.Engl.J.Med. 335:1363, 1996
90. Abbott AM, Bueno R, Pedrini MT, et al: Insulin-like growth factor I receptor gene structure. J.Biol.Chem. 267:10759, 1992
91. Ullrich A, Gray A, Tam AW, et al: Insulin-like growth factor I receptor primary structure: comparison with insulin receptor suggests structural determinants that define functional specificity. EMBO J. 5:2503, 1986
92. Beitner-Johnson D, LeRoith D: Insulin-like growth factor-I stimulates tyrosine phosphorylation of endogenous c-Crk. J.Biol.Chem. 270:5187, 1995
93. Sawada K, Krantz SB, Dessypris EN, et al: Human colony-forming units-erythroid do not require accessory cells, but do require direct interaction with insulin-like growth factor I and/or insulin for erythroid development. J.Clin.Invest. 83:1701, 1989
94. Correa PN, Axelrad AA: Production of erythropoietic bursts by progenitor cells from adult human peripheral blood in an improved serum-free medium: role of insulinlike growth factor 1. Blood 78:2823, 1991
95. Correa PN, Eskinazi D, Axelrad AA: Circulating erythroid progenitors in polycythemia vera are hypersensitive to insulin-like growth factor-1 in vitro: Studies in an improved serum-free medium. Blood 83:99, 1994
96. Mirza AM, Correa PN, Axelrad AA: Increased basal and induced tyrosine phosphorylation of the

insulin-like growth factor I receptor b subunit in circulating mononuclear cells of patients with polycythemia vera. Blood 86:877, 1995

97. Rodriguez-Tarduchy G, Collins MK, Garcia I, et al: Insulin-like growth factor-I inhibits apoptosis in IL-3- dependent hemopoietic cells. J.Immunol. 149:535, 1992

98. Adachi S, Kubota M, Lin YW, et al: *In vivo* administration of granulocyte colony-stimulating factor promotes neutrophil survival *in vitro*. Eur.J.Haematol. 53:129, 1994

99. Wong GG, Witek JAS, Temple PA, et al: Human GM-CSF: molecular cloning of the complementary DNA and purification of the natural and recombinant proteins. Science 228:810, 1985

100. Le Beau MM, Pettenati MJ, Lemons RS, et al: Assignment of the GM-CSF, CSF-1, and FMS genes to human chromosome 5 provides evidence for linkage of a family of genes regulating hematopoiesis and for their involvement in the deletion (5q) in myeloid disorders. Cold Spring Harbor Symp.Quant.Biol. LI:899, 1986

101. Gasson JC, Weissbart RH, Kaufman SE, et al: Purified human granulocyte-macrophage colony-stimulating factor: direct action on neutrophils. Science 226:1339, 1984

102. Kleinerman ES, Knowles RD, Lachman LB, et al: Effect of recombinant granulocyte/macrophage colony-stimulating factor on human monocyte activity *in vitro* and following intravenous administration. Cancer Res. 48:2604, 1988

103. Cannistra SA, Vellenga E, Groshek P, et al: Human granulocyte-monocyte colony-stimulating factor and interleukin 3 stimulate monocyte cytotoxicity through a tumor necrosis factor-dependent mechanism. Blood 71:672, 1988

104. Lopez AF, Williamson DJ, Gamble JR, et al: Recombinant human granulocyte-macrophage colony-stimulating factor stimulates in vitro mature human neutrophil and eosinophil function, surface receptor expression, and survival. J.Clin.Invest. 78:1220, 1986

105. Vadas MA, Nicola NA, Metcalf D: Activation of antibody-dependent cell-mediated cytotoxicity of human neutrophils and eosinophils by separate colony-stimulating factors. J.Immunol. 130:795, 1983

106. Vadhan-Raj S, Buescher S, Broxmeyer HE, et al: Stimulation of myelopoiesis in patients with aplastic anaemia by recombinant human granulocyte-macrophage colony-stimulating factor. N.Engl.J.Med. 319:1628, 1988

107. Ferrero D, Tarella C, Badoni R, et al: Granulocyte-macrophage colony-stimulating factor requires interaction with accessory cells or granulocyte-colony stimulating factor for full stimulation of human myeloid progenitors. Blood 73:402, 1989

108. Lieschke GJ, Dunn AR: Granulocyte colony-stimulating factor (G-CSF)-deficient mice, in Durum SC, Muegge K (eds): Cytokine knockouts, Totawa, Humana Press, 1998, p 435

109. Dunn AR, Lieschke GJ: Granulocyte-macrophage colony-stimulating factor (G-CSF)-deficient mice, in Durum SK, Muegge K (eds): Cytokine knockouts, Totawa, N.J., Human Press, 1998, p 401

110. Lindemann A, Riedel D, Oster W, et al: Granulocyte/macrophage colony-stimulating factor induces interleukin 1 production by human polymorphonuclear neutrophils. J.Immunol. 140:837, 1988

111. Bagby GC: Interleukin 1 and hematopoiesis. Blood Rev. 3:152, 1989

112. Simmers RN, Webber LM, Shannon MF, et al: Localization of the G-CSF gene on chromosome 17 proximal to the breakpoint in the t(15;17) in acute promyelocytic leukemia. Blood 70:330, 1987

113. Sieff CA: Hematopoietic Growth Factors. J.Clin.Invest. 79:1549, 1987

114. Clark SC, Kamen R: The human hematopoietic colony-stimulating factors. Science 236:1229, 1987

115. Metcalf D: The molecular biology and functions of the granulocyte-macrophage colony-stimulating factors. Blood 67:257, 1986

116. Uzumaki H, Okabe T, Sasaki N, et al: Characterization of receptor for granulocyte colony-stimulating factor on human circulating neutrophils. Biochem.Biophys.Res.Commun. 156:1026, 1988

117. Nathan CF: Respiratory burst in adherent human neutrophils: Triggering by colony-stimulating factors CSF-GM and CSF-G. Blood 73 :301, 1989

118. Vellenga E, Rambaldi A, Ernst TJ, et al: Independent regulation of M-CSF and G-CSF gene expression in human monocytes. Blood 71:1529, 1988

119. Koeffler HP, Gasson J, Ranyard J, et al: Recombinant human TNF alpha stimulates production of granulocyte colony-stimulating factor. Blood 70:55, 1987

120. Larsen A, Davis T, Curtis BM, et al: Expression cloning of a human granulocyte colony-stimulating factor receptor: a structural mosaic of hematopoietin receptor, immunoglobulin, and fibronectin

domains. J.Exp.Med. 172:1559, 1990

121. Bodine DM, Crosier PS, Clark SC: Effects of hematopoietic growth factors on the survival of primitive stem cells in liquid suspension culture. Blood 78: 914, 1991

122. Ikebuchi K, Ihle JN, Hirai Y, et al: Synergistic factors for stem cell proliferation: Further studies of the target stem cells and the mechanism of stimulation by interleukin-1, interleukin-6, and granulocyte colony- stimulating factor. Blood 72:2007, 1988

123. Dong F, Brynes RK, Tidow N, et al: Mutations in the gene for the granulocyte colony-stimulating-factor receptor in patients with acute myeloid leukemia preceded by severe congenital neutropenia [see comments]. N.Engl.J.Med. 333:487, 1995

124. Hammond WP, Csiba E, Canin A, et al: Chronic neutropenia. A new canine model induced by human granulocyte colony-stimulating factor. J.Clin.Invest. 87:704, 1991

125. Beck G, Habicht GS: Isolation and characterization of a primitive interleukin-1-like protein from an invertebrate, Asterias forbesi. Proc.Natl.Acad.Sci.USA 83:7429, 1986

126. Asson-Batres MA, Spurgeon SL, Diaz J, et al: Evolutionary conservation of the AU-rich 3' untranslated region of messenger RNA. Proc.Natl.Acad.Sci.USA 91:1318, 1994

127. Yoshida H, Hayashi S-I, Kunisada T, et al: The murine mutation osteopetrosis is in the coding region of the macrophage colony stimulating factor gene. Nature 345:442, 1990

128. Morris SW, Valentine MB, Shapiro DN, et al: Reassignment of the human CSF1 gene to chromosome 1p13-p21. Blood 78:2013, 1991

129. Ralph P, Warren MK, Nakoinz I, et al: Biological properties and molecular biology of the human macrophage growth factor, CSF-1. Immunobiology 172:194, 1986

130. Warren MK, Ralph P: Macrophage growth factor CSF-1 stimulates human monocyte production of interferon, tumor necrosis factor, and colony-stimulating activity. J.Immunol. 137:2281, 1986

131. Mufson RA, Aghajanian J, Wong G, et al: Macrophage colony-stimulating factor enhances monocyte and macrophage antibody-dependent cell-mediated cytotoxicity. Cell.Immunol. 119:182, 1989

132. Cheers C, Hill M, Haigh AM, et al: Stimulation of macrophage phagocytic but not bactericidal activity by colony-stimulating factor 1. Infect.Immun. 57:1512, 1989

133. Segal GM, McCall E, Stueve T, et al: Interleukin 1 stimulates endothelial cells to release multilineage human colony-stimulating activity. J.Immunol. 138:1772, 1987

134. Lagasse E, Weissman IL: Enforced expression of Bcl-2 in monocytes rescues macrophages and partially reverses osteopetrosis in *op/op* mice. Cell 89:1021, 1997

135. Clutterbuck EJ, Hirst EMA, Sanderson CJ: Human interleukin-5 (IL-5) regulates the production of eosinophils in human bone marrow cultures: Comparison and interaction with IL-1, IL-3, IL-6, and GMCSF. Blood 73:1504, 1989

136. Campbell HD, Tucker WQJ, Hort Y, et al: Molecular cloning, nucleotide sequence, and expression of the gene encoding human eosinophil differentiation factor (interleukin 5). Proc.Natl.Acad.Sci.USA 84:6629, 1987

137. Clutterbuck EJ, Sanderson CJ: Human eosinophil hematopoiesis studied in vitro by means of murine eosinophil differentiation factor (IL5): production of functionally active eosinophils from normal human bone marrow. Blood 71:646, 1988

138. Yokota T, Coffman RL, Hagiwara H, et al: Isolation and characterization of lymphokine cDNA clones encoding mouse and human IgA-enhancing factor and eosinophil colony-stimulating factor activities: relationship to interleukin 5. Proc.Natl.Acad.Sci.USA 84:7388, 1987

139. Sutherland GR, Baker E, Callen DF, et al: Interleukin-5 is at 5q31 and is deleted in the 5q-syndrome. Blood 71:1150, 1988

140. Coffman RL, Seymour BWP, Hudak S, et al: Antibody to interleukin-5 inhibits helminth-induced eosinophilia in mice. Science 245:308, 1989

141. Nishinakamura R, Miyajima A, Mee PJ, et al: Hematopoiesis in mice lacking the entire granulocyte-macrophage colony-stimulating factor/interleukin-3/interleukin-5 functions. Blood 88:2458, 1996

142. Mosmann TR, Bond MW, Coffman RL, et al: T-cell and mast cell lines respond to B-cell stimulatory factor 1. Proc.Natl.Acad.Sci.USA 83:5654, 1986

143. Mazur EM, Cohen JL, Bogart L, et al: Recombinant gibbon interleukin-3 stimulates megakaryocyte colony growth in vitro from human peripheral blood progenitor cells. J.Cell Physiol. 136:439, 1988

144. Kavnoudias H, Jackson H, Ettlinger K, et al: Interleukin 3 directly stimulates both megakaryocyte progenitor cells and immature megakaryocytes. Exp.Hematol. 20:43, 1992

145. Ishibashi T, Kimura H, Uchida T, et al: Human interleukin 6 is a direct promoter of maturation of megakaryocytes *in vitro*. Proc.Natl.Acad.Sci.USA 86:5953, 1989

146. Ishibashi T, Kimura H, Shikama Y, et al: Interleukin-6 is a potent thrombopoietic factor in vivo in mice. Blood 74:1241, 1989

147. Paul SR, Bennett F, Calvetti JA, et al: Molecular cloning of a cDNA encoding interleukin 11, a stromal cell-derived lymphopoietic and hematopoietic cytokine. Proc.Natl.Acad.Sci.USA 87:7512, 1990

148. Weich NS, Wang AL, Fitzgerald M, et al: Recombinant human interleukin-11 directly promotes megakaryocytopoicsis in vitro. Blood 90:3893, 1997

149. Metcalf D: The leukemia inhibitory factor (LIF). Int.J.Cell Cloning 9:95, 1991

150. Briddell RA, Bruno E, Cooper RJ, et al: Effect of *c-kit* ligand on in vitro human megakaryocytopoiesis. Blood 78:2854, 1991

151. Ishibashi T, Koziol JA, Burstein SA: Human recombinant erythropoietin promotes differentiation of murine megakaryocytes in vitro . J Clin.Invest. 79:286, 1987

152. Gurney AL, Kuang WJ, Xie MH, et al: Genomic structure, chromosomal localization, and conserved alternative splice forms of thrombopoietin. Blood 85:981, 1995

153. Chang MS, McNinch J, Basu R, et al: Cloning and characterization of the human megakaryocyte growth and development factor (MGDF) gene. JBC 270:511, 1995

154. McCarty JM, Sprugel KH, Fox NE, et al: Murine thrombopoietin mRNA levels are modulated by platelet count. Blood 86:3668, 1995

155. Nagata Y, Shozaki Y, Nagahisa H, et al: Serum thrombopoietin level is not regulated by transcription but by the total counts of both megakaryocytes and platelets during thrombocytopenia and thrombocytosis. Thromb.Haemost. 77:808, 1997

156. Nomura S, Ogami K, Kawamura K, et al: Cellular localization of thrombopoietin mRNA in the liver by in situ hybridization. Experimental Hematology 25:565, 1997

157. Vigon I, Florindo C, Fichelson S, et al: Characterization of the murine Mpl proto-oncogene, a member of the hematopoietic cytokine receptor family: molecular cloning, chromosomal location and evidence for a function in cell growth. Oncogene 8:2607, 1993

158. Vigon I, Mornon JP, Cocault L, et al: Molecular cloning and characterization of MPL, the human homolog of the v-mpl oncogene: identification of a member of the hematopoietic growth factor receptor superfamily. Proc.Natl.Acad.Sci.U.S.A. 89:5640 , 1992

159. Peck-Radosavljevic M, Zacherl J, Meng YG, et al: Is inadequate thrombopoietin production a major cause of thrombocytopenia in cirrhosis of the liver? Journal of Hepatology 27:127, 1997

160. Martin TG3, Somberg KA, Meng YG, et al: Thrombopoietin levels in patients with cirrhosis before and after orthotopic liver transplantation. Ann.Intern.Med. 127:285, 1997

161. Fielder PJ, Gurney AL, Stefanich E, et al: Regulation of thrombopoietin levels by c-mpl-mediated binding to platelets. Blood 87:2154, 1996

162. Emmons RV, Reid DM, Cohen RL, et al: Human thrombopoietin levels are high when thrombocytopenia is due to megakaryocyte deficiency and low when due to increased platelet destruction. Blood 87:4068, 1996

163. Ulich TR, Del Castillo J, Yin S, et al: Megakaryocyte growth and development factor ameliorates carboplatin-induced thrombocytopenia in mice. Blood 86:971, 1995

164. Kuter DJ, Rosenberg RD: The reciprocal relationship of thrombopoietin (c-Mpl ligand) to changes in the platelet mass during busulfan-induced thrombocytopenia in the rabbit. Blood 85:2720, 1995

165. Shivdasani RA, Fielder P, Keller GA, et al: Regulation of the serum concentration of thrombopoietin in thrombocytopenic NF-E2 knockout mice. Blood 90:1821, 1997

166. Carver-Moore K, Broxmeyer HE, Luoh S, et al: Low levels of erythroid and myeloid progenitors in thrombopoietin- and c-*mpl*-deficient mice. Blood 88:803, 1996

167. Alexander WS, Roberts AW, Nicola NA, et al: Deficiencies in progenitor cells of multiple hematopoietic lineages and defective megakaryocytopoiesis in mice lacking the thrombopoietic receptor c-Mpl. Blood 87:2162, 1996

168. Gurney AL, Carver-Moore K, De Sauvage FJ, et al: Thrombocytopenia in c-mpl-deficient mice. Science 265:1445, 1994

169. Kimura S, Roberts AW, Metcalf D, et al: Hematopoietic stem cell deficiencies in mice lacking c-Mpl, the receptor for thrombopoietin. Proc.Natl.Acad.Sci.U.S.A 95:1195, 1998

170. Solar GP, Kerr WG, Zeigler FC, et al: Role of c-mpl in early hematopoiesis. Blood 92:4, 1998

171. Rasko JE, Basser RL, Boyd J, et al: Multilineage mobilization of peripheral blood progenitor cells in humans following administration of PEG-rHuMGDF. Br.J.Haematol. 97:871, 1997

172. Vadhan-Raj S, Murray LJ, Bueso-Ramos C, et al: Stimulation of megakaryocyte and platelet production by a single dose of recombinant human thrombopoietin in patients with cancer [see comments]. Ann.Int.Med. 126:673, 1997

173. O'Malley CJ, Rasko JE, Basser RL, et al: Administration of pegylated recombinant human megakaryocyte growth and development factor to humans stimulates the production of functional platelets that show no evidence of in vivo activation. Blood 88:3288, 1996

174. McKinley D, Wu Q, Yang-Feng T, et al: Genomic sequence and chromosomal location of human interleukin-11 gene (IL11). Genomics 13:814, 1992

175. Kawashima L, Ohsumi L, Mita-Honjo K, et al: Molecular cloning of cDNA encoding adipogenesis inhibitory factor and identity with interleukin-11. FEBS Lett. 283:199, 1991

176. Suzow J, Friedman AD: The murine myeloperoxidase promoter contains several functional elements, one of which binds a cell type-restricted transcription factor, myeloid nuclear factor 1 (MyNF1). Mol.Cell.Biol. 13:2141, 1993

177. Yin T, Taga T, Tsang ML, et al: Involvement of IL-6 signal transducer gp130 in IL-11-mediated signal transduction. J.Immunol. 151:2555, 1993

178. Yin T, Miyazawa K, Yang Y-C: Characterization of interleukin-11 receptor and protein tyrosine phosphorylation induced by interleukin-11 in mouse 3T3-L1 cells. J.Biol.Chem. 267:8347, 1992

179. Paul SR, Schendel P: The cloning and biological characterization of recombinant human interleukin 11. Int.J.Cell Cloning 10:135, 1992

180. Teramura M, Kobayashi S, Hoshino S, et al: Interleukin-11 enhances human megakaryocytopoiesis in vitro. Blood 79:327, 1992

181. Neben TY, Loebelenz J, Hayes L, et al: Recombinant human interleukin-11 stimulates megakaryocytopoiesis and increases peripheral platelets in normal and splenectomized mice. Blood 81:901, 1993

182. Hangoc G, Yin T, Cooper S, et al: In vivo effects of recombinant interleukin-11 on myelopoiesis in mice. Blood 81:965, 1993

183. Nandurkar HH, Robb L, Tarlinton D, et al: Adult mice with targeted mutation of the interleukin-11 receptor (IL11Ra) display normal hematopoiesis. Blood 90:2148, 1997

184. Kondo M, Weissman IL, Akashi K: Identification of clonogenic common lymphoid progenitors in mouse bone marrow. Cell 91:661, 1997

185. Sutherland GR, Baker E, Fernandez KEW, et al: The gene for human interleukin 7 *(IL7)* is at 8q12-13. Hum.Genet. 82:371, 1989

186. Namen AE, Lupton S, Hjerrild K, et al: Stimulation of B-cell progenitors by cloned murine interleukin-7. Nature 333:571, 1988

187. Watanabe M, Ueno Y, Yajima T, et al: Interleukin 7 is produced by human intestinal epithelial cells and regulates the proliferation of intestinal mucosal lymphocytes. J.Clin.Invest. 95:2945, 1995

188. Goodwin RG, Lupton S, Schmierer A, et al: Human interleukin 7: Molecular cloning and growth factor activity on human and murine B-lineage cells. Proc.Natl.Acad.Sci.USA 86:302, 1989

189. Takeda S, Gillis S, Palacios R: *In vitro* effects of recombinant interleukin 7 on growth and differentiation of bone marrow pro-B- and pro-T-lymphocyte clones and fetal thymocyte clones. Proc.Natl.Acad.Sci.USA 86:1634, 1989

190. Digel W, Schmid M, Heil G, et al: Human interleukin-7 induces proliferation of neoplastic cells from chronic lymphocytic leukemia and acute leukemias. Blood 78:753, 1991

191. Veiby OP, Borge OJ, Mårtensson A, et al: Bidirectional effect of interleukin-10 on early murine B- cell development: Stimulation of flt3-ligand plus interleukin- 7-dependent generation of CD19⁻ ProB cells from uncommitted bone marrow progenitor cells and growth inhibition of CD19⁺ ProB cells. Blood 90:4321, 1997

192. Dokter WHA, Sierdsema SJ, Esselink MT, et al: IL-7 enhances the expression of IL-3 and granulocyte-macrophage- CSF mRNA in activated human T cells by post-transcriptional mechanisms. J.Immunol. 150:2584, 1993

193. Alderson MR, Tough TW, Ziegler SF, et al: Interleukin 7 induces cytokine secretion and tumoricidal activity by human peripheral blood monocytes. J.Exp.Med. 173:923, 1991

194. Standiford TJ, Strieter RM, Allen RM, et al: IL-7 up-regulates the expression of IL-8 from resting and stimulated human blood monocytes. J.Immunol. 149:2035, 1992

195. von Freeden-Jeffry U, Vieira P, Lucian LA, et al: Lymphopenia in interleukin (IL)-7 gene-deleted mice identifies IL-7 as a nonredundant cytokine. J.Exp.Med. 181:1519, 1995

196. Peschon JJ, Gliniak BC, Morrissey P, et al: Lymphoid development and function in IL-7R-deficient mice, in Durum SC, Muegge K (eds): Cytokine knockouts, Totowa, N.J., Humana Press, 1998, p

197. Seigel LJ, Harper ME, Wong-Staal F, et al: Gene for T-cell growth factor: location on human chromosome 4q and feline chromosome B1. Science 223:175, 1984

198. Smith KA: Interleukin-2: Inception, impact, and implications. Science 240:1169, 1988

199. Taniguchi T, Minami Y: The IL-2/IL-2 receptor system: a current overview. Cell 73:5, 1993

200. Smith KA: The interleukin 2 receptor. Adv.Immunol. 42:165, 1989

201. Hayashida K, Kitamura T, Gorman DM, et al: Molecular cloning of a second subunit of the receptor for human granulocyte-macrophage colony-stimulating factor (GM-CSF): reconstitution of a high-affinity GM-CSF receptor. Proc.Natl.Acad.Sci.USA 87:9655, 1990

202. Takeshita T, Asao H, Ohtani K, et al: Cloning of the t chain of the human IL-2 receptor complex. Science 257:379, 1992

203. Farrar WL, Cleveland JL, Beckner SK, et al: Biochemical and molecular events associated with interleukin 2 regulation of lymphocyte proliferation. Immunol.Rev. 92:49, 1986

204. Purkerson JM, Newberg M, Wise G, et al: Interleukin 5 and interleukin 2 cooperate with interleukin 4 to induce IgG1 secretion from anti-Ig-treated B cells. J.Exp.Med. 168:1175, 1988

205. Fotedar R, Diener E: The role of recombinant IL-2 and IL-1 in murine B cell differentiation. Lymphokine Res. 7:393, 1988

206. Matsui K, Nakanishi K, Cohen DI, et al: B cell response pathways regulated by IL-5 and IL-2. Secretory mH chain-mRNA and J chain mRNA expression are separately controlled events. J.Immunol. 142:2918, 1989

207. Ben Aribia MH, Leroy E, Lantz O, et al: rIL-2-induced proliferation of human circulating NK cells and T lymphocytes: synergistic effects of IL-1 and IL-2. J.Immunol. 139:443, 1987

208. Schorle H, Holtschke T, Hunig T, et al: Development and function of T cells in mice rendered interleukin- 2 deficient by gene targeting. Nature 352:621, 1991

209. Sadlack B, Lohler J, Schorle H, et al: Generalized autoimmune disease in interleukin-2-deficient mice is triggered by an uncontrolled activation and proliferation of CD4+ T cells. Eur.J.Immunol. 25:3053, 1995

210. Horak I: Immunodeficiency in IL-2-knockout mice. Clin.Immunol.Immunopathol. 76:S172, 1995

211. Mohamadzadeh M, Takashima A, Dougherty I, et al: Ultraviolet B radiation up-regulates the expression of IL-15 in human skin. JI 155:4492, 1995

212. Grabstein KH, Eisenman J, Shanebeck K, et al: Cloning of a T cell growth factor that interacts with the beta chain of the interleukin-2 receptor. Science 264:965, 1994

213. Anderson DM, Johnson L, Glaccum MB, et al: Chromosomal assignment and genomic structure of Il15. Genomics 25:701, 1995

214. Mrozek E, Anderson P, Caligiuri MA: Role of interleukin-15 in the development of human CD56+ natural killer cells from CD34+ hematopoietic progenitor cells. Blood 87:2632, 1996

215. Carson WE, Fehniger TA, Haldar S, et al: A potential role for interleukin-15 in the regulation of human natural killer cell survival. J.Clin.Invest. 99:937, 1997

216. Agostini C, Trentin L, Sancetta R, et al: Interleukin-15 triggers activation and growth of the CD8 T-cell pool in extravascular tissues of patients with acquired immunodeficiency syndrome. Blood 90:1115, 1997

217. Jullien D, Sieling PA, Uyemura K, et al: IL-15, an immunomodulator of T cell responses in intracellular infection. JI 158:800, 1997

218. Quinn LS, Haugk KL, Grabstein KH: Interleukin-15: a novel anabolic cytokine for skeletal muscle. Endocrinology 136:3669, 1995

219. Angiolillo AL, Kanegane H, Sgadari C, et al: Interleukin-15 promotes angiogenesis in vivo. Biochem.Biophys.Res.Commun. 233:231, 1997

220. Le Beau MM, Lemons RS, Espinosa R, III, et al: Interleukin-4 and interleukin-5 map to human chromosome 5 in a region encoding growth factors and receptors and are deleted in myeloid leukemias with a del(5q). Blood 73:647, 1989

221. Sutherland GR, Baker E, Callen DF, et al: Interleukin 4 is at 5q31 and interleukin 6 is at 7p15. Hum.Genet. 79:335, 1988

222. Van Leeuwen BH, Martinson ME, Webb GC, et al: Molecular organization of the cytokine gene cluster, involving the human IL-3, IL-4, IL-5, and GM-CSF genes, on human chromosome 5. Blood 73:1142, 1989

223. Yokota T, Otsuka T, Mosmann T, et al: Isolation and characterization of a human interleukin cDNA clone homologous to mouse B-cell stimulatory factor 1, that expresses B-cell and T-cell-stimulating activities. Proc.Natl.Acad.Sci.USA 83:1, 1986

224. Arai N, Nomura D, Villaret D, et al: Complete nucleotide sequence of the chromosomal gene for human IL-4 and its expression. J.Immunol. 142:274, 1989

225. Lewis DB, Prickett KS, Larsen A, et al: Restricted production of interleukin 4 by activated human T cells. Proc.Natl.Acad.Sci.USA 85:9743, 1988

226. Wieser M, Bonifer R, Oster W, et al: Interleukin-4 induces secretion of CSF for granulocytes and CSF for macrophages by peripheral blood monocytes. Blood 73:1105, 1989

227. Peschel C, Green I, Paul WE: Interleukin-4 induces a substance in bone marrow stromal cells that reversibly inhibits factor-dependent and factor-independent cell proliferation. Blood 73:1130, 1989

228. Vieira P, de Waal-Malefyt R, Dang M-N, et al: Isolation and expression of human cytokine synthesis inhibitory factor cDNA clones: Homology to Epstein-Barr virus open reading frame BCRFI. Proc.Natl.Acad.Sci.USA 88:1172 , 1991

229. Moore KW, O'Garra A, Malefyt Rd, et al: Interleukin-10. Annu.Rev.Immunol. 11:165, 1993

230. Kim JM, Brannan CI, Copeland NG, et al: Structure of the mouse IL-10 gene and chromosomal localization of the mouse and human genes. J.Immunol. 148:3618, 1992

231. Gazzinelli RT, Wysocka M, Hieny S, et al: In the absence of endogenous IL-10, mice acutely infected with Toxoplasma gondii succumb to a lethal immune response dependent on CD4+ T cells and accompanied by overproduction of IL-12, IFN- gamma and TNF-alpha. J.Immunol. 157:798, 1996

232. Berg DJ, Davidson N, Kuhn R, et al: Enterocolitis and colon cancer in interleukin-10-deficient mice are associated with aberrant cytokine production and CD4(+) TH1- like responses. J.Clin.Invest. 98:1010, 1996

233. Fiorentino DF, Bond MW, Mosmann TR: Two types of mouse helper T cells. IV. Th2 clones secrete a factor that inhibits cytokine production by Th1 clones. J.Exp.Med. 170:2081, 1989

234. Kobayashi M, Fitz L, Ryan M, et al: Identification and purification of natural killer cell stimulatory factor (NKSF), a cytokine with multiple biologic effects on human lymphocytes. J.Exp.Med. 170:827, 1989

235. Podlaski FJ, Nanduri VB, Hulmes JD, et al: Molecular characterization of interleukin 12. Arch.Biochem.Biophys. 294:230, 1992

236. Wolf SF, Temple PA, Kobayashi M, et al: Cloning of cDNA for natural killer cell stimulatory factor, a heterodimeric cytokine with multiple biologic effects on T and natural killer cells. J.Immunol. 146:3074, 1991

237. Gubler U, Chua AO, Schoenhaut DS, et al: Coexpression of two distinct genes is required to generate secreted bioactive cytotoxic lymphocyte maturation factor. Proc.Natl.Acad.Sci.USA 88:4143, 1991

238. Yamamoto K, Kobayashi H, Miura O, et al: Assignment of IL12RB1 and IL12RB2, interleukin-12 receptor beta 1 and beta 2 chains, to human chromosome 19 band p13.1 and chromosome 1 band p31.2, respectively, by in situ hybridization . Cytogenet.Cell Genet. 77:257, 1997

239. Chua AO, Wilkinson VL, Presky DH, et al: Cloning and characterization of a mouse IL-12 receptor-beta component. J.Immunol. 155:4286, 1995

240. Magram J, Sfarra J, Connaughton S, et al: IL-12-deficient mice are defective but not devoid of type 1 cytokine responses. Ann.N.Y.Acad.Sci. 795:60, 1996

241. Mattner F, Magram J, Ferrante J, et al: Genetically resistant mice lacking interleukin-12 are susceptible to infection with Leishmania major and mount a polarized Th2 cell response. Eur.J.Immunol. 26:1553, 1996

242. Morgan JG, Dolganov GM, Robbins SE, et al: The selective isolation of novel cDNAs encoded by the regions surrounding the human interleukin 4 and 5 genes. Nucleic Acids Res. 20:5173, 1998

243. Obiri NI, Debinski W, Leonard WJ, et al: Receptor for interleukin 13. Interaction with interleukin 4 by a mechanism that does not involve the common gamma chain shared by receptors for interleukins 2, 4, 7, 9, and 15. JBC 270:8797, 1995

244. Zurawski SM, Vega F, Jr., Huyghe B, et al: Receptors for interleukin-13 and interleukin-4 are complex and share a novel component that functions in signal transduction. EMBO J. 12:2663, 1993

245. Montaner LJ, Doyle AG, Collin M, et al: Interleukin 13 inhibits human immunodeficiency virus type 1 production in primary blood-derived human macrophages in vitro. J.Exp.Med. 178:743, 1993

246. Hatch WC, Freedman AR, Boldt-Houle DM, et al: Differential effects of interleukin-13 on cytomegalovirus and human immunodeficiency virus infection in human alveolar macrophages. Blood 89:3443, 1997

247. Zurawski G, De Vries JE: Interleukin 13 elicits a subset of the activities of its close relative interleukin 4. Stem Cells 12:169, 1994

248. De Waal Malefyt R, Abrams JS, Zurawski SM, et al: Differential regulation of IL-13 and IL-4 production by human CD8+ and CD4+ Th0, Th1 and Th2 T cell clones and EBV-transformed B cells. Int.Immunol. 7:1405, 1995

249. Muchamuel T, Menon S, Pisacane P, et al: IL-13 protects mice from lipopolysaccharide-induced lethal endotoxemia: correlation with down-modulation of TNF-alpha, IFN- gamma, and IL-12 production. JI 158:2898, 1997

250. Maciaszek JW, Parada NA, Cruikshank WW, et al: IL-16 represses HIV-1 promoter activity. JI 158:5, 1997

251. Smirnov DV, Smirnova MG, Korobko VG, et al: Tandem arrangement of human genes for interleukin-4 and interleukin-13: resemblance in their organization. Gene 155:277, 1995

252. Minty A, Chalon P, Derocq J-M, et al: Interleukin-13 is a new human lymphokine regulating inflammatory and immune responses. Nature 362:248, 1993

253. Krishnaswamy G, Lakshman T, Miller AR, et al: Multifunctional cytokine expression by human mast cells: regulation by T cell membrane contact and glucocorticoids. J.Interferon.Cytokine.Res. 17:167, 1997

254. Li H, Sim TC , Alam R: IL-13 released by and localized in human basophils. JI 156:4833, 1996

255. Ambrus JL, Jr., Jurgensen CH, Brown EJ, et al: Purification to homogeneity of a high molecular weight human B cell growth factor; demonstration of specific binding to activated B cells; and development of a monoclonal antibody to the factor. J Exp.Med 162:1319, 1985

256. Vazquez A, Gerard JP, Olive D, et al: Different human B cell subsets respond to interleukin 2 and to a high molecular weight B cell growth factor (BCGF). Eur.J.Immunol. 16:1503, 1986

257. Ambrus JL, Jr., Fauci AS: Human B lymphoma cell line producing B cell growth factor. J.Clin.Invest. 75:732, 1985

258. Uckun FM, Fauci AS, Heerema NA, et al: B-cell growth factor receptor expression and B-cell growth factor response of leukemic B cell precursors and B lineage lymphoid progenitor cells. Blood 70:1020, 1987

259. Uckun FM, Fauci AS, Chandan-Langlie M, et al: Detection and characterization of human high molecular weight B cell growth factor receptors on leukemic B cells in chronic lymphocytic leukemia. J Clin Invest. 84:1595, 1989

260. Ford R, Tamayo A, Martin B, et al: Identification of B-cell growth factors (interleukin-14; high molecular weight-B-cell growth factors) in effusion fluids from patients with aggressive B-cell lymphomas. Blood 86:283, 1995

261. Delfraissy JF, Wallon C, Vazquez A, et al: B cell hyperactivity in systemic lupus erythematosus: selectively enhanced responsiveness to a high molecular weight B cell growth factor. Eur.J.Immunol. 16:1251, 1986

262. Cruikshank WW, Lim K, Theodore AC, et al: IL-16 inhibition of CD3-dependent lymphocyte activation and proliferation. JI 157:5240, 1996

263. Zhang YJ, Center DM, Wu DMH, et al: Processing and activation of pro-interleukin-16 by caspase-3. J Biol Chem. 273 :1144, 1998

264. Scala E, D'Offizi G, Rosso R, et al: C-C chemokines, IL-16, and soluble antiviral factor activity are increased in cloned T cells from subjects with long-term nonprogressive HIV infection. JI 158:4485, 1997

265. Lim KG, Wan HC, Bozza PT, et al: Human eosinophils elaborate the lymphocyte chemoattractants. IL- 16 (lymphocyte chemoattractant factor) and RANTES. JI 156:2566, 1996

266. Rumsaeng V, Cruikshank WW, Foster B, et al: Human mast cells produce the CD4+ T lymphocyte chemoattractant factor, IL-16. JI 159:2904, 1997

267. Rottenberg ME, Riarte A, Sporrong L, et al: Outcome of infection with different strains of Trypanosoma cruzi in mice lacking CD4 and/or CD8. Immunol.Lett. 45: 53, 1995

268. Maciaszek JW, Parada NA, Cruikshank WW, et al: IL-16 represses HIV-1 promoter activity. J.Immunol. 158:5, 1997

269. Gao M, Tsuchie H, Detorio MA, et al: Interleukin-16 does not suppress HIV-1 replication in naturally infected peripheral blood mononuclear cells [letter]. AIDS 11:538, 1997

270. Zhou P, Goldstein S, Devadas K, et al: Human CD4+ cells transfected with IL-16 cDNA are resistant to HIV-1 infection: inhibition of mRNA expression. Nature Medicine 3:659, 1997

271. Koike K, Ogawa M, Ihle HN, et al: Recombinant murine granulocyte-macrophage (GM) colony-stimulating factor supports formation of GM and multipotential blast cell colonies in culture:

comparison with the effects of interleukin-3. J.Cell.Physiol. 131:458, 1987

272. Bot FJ, Dorssers L, Wagemaker G, et al: Stimulating spectrum of human recombinant multi-CSF (IL-3) on human marrow precursors: importance of accessory cells. Blood 71:1609, 1988

273. Tomonaga M, Golde DW, Gasson JC: Biosynthetic (recombinant) human granulocyte-macrophage colony-stimulating factor: effect on normal bone marrow and leukemic cell lines. Blood 67:31, 1986

274. Kaushansky K, O'Hara PJ, Berkner K, et al: Genomic cloning, characterization, and multilineage growth-promoting activity of human granulocyte-macrophage colony-stimulating factor. Proc.Natl.Acad.Sci.USA 83:3101 , 1986

275. Galli SJ, Zsebo KM, Geissler EN: The kit ligand, stem cell factor. Adv.Immunol. 55:1, 1994

276. Lyman SD: Biology of flt3 ligand and receptor. Int.J.Hematol. 62:63, 1995

277. Kobayashi M, Laver JH, Kato T, et al: Thrombopoietin supports proliferation of human primitive hematopoietic cells in synergy with steel factor and/or interleukin-3. Blood 88:429, 1996

278. Kaushansky K: Thrombopoietin: More than a lineage-specific megakaryocyte growth factor. Stem Cells 15 Suppl. 1:97, 1997

279. Metcalf D: The molecular control of cell division, differentiation commitment and maturation in haemopoietic cells. Nature 339:27, 1989

280. Niemeyer CM, Sieff CA, Mathey-Prevot B, et al: Expression of human interleukin-3 (multi-CSF) is restricted to human lymphocytes and T-cell tumor lines. Blood 73:945, 1989

281. Wodnar-Filipowicz A, Heusser CH, Moroni C: Production of the haemopoietic growth factors GM-CSF and interleukin-3 by mast cells in response to IgE receptor-mediated activation. Nature 339:150, 1989

282. Farrar WL, Vinovour M, Hill JM: In situ hybridization histochemistry localization of interleukin-3 mRNA in mouse brain. Blood 73:137, 1989

283. Davignon J-L, Kimoto M, Kindler V, et al: Selective production of interleukin 3 (IL3) and granulocyte-macrophage colony-stimulating factor (GM-CSF) *in vitro* by murine L3T4[+] T cells: Lack of spontaneous IL3 and GM-CSF production by Ly-2[-]/L3T4[-] *lpr* subset. Eur.J.Immunol. 18:1367, 1988

284. Kelso A, Gough NM: Coexpression of granulocyte-macrophage colony-stimulating factor, gamma interferon, and interleukins 3 and 4 is random in murine alloreactive T-lymphocyte clones. Proc.Natl.Acad.Sci.USA 85:9189, 1988

285. Bickel M, Tsuda H, Amstad P, et al: Differential regulation of colony-stimulating factors and interleukin 2 production by cyclosporin A. Proc.Natl.Acad.Sci.USA 84:3274, 1987

286. Sieff CA, Niemeyer CM, Nathan DG, et al: Stimulation of human hematopoietic colony formation by recombinant gibbon multi-colony-stimulating factor or interleukin 3. J.Clin.Invest. 80:818, 1987

287. Migliaccio G, Migliaccio AR, Adamson JW: In vitro differentiation of human granulocyte/macrophage and erythroid progenitors: Comparative analysis of the influence of recombinant human erythropoietin, G-CSF, GM-CSF, and IL-3 in serum-supplemented and serum-deprived cultures. Blood 72:248, 1988

288. Migliaccio G, Migliaccio AR, Visser JWM: Synergism between erythropoietin and interleukin-3 in the induction of hematopoietic stem cell proliferation and erythroid burst colony formation. Blood 72:944, 1988

289. Lopez AF, Dyson PG, To LB, et al: Recombinant human interleukin-3 stimulation of hematopoiesis in humans: Loss of responsiveness with differentiation in the neutrophilic myeloid series. Blood 72:1797, 1988

290. Broxmeyer HE, Williams DE, Hangoc G, et al: The opposing actions in vivo on murine myelopoiesis of purified preparations of lactoferrin and the colony stimulating factors. Blood Cells 13:31, 1987

291. Dao MA, Pepper KA, Nolta JA: Long-term cytokine production from engineered primary human stromal cells influences human hematopoiesis in an in vivo xenograft model. Stem Cells 15:443, 1997

292. Mach N, Lantz CS, Galli SJ, et al: Involvement of interleukin-3 in delayed-type hypersensitivity. Blood 91:778, 1998

293. Hannum C, Culpepper J, Campbell D, et al: Ligand for FLT3/FLK2 receptor tyrosine kinase regulates growth of haematopoietic stem cells and is encoded by variant RNAs. Nature 368:643, 1994

294. Lyman SD, Jacobsen SEW: c-kit ligand and flt3 ligand: stem/progenitor cell factors with

overlapping yet distinct activities. Blood 91:1101, 1998

295.   Agnes F, Shamoon B, Dina C, et al: Genomic structure of the downstream part of the human FLT3 gene: exon/intron structure conservation among genes encoding receptor tyrosine kinases (RTK) of subclass III. Gene 145:283, 1994

296.   Rosnet O, Schiff C, Pebusque MJ, et al: Human FLT3/FLK2 gene: cDNA cloning and expression in hematopoietic cells. Blood 82:1110, 1993

297.   Lyman SD, James L, Zappone J, et al: Characterization of the protein encoded by the flt3 (flk2) receptor-like tyrosine kinase gene. Oncogene 8:815, 1993

298.   Lyman SD, James L, Escobar S, et al: Identification of soluble and membrane-bound isoforms of the murine flt3 ligand generated by alternative splicing of mRNAs. Oncogene 10:149, 1995

299.   Lyman SD, James L, Johnson L, et al: Cloning of the human homologue of the murine flt3 ligand: A growth factor for early hematopoietic progenitor cells. Blood 83:2795, 1994

300.   Wodnar-Filipowicz A, Lyman SD, Gratwohl A, et al: Flt3 ligand level reflects hematopoietic progenitor cell function in aplastic anemia and chemotherapy-induced bone marrow aplasia. Blood 88:4493, 1996

301.   Lyman SD, James L, Bos TV, et al: Molecular cloning of a ligand for the flt3/flk-2 tyrosine kinase receptor: a proliferative factor for primitive hematopoietic cells. Cell 75:1157, 1993

302.   Broxmeyer HE, Lu L, Cooper S, et al: Flt3 ligand stimulates/costimulates the growth of myeloid stem/progenitor cells. Experimental Hematology 23:1121, 1995

303.   Piacibello W, Fubini L, Sanavio F, et al: Effects of human FLT3 ligand on myeloid leukemia cell growth: Heterogeneity in response and synergy with other hematopoietic growth factors. Blood 86: 4105, 1995

304.   Jacobsen SE, Okkenhaug C, Myklebust J, et al: The FLT3 ligand potently and directly stimulates the growth and expansion of primitive murine bone marrow progenitor cells in vitro: synergistic interactions with interleukin (IL) 11, IL-12, and other hematopoietic growth factors. J.Exp.Med. 181:1357, 1995

305.   Hirayama F, Lyman SD, Clark SC, et al: The *flt3* ligand supports proliferation of lymphohematopoietic progenitors and early B-lymphoid progenitors. Blood 85:1762, 1995

306.   Shah AJ, Smogorzewska EM, Hannum C, et al: Flt3 ligand induces proliferation of quiescent human bone marrow CD34$^+$CD38$^-$ cells and maintains progenitor cells in vitro. Blood 87:3563, 1996

307.   Haylock DN, Horsfall MJ, Dowse TL, et al: Increased recruitment of hematopoietic progenitor cells underlies the ex vivo expansion potential of FLT3 ligand. Blood 90:2260, 1997

308.   Yonemura Y, Ku H, Lyman SD, et al: In vitro expansion of hematopoietic progenitors and maintenance of stem cells: comparison between FLT3/FLK-2 ligand and KIT ligand. Blood 89:1915, 1997

309.   Dooley DC, Xiao M, Oppenlander BK, et al: Flt3 ligand enhances the yield of primitive cells after ex vivo cultivation of CD34$^+$ CD38^{dim} cells and CD34$^+$ CD38^{dim} CD33^{dim} HLA-DR$^+$ cells. Blood 90:3903, 1997

310.   Veiby OP, Jacobsen FW, Cui L, et al: The flt3 ligand promotes the survival of primitive hemopoietic progenitor cells with myeloid as well as B lymphoid potential. Suppression of apoptosis and counteraction by TNF-alpha and TGF- beta. JI 157:2953, 1996

311.   Hudak S, Hunte B, Culpepper J, et al: FLT3/FLK2 ligand promotes the growth of murine stem cells and the expansion of colony-forming cells and spleen colony-forming units. Blood 85: 2747, 1995

312.   Ohishi K, Katayama N, Itoh R, et al: Accelerated cell-cycling of hematopoietic progenitors by the flt3 ligand that is modulated by transforming growth factor-beta. Blood 87:1718, 1996

313.   Mackarehtschian K, Hardin JD, Moore KA, et al: Targeted disruption of the flk2/flt3 gene leads to deficiencies in primitive hematopoietic progenitors. Immunity 3:147, 1995

314.   Yang Y-C: Human interleukin-9: a new cytokine in hematopoiesis. Leuk.Lymphoma 8:441, 1992

315.   Renaud J-C, Houssiau F, Druez C, et al: Interleukin-9. Int.Rev.Exp.Pathol. 34:99, 1993

316.   Mock BA, Krall M, Kozak CA, et al: *IL9* maps to mouse chromosome 13 and human chromosome 5. Immunogenetics 31:265, 1990

317.   Kelleher K, Bean K, Clark SC, et al: Human interleukin-9: Genomic sequence, chromosomal location, and sequences essential for its expression in human T-cell leukemia virus (HTLV)-I-transformed human T cells. Blood 77:1436, 1991

318.   Van Snick J, Goethals A, Renauld J-C, et al: Cloning and characterization of a cDNA for a new mouse T cell growth factor (P40). J.Exp.Med. 169:363, 1989

319.   Renauld J-C, Goethals A, Houssiau F, et al: Human P40/IL-9: Expression in activated CD4$^+$ T

cells, genomic organization, and comparison with the mouse gene. J.Immunol. 144:4235, 1990

320. Monteyne P, Renauld JC, Van Broeck J, et al: IL-4-independent regulation of in vivo IL-9 expression. J.Immunol. 159:2616, 1997

321. Renauld J-C, Druez C, Kermouni A, et al: Expression cloning of the murine and human interleukin 9 receptor cDNAs. Proc.Natl.Acad.Sci.USA 89:5690, 1992

322. Donahue RE, Yang Y-C, Clark SC: Human P40 T-cell growth factor (interleukin-9) supports erythroid colony formation. Blood 75:2271, 1990

323. Holbrook ST, Ohls RK, Schibler KR, et al: Effect of interleukin-9 on clonogenic maturation and cell-cycle status of fetal and adult hematopoietic progenitors. Blood 77:2129, 1991

324. Ferguson-Smith AC, Chen YF, Newman MS, et al: Regional localization of the interferon-beta 2/B-cell stimulatory factor 2/hepatocyte stimulating factor gene to human chromosome 7p15-p21. Genomics 2:203, 1988

325. Yamasaki K, Taga T, Hirata Y, et al: Cloning and expression of the human interleukin-6 (BSF-2/IFNb 2) receptor. Science 241:825, 1988

326. May LT, Ghrayeb J, Santhanam U, et al: Synthesis and secretion of multiple forms of b_2-interferon/B-cell differentiation factor 2/hepatocyte-stimulating factor by human fibroblasts and monocytes. J.Biol.Chem. 263:7760, 1988

327. May LT, Torcia G, Cozzolino F, et al: Interleukin-6 gene expression in human endothelial cells: RNA start sites, multiple IL-6 proteins and inhibition of proliferation. Biochem.Biophys.Res.Commun. 159:991, 1989

328. Horii Y, Muraguchi A, Suematsu S, et al: Regulation of BSF-2/IL-6 production by human mononuclear cells: Macrophage-dependent synthesis of BSF-2/IL-6 by T cells. J.Immunol. 141:1529, 1988

329. Walther Z, May LT, Sehgal PB: Transcriptional regulation of the interferon-b2/B cell differentiation factor BSF-2/hepatocyte-stimulating factor gene in human fibroblasts by other cytokines. J.Immunol. 140:974, 1988

330. Jirik FR, Podor TJ, Hirano T, et al: Bacterial lipopolysaccharide and inflammatory mediators augment IL-6 secretion by human endothelial cells. J.Immunol. 142:144, 1989

331. Caracciolo D, Clark SC, Rovera G: Human interleukin-6 supports granulocytic differentiation of hematopoietic progenitor cells and acts synergistically with GM-CSF. Blood 73:666, 1989

332. Wong GG, Witek-Giannotti JS, Temple PA, et al: Stimulation of murine hemopoietic colony formation by human IL-6. J.Immunol. 140:3040, 1988

333. Levy Y, Tsapis A, Brouet J-C: Interleukin-6 antisense oligonucleotides inhibit the growth of human myeloma cell lines. J.Clin.Invest. 88:696, 1991

334. Rieckmann P, D'Alessandro F, Nordan RP, et al: IL-6 and tumor necrosis factor-alpha. Autocrine and paracrine cytokines involved in B cell function. J.Immunol. 146:3462, 1991

335. Emilie D, Devergne O, Raphael M, et al: Production of interleukin-6 in high grade B lymphomas. Curr.Top.Microbiol.Immunol. 182:349, 1992

336. Klein B, Zhang XG, Jourdan M, et al: Interleukin-6 is a major myeloma cell growth factor in vitro and in vivo especially in patients with terminal disease. Curr.Top.Microbiol.Immunol. 166:23, 1990

337. Kopf M, Ramsay A, Brombacher F, et al: Pleiotropic defects of IL-6-deficient mice including early hematopoiesis, T and B cell function, and acute phase responses. Ann.N.Y.Acad.Sci. 762:308, 1995

338. Xing Z, Gauldie J, Cox G, et al: IL-6 is an antiinflammatory cytokine required for controlling local or systemic acute inflammatory responses. J.Clin.Invest. 101:311, 1998

339. Thornberry NA: Interleukin-1b converting enzyme. Methods Enzymol. 244:615, 1994

340. Ridgway D, Borzy MS, Bagby GC: Granulocyte macrophage colony stimulating activity production by cultured human thymic non-lymphoid cells is regulated by endogenous interleukin-1. Blood 72:1230, 1988

341. Goeddel DV, Aggarwal BB, Gray PW, et al: Tumor necrosis factors: gene structure and biological activities, in AnonymousMolecular Biology of Homo Sapiens, Cold Spring Harbor, Cold Spring Harbor Laboratory, 1986, p 597

342. Spies T, Blanck G, Bresnahan M, et al: A new cluster of genes within the human major histocompatibility complex. Science 243:214, 1989

343. Roodman GD: Mechanisms of erythroid suppression in the anemia of chronic disease. Blood Cells 13:171, 1987

344. Maciejewski JP, Weichold FF, Young NS: HIV-1 suppression of hematopoiesis in vitro mediated

by envelope glycoprotein and TNF-alpha. J.Immunol. 153:4303, 1994

345. Vogel SN, Douches SD, Kaufman EN, et al: Induction of colony stimulating factor in vivo by recombinant interleukin 1 alpha and recombinant tumor necrosis factor alpha 1. J.Immunol. 138:2143, 1987

346. Kaushansky K, Broudy VC, Harlan JM, et al: Tumor necrosis factor-a and tumor necrosis factor-b (lymphotoxin) stimulate the production of granulocyte-macrophage colony-stimulating factor, macrophage colony-stimulating factor, and IL-1 in vivo. J.Immunol. 141:3410, 1988

347. Moldawer LL, Marano MA, Wei H, et al: Cachectin/tumor necrosis factor-a alters red blood cell kinetics and induces anemia in vivo. FASEB J. 3:1637, 1989

348. Hsu D-H, De Waal Malefyt R, Fiorentino DF, et al: Expression of interleukin-10 activity by Epstein-Barr virus protein BCRF1. Science 250:830, 1990

349. Yao Z, Spriggs MK, Derry JMJ, et al: Molecular characterization of the human interleukin (IL)-17 receptor. Cytokine. 9:794, 1997

350. Yao Z, Fanslow WC, Seldin MF, et al: Herpesvirus Saimiri encodes a new cytokine, IL-17, which binds to a novel cytokine receptor. Immunity. 3:811, 1995

351. Fossiez F, Djossou O, Chomarat P, et al: T cell interleukin-17 induces stromal cells to produce proinflammatory and hematopoietic cytokines [see comments]. J.Exp.Med. 183:2593, 1996

352. Stoll S, Müller G, Kurimoto M, et al: Production of IL-18 (IFN-gamma-inducing factor) messenger RNA and functional protein by murine keratinocytes. J.Immunol. 159:298, 1997

353. Gu Y, Kuida K, Tsutsui H, et al: Activation of interferon-gamma inducing factor mediated by interleukin-1b converting enzyme. Science 275:206, 1997

354. Ghayur T, Banerjee S, Hugunin M, et al: Caspase-1 processes IFN-gamma-inducing factor and regulates LPS-induced IFN-gamma production. Nature 386:619, 1997

355. Parnet P, Garka KE, Bonnert TP, et al: IL-1Rrp is a novel receptor-like molecule similar to the type I interleukin-1 receptor and its homologues T1/ST2 and IL-1R AcP. JBC 271:3967, 1996

2. The Interaction of Cytokines with Stem Cell and Stromal Cell Physiology

Paul J. Simmons, David N. Haylock,
Jean-Pierre Levesque, Andrew CW Zannettino

Introduction

It is now well established that cellular interactions between primitive haemopoietic progenitor cells (HPC) and the stromal tissue of the bone marrow (BM) play a central role in regulating haemopoiesis. Despite considerable research efforts, the precise molecular mechanisms responsible for this control remain to be fully defined. Nevertheless, from these studies has emerged the general consensus that at least two classes of molecules including haemopoietic growth factors (HGF) and members of several cell adhesion molecule (CAM) superfamilies contribute to the regulation of haemopoiesis although the exact contribution made by each class of molecule remains to be determined. There are abundant data derived from studies performed in vitro and in vivo demonstrating HGF as potent regulators of HPC survival, growth and differentiation. The exact contribution made by CAMs is less well understood but emerging evidence derived from studies performed both in the haemopoietic and other systems clearly demonstrate that in addition to their well documented pro-adhesive functions, CAMs, like cytokine receptors, are also signalling molecules. Such observations therefore support the notion that in addition to their well documented role in initiating and maintaining contact between HPC and stromal cells, CAMs may also participate more directly in the growth and development of primitive HPC. In support of this proposal are recent data which demonstrate the considerable functional overlap and interdependence between the HGF and CAM families as demonstrated, for example, by the capacity of HGF to regulate the functional properties of CAMs on primitive HPC. Haemopoiesis may therefore be considered as a process which is intimately regulated by signals provided to developing haemopoietic cells by their surrounding microenvironment both by stromal cell-HPC cell interactions mediated by various CAMs and also through the action of specific HGF following binding to their cognate cell surface receptors. Such observations imply a key role for cytokines and growth factors as orchestrators of physiological interactions between the primitive haemopoietic and stromal cell compartments of the bone marrow. In this article, our intention is to briefly review the contribution of both classes of molecule to the regulation of haemopoiesis. The underlying theme we will explore is the importance of both classes of molecules and how by exploiting knowledge of the interplay between the two this may result in an enhanced ability to manipulate the ex vivo growth of primitive haemopoietic cells for various cellular therapies.

The Pleiotropic Actions of Cytokines on Haemopoietic Progenitor Cells

As reviewed in detail by Metcalf [1], cytokines exhibit pleiotropic biological activities including the ability to prevent the death of haemopoietic progenitor cells (HPC) by suppressing apoptosis [2], stimulation of cell proliferation and activation of mature cell function [3-5]. In addition, the colony-stimulating factors (CSF's) display a high degree of redundancy, at least in in-vitro clonogenic assays. For example, each of the four colony-stimulating factors, granulocyte-CSF (G-CSF), granulocyte-macrophage-CSF (GM-CSF), macrophage-CSF (M-CSF) and interleukin-3 (IL-3) were found to stimulate the formation of distinctive types of colonies [6,7]. However, it was noted that more than one cytokine could stimulate the formation of what appeared to be the same type of colony. This was best illustrated by generation of small neutrophilic colonies by G-CSF, GM-CSF, IL-3, stem cell factor (SCF) and IL-6. A similar situation also exists with regard to factors which stimulate or potentiate the formation of megakaryocyte and eosinophil colonies [8].

In vitro clonogenic assays have also provided a particularly valuable means for investigating interactions between haemopoietic regulators because two distinct parameters can be distiguished: alterations in colony *size* and alteration in colony *number*. The term *synergy* is used to define the situation where two or more regulators, acting on the same precursor cell induce a greater number of progeny. The second event, where two or more regulators promote increased numbers of precursors to proliferate is termed *recruitment*. Increased recruitment is considered to be an indication that some progenitors require simultaneous stimulation by two or more factors before being able to respond. Many studies have provided evidence of both synergistic interactions and increased recruitment of both mouse and human HPC when cultured with combinations of CSF or HGF [9-15]. Clonogenic assay of human BM also demonstrated synergy between IL-3 and GM-CSF [16] and also between M-CSF and GM-CSF [17] which was evident by the presence of so-called high proliferative potential (HPP) colonies. Subsequent studies demonstrated that HPP colony- forming cells (HPP-CFC) could be further divided according to their growth factor requirements [18] and for the first time suggested that multiple HGF are required to induce proliferation of primitive HPC [19]. As detailed below, subsequent studies based on a more sophisticated analysis of the responses of immunophentypically defined subpopulations of murine and human HPC to HGF have confirmed and extended these observations. Indeed it is now generally accepted that an implicit feature of the biology of hierarchically primitive haemopoietic cells is their apparent obligatory requirement for stimulation by multiple cytokines in order to initiate proliferation. Although poorly understood as yet at the molecular or biochemical level, this feature of primitive haemopoietic cells is of central importance to our ability to successfully manipulate the growth of haemopoietic tissues in vitro for use in various cellular therapies.

The Use of Cytokines to Manipulate the Growth of Haemopoietic Progenitors Ex-Vivo

Currently, there is great interest in the development of effective strategies for the manipulation of hematopoietic progenitor and stem cells for therapeutic purposes [20].

Proposed initiatives include the generation of committed progenitor cells or myeloid precursors for transplantation [21,22] and also use of HPC as vehicles for gene therapy [23,24]. Many investigators have chosen cytokine dependent, stroma-free culture systems which eliminate the highly variable and poorly defined influences of stromal cell interactions on growth of HPC, thereby ensuring a more defined growth environment through provision of exogenous cytokines and growth factors to stimulate cell proliferation and control differentiation. The identity and particular combination of cytokines used in these ex vivo culture systems to a large extent dictates the nature of the cellular product generated. For example, we and several other groups have demonstrated that the combination of interleukin-3 (IL-3), IL-6, granulocyte-colony stimulating factor (G-CSF) and stem cell factor (SCF) (36GS) provides a very effective means of producing neutrophil granulocyte postprogenitors [25,26] while combinations involving tumour necrosis factor alpha (TNFα), granulocyte-macrophage colony-stimulating factor (GM-CSF) and IL-4 are commonly used for the ex vivo generation of dendritic cells [27,28]. The proposed clinical applications of these ex-vivo expanded cells as adjunct populations in the treatment of neutropaenia post transplant and in immunotherapies, respectively, are such that the maintenance of transplantable haemopoietic stem cells following culture in these HGF combinations is of secondary concern only. This is quite distinct from applications such as retroviral mediated gene therapy or expansion of umbilical cord blood progenitors where the survival of such cells is of paramount importance.

Accordingly, there is considerable interest in identifying those HGF which influence the survival, proliferation and development of transplantable hematopoietic stem cells and their immediate progeny in vitro. In addressing this question significant contributions have been made by groups who developed culture systems for identifying precursors of HPC (Pre-CFU) [29-34]. Collectively, these studies demonstrated that early haemopoietic precursors proliferate and differentiate in response to IL-1 or IL-6 in synergy with IL-3 while progressively more committed populations of HPC responded preferentially to GM-CSF, G-CSF and M-CSF. Similar investigations, using so-called delta or Pre-CFU assays were performed with human bone marrow CD34+ cells [32]. In this assay system the generation of nascent CFU-GM serves as an index of precursors to CFU-GM. Hierarchically primitive progenitor cells identified as Pre-CFU were CD34[+] and found to lack detectable markers for T-cell, B-Cell, natural killer cell, and myeloid lineages. The generation of nascent CFU-GM from 4-HC[RESISTANT] CD34+ cells was highly dependent on the cytokine(s) used for culture: IL-3, when used alone was consistently better than either IL-1 or IL-6, while the combination of IL-1 + IL-3 was better than any single cytokine or any other 2 cytokine combination tested [32]. Muench et al [36] and Haylock et al[34] analysed the effects of various combinations of HGF including IL-1, IL-3, IL-6, GM-CSF, G-CSF and SCF on the stimulation of either post 5-FU BM or mobilised CD34[+] cells, respectively. These studies, based on Pre-CFU assays, substantiated the roles of IL-1, IL-6 and SCF as regulators of primitive HPC and demonstrated that maximal generation of myeloid progenitor cells from CD34[+] pre-CFU cells in this in vitro culture system required stimulation by a combination of both early and late-acting cytokines [35-39].

Proliferation of Primitive HPC: The Multi-Factor Paradigm

To date, relatively few studies have attempted to systematically define the contribution of cytokines either as single agents or in combination to the maintenance and/or proliferation of primitive human HPC in vitro. The major consideration here, as previously noted, is that primitive hematopoietic progenitors in vitro exhibit an almost obligatory requirement for stimulation by multiple synergistic HGF in order to elicit proliferation [1,29,40]. Of those HGF shown to have activity in this respect, several including IL-1, IL-6, IL-11, IL-12, leukaemia inhibitory factor (LIF) and SCF are regar_ed as synergistic HGF which act to enhance the stimulatory activity of other HGF such as IL-3, the colony-stimulating factors or erythropoietin (EPO) and exhibit little or no effect alone on proliferation in vitro [41-44]. A second major consideration is that primitive human haemopoietic progenitors (Pre-CFU) with candidate stem cell properties are quiescent and represent a very minor subpopulation of CD34[+] cells [33] and thus assessment of the cytokine requirements of the bone marrow CD34+ population as a whole is unlikely to provide valuable insights into the growth factor requirements of these rare cells.

To circumvent this problem several laboratories including our own have developed single cell pre-CFU assays in which the response of phenotypically defined subpopulations of HPC to single cytokines or various combinations thereof can be assayed in vitro under stromal cell free, serum deprived culture conditions. Under these conditions, growth is absolutely dependent on provision of exogenous cytokines. Such assays thus provide a powerful and unambiguous means to simultaneously monitor several parameters of cytokine action including effects on survival or death due to the induction of apoptosis, the rate of recruitment into division, proliferative rate and potential and the capacity for differentiation into multiple haemopoietic lineages. A recent report from this laboratory [45] employed this single cell assay to examine the mechanisms underlying the potent proliferative stimulus to bone marrow derived HPC provided by the ligand for the flt3/flk2 receptor tyrosine kinase (Flt3L) [46]. Addition of Flt3L to the above mentioned combination of 36GS was shown to markedly enhance myeloid cell production from CD34[+]CD38[-] cells, a phenotype highly enriched in primitive HPC [33]. This response was demonstrated to be due both to an increase in the proportion of primitive HPC that divide and to the enhanced rate and proliferative potential of the recruited cells. The combination of 36GS+Flt3L (36GSF) was also highly effective at initiating cell division in CD34[+] 4-HC[RESISTANT] HPC and in a more deeply quiescent population of CD34+CD38- cells identified by their low retention of Rhodamine 123. Significantly, this response of primitive HPC is in direct contrast to committed HPC which divide and proliferate in single or minimal combinations of HGF including G-CSF, IL-3, GM-CSF or IL-3+SCF. The apparent preferential synergistic action of Flt3L on primitive HPC is supported by the studies of Shah et al [47] who demonstrated similar results with single CD34+CD38- cells cultured on preformed irradiated BM stromal cells supplemented with HGF and by the work of Petzer et al [48,49] who demonstrated that Flt3L alone or in combination with other HGF including SCF, IL-3, IL-6, G-CSF and β-NGF resulted in expansion of primitive long-term culture initiating cells (LTC-IC) within the CD34+CD38- cell population.

A Key Role for Thrombopoietin in the Biology of Primitive HPC

Recently, several studies have described a key role for thrombopoietin (TPO)[50] or megakaryocyte growth and development factor (MGDF)[51], the ligand for the *c-Mpl* proto-oncogene in maintaining survival and inducing division of primitive HPC. Although initially considered to be a lineage specific factor affecting the proliferation and maturation of megakaryocytes, recent studies including the administration of TPO to myeloablated and non-human primates [52,53] and the impaired hematopoiesis observed in *c-Mpl* knockout mice [54] strongly suggest that TPO/MGDF also acts on primitive HPC. This notion is supported by an increasing number of reports. Ramsfjell et al described the synergistic interaction of TPO with SCF and Flt3L on lineage negative, Sca-1$^+$ murine bone marrow progenitor cells [55]. In the report by Borge et al, TPO, when used as a single factor was found to support survival of 22% of single CD34$^+$CD38$^-$ cells when cultured for 5 days under stroma-free serum deplete conditions, which was significantly better than with IL-3, SCF or Flt3L [56]. This effect of TPO was attributed to its ability to suppress apoptosis and is consistent with an earlier report by Ritchie et al who described TPO as being able to suppress apoptosis and promote survival of the

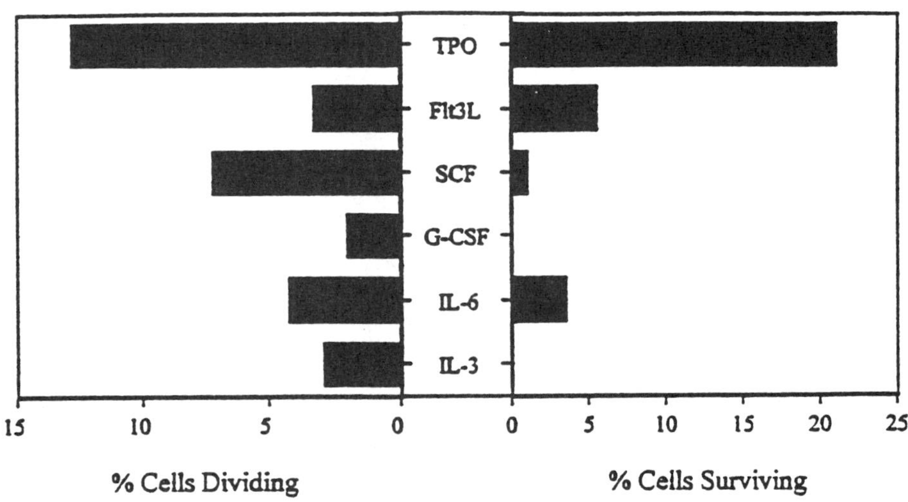

Figure 1. TPO/MGDF Preferentially promotes the Survival of Primitive CD34$^+$CD38$^-$ HPC. Single CD34+CD38- cells were cultured for 14 days in serum free medium in the presence of the indicated factors. Any proliferative response was scored on day 14. A combination of all six cytokines (36GSFT) was added to all wells containing single cells on day 14 and proliferation (as a measure of survival) measured after a further 7 days.

factor-dependent cell line MO7e [57]. Additional evidence for the role of TPO as a survival factor for CD34+CD38- adult BM cells was observed by Haylock et al [58] who incubated cells in single cytokines for 14 days then cultured with a combination of 6 cytokines to identify residual viable cells.

In these experiments TPO was able to support survival of 21% of CD34+CD38- cells (Fig 1). In more recent studies, Ramsfjell et al reported that Thrombopoietin synergises with SCF, Flt3L or IL-3 to potently enhance clonogenic growth of CD34+CD38- cells [59]. These data are supported by our own studies investigating the ability of different HGF combinations to induce division of single adult BM CD34+CD38- cells. As depicted in figure 2, the addition of TPO to a combination of 36GSF results in division of 92% of these cells during 14 days culture in pre-CFU media. Remarkably, when cultured in 36GSFT, 33.7% of dividing CD34+CD38- cells were capable of at least 12 divisions, producing more than 4,096 cells and 2.6% of cells produced 15,000 cells or more. In subsequent cultures of 1,000 CD34+CD38- cells, followed for 10 weeks we observed a 64-271 x 10^6 fold expansion of total nucleated cells and a 270,000 fold expansion of CD34+ cells. At 7 and 14 days, 75% and 45% of CD34+ lacked detectable expression of CD38. Thereafter, despite the proportion of CD34+CD38- cells decreasing there was an absolute increase of 570 fold in CD34+CD38- cells at 4 weeks. Moreover, 35.4% and 9.4% of CD34 cells co-expressed the Thy-1 antigen (an additional characteristic of primitive HPC) at 7 and 14 days of culture, respectively.

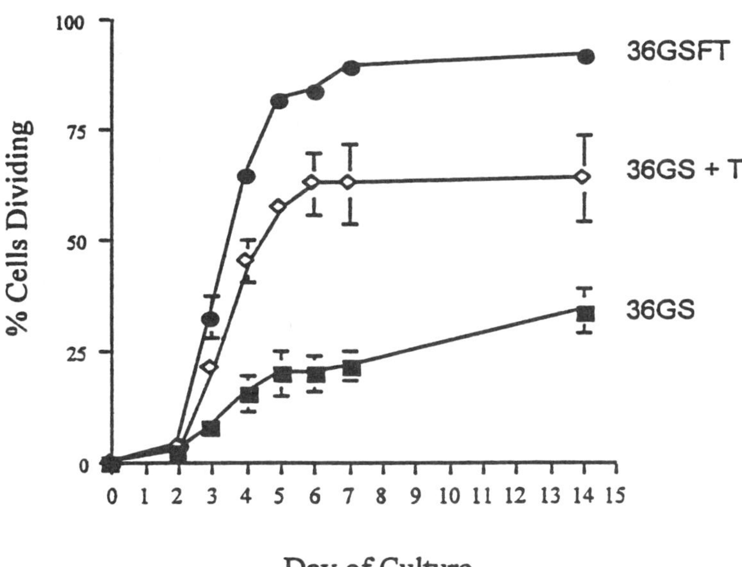

Figure 2. Recruitment of CD34+CD38- HPC into division by combinations of cytokines. Single CD34+CD38- cells were deposited in wells containing serum deprived medium and the indicated combinations of cytokines (see text for details). The proportion of single cells induced to divide over time is shown. Maximal recruitment requires stimulation by a combination of all 6 cytokines.

Collectively these data, together with those of Borge et al and Ramsfjell et al and the impaired haemopoiesis observed in the c-mpl knockout mouse [54] provides convincing evidence that TPO, in addition to its well documented role as a regulator of platelet mass, also has a critical role in supporting the survival and proliferation of primitive HPC.

Additional evidence that signalling through c-mpl may have an important role in amplification of the primitive HSC pool comes from the work of Goncalves et al who enforced expression of mpl in murine stem cells and observed proliferation and differentiation of progenitors of several lineages but without preferential differentiation toward megakaryocytopoiesis [60]. The notion of TPO acting as a potent stem cell stimulator and acting synergistically with other cytokines is strongly supported by recent studies performed with umbilical cord blood CD34[+] cells [61,62]. Piacibello et al reported that the combination of TPO and Flt3L, in the absence of stromal cells resulted in a considerable amplification in the total number of HPC and a concordant increase in the absolute numbers of cells exhibiting a CD34+CD38- phenotype, characteristic of candidate HSC in adult human BM. Moreover, cell generation was sustained for more than 6 months under these culture conditions without any apparent sign of diminution over time. As cited by these authors, the clinical applications of this study are potentially very exciting: transplantation of adults would become possible if CB HPC could be readily expanded. Exciting though these observation are, caution should nevertheless be exercised in interpreting these data since expansion of a primitive cell phenotype does not necessarily equate with expansion of transplantable HSC number, as clearly demonstrated by Lansdorp and colleagues in the mouse [63].

Cytokine-Supported Haemopoiesis: A Role for Stromal Cell Interactions?

Collectively, the studies reviewed above suggest that primitive HPC including those with the phenotypic properties of haemopoietic stem cells can be induced to proliferate in vitro in the presence of cytokines alone. In accord with this, Verfaillie and colleagues have recently shown that maintenance of long-term culture-initiating cells (LTC-IC) in human long term marrow cultures can occur both in the absence of direct physical contact with marrow stromal cells and, moreover, when cells are cultured in either conditioned medium from marrow stromal cells or in a combination of recombinant cytokines added at the concentrations typically measured in the stromal cell conditioned medium [64,65]. What then for stromal cell-stem cell interactions in regulating responses of primitive HPC; are such interactions redundant in cytokine dependent stromal free culture systems? This issue was highlighted by Rowley et al who showed that generation of nascent CFC from a 4HC-resistant, highly immature population of CD34[+]lineage[-] cells required interaction with an irradiated allogeneic stromal layer in addition to IL-1+IL-3+IL-6+G-CSF+GM-CSF+SCF [66]. This study thus suggests that despite use of this potent combination of 6 cytokines, very primitive haemopoietic cell populations in vitro still require additional signals provided by the stromal layer to stimulate optimal production of nascent CFC. These signals may be mediated by as yet identified cytokines produced and/or presented by the stromal layer or by specific adhesive interactions between primitive HPC and stromal cells, or through a combination of both.

Such considerations formed the basis of a method for large scale expansion of human HPC from BM mononuclear cells (MNC). Bioreactors were innoculated, then incubated for one day without perfusion to facilitate stromal layer attachment [67]. Growth of HPC in this culture system was dependent on generation of the autologous stromal layer. In a subsequent study performed with cord blood MNC, expansion of LTC-IC was only achieved when exogeneous IL-3, IL-6 and SCF was added to the perfusion bioreactor culture [68], indicating that despite contact with stromal cells, primitive HPC required additional cytokines to either allow survival or promote division. Clearly, a bioreactor culture is a complex system which could not be used to investigate the influence of single HGF or cell adhesive interactions on growth of HPC. However these observations do highlight the need for a more comprehensive analysis of how HGF and adhesion to defined substrates affect the survival, recruitment and proliferation of defined HPC populations.

Further underscoring the necessity for greater understanding of the precise contribution made by adhesive interactions to the physiology of haemopoietic stem cells is the notion that exposure of HSC to cytokines in vitro may alter their subsequent ability to engraft. Does culture of HSC with cytokines in the absence of marrow stromal cells result in the loss of stem cell viability or potential ? Alternatively, do such culture conditions result in a change in their capacity to either home to the bone marrow or remain within the BM microenvironment or both? The most comprehensive data supporting this concept comes from Quesenberry and colleagues [69-73]. In an initial study reported by Stewart et al[72] bone marrow collected from 5FU treated mice showed markedly defective engraftment when transplanted into nonmyeloablated hosts. These findings were confirmed by Ramshaw et al [73,74] and were somewhat surprising given that they and others [75,76] demonstrated that post 5FU BM competed effectively with normal marrow in irradiated hosts and contributed to long term haemopoiesis. These results were in part explained by the different microenvironment of the two models. The irradiated hosts were more likely to have localised damage within the microenvironment which would facilitate entry of HSC whereas nonablated mice would have an intact marrow stromal cell-endothelial cell interface. The data also suggested that the defect may be related to stem cell cycle status, with actively cycling stem cells displaying impaired engraftment in unprepared hosts.

A subsequent study showed that murine BM cells expanded in culture with IL-3, IL-6, IL-11 and SCF also have an engraftment defect[69]. Additional evidence that preincubation of HPC with HGF reduces seeding to the BM was provided by van der Loo et al [77]. In this particular study a 2-3 hour incubation with IL-3 or a combination of IL-3, IL-12 and SCF led to a substantial decrease in seeding of all haemopoietic subsets measured, both in the spleen and bone marrow. More recently, retrovirally transduced murine HPC were found to be less effective than non-transduced HPC in contributing to long-term stable engraftment [71]. It was proposed that incubation of HPC with IL-3, IL-6, IL-11 and SCF although stimulating progression through S phase and facilitating retroviral transduction also impaired homing or lodgment of these cells to the BM. In contrast to these reports, the studies of Bodine[78] and Neben[79] suggest that exposure of primitive HPC may enhance engraftment. Bodine et al who showed that in vitro exposure of marrow cells to IL-3, IL-6, and SCF for 6 days augmented in vivo repopulation in W/W^V animals several fold. Similarly, Neben et al reported that culture of murine bone marrow with the same combination of cytokines (IL-3, IL-6, IL-11 and SCF) for 6 days improved repopulating ability in myeloablated hosts by four fold.

There is clearly a need for more detailed investigation of this phenomenon and of the underlying mechanisms involved. Changes in the homing/lodgement and retention of primitive HPC within the BM micoenvironment could include alteration in the function of particular cell adhesion molecules as a direct consequence of signalling through cytokine receptors. This possibility is suggested by recent observations demonstrating changes in the adhesive properties of human BM derived CD34[+] cells following in vitro exposure to cytokines. Specifically, several cytokines, in particular SCF, IL-3 and GM-CSF resulted in the transient activation of the two β1 integrins VLA-4 and VLA-5 and subsequent increased adhesion to fibronectin [80,81] and VCAM-1 (Levesque and Haylock unpublished data). In a subsequent report, Schofield et al demonstrated that low levels of IL-3 result in a significant reduction in the adhesion of CD34[+] cells to the alternatively spliced IIICS region of fibronectin, which can be attributed to a change in the activation state of VLA-4 [82].

Adhesive Interactions and Their Role in Haemopoietic Regulation

These data highlight the importance of adhesive interactions in the regulation of haemopoiesis. Although the importance of HPC-stroma and HPC-ECM interactions have been very extensively documented, exactly how these interactions contribute to haemopoiesis is much less well understood. Although this has not been studied extensively in HPC, there is abundant evidence in non-haemopoietic tissues that cell adhesion molecules (CAMs) of the type expressed by HPC participate in a large variety

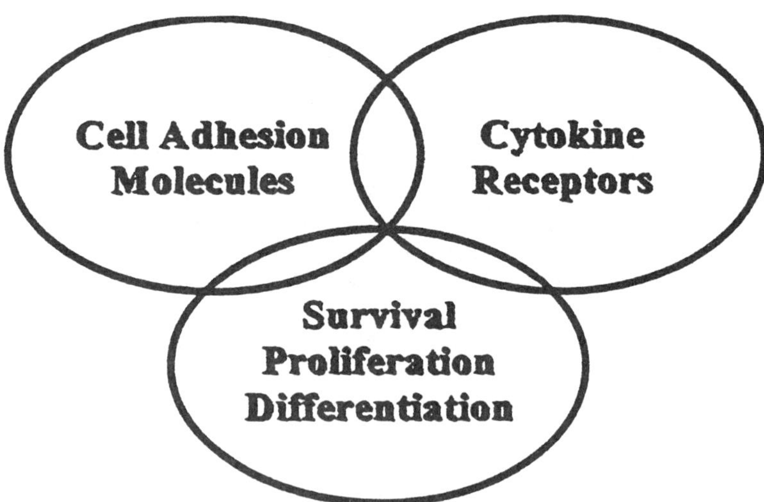

Figure 3. The Concept of Functional Overlap and Interdependence between Cell Adhesion Molecules and Cytokines/Cytokine Receptors

of signal transduction events important not only for regulating cell adhesion and motility but also cell growth [83-86] apoptosis [87] and specific gene regulation [88]. Furthermore, signals generated locally by CAMs can interact with classical signal transduction pathways to help control cell growth and differentiation.

The signal transducing properties demonstrated in other cellular systems for many of the CAMs expressed by HPC has consequently led to the concept that in addition to supporting the attachment of HPC to marrow stromal elements, these molecules may also play a more direct role in regulating HPC survival and development. This coupling between physical aspects of cell adhesion and developmental signaling thus provides a mechanism to tightly integrate adhesive interactions of haemopoietic cells within the BM with cell growth, differentiation and development, a coordination that is essential to maintain a correct balance between the complex interacting processes of proliferation, differentiation, maturation and programmed cell death (Fig 3).

The importance of this functional overlap and mutual interdependence between the cytokine/cytokine receptor and cell adhesion superfamilies as illustrated in figure 3, while perhaps better appreciated in other cellular systems, is probabaly no less important in the hamopoietic system. In considering the implications of this interplay, this raises the possibility that many of the deficiencies which are becoming evident in stroma-free, cytokine driven suspension culture systems now commonly used to 'expand' haemopoietic tissues in vitro may be due to the inability of primitive HPC to participate in the type of adhesive interactions they experience within the stromal cell microenvironment of the bone marrow in vivo. Therefore, can such systems be improved by selectively incorporating some of the missing components, for example ECM molecules or stromal cell adhesion molecules ? Such studies are currently in their infancy but recent observations based on an examination of the role of two classes of cell adhesion molecules expressed by HPC, namely integrins and sialomucins suggest the probable benefits of this approach in the long term.

The Crosstalk between β1-Integrins and Cytokine Receptors

The dominant role played by members of the β1 integrin superfamily, in particular CD49d/CD29 (VLA-4 or α4β1 integrin)[89-92] in mediating HPC-stromal cell adhesive interactions both in vitro and in vivo is well documented. Beta 1 integrins are expressed on quiescent HSC as non-active, non-ligand binding receptors. However, exposure of HSC to cytokines which stimulate their growth, such as IL-3, GM-CSF, G-CSF, IL-6, SCF,[80,81] Flt3-L and TPO (Lévesque and Haylock, unpublished observations) activate transiently and very selectively both VLA-4 and VLA-5, promoting HSC attachment to fibronectin and VCAM-1. Interestingly, the affinity of the other β1 integrins expressed by HPC and HSC, VLA-2 and VLA-6, is unaffected [80] and cytokines with the capacity to stimulate the adhesive properties of these integrins have yet to be identified. This effect of cytokines on VLA-4 and VLA-5 function is mediated by a genuine activation of these two integrins since their expression at the cell surface is not altered during the period of cytokine exposure [80] and additionally, is accompanied by the specific expression of β1 integrin activation-related epitopes [93]. Evidence for cross-talk between β1 integrin and mitogenic cytokine receptors is provided by the fact that combinations of mitogenic cytokines that synergize to induce proliferation of human CD34[+] HPCs also enhanced VLA-4/VLA-5-mediated adhesion HPCs to the same extent [81]. The strong correlation between these two events suggests that there is a functional and molecular link between cytokine-dependent activation β1 integrin-mediated adhesion and induction of proliferation [81]. Based upon these findings, a two step model was proposed in which 1) integrin activation by an "inside-out" signaling generated by cytokine receptor ligation is followed 2) by the generation of a secondary signal or "outside-in" signal resulting from the ligation of VLA-4 and VLA-5 to their adhesive ligands [81].

Whether the outside-in signal generated by ligated VLA-4 and VLA-5 cooperates with or antagonizes the mitogenic signal generated by cytokines receptors is currently unclear. Some authors have reported that enforcing cell attachment to fibronectin with function activating anti-human β1 integrin monoclonal antibodies results in an inhibition of HPC cycling [96]. These results should however be interpreted with caution since they may not reflect the physiological situation. Indeed, unlike physiological inside-out activation of integrins which is transient,[80] enforced adhesion by function activating anti-human β1 integrin monoclonal antibody is stable and cannot be regulated during cell cycle (JP Lévesque, unpublished observations) and may therefore inhibit cytokinesis resulting in cell death. In contrast, several recent reports have documented quite the opposite observation, demonstrating a significant enhancement of the growth of HPC in vitro as a consequence of β1-integrin-mediated adhesion to fibronectin [94,95]. In further support of the above model, studies in a number of cell systems and in hemopoietic cell lines have clearly demonstrated a spatial and functional convergence of the transduction pathways activated by mitogenic cytokine receptors and by integrin-mediated outside-in signalling [97-99]. For example, both classes of receptor result in the activation of similar transducers such as MAP kinases [100-102], the protooncogene vav [103] and the adaptor Grb2[104]. Moreover, integrin-mediated adhesion is a necessary step for the synthesis of some cyclins and the activity of cell cycle dependent kinases [83-86].

Outside-In Signalling Through Mucin-Like Molecules On HPC: Negative Regulators Of Haemopoiesis?

The sialomucins represent an emerging class of cell adhesion molecules. Many members of this superfamily including CD34, CD43 and CD162/PSGL-1, the counter-receptor for P-selectin are expressed at high levels by primitive human haemopoietic cells (reviewed in [112]). A series of recent reports suggest that outside-in signalling in HPC can also be directly mediated by mucin-like molecules. For example, constitutive expression of the full length splice variant of CD34 in murine M1 cells was shown to inhibit cytokine induced differentiation [105]. Antibody crosslinking of CD43 resulted in the induction of apoptosis in human CD34[+] HPC. Multipotential progenitors (CFU-GEMM) and erythroid progenitors (BFU-E) were substantially more sensitive to CD43-induced apoptosis than myeloid progenitors (CFU-GM)[106]. Although expressing CD43 at high level, candidate HSC were apparently refractory to the apoptosis inducing effects of the anti-CD43 antibody [107]. Similarly, recent studies from this laboratory demonstrate that adhesion of CD34[+] cells to P-selectin mediated by PSGL-1 markedly inhibits haemopoiesis in stromal cell-free, cytokine supported culture. This response appears to be due both to the induction of apoptosis in a subpopulation of primitive CD34+CD38- cells and to a slowing of the proliferation rate of the more mature CD34+CD38+ subpopulation (Zannettino et al, manuscript submitted). Of note, the hierarchically most primitive HPC within the CD34+CD38- subpopulation are not induced to undergo apoptosis but remain viable and can be recruited into division once removed from the P-selectin coated surface. Thus adhesion of primitive HPC to P-selectin results in a reversible cytostatic effect. These studies therefore imply a key role for the PSGL-1 sialomucin as a signalling molecule on primitive human HPCs.

Thus, mucin-like molecules on HPC appear to be negative regulators of haemopoiesis. The question of whether the growth inhibitory properties of these molecules occurs in vivo requires further study. In the case of PSGL-1, some clues are provided by the phenotype of mice deficient in CD62P and CD62E. CD62P[-/-] mice demonstrate increased numbers of megakaryocyte progenitors in the bone marrow [108]. Moreover, mice doubly deficient in CD62P and CD62E exhibit an extreme leukocytosis and abnormally elevated HPC numbers [109]. A similar phenotype was recently reported for mice deficient in $\alpha(1,3)$ fucosyltransferase Fuc-TVII, an enzyme required for selectin ligand biosynthesis [110]. Given the susceptibility of the CD62P/E[-/-] mice to opportunistic bacterial infections, the raised leukocte counts may in part be driven by infection. However, even neonatal animals exhibited a leukocytosis suggesting that this is a direct consequence of the absence of both selectins. This raises the intriguing possibility that the unanticipated role of the two endothelial selectins in regulating leukocyte homeostasis may be due to negative regulation of HPC by interactions between selectins and their ligands. One possible role of these mucin-mediated interactions in vivo might be as a powerful negative regulatory mechanism to dampen excessive expansion of HPC. Alternatively, mucin-like molecules may deliver a positive proliferative stimulus to HPC if combined with an appropriate, as yet unknown, stimulus. This hypothesis is suggested by studies with CD43 antibody which provides a costimulatory proliferative stimulus to T cells [111] in contrast to its ability to induce apoptosis of HPC. Thus in the absence of this additional stimulus, CD43-mediated signalling in HPC could result to the elimination of these improperly activated cells through the induction of apoptosis. Other scenarios are clearly possible but for the present additional studies will be required to elucidate both the phsiological significance of these observations and the signal transduction pathways involved.

Although we currently lack understanding of the precise mechanisms involved, the studies briefly reviewed above clearly illustrate how these two classes of CAMs, the integrins and sialomucins, affect the growth and development of primitive haemopoietic cells in vitro. In addition these observations also serve as powerful examples of the interplay between cytokines, cell adhesion receptors and the various adhesive ligands exhibited by the stromal tissue of the bone marrow. Moreover, by exploiting this knowledge these studies also raise raise the possibility of identifying improved means to manipulate the growth of primitive HPC in cytokine driven ex-vivo culture systems, either by enhancing their recruitment and proliferation or perhaps by inducing quiesence as a means of facilitating their subsequent engraftment.

Concluding Comments

Accumulating data indicate that it is now possible, with just cytokines, to induce division of most if not all cells with a putative HSC phenotype. The key growth factors required for this include SCF, FLT3L and TPO/MGDF. Perhaps the most significant question is whether it will be possible to expand the absolute numbers of stem cells in any given source of haemopoietic tissue while retaining their full biological potential and transplantability ? This issue may be addressed in part, by analysis of the outcome of transplantation studies in immunocompromised animal models such as the NOD-SCID mouse system. At present the data indicate that for human HPC we have yet to convincingly demonstrate expansion of cells with true repopulating stem cell properties in suspension culture systems supported by cytokines alone. We suggest based on a consideration of the complex nature of stromal cell environment in which stem cells normally reside, that future methodologies designed to expand such cells incorporate not only cytokines but also components of stromal cells that support the adhesion of stem cells.

References

1.   Metcalf D. Hematopoietic regulators: Redundancy or subtlety? Blood 82: 3515-3523, 1993.
2.   Metcalf D. Effects of GM-CSF deprivation on precursors of granulocytes and macrophages. J .Cell .Physiol. 112: 411, 1982.
3.   Gasson JC, Weisbart RH, Kaufman SE et al. Purified human granulocyte-macrophage colony-stimulating factor: direct action on neutrophils. Science 226: 1339, 1984.
4.   Weisbart RH, Golde DW, Clarke SC et al. Human granulocyte-macrophage colony-simulating factor is a neutrophil activator. Nature 314: 361, 1985.
5.   Stanley IR, Burgess AW. GM-CSF stimulates the synthesis of membrane and nuclear proteins in murine neutrophils. J Cell Biochem 23: 241, 1983.
6.   Metcalf D, Burgess AW, Johnson GR et al. In vitro actions on hemopoietic cells of recombinant murine GM-CSF purified after production in Eschericia coli: comparison with purified native GM-CSF. J.Cell. Physiol. 128: 421, 1986 .
7.   Metcalf D, Nicola NA. The clonal proliferation of normal mouse hemopoietic cells: enhancement and suppression by CSF combinations. Blood 79: 2861, 1992.
8.   Rennick D, J. J, Yang G et al. Interleukin-6 interacts with interleukin-4 and other hematopopietic growth factors to selectively enhance the growth of megakaryocytic, erythroid, myeloid and multipotent progenitor cells. Blood 73: 1828, 1989.
9.   Metcalf D, Begley CG, Johnson GR et al. Biological properties in vitro of a recombinant human granulocyte-macrophage colony stimulating factor. Blood 67: 37-45, 1986.
10.   Sieff CA, Ekern SC, Nathan DG et al. Combinations of recombinant colony-stimulating factors are required for optimal hematopoietic differentiation in serum-deprived culture. Blood 73: 688-693, 1989.
11.   Sonada Y, Yang Y-C, Wong GG et al. Analysis in serum-free culture of the targets of recombinant human hemopoietic growth factors: interleukin-3 and granulocyte/macrophage colony stimulating factors are specific for early developmental stages. Proc Natl Acad Sci USA 85: 4360, 1988.
12.   Williams DE, Hangoc G, Cooper S et al. The effects of purified recombinant murine interleukin-3 and/or purified natural murine CSF-1 in vivo on the proliferation of murine high-and low-proliferative potential colony-forming cells: demonstration of in vivo synergism. Blood 70: 401-403, 1987.
13.   Migliaccio G, A.R. M, Visser JWM. Synergism between erythrpoietin and interleukin-3 in the induction of hematopoietic stem cell proliferation and erythroid burst colony formation. Blood 72: 944, 1988 .

14.   McNeice IK, Robinson BE, Quesenberry PJ. Stimulation of murine colony-forming cells with high proliferative potential by the combination of GM-CSF and CSF-1. Blood 72: 191-195, 1988 .

15.   Bartelmez SH, Bradley TR, Bertoncello I et al. Interleukin 1 plus interleukin 3 plus colony stimulating factor are essential for clonal proliferation of primitive myeloid bone marrow cells. Exp Hematol 17: 240, 1989.

16.   McNeice IK, Stewart FM, Deacon DM et al. Detection of human CFC with a high proliferative potential. Blood 74: 609-612, 1989

17.   Falk LA, Vogel SN. Granulocyte-macrophage colony stimulating factor (GM-CSF) and macrophage colony stimulating factor (CSF-1) synergise to stimulate progenitor cells with high proliferative potential. J. Leuk. Biol. 44: 455-464, 1988 .

18.   McNeice IK, Bradley TR, Kreigler AB et al. Subpopulations of mouse bone marrow high proliferative potential colony forming cells (HPP-CFC). Exp. Hematol. 14: 856-860, 1986.

19.   McNeice IK, Bertoncello I, Breigler AB et al. Colony-forming cells with high proliferative potential (HPP). Int. J. Cell Cloning 8: 146-160, 1990.

20.   Emerson S. Ex vivo expansion of hematopoietic precursors, progenitors, and stem cells: The next generation of cellular therapies. Blood 87: 3082, 1996

21.   Brugger W, Heimfeld S, Berenson RJ, et al. Reconstitution of hematopoiesis after high-dose chemotherapy by autologous progenitor cells generated ex vivo. New England Journal of Medicine 333: 283, 1995

22.   Williams SF, Lee WJ, Bender JG, et al. Selection and expansion of peripheral blood CD34+ cells in autologous stem cell transplantation for breast cancer. Blood 87: 1687, 1996.

23.   Cassel A, Cottler-Fox M, Doren S, Dunbar C. Retroviral-mediated gene transfer into CD34-enriched human peripheral blood stem cells. Exp. Hematol. 21: 585, 1993

24.   Nolta JA, Crooks GM, Overell RW, et al. Retroviral vector-mediated gene transfer into primitive human hematopoietic progenitor cells: Effects of mast cell growth factor (MGF) combined with other cytokines. Exp.Hematol. 20: 1065, 1992

25.   Makino S, Haylock DN, Dowse T, et al. Ex-vivo culture of peripheral blodd CD34+ cells: effect of haemopoietic growth factors on the production of neutrophilic precursors. J. Hematotherapy 6: 475, 1997

26.   Purdy MH, Hogan CJ, Hami L, et al. Large volume ex-vivo expansion of CD34-positive hematopoietic progenitor cells for transplantation. J.Hematotherapy. 4: 515, 1995.

27.   Caux C, Vanbervliet B, Massacrier C, et al. CD34+ hematopoietic progenitors from human cord blood differentiate along two independent dendritic cell pathways in response to GM-CSF and TNFα. J.Exp. Med. 184:695, 1996.

28.   Rosenzwajg M, Camus S, Guigon M, Gluckman JC. The influence of interleukin (IL)-4, IL-13 and Flt3 ligand on human dendritic cell differentiation from cord blood CD34+ progenitor cells. Exp. Hematol 26: 63, 1998

29.   Brandt J, Srour EF, Van Besien K: Cytokine-dependent long-term culture of highly enriched precursors of hemopoietic progenitor cells from human bone marrow. J Clin Invest 86: 932, 1990

30.   Iscove NN, Shaw AR, Keller G. Net increase of pluripotential hematopoietic precursors in suspension culture to IL-1 and IL-3. J Immunol 142: 2332, 1989.

31.   Muller-Sieberg CE, Townsend K, Weismann IL et al. Proliferation and differentiation of highly enriched mouse hematopoietic stem and progenitor cells in response to defined growth factors. J Exp Med 167: 1825, 1988.

32.   Smith C, Gasparetto C, Collins N et al. Purification and partial characterisation of a human hematopoietic precursor population. Blood 77: 2122, 1991.

33.   Terstappen LWMM, Huang SM, Safford M et al. Sequential generations of hematopoietic colonies dereived from single nonlineage-committed CD34+CD38- progenitor cells. Blood 77: 1218, 1991.

34.   Haylock DN, To LB, Dowse TL et al. Ex vivo expansion and maturation of peripheral blood CD34+ cells into the myeloid lineage. Blood 80: 1405-1412, 1992.

35.   Williams N, Bertoncello I, Kavnoudias H et al. Recombinant rat stem cell factor stimulates the amplification and differentiation of fractionated mouse stem cell populations. Blood 79: 634, 1992.

36.   Muench MO, Schneider JG, Moore MAS. Interactions among colony-stimulating factors, IL-1b, IL-6, and Kit-ligand in the regulation of primitive murine hematopoietic cells. Exp Hematol 20: 339, 1992

37.   Musashi M, Yang Y-C, Paul SR et al. Direct and synergistic effects of interleukin 11 on murine hemopoiesis in culture. Proc Natl Acad Sci USA 88: 765-769, 1991 .

38.   Mayani H, Dragowska W, Lansdorp PM. Cytokine-induced selective expansion and maturation of

erythroid versus myeloid progenitors from purified cord blood precursor cells. Blood 81: 3252-3258, 1993.

39. Bodine DM, Crosier PS, Clark SC. Effects of hematopoietic growth factors on the survival of primitive stem cells in liquid suspension culture. Blood 78: 914-920, 1991.

40. Leary AG, Zeng HQ, Clark SC, Ogawa M. Growth factor requirements for survival in Go and entry into the cell cycle of primitive human hemopoietic progenitors. Proc. Natl. Acad. Sci. USA 89: 4013, 1992

41. Muench MO, Scneider JG, Moore MAS. Interactions among colony-stimulating factors IL-1b, IL-6 and kit-ligand in the regulation of primitive murine hemopoietic cells. Exp. Hematol. 20: 339, 1992

42. Musashi M, Yang Y-C, Paul SR, Clark SC, Sudo T, Ogawa M: Direct and synergistic effects of interleukin 11 on murine hemopoiesis in culture. Proc. Natl. Acad. Sci. USA 88: 765-769, 1991

43. Bernstein ID, Andrews RG, Zsebo KM. Recombinant human stem cell factor enhances the formation of colonies by CD34+ and CD34+lin- cells and the generation of colony-forming cell progeny from CD34+lin- cells cultured with interleukin-3, granulocyte colony-stimulating factor, or granulocyte-macrophage colony-stimulating factor. Blood 77: 2316, 1991

44. McNiece IK, Langley KE, Zsebo KM: Recombinant human stem cell factor synergises with GM-CSF, G-CSF, IL-3 and EPO to stimulate human progenitor cells of the myeloid and erythroid lineages. Exp. Hematol. 19: 226, 1991

45. Haylock DN, Horsfall M, Dowse TL, et al. Increased recruitment of hematopoietic progenitor cells underlies the ex vivo expansion potential of FLT3 ligand. Blood 90: 2260-2272, 1997

46. Lyman SD, James L, Johnson L, et al. Cloning of the human homologue of the murine flt3 Ligand: A growth factor for early hematopoietic progenitor cells. Blood 83: 2795, 1994

47. Shah AJ, Smogorzewska EM, Hannum C et al. Flt3 ligand induces proliferation of quiescent human bone marrow CD34+CD38- cells and maintains progenitor cells in vitro. Blood 87: 3563-3570, 1996.

48. Petzer AL, Hogge DE, Lansdorp PM et al. Self-renewal of primitive human hematopoietic cells (long-term-culture-initiating cells) in invitro and their expansion in defined medium. Proc Natl Acad Sci USA 93: 1470-1474, 1996.

49. Petzer AL, Zandstra PW, Piret JM et al. Differential cytokine effects on primitive (CD34+CD38-) human hematopoietic cells: novel responses to Flt3-ligand and thrombopoietin. J Exp Med 183: 2551-2558, 1996.

50. Kaushansky K, Lok S, Holly RD, et al. Promotion of megakaryocyte progenitor expansion and differentiation by the c-Mpl ligand thrombopoeitin. Nature 369: 568, 1994.

51. Bartley TD, Bogenberger J, Hunt P, et al. Identification and cloning of a megakaryocyte growth and development factor that is a ligand for the cytokine receptor Mpl. Cell 77: 1117-1124, 1994

52. Hokom MM, Lacey D, Kinstler OB, et al. Pegylated megakaryocyte growth and development factor abrogates the lethal thrombocytopenia associated with carboplatin and irradiation in mice. Blood 86:4486,1995

53. Farese AM, Hunt P, Grab LB, MacVittie TJ: Combined administration of recombinant human megakaryocyte growth and development factor and granulocyte colony-stimulating factor enhances multilineage hematopoietic reconstitution in nonhuman primates after radiation-induced marrow aplasia. J Clin Invest 97:2145, 1996

54. Alexander WS, Roberts AW, Nicola NA, Li R, Metcalf D. Deficiencies in progenitor cells of multiple hematopoietic lineages and defective megakaryopoiesis in mice lacking the thrombopoietic receptor c-Mpl. Blood 87: 2162, 1996.

55. Ramsfjell V, Borge OJ, Veiby OP, et al. Thrombopoietin, but not erythropoietin, directly stimulates multilineage growth of primitive murine bone marrow progenitor cells in synergy with early acting cytokines: distinct interactions with the ligands for c-kit and FLT3. Blood 88: 4481, 1996.

56. Borge OJ, Ramsfjell V, Cui L et al. Ability of early acting cytokines to directly promote survival and suppress apoptosis of human primitive CD34+CD38- bone marrow cells with multilineage potential at the single-cell level: key role of thrombopoietin. Blood 90: 2282-2292, 1997.

57. Ritchie A, Vadhan-Raj S, Broxmeyer HE. Thrombopoietin suppresses apoptosis and behaves as a survival factor for the human growth factor-dependent cell line MO7e. Stem Cells 14: 157, 1996.

58. Haylock DN, Nuitta S, Wyatt J, et al. Survival and recruitment of primitive human haemopoietic progenitor cells in vitro: The essential role of megakaryocyte growth and development factor. (Manuscript submitted).

59. Ramsfjell V, Borge OJ, Cui L et al. Thrombopoietin directly and potently stimulates multilineage growth and progenitor expansion from primitive (CD34+CD38-) human bone marrow progenitor cells: distinct and key interactions with the ligands for c-kit and flt3, and inhibitory effects of TGF-

beta and TNF-alpha. J Immunology 158: 5169-5177, 1997.

60. Goncalves F, Lacout C, Villeval J-L et al. Thrombopoietin does not induce lineage-restricted commitment of Mpl-r expressing pluripotent progenitors but permits their complete erythroid and megakaryocytic differentiation. Blood 89: 3544-3553, 1997.

61. Ohmizono Y, Sakabe H, Kimura T et al. Thrombopoietin augments ex vivo expansion of human cord blood-derived hematopoietic progenitors in combination with stem cell factor and flt3 ligand. Leukaemia 11: 524-530, 1997.

62. Piacibello W, Sanavio F, Severino A et al. Extensive amplification and self-renewal of human primitive hematopoietic stem cells from cord blood. Blood 89: 2644-2653, 1997.

63. Rebel VI, Dragowska W, Eaves CJ et al. Amplification of Sca-1+Lin-WGA+ cells in serum-free cultures containing steel factor, interleukin-6, and erythropoietin with maintenance of cells with long-term in vivo reconstituting potential. Blood 83: 128-136, 1994.

64. Verfaille CM, Catanzarro PM, Li W-N. Macrophage inflammatory protein 1α, interleukin 3 and diffusible marrow stromal factors maintian human hematopoietic stem cells for at least eight weeks in vitro. J Exp Med 179: 643-649, 1994.

65. Verfaille CM. Soluble factor(s) produced by human bone marow stroma increase cytokine-induced proliferation and maturation of primitive hematopoietic progenitors while preventing their terminal differentiation. Blood 82: 2045-2053, 1993.

66. Rowley SD, Brashem-Stein C, Andrews R et al. Hematopoietic precursors resistant to treatment with 4-hydroxyperoxyxcylophosphamide: requirement for an interaction with marrow stroma in addition to hematopoietic growth factors for maximal generation of colony-forming activity. Blood 82: 60-65, 1993.

67. Koller MR, Emerson SG, Palsson BO. Large-scale expansion of human stem cell and progenitor ells from bone marrow mononuclear cells in continuous perfusion cultures. Blood 82: 378-384, 1993.

68. Koller MR, Bender JG, Miller WM et al. Expansion of primitive human hematopoietic progenitors in a perfusion bioreactor system with IL-3, IL-6, and stem cell factor. Biotechnology 11: 358-363, 1993.

69. Peters SO, Kittler HS, Ramshaw PJ et al. Murine marrow cells expanded in culture with IL-3, IL-6, IL-11, and SCF acquire an engraftment defect in normal hosts. Exp Hematol 23: 461-469, 1995.

70. Peters SO, Kittler ELW, Ramshaw HS et al. Ex vivo expansion of murine marrow cells with interleuki-3 (IL-3), IL-6, IL-11, and stem cell factor leads to impaired engraftment in irradiated hosts. Blood 87: 30-37, 1996.

71. Kittler ELW, Peters SO, Crittenden RB et al. Cytokine-facilitated transduction leads to low-level engraftment in non-ablated hosts. Blood 90: 865-872, 1997.

72. Stewart FM, Crittenden RB, Lowry PA et al. Long-term engraftment of normal and post-5-fluorouracil murine bone marrow into normal nonmyeloablated mice. Blood 81: 2566, 1993.

73. Ramshaw HS, Rao SS, Crittenden RB et al. Engraftment of bone marrow cells into normal unprepared hosts: effects of 5-fluorouracil and cell cycle status. Blood 86: 924-929, 1995.

74. Ramshaw HS, Li P, Haylock DN et al. Increased recruitment of primitive haemopoietic progenitor cells by Flt3 ligand leads to enhanced rates of retroviral transduction. Exp Hematol 24: 1058, 1996.

75. Lerner C, Harrison DE. 5-fluorouracil spares hemopoietic stem cells responsible for long-term repoulation. Exp Hematol 18: 114, 1990.

76. Harrison DE, Lerner CP. Most primitive hematopoietic stem cells are stimulated to cycle rapidly after treatment with 5-fluorouracil. Blood 78: 1237, 1991 .

77. van der Loo JCM, Ploemacher RE. Marrow- and spleen-seeding efficiencies of all murine hematopoietic stem cell subsets are decreased by preincubation with hematopoietic growth factors. Blood 85: 2598-2606, 1995.

78. Bodine DM, Orlic D, Birkett NC et al. Stem cell factor increases colony-forming unit-spleen number in vitro in synergy with interleukin-6, and in vivo in Sl'sld mice as a single factor. Blood 79: 913, 1992.

79. Neben S, Donaldson D, Sieff C et al. Synergistic effects of interleukin 11 with other growth factors on the expansion of murine hematopoietic progenitors and maintenance of stem cells in liquid cultures. Exp Hematol 22: 553, 1994.

80. Lévesque JP, Leavesley DI, Niutta S et al. Cytokines increase human hemopoietic cell adhesiveness by activation of very late antigen (VLA)-4 and VLA-5 integrins. J Exp Med 181: 1805-1815, 1995.

81. Lévesque J, Haylock D, Simmons P. Cytokine regulation of proliferation and cell adhesion are correlated events in human CD34+ hemopoietic progenitors. Blood 88: 1168-1176, 1996.

82. Schofield KP, Rushton G, Humphries MJ et al. Influence of interleukin-3 and other growth factors

on a4b1 integrin-mediated adhesion and migration of human hematopoietic progenitor cells. Blood 90: 1858-1866, 1997.

83. Fang F, Orend G, Watanabe N et al. Dependence of cyclinE-cdk2 kinase activity on cell anchorage. Science 271: 499-502, 1996.

84. Hansen LK, Mooney DJ, Vacanti JP et al. Integrin binding and cell spreading on extracellular matrix act at different points in the cell cycle to promote hepatocyte growth. Mol Biol Cell 5: 967-975, 1994.

85. Symington BE. Growth signalling through the alpha5beta1 fibronectin receptor. Biochem Biophys Res Comm 208: 136-134, 1995.

86. Zhu X, Ohtsubo M, Bohmer RM et al. Adhesion-dependent cell cycle progression linked to the expression of cyclin D1, activation of cyclin E-cdk2, and phosphorylation of the retinoblastoma protein. J Cell Biol 133: 391-403, 1996.

87. Zhang Z, Vuori K, Reed JC et al. The $\alpha5\beta1$ integrin supports survival of cells on fibronectin and up-regulates Bcl-2 expression. Proc Natl Acad Sci USA 92: 6161-6165, 1995.

88. Yurochko AD, Liu DY, Eierman D et al. Integrins as a primary signal transduction molecule regulating monocyte immediate-early gene induction. Proc Natl Acad Sci USA 89: 9034-9038, 1992.

89. Miyake K, Weissman IL, Greenberger JS et al. Evidence for a role of the integrin VLA-4 in lympho-hemopoiesis. J Exp Med 173: 599-607, 1991.

90. Simmons PJ, Masinovsky B, Longenecker BM et al. Vascular-cell adhesion molecule-1 expressed by bone marrow stromal cells mediated the binding of hematopoietic progenitor cells. Blood 80: 388-395, 1992.

91. Williams DA, Rios M, Stephens C et al. Fibronectin and VLA-4 in hæmopoietic stem cell-microenvironment. Nature 352: 438-441, 1991.

92. Hirsch E, Iglesias A, Potocnik AJ et al. Impaired migration but not differentiation of haemopoietic stem cells in the absence of $\beta1$ integrins. Nature 380: 171-175, 1996.

93. Takamatsu Y, Simmons PJ, Lévesque JP. Dual control by divalent cations and mitogenic cytokines of $\alpha4\beta1$ and $\alpha5\beta1$ integrin affinity on human hemopoietic cells. Cell Adhes Commun 1997 (In press)

94. Schofield KP, Humphries MJ, de Wynter E, Testa N, Gallagher JT. The effcet of alpha4 beta-integrin binding sequences of fibronectin on growth of cells from human hematopoietic progenitors. Blood 91: 3230, 1998.

95. Yokota T, oritani K, Mitsui H, Aoyama K, Ishikawa J, Sugahara H, Matsumura I, Tsai S, Tomiyama Y, Kanakura Y, Matsuzawa Y. Growth supporting activities of fibronectin on hematopoietic stem/progenitor cells in vitro: structural requirements for fibronectin activities of CS1 and cell binding domains. Blood 91: 3263, 1998

96. Hurley RW, McCarthy JB, Verfaillie CM. Direct adhesion to bone marrow stroma via fibronectin receptors inhibits hematopoietic progenitor proliferation. J Clin Invest 96: 511-519, 1995.

97. Miyamoto S, Teramoto H, Coso OA et al. Integrin function: molecular hierarchies of cytoskeletal and signalling molecules. J Cell Biol 131: 791-805, 1995.

98. Plopper G. Convergence of integrin and growth factor receptor signalling pathways with the focal adhesion complex. Mol Biol Cell 6: 1349-1365, 1995.

99. Assoian R. Anchorage-dependent cell cycle progression. J Cell Biol 136: 1-4, 1997.

100. Chen Q, Kinch MS, Lin TH et al. Integrin-mediated cell adhesion activates mitogen-activated protein kinases. J Biol Chem 269: 26602-26605, 1994.

101. Morino N, Mimura T, Hamasaki K et al. Matrix/integrin interaction activates the mitogen-activated protein kinase, p44^{erk-1} and p42^{erk-2}. J Biol Chem 270: 269-273, 1995.

102. Renshaw MW, Ren XD, Schwartz MA. Growth factor activation of MAP kinase requires cell adhesion. EMBO J 16: 5592-5599, 1997.

103. Gotoh A, Takahira H, Gaehlen RL et al. Cross-lonking of integrins induces tyrosine phosphorylation of the proto-oncogene product vav and the protein tyrosine kinase syk in human factor-dependent myeloid cells. Cell Growth Different 8: 721-729, 1997.

104. Schlaepfer DD, Hanks SK, Hunter T et al. Integrin-mediated signal transduction linked to ras pathway by GRB2 binding to focal adhesion kinase. Nature 372: 786-791, 1994.

105. Fackler M, Krause D, Smith O et al. Full length but not truncated CD34 inhibits hematopoietic cell differentaition of M1 cells. Blood 85: 3040-3047, 1995.

106. Bazil V, Brandt J, Tsukamoto A et al. Apoptosis of human hematopoietic progenitor cells induced by crosslinking of surface CD43, the major sialoglycoprotein of leukocytes. Blood 86: 502-511, 1995.

107. Bazil V, Brandt J, Chen S et al. A monoclonal antibody recognizing CD43 (leukosialin) initiates apoptosis of human hematopoietic progenitor cells but not stem cells. Blood 87: 1272-1281, 1996.
108. Banu N, Groopman JE, Frenette PS et al. Role of P-selectin and E-selectin in megakaryocytopoiesis. Blood 86: 284a, 1995.
109. Frenette PS, Mayadas TN, Rayburn H et al. Susceptibility to infection and altered hematopoieis in mice deficient in both P- and E-selectins. Cell 84: 563-574, 1996.
110. Maly P, al e. The a(1,3) fucosyltransferase Fuc-TVII controls leokocyte trafficking through an essential role in L-, E- and P-selectin ligand biosynthesis. Cell 86: 643-653, 1996.
111. Park JK, Rosenstein YJ, Remold-O'Donnell et al. Enhancement of T-cell activation by the CD43 molecule whose expression in defective in Wiskott-Aldrich syndrome. Nature 350: 706-710, 1991.
112. Simmons PJ, Lévesque JP, Zannettino ACW. Cell adhesion molecules and their role in regulating haemopoiesis. Baillère's Clin Hematol 10: 485-505, 1997.

3. The Interaction of Cytokines with T cell and Natural Killer Cell Physiology.

Richard A. Carter, Edmund K. Waller

Introduction

The development and differentiation of lymphocytes are regulated by the local microenvironment in the thymus, bone marrow and intestinal epithelium. Mice engineered to lack the transcription factor Ikaros develop normal myeloid and erythroid cells, but lack lymphoid cells[1], implying the existence of a 'lymphoid stem cell' restricted to T, B, or NK cell lineage specific differentiation. Experimental evidence suggests that cytokines act both to regulate differentiation of lymphoid progenitors and to activate and expand mature lymphocyte populations. A unidirectional model for lymphoid differentiation suggests that lineage commitment is driven by exposure of stem cells to lineage-specific cytokines. The availability of recombinant cytokines that regulate lymphoid differentiation and function has led to their clinical application in enhancing anti-tumor immunity and immune reconstitution in the setting of bone marrow transplantation. A discussion of the effect of cytokines on T cell and Natural Killer cell differentiation and function will be the subject of this review. B cell differentiation has been reviewed elsewhere[2].

Monoclonal antibodies to a variety of lineage-specific human cell surface antigens and model systems of human T cell and NK cell development have defined the events of T cell and NK cell differentiation. Terstappen and Picker used flow cytometry to provide a detailed description of the T cell intermediates between undifferentiated stem cells and mature T cells in the human thymus and bone marrow microenvironments[3]. The availability of immunodeficient SCID mice that can be engrafted with human lymphoid tissue[4], has helped elucidate the pathways of human lymphoid differentiation *in vivo*[5]. In addition, fetal thymic organ culture (FTOC) systems have allowed a parallel *in-vitro* analysis of the development of human T and NK cells. These experimental systems and the recent development of cytokine deficient 'knockout mice' has led to a conceptual model for the development of early thymocytes with key branch points regulated by specific cytokines.

T cell development Pathway

The thymus is the principal site of T cell development. The human thymus begins to form in week 7 of gestation[6]. Shortly thereafter, T cell progenitors migrate to the thymus from the fetal liver and yolk sac. It is unclear if these early cells are true pluripotent stem cells or if they are lymphoid progenitors restricted to T cell development prior to reaching the thymus. The thymus does not develop fully differentiated cortical and medullary regions until week 15 of gestation. The thymic environment includes epithelial components and mesenchymal cells located in the capsule, blood vessels and interlobular septae[6,7]. Anderson[8,9] has demonstrated that these mesenchymal and epithelial cells are necessary for murine T cell development. Exactly how cells of the microenvironment effect stem cells is unknown, however a likely mechanism is through the local secretion of cytokines in a paracrine manner. If T cell development is blocked, the development of the thymus stops after the appearance of the cortex[10], suggesting that the developing and phenotypically mature T cells play a role in the development of the thymic medulla.

The development of T cells has been extensively studied in mice[11] leading to a conceptual model in which thymic progenitors progress in a stepwise fashion from the $CD3^-,CD4^-,CD8^-$ triple negative (TN) progenitor through a $CD4^+,CD8^+$ double positive (DP) intermediate to the single positive (SP) differentiated $CD4^+$ and $CD8^+$ thymocytes which enter the peripheral circulation (See figure 1). The earliest thymic progenitors express low levels of CD4 and are capable of giving rise to T cells, B cells and NK cells, but not myeloid cells[12]. The fact that these cells are not committed to the T cell lineage until they reach the thymus suggests that the thymic microenvironment favors T cell commitment. As $CD4^{lo}$ thymocytes lose CD4 expression and become TN thymocytes, they commit to T cell development. This process can be further described by the pattern of CD44 and CD25 expression on thymic progenitors in mice. TN cells can be divided into $CD44^+CD25^+$ c-kit $^+$ TN pro-T cells and $CD44^-CD\ 25^+$ c-kit^{lo} pre-T cells [13]. This distinction is important because pro-T cells respond to IL-7 while the later cells do not. *In vivo* injection of antibodies to IL-7 results in decreased thymic cellularity[14] with normal thymic subpopulations of TN, DP, and SP thymocytes suggesting that IL-7 is important in expansion but not differentiation of T cell progenitors.

In murine T cell development, a critical juncture occurs prior to the differentiation of the DP cell and prior to the rearrangement of the ß chain of the T cell receptor (TCR)[15][16]. Knockout mice deficient for the gene which codes for the ß chain are unable to produce DP cells[17]. Similar data have been obtained from mice lacking recombination-activating genes (RAG) and SCID mice[18][19][20]. Replacement of the gene coding for the ß chain of the TCR leads to normal development of DP cells[17][21][22][23].

Efforts have been made to apply this model to human T cell development. Waller, et al, examined human T cell development by injecting fetal thymic progenitor populations into human thymic xenografts in SCID-hu mice and developed the schema shown in Figure 2. In this model, $(CD3^-4^-8^-)$ triple negative (TN) thymic progenitors were isolated by fluorescence activated cell sorters, fluorescently labeled on the cell surface using PKH2 (a membrane label), and injected intrathymically into heterologous human thymic xenografts in SCID-hu mice[5]. Analysis of thymic xenografts demonstrated a sequential appearance of fluorescently labeled $CD34^+8^-$, $CD34^+8^+$ and $CD3^+4^+8^+$ cells. In addition, FACS isolated and fluorescently labeled CD34 8 cells injected intrathymically differentiated into $CD4^+8^+$ cells. Cycling $CD4^+8$ cells subsequently differentiated into mature $CD4^+$ and CD8 single positive T cells expressing high levels of CD3.

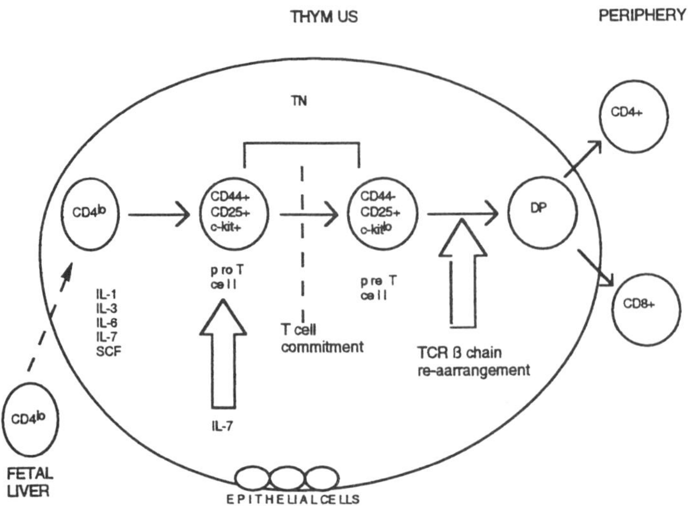

Figure 1: Model of Murine Intrathymic T cell development. TN = 'Triple Negative' CD3- CD4- CD8-. DP= 'Double Positive' CD4+ CD8+.

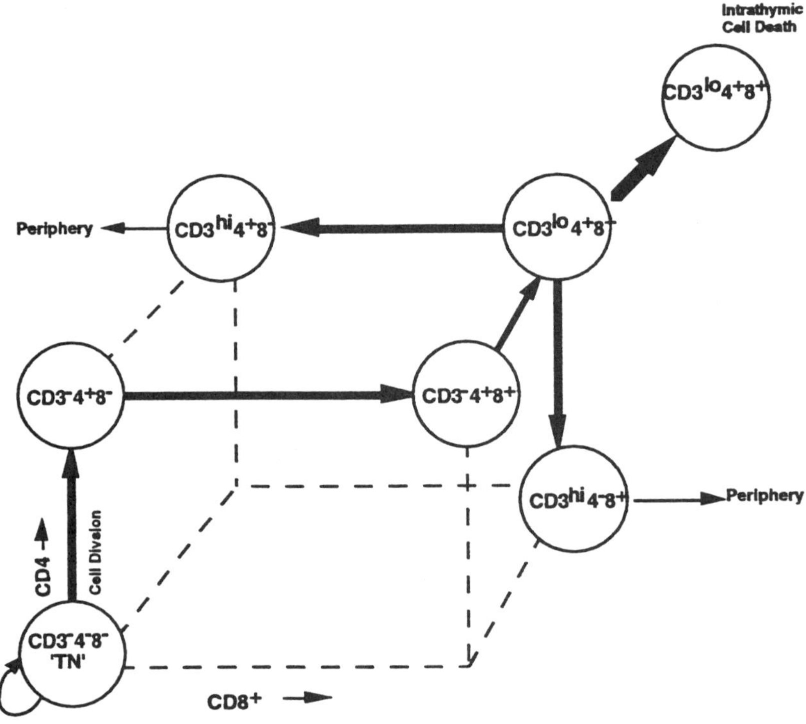

Figure 2. Model for Human intrathymic T cell development based on the SCID-hu mouse[5].

Human Natural Killer Cell development

The irreversible commitment to the B or T cell lineage is marked by re-arrangements of immunoglobulin (Ig) and T cell receptor (TCR) genes. In contrast, NK cells likely represent a lineage distinct from T cells and B cells because they develop normally in RAG-2 deficient mice and SCID mice that lack the ability to re-arrange TCR and Ig genotypes[19,27]. The human NK cell does not re-arrange Ig or TCR genes[24], lacks expression of CD3ϵ, but usually expresses CD16 and/or CD56 and is cytokine to some tumors and virally infected cells. The cytotoxicity of NK cells is triggered by the failure to recognize 'self' type MHC[25,26]. Unlike T cells, NK can recognize their target in the absence of the MHC. Fetal NK cells can lyse NK sensitive targets, and in the presence of interferon or IL-2, they will lyse otherwise resistant targets, including virally infected cells [28][29][30]. Fetal NK cells also produce regulating cytokines including gamma-interferon, granulocyte-macrophage colony stimulating factor and tumor-necrosis factor 2 [25].

Although TCR gene re-arrangement separates NK and T cells, these lineages share many surface markers[31], suggesting that they are related in ontogeny. Anecdotal evidence in human SCID patients also supports the hypothesis of a common precursor. SCID patients with normal B and myeloid development, but who lack both T and NK cells have been described[32], as well as a patient who has T and B cells but lacked NK cells[33]. These observations imply that NK differentiation is related to but distinct from T cell development. While T cells undergo differentiation and education in the thymus, NK cells develop normally in athymic nude mice [34] and are present in a high proportion relative to T cells in the bone marrow, suggesting that this is the site of NK cell development. Although NK cells can be found in low frequency in the human thymus [35], it is unclear if these cells are have developed intrathymically or represent transient emigrants from the peripheral circulation.

The Role of cytokines in NK/ T cell development

The observation that cytokines can induce myeloid differentiation has led to the clinical use of GM-CSF and G-CSF to accelerate myelopoiesis following chemotherapy induced aplasia [36]. Intense interest surrounds finding cytokines that favor stem cell commitment and differentiation to the lymphoid lineage in order to reverse immunodeficiencies caused by HIV infection or chemo-radiation or to augment immune responses in cancer patients. IL-2 and IL-4 are known to promote differentiation of stem cells into phenotypically mature T cell *in vitro*[37][38][39][40]. These cytokines do not appear to be essential to T cell development, however, because patients deficient in IL-2 develop normal numbers of CD4$^+$ and CD8$^+$ cells [41][42][43]. Excluding the occasional experiment of nature, most of the information concerning cytokines in T cell development comes from experiments involving antibodies to specific cytokines added to FTOC systems and knockout mice. Knockouts of the IL6 and interferon gamma genes suggest that these cytokines are not essential [44][45]. IL-2 and IL-4 knockout mice develop a normal thymus and mature T cells[46][47][48]. The results of these experiments correlate well and are extensively reviewed by Zlotnick and Moore[11]. The mouse knockout experiments are limited because when the thymus develops in the absence of a given cytokine, other cytokines may compensate leading to normal T cell development. Despite this, knockout mouse experiments suggest that IL-7 is crucial to T cell development (See Table 1).

Table 1: Summary of experiments involving cytokine knockout mice.

CYTOKINE	T CELL DEVELOPMENT	REFERENCE
IL-2	Normal	46
IL-2 Receptor gamma chain	Decrease in T cells Absence of NK cells	49
IL-4	Normal T cell development Absent Th2 response upon stimulation.	47 50
IL-6	Normal	51
IL-7	Severely decreased thymic cellularity. Decrease in gamma delta T cells.	52 53
IL-7R alpha	Severely decreased thymic cellularity, differentiation block at CD4^{lo}	54
IL-8R	Normal	55
IL-10	Normal	56
IFN gamma	Normal	57
IFNgamma receptor	Normal	45
GM-CSF	Normal	58
Lymphotoxin	Normal	59

Data are emerging that suggest IL-7 may also be crucial in human T cell development. Plum, et al, developed a human/ murine chimeric fetal thymic organ culture system by injecting human CD34$^+$ stem cells into the thymic glands of SCID mice[60]. Monoclonal antibodies to either IL-7 or the alpha chain of the IL-7 receptor produced a profound decrease in thymic cellularity. Further analysis revealed that few thymic precursors were able to progress to the double positive stage (see Figure 1). Here again, experiments of nature are instructive.

X-linked Severe Combined Immunodeficiency (SCIDX1) is characterized by poor T and NK cell function. The defect in SCIDX1 maps to region q13.1 on the X chromosome and implies an essential role for specific cytokines in the development of T and NK cells[61 62 63 64]. This defect affects the interleukin-2 receptor gamma chain (aka the gamma-c gene), which is shared by IL-2, IL4, IL7 and IL15 [65 66 67 68 69]. In addition, IL-7 has been demonstrated to support the growth of human TN thymocyte precursors *in vitro* [70,71,72,73], and is a potent stimulatory factor for T cells [74,75]. Neutralizing antibodies to IL-7 added to fetal thymic organ culture prevent T cell development [76]. IL-7 enhances the expression of interferon gamma in activated T cells independent of IL-12, suggesting that it is an may serve as an intermediate cytokine in triggering a Th1 response[77]. In murine models, IL-7 mobilizes stem cells into the peripheral blood[78]. Finally, IL-7 has been found to accelerate reconstitution of the thymus following syngeneic bone marrow transplant in mice[79], an approach which could translate into clinical trials.

The influence of cytokines on NK cell development is not well understood. Caligiuri suggests that NK cells can be sustained by IL-15, but not by TNF alpha, IL1 ß, IL-4, IL-7, IL-9, IL-10, IL-12, or IL -13. Bone marrow stromal cells secrete IL15 which can maintain NK cells in culture systems free of stroma cells, perhaps via expression of bcl-2[80]. When combined with stem cell factor and IL-2, IL-7 favors the development of thymic precursors into CD56+ NK cells. [81].

Cytokines in post-thymic T cell/NK cell activation and expansion.

Just as the intrathymal development of T cells is described by phenotypic changes, activation and expansion of post-thymic T cells has been described based on observations concerning surface molecules. Initially, naive T cells which leave the thymus are identified by expression the high molecular weight isoform of the surface molecule CD45, CD45RA. These cells also express L- selection, a surface molecule associated with the tendency to migrate to lymph nodes. When exposed to antigens, T cell activation is associated with reciprocal loss of CD45RA expression and the expression of the low molecular weight isoform, CD45RO. Activated CD45RO+ T cells are the effector T cell population, which mediate antigen specific immune response via cytokine secretion [82] [83]. In the absence of further stimulation, activated T cells lose CD45RO expression and revert the naive phenotype [84] [85] [86].

IL-2 is central to the activation, proliferation, and survival of post-thymic T cells and NK cells. IL-2 is secreted by activated T cells and acts as an autocrine and paracrine growth factor [11,38] . Local production of IL-2 in the vicinity of T cells that have encountered special antigen particles presented by antigen resenting cells expressing stimulatory molecules leads to the proliferation of antigen specific T cells and the development of the immune response to predominance of cellular (cytokine) effectors versus synthesis of humoral (antibody) effectors depends upon the interplay of a number of additional cytokines with IL-2 on the antigen activated T cell. The CD4, 'T-helper response' is defined as either Th1 or Th2 (see figure 3). The Th1 subset produces IL-2, IL-12 and IFN gamma [87] [88] and stimulates a delayed type hypersensitivity or cell mediated immunity. Th2 lymphocytes produce IL-4, IL-5, and IL-10, and promote humoral response and allergic type reactions involving mast cells and eosinophils[89] [90]. Macrophages exposed to bacterial antigens generate IL-12[91] [92] [93] and trigger Th1 response, whereas IL4 produced by mast cells and NK cell triggers a Th2 response[89]. The commitment of an antigen specific CD4+ T cell (Th0) to the Th1 or Th2 pathway depends upon its exposure to the cytokines specific to these lineages during the activation phase. The regulation of Th1 versus Th2 commitment is directed by cytokines secreted into the local microenvironment by cells of the innate immune response, specifically macrophages which secrete IL-12 and mast cells which secrete IL-4.

Clinical Applications of Cytokines in Bone Marrow Transplantation

<u>Graft -vs-Host Disease</u>. Experimental evidence suggests that inflammatory cytokines play a central role in the pathogenesis of Graft-vs-Host disease[94] (GVHD). Ferrara's cytokine theory of GVHD involves three steps[95]. The pre-transplant conditioning

regimen induces tissue damage in host tissues which leads to the release of inflammatory cytokines tumor necrosis factor and Interleukin-1. In the autologous setting, this is a self limited cause of fever and rash, as has been previously described as the 'autoaggressive syndrome' [96]. These cytokines increase the expression of HLA molecules on the surface of host cells. In the allogeneic setting, the cytokine dysregulation proceeds to the second step and mature T cells of donor origin recognize HLA molecules which have been up-regulated by exposure to pro-inflammatory cytokines. In the third step, the efferent arm of GVHD is characterized by activated T cells that proliferate and secrete either IL-2 and IFN gamma, leading to an inflammatory Th1 response stimulating donor mononuclear cells to secrete IL-1 and TNF alpha causing further tissue damage and an acute GVHD response. Alternatively, T cell production of IL4 and IL10 leads to a Th2 response and can produce chronic GVHD[97].

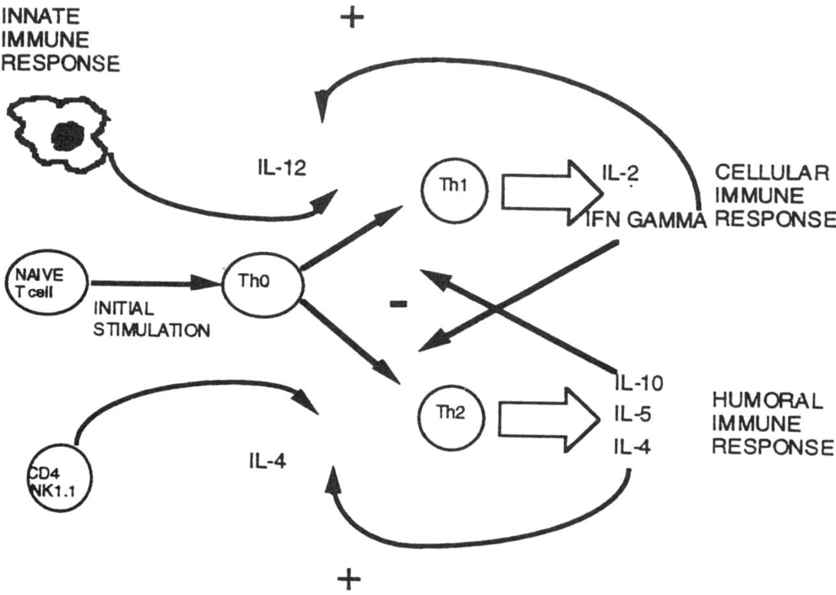

Figure 3. Role of cytokines in directing specific T helper subsets.

The importance of tumor necrosis factor α in graft-vs-host disease was first described by Piguet et al[98]. Subsequently, Nestel, et al. demonstrated that macrophages in mice with GVHD were primed to release TNF alpha, and that this effect could be blocked with anti-TNF alpha antiserum[99]. In both a retrospective review and a prospective analysis of transplant patients, Holler et al described a relationship between increased serum TNF alpha levels and the complications of veno-occlusive disease and GVHD [100]. These observations have led to several clinical trials. Holler, et al. demonstrated a delay in the onset of acute GVHD in patients given a monoclonal antibody neutralizing tumor necrosis factor alpha following the preparative regimen[101]. However, a phase III trial of pentoxifylline, which is known to down regulate TNF alpha *in vitro,* failed to show any decrease in GVHD or veno-occlusive disease[102]. A partial response was observed when an monoclonal antibody to TNF alpha was used to treat severe GVHD disease in a phase II trial[103].

Animal data suggests that Interleukin 1 also plays a key role in the cytokine dysregulation of acute GVHD. Abhyankar, et al. used reverse transcriptase-polymerase chain reaction (RT-PCR) to demonstrate elevation of messenger RNA coding for interleukin 1 alpha in the spleen and skin of animals who died of GVHD[104], moreover, GVHD was significantly decreased in animals that received an IL-1 receptor antagonist[105]. A phase I trial of an interleukin 1 receptor antagonist in patients with steroid resistant acute GVHD, revealed a partial response, suggesting efficacy for this treatment approach[106].

Despite evidence that the number of host specific interleukin-2 producing T cells predicts for acute GVHD[107 108], efforts to antagonize IL-2 production using a monoclonal antibody as prophylaxis for acute GVHD have been unsuccessful[109]. The administration of exogenous IL-2 in a murine model paradoxically reduces GVHD[110 111], perhaps by inhibition of IFN gamma[112]. However, this approach may prove to be too toxic for patients[113 114]. IL2 is potentially useful for treating lymphoma patients post autologous transplant[115], but not as consolidation for ALL patients post autologous transplant[116].

Alpha interferon is used prior to allogeneic transplant in the management of CML and as an immunologic adjuvant following autologous transplant in patients with non-Hodgkin's lymphoma and multiple myeloma. Initially a report suggested that CML patients undergoing transplant who had previously been treated with alpha interferon did not have any increase in GVHD[117]. Recently, however, data has emerged that prior pre-treatment with interferon alpha predisposes recipients of allogeneic BMT to GVHD, especially in the matched-unrelated donor setting[118 119]. The role of alpha interferon in the adjuvant setting following autologous peripheral stem cell transplantation is poorly defined, although randomized studies of adjuvant alpha interferon following standard chemotherapy have demonstrated a survival benefit.

The role of gamma interferon in the pathogenesis of GVHD is better understood. In a murine model of GVHD, interferon gamma given post transplant was found to prevent GVHD, perhaps by down-regulating interferon gamma secreting T cells[120]. Interferon gamma increases expression of MHC class I and II molecules[121]. In the setting of acute GVHD, this may make target tissues more sensitive to T cell mediated killing[122]. Monoclonal antibodies to IFN gamma were found to block GVHD of the gut epithelium in a murine model[123].

Cytokine patterns differ in acute and chronic GVHD in a manner consistent with the Th1 Th2 paradigm[124 125]. *In vitro* study of lymphocytes from animals with chronic GVHD confirms this observation[126]. The type 1 cytokines, IL-2 and IFN gamma, are found early in the cytokine cascade and activate mononuclear phagocytes. Interferon gamma upregulates MHC class II expression on macrophages[127] and primes them to release the proinflammatory cytokines TNF alpha and IL-1 when stimulated with bacterial lipopolysaccharide[128 129 130]. In a murine model, IL-2 causes macrophages to produce TNF alpha, whereas IL-4 causes down-regulation of TNF alpha secretion[131]. Conversely, the type 2 cytokines, IL-4 and IL-10, occur later in GVHD and inhibit macrophages from producing inflammatory cytokines and down regulate macrophage response to lipopolysaccharide[131 132]. IL-4 also favors secretion of IL-1 receptor antagonist which blocks the action of IL-1[133]. Type 2 cytokines block the production of type 1 cytokines[134]. Type 1 and Type 2 cytokines have opposite effects on CD 8+ cytotoxic T cells. IL-2 is a critical trigger for the cytotoxic T cell response[135]. The importance of the functional distinction between type 1 and type 2 cytokines or the Th1 vs Th2 response is demonstrated by study of the protozoal infection cutaneous Leishmania major. This infection is poorly controlled by a Th2 response, but can be cured by a Th1 response[136]. Clearly, the ability to shift from a type 1 response to a type 2 response has potential clinical benefit in interrupting the cytokine cascade that leads to acute graft-versus-host disease[94].

Interleukin 6 and 8 have been implicated as possible causative factors in complications following transplant. High interleukin 6 levels have been reported in patients with hepatorenal syndrome following allogeneic transplant[137]and autologous transplant[138]. In addition, IL-6 levels have been correlated to lymphoproliferative disorders following transplant[139]. One report describes elevated IL-8 levels in patients with GVHD following transplant for ß Thalassemia[140].

Future directions.

Recently, a new member of the tyrosine kinase receptor family was described, the flt3 receptor [141] [142]. Subsequently, the ligand for this receptor was described[143] [144] and has stimulated intense interest. Flt-3 appears to stimulate very early myeloid precursors with no effect on erythroid or megakaryocytic development. Flt-3 ligand increases bone marrow cellularity when given to primates[145], and in a murine model engineered to overexpress flt-3 ligand by retro-viral vector mediated gene transfer, lymphocytes, neutrophils and monocytes were significantly increased[146]. Although it only weakly stimulates hematopoietic progenitors when used alone, flt-3 has a significant synergistic effect when given in conjunction with other cytokines, including IL3, Il6, IL-7, IL-10, IL-11, GM-CSF, and G-CSF[147] [148] [149] [150]. Because it has no significant effect on mast cells, flt-3 is not limited by the toxicities that plagued the clinical trials with steel factor. Flt-3 appears to expand the number of long-term culture-initiating cells allowing *ex-vivo* expansion of stem cells in the absence of stromal cells[151]. Flt-3 may prove useful in gene therapy by inducing primitive stem cells to cycle, making them targets for gene transduction. In murine models of melanoma and lymphoma, Flt-3 has been shown to inhibit tumor growth, perhaps through the activation of dendritic cells[152].

Current research programs attempt to use cytokines for *ex vivo* expansion of large numbers of pluripotent hematopoietic progenitor cells[153]. As the concepts of graft engineering and adoptive immunotherapy become more advanced, there seems also to be potential benefit to the *ex vivo* expansion of different lymphocyte populations that could be added to enriched or expanded hematopoietic progenitor cells. Expanded populations of Natural Killer cells have potential clinical benefit in the treatment of chronic myeloid leukemia[154] [155]. Another interesting conceptual approach would be to obtain sensitized lymphocytes from lymph nodes which drain tumor sites, expand them *ex vivo* under conditions which favor intra-cellular signal transduction, and re-inject them as a form of immunotherapy. Baldwin et al, have demonstrated the efficacy of this approach in a rat glioma model[156]. The ability to administer expanded autologous T cells has the potential to reverse the immunodeficiency associated with HIV disease[157]. Further definition of cytokine function will be crucial to further the application of adoptive immunotherapy to treat patients with cancer and HIV infection.

References

1.   Georgopoulos K, Bigby M, Wang J-H, et al: The Ikaros gene is required for the development of all lymphoid lineages. Cell 79:143, 1994
2.   Duchosal MA: B-cell development and differentiation. [Review] [146 refs]. Seminars in Hematology 341:(Suppl 1)2-12, 1997
3.   Terstappen LW, Huang S, Picker LJ: Flow cytometric assessment of human T-cell differentiation in thymus and bone marrow. Blood 79:(3)666-77, 1992
4.   McCune JM, Namikawa R, Kaneshima H, et al: The SCID-hu mouse: murine model for the analysis of human hematolymphoid differentiation and function. Science. 241:1632-1639, 1988
5.   Kraft DL, Weissman IL, E.K.Waller: Differentiation of CD3-4-8- human fetal thymocytes in vivo: characterization of a CD3-4+8- intermediate. J. Exp. Med. 178:265-277, 1993
6.   Haynes B: The human thymic microenvironment. Adv Immunol 36:87, 1984
7.   Boyd RL, Tucek CL, Godfrey DI, et al. The thymic microenvironment. Immunol Today 14:445, 1993.
8.   Anderson G, Owen JT, Moore NC, Jenkinson EJ: Thymic epithelial cells provide unique signals for positive selection of CD4+CD8+ thymocytes in vitro. J Exp Med 179:2027, 1994.
9.   Anderson G, Jenkinson EJ, Moore NC, Owen JJT: MHC class II MHC-positive epithelium and mesenchyme cells are both required for T cell development in the thymus. Nature 362:70, 1993.
10. Spits H, Lanier L, Phillips J: Development of Human T and Natural Killer Cells. Blood 85:(10)2654-2670, 1995
11. Zlotnick A, Moore T: Cytokine production and requirements during T-cell development. Current Opinion in Immunology 7:206-213, 1995
12. Wu L, Antica M, Johnson GR, et al: Developmental potential of the earliest precursor cells from the adult mouse thymus. J Exp Med 174:1617-27, 1991
13. Moore TA, Zlotnik A: T-cell Lineage Commitment and Cytokine Responses of Thymic Progenitors. Blood 86:(5)1850-1860, 1995
14. Grabstein KH, Waldschmidt TJ, Finkleman FD, et al: Inhibition of murine B and T lymphopoiesis in vivo by an anti-interleukin 7 monoclonal antibody. J Exp Med 178:257, 1993
15. Von Boehmer H: Positive selection of lymphocytes. Cell 76:219, 1994
16. Palmer DB, Hayday A, Owen MJ: Is TCR ß expression an essential event in early thymocyte development? Immunology Today 14:460, 1993
17. Mombaerts P, Clarke AR, Hooper ML, Tonegawa S: Mutations in T cell receptor genes alpha and beta block thymocyte development at different stages. Nature 360:225-31, 1992
18. von Boehmer H: Development biology of T cells in T cell receptor transgenic mice. Ann Rev Immunol 8:531, 1990
19. Shinkai Y, Rathbun G, Lam KP, al e: RAG-2-deficient mice lack mature lymphocytes owing to inability to initiate V(D)J rearrangement. Cell 68:855-867, 1992
20. Mombaerts P, Iacomini J, Johnson RS, et al: RAG-1 deficient mice have no have no mature B and T lymphocytes. Cell 68:(5)869-77, 1992
21. Kishi H, Borgulya P, Scott B, et al: Surface expression of ß T cell receptor (TCR) chain in the absence of other TCR or CD3 proteins on immature T cells. EMBO journal 10:93, 1990
22. Groettrup M, Baron A, Griffiths G, et al: T cell receptor ß chain homodimers on the surface of immature but not mature alpha, gamma, and delta chain deficient T cell lines. EMBO Journal 11:2735-2745, 1992
23. Shinkai Y, Koyasu S, Nakayama KI, et al: Restoration of T cell development in RAG-2 deficient mice by functional TCR transgenes. Science 259:822, 1993
24. Lanier LL, Phillips JH, Hackett JJ, et al: Journal of Immunology 137:2735-2739, 1986
25. Phillips JH, Hori T, Nagler A, et al: Ontogeny of human natural killer (NK) cells: fetal NK cells mediate cytolytic function and express cytoplasmic CD3 epsilon, delta proteins. J Exp Med 175:1055-1066, 1992
26. Ljunggren HG, Karre K: Host resistance directed selectively against H-2-deficient lymphoma

variants. Analysis of the mechanism. J Exp Med 162:(6)1745-59, 1985

27. Hackett JJ, Bosma GC, Bosma MJ, et al: Transplantable progenitors of natural killer cells are distinct from those of T and B lymphocytes. Proc Natl Acad Sci USA 83:3427-3431, 1986

28. Trinchieri G, Santoli D: Anti-viral activity induced by culturing lymphocytes with tumor-derived or virus-transformed cells. Enhancement of human natural killer cell activity by interferon and antagonistic inhibition of susceptibility of target cells to lysis. J Exp Med 147:1314-1333, 1978

29. Trinchieri G, Matsumoto-Kobayashi M, Clark SC, et al: Response of resting human peripheral blood natural killer cells to interleukin-2. J Exp Med 160:1147-1169, 1984

30. Welsh RMJ, Hallenbrook LA: Effect of virus infections on target cell susceptibility to natural killer cell mediated lysis. J Immunol 124:2491-2497, 1980

31. Lanier LL, Spits H, Phillips JH: The developmental relationship between NK cells and T cells. Immunology Today 13:(10)392-395, 1992

32. Bacchetta R, Vanderkerckhove BAE, Touraine J-L, et al: Chimerism and tolerance to host and donor in severe combined immunodeficiencies transplanted with fetal liver stem cells. J Clin Invest 91:1067, 1993

33. Biron CA, Byron KS, Sullivan JL: Severe herpes virus infections in an adolescent without natural killer cells [see comments]. N Eng J Med 320:1731-1735, 1989

34. Herberman RB, Nunn ME, Holden HT, et al: Augmentation of natural cytotoxic reactivity of mouse lymphoid cells against syngeneic and allogeneic target cells. Int J Cancer 16:2309-239, 1975

35. Mingari MC, Poggi A, Biassoni R, et al: In vitro proliferation and cloning of CD3- CD16+ cells from human thymocyte precursors. J Exp Med 174:21-26, 1991

36. Sheridan WP, Begley CG, Juttner CA, et al: Effect of peripheral-blood progenitor cells mobilized by filgrastim (G-CSF) on platelet recovery after high-dose chemotherapy. Lancet 339:640-4, 1992

37. Toribio ML, De La Hera A, Borst J, et al: Involvement of the interleukin 2 pathway in the rearrangement and expression of both alpha beta and gamma delta T cell receptor genes in human T cell precursors. J Exp Med 168:2231, 1988

38. Toribio ML, Alonso JM, Barcena A, et al: Human T cell precursors: Involvement of the IL-2 pathway in the generation of mature T cells. Immunology Reviews 104:55, 1988

39. Barcena A, Torbio ML, Pezzi L, Martinez C: A role for interleukin 4 in the differentiation of mature T cell receptor gamma delta cells from human intrathymic T cell precursors. J Exp Med 172:(2)439-46, 1990

40. Denning SM, Kurtzburg J, Leslie DS, Haynes BF: Human postnatal CD4-CD8-CD3- thymic precursors differentiate in vitro into T cell receptor delta-bearing cells. 142 2988, 1989

41. Weinburg K, Parkman R: Severe combined immunodeficiency due to a specific defect in the production of interleukin-2. New England Journal of Medicine 322:1718, 1990

42. Pahwah R, Chatila T, Paradise C, Day NK, Geha R, Schwartz SA: Recombinant interleukin-2 therapy in severe combined immunodeficiency disease. Proc Natl Acad Sci USA 86:5069, 1990

43. DiSanto JP, Keever CA, Small T, Nichols GL, O'Reilly RJ, Flomenburg N: Absence of interleukin 2 production in a severe combined immunodeficiency disease syndrome with T cells. J Exp Med 171:1697, 1990

44. Poli V, Balena R, Fattori E, et al: Interleukin-6 deficient mice are protected from bone loss caused by estrogen depletion. EMBO Journal 13:1189, 1994

45. Huang S, Hendriks W, Althage A, et al: Immune response in mice that lack the interferon gamma receptor. Science 259:1742, 1993

46. Schorle H, Holtschke T, Hunig T, et al: Development and function of T cells in mice rendered interleukin-2 deficient by gene targeting. Nature 352:621, 1991

47. Kuhn R, Rajewski K, Muller W: Generation and analysis of interleukin-4 deficient mice. Science 254:707, 1991

48. Sadlack B, Kuhn R, Schorle H, et al: Development and Proliferation of lymphocytesin mice deficient for both interleukins-2 and -4. European Journal of Immunology 24:281, 1994

49. DiSanto JP, Muller W, Guy-Grand D, et al: Lymphoid development in mice with a targeted deletion of the interleukin 2 receptor gamma chain. Proc Natl Acad Sci USA. 99:(2)377-381, 1995

50. Kopf M, Le Gros G, Bachmann M, et al: Disruption of the murine IL-4 gene blocks Th2 cytokine responses. Nature 362:(6417)245-8, 1993

51. Kopf M, Baumann H, Freer G, et al: Impaired immune and acute-phase responses in interleukin-6-deficient mice. Nature 368:(6469)339-42, 1994

52. Moore T, von Freeden-Jeffry U, Murray R, Zlotnik A: Inhibition of gamma delta T cell development and early thymocyte maturation in IL-7 -/- mice. J Immunol 157:(6)2366-73, 1996

53.   von Freeden-Jeffry U, Vieira P, Lucian LA, et al: Lymphopenia in interleukin (IL)-7 gene-deleted mice identifies IL-7 as a nonredundant cytokine. J Exp Med 181:(4)1519-26, 1995

54.   Peschon JJ, Morissey PJ, Grabstein KH, et al: Early lymphocyte expansion is severely impaired in interleukin 7 receptor deficient mice. J Exp Med 180:1955-1960, 1994

55.   Cacalano G, Lee J, Kikly K, et al: Neutrophil and B cell expansion in mice that lack the murine IL-8 receptor homolog [see comments][published erratum appears in Science 1995 Oct 20;270(5235):365]. Science 265:(5172)682-4, 1994

56.   Kuhn R, Lohler J, Rennick D, et al: Interleukin-10-deficient mice develop chronic enterocolitis [see comments]. Cell 75:(2)263-74, 1993

57.   Dalton DK, Pitts-Meek S, Keshav S, et al: Multiple defects of immune cell function in mice with disrupted interferon-gamma genes [see comments]. Science 259:(5102)1739-42, 1993

58.   Stanley E, Lieschke GJ, Grail D, et al: Granulocyte/macrophage colony-stimulating factor-deficient mice show no major perturbation of hematopoiesis but develop a characteristic pulmonary pathology. Proc Natl Acad Sci USA 91:(12)5592-6, 1994

59.   De Togni P, Goellner J, Ruddle NH, et al: Abnormal development of peripheral lymphoid organs in mice deficient in lymphotoxin [see comments]. Science 264:(5159)703-7, 1994

60.   Plum J, De Smedt M, Leclercq G, et al: Interleukin-7 is a critical growth factor in early human T-cell development. Blood 88:(11)4239-45, 1996

61.   Voss SD, Hong R, Sondel PM: Severe Combined Immunodeficiency, interleukin-2 (IL-2), and the IL-2 receptor: Experiments of nature continue to pave the way. Blood 83:626, 1994

62.   de Saint Basile GD, Arveiler B, Oberle I, et al: Close linkage of the locus for X-chromosome linked severe combined immunodeficiency to polymorphic DNA markers in Xq11-Xq13. Proceedings of the National Academy of Sciences of the United States of America 84:7576, 1987

63.   Noguchi M, Yi H, Rosenblatt HM, et al: Interleukin-2 receptor gamma chain mutation results in X linked severe combined immunodeficiency in humans. Cell 73:147, 1993

64.   Puck JM, Deschenes SM, Porter JC, et al: The Interleukin-2 receptor gamma chain mutation maps to Xq13.1 and is mutated in X-linked, SCIDX1. Human Molecular Genetics 2:1099, 1993

65.   Kondo M, Takeshita T, Higuchi M, et al: Functional participation of the IL-2 receptor gamma chain in IL-7 receptor complexes. Science 263:1453-4, 1994

66.   Kondo M, Takeshita T, Ishii N, et al: Sharing of the interleukin-2(IL-2) receptor gamma chain between receptors for IL-2 and IL-4. Science 262:1874-1877, 1993

67.   Noguchi M, Nakamura Y, Russell SM, et al: Interleukin-2 receptor gamma chain: A functional component of the interleukin-7 receptor. Science 262:1877-80, 1993

68.   Russell SM, Keegan AD, Harada N, et al: Interleukin-2 receptor gamma gene: A functional component of the interleukin-4 receptor. Science 262:1880-3, 1993

69.   Grabstein KH, Eisenman J, Shanebeck K, et al: Cloning of a T cell growth factor that interacts with the ß chain of the interleukin-2 receptor. Science 264:965, 1994

70.   Schmitt C, Ktorza S, Sarun S, et al: CD34 expressing human thymocyte precursors proliferate in response to IL-7 but have lost myeloid differentiation potential. Blood 82:3675, 1993

71.   Hori T, Cupp J, Wrighton N, Lee F, Spits H: Identification of a novel human thymocyte subset with a phenotype of CD3-,CD4+,CDå+ß-:Possible progeny of the CD3-,CD4-,CD8- subset. Journal of Immunology 146:4078-84, 1991

72.   Groh V, Fabbi M, Strominger JL: Maturation or differentiation of human thymocyte precursors *in vitro?* Proceedings of the National Academy of Sciences of the United States of America 87:5973, 1990

73.   Morrissey PJ, Goodwin RG, Nordan RP, et al: Recombinant interleukin 7, pre-B cell growth factor, has costimulatory activity on purified mature T cells. J Exp Med 169:707-16, 1989

74.   Welch PA, Namen AE, Goodwin RG, et al: Human IL-7, A novel T cell growth factor. Journal of Immunology 143:3562, 1989

75.   Armitage RJ, Namen AE, Sassenfield HM, Grabstein KH: Regulation of human T cell proliferation by IL-7. Journal of Immunology 144:938, 1990

76.   Wiles MV, Ruiz P, Imhof BA: Interleukin-7 expression during mouse thymus development. European Journal of Immunology 22:1037, 1992

77.   Komschlies KL, Grzegorzewski KJ, Wiltrout RH: Diverse immunological and hematological effects of interleukin 7: implications for clinical application. [Review] [138 refs]. Journal of Leukocyte Biology 58:(6)623-33, 1995

78.   Grzegorzewski KJ, Komschlies KL, Jacobsen SE, et al: Mobilization of long-term reconstituting hematopoietic stem cells in mice by recombinant human interleukin 7. J Exp Med 181:(1)369-74,

1995

79. Bolotin E, Smogorzewska M, Smith S, et al: Enhancement of thymopoiesis after bone marrow transplant by in vivo interleukin-7. Blood 88:(5)1887-94, 1996

80. Carson WE, Fehniger TA, Haldar S, et al: A potential role for interleukin-15 in the regulation of human natural killer cell survival. Journal of Clinical Investigation 99:(5)937-43., 1997

81. Silva MR, Hoffman R, Srour EF, Ascensoa JL: Generation of human natural killer cells from immature progenitors does not require marrow stromal cells. Blood 84:841, 1994

82. Bell E: Function of CD4 T cell subsets in vivo: expression of CD45R isoforms. Seminars in Immunology 4:43-50, 1992

83. Michie C, McLean A, Alcock C, Beverley P: Lifespan of human lymphocyte subsets defined by CD45 isoforms. Nature 360:264-5, 1992

84. Rothstein D, Yamada A, Schlossman S, Morimoto C: Cyclic regulation of CD45 isoform expression in a long term human CD4+CD45RA+ T cell line. Journal of Immunology. 146(4):1175-83, 1991 Feb 15. 146:1175-83, 1991

85. Warren H, Skipsey L: Loss of activation-induced CD45RO with maintenance of CD45RA expression during prolonged culture of T cells and NK cells. Immunology 74:78-85, 1991

86. Sarawar S, Sparshott S, Sutton P, et al: Rapid re-expression of CD45RC on rat CD4 T cells in vitro correlates with a change in function. European Journal of Immunology 23:103-9, 1993

87. Mosmann TR, Cherwinski H, Bond MW, et al: Two types of murine helper T cell clone. I. Definition according to profiles of lymphokine activities and secreted proteins. Journal of Immunology 136:2348, 1986

88. Mosmann TR, Coffman RL: Heterogeneity of cytokine secretion patterns and functions of helper T cells. Advances in Immunology 46:111-147, 1989

89. Maggie E, Parronchi P, Manetti R, et al: Reciprocal Regulatory Effects of IFN-gamma and IL-4 on the *in Vitro* Development of Human Th1 and Th2 Clones. Journal of Immunology 148:2142-2147, 1992

90. Abesira-Amar O, Gilbert M, Joliy M, et al: IL-4 plays a role in the Differential Development of Th0 into Th1 and Th2 Cells. Journal of Immunology 148:3820-3829, 1992

91. Hsieh C-S, Macatonia SE, Tripp CS, et al: Development of Th1 CD4+ T cells through IL-12 produced by *Listeria*-induced macrophages. Science 260:547-549, 1993

92. Seder RA, Gazzinelli R, Sher A, Paul WE: IL-12 acts directly on CD4+ T cells to enhance priming for IFN-γ production and diminishes IL-4 inhibition of such priming. Proceedings of the National Academy of Sciences 90:10188-10192, 1993

93. Manetti R, Parronchi P, Giudizi MG, et al: Natural killer cell stimulatory factor (interleukin 12 [IL-12]) induces T helper type 1 (Th1)-specific immune responses and inhibits the development of IL-4 producing Th cells. J Exp Med 177:1199-1204, 1993

94. Ferrara JL, Cooke KR, Pan L, Krenger W: The Immunopathology of acute graft-versus-host-disease. Stem Cells 14:(5)473-89, 1996

95. Ferrara JL: Cytokines other than growth factors in bone marrow transplantation. Current Opinion in Oncology 6:127-134, 1994

96. Moreb JS, Kubilis PS, Mullins DL, et al: Increased frequency of autoaggression syndrome associated with autologous stem cell transplantation in breast cancer patients. Bone Marrow Transplantation 19:(2)101-6, 1997

97. Krenger W, Ferrara JL: Graft-versus-host disease and the Th1/Th2 paradigm. Immunologic Research 15:(1)50-73, 1996

98. Piguet PF, Grau GE, Allet B, Vassalli PJ: Tumor Necrosis Factor/Cachectin Is an Effector of Skin and Gut Lesions of the Acute Phase of Graft-Versus-Host Disease. J Exp Med 166:1280-1289, 1987

99. Nestel FP, Price KS, Seemayer TA, Lapp WS: Macrophage priming and Lipopolysaccharide-Triggered Release of Tumor Necrosis Factor Alpha During Graft-Versus-Host Disease. J Exp Med 175:405-413, 1992

100. Holler E, Kolb HJ, Hintermeier-Knabe R, et al: Role of Tumor Necrosis Alpha in Acute Graft-Versus-Host Disease and Complications Following Allogeneic Bone Marrow Transplantation. Transplant Proceedings 25:1234-1236, 1993

101. Holler E, Kolb HJ, Mittermuller J, et al: Modulation of acute graft-versus-host-disease after allogeneic bone marrow transplantation by tumor necrosis factor alpha (TNF alpha) release in the course of pretransplant conditioning: role of conditioning regimens and prophylactic application of a monoclonal antibody neutralizing human TNF alpha (MAK 195F). Blood 86:(3)890-899, 1995

102. Attal M, Huguet F, Rubie H, et al: Prevention of Regimen-Related Toxicities After Bone Marrow

Transplantation by Pentoxifylline: A Prospective Randomized Trial. Blood 82:732-736, 1993

103. Herve P, Flesch M, Tiberghien P, et al: Phase I-II Trial of a Monoclonal Anti-Tumor Necrosis Factor Alpha Antibody for the treatment of Refractory Severe Acute Graft-Versus-Host Disease. Blood 79:3362-3368, 1992

104. Abhyankar S, Gilliland DG, Ferrara JL: Interleukin-1 is a critical effector molecule during cytokine dysregulation in graft versus host disease to minor histocompatibility antigens. Transplantation 56:(6)1518-23., 1993

105. McCarthy PL, Abhyankar S, Newben S, et al: Inhibition of interleukin-1 by an interleukin-1 receptor antagonist prevents graft-versus-host disease. Blood 78:(8)1915-8, 1991

106. Ferrara JL, Weinstein HJ, Guinan EC, et al: Phase I/II Trial of Recombinant Human IL-1 Receptor Antagonist (IL-1ra) for Steroid Resistant GVHD [Abstract]. Blood 80:270, 1992

107. Theobald M, Nierle T, Bunjes D, et al: Host-specific interleukin-2-secreting donor T-cell precursors as predictors of acute graft-versus-host disease in bone marrow transplantation between HLA-identical siblings [see comments]. New England Journal of Medicine 328:(20)1497-8, 1992

108. Schwarer AP, Jiang YZ, Brookes PA, et al: Frequency of anti-recipient alloreactive helper T-cell precursors in donor blood and graft-versus-host disease after HLA-identical sibling bone-marrow transplantation. Lancet 341:(8839)203-05, 1993

109. Belanger C, al. e: Use of an anti-interleukin 2 receptor monoclonal antibody for GvHD prophylaxis in unrelated bone marrow transplantation. GEGMO Group. Bone Marrow Transplant 11:(Suppl 1)112-3, 1993

110. Sykes M, Romick ML, Hoyles KA, et al: In vivo administration of interleukin 2 plus T cell-depleted syngeneic marrow prevents graft-versus-host disease mortality and permits alloengraftment. J Exp Med 171:(3)645-58, 1990

111. Sykes M, Abraham VS, Harty MW, et al: IL-2 reduces graft-versus-host disease and preserves a graft-versus-leukemia effect by selectively inhibiting CD4+ T cell activity. J Immunol 150:(1)197-205, 1993

112. Szebini J, Wang MG, Pearson DA, et al: IL-2 inhibits early increases in serum gamma interferon levels associated with graft-versus-host-disease. Transplantation 58:(12)1385-93, 1994

113. Weisdorf DJ, Anderson PM, Blazar BR, et al: Interleukin 2 immediately after autologous bone marrow transplantation for acute lymphoblastic leukemia--a phase I study. Transplantation 55(1):61-66, 1993.

114. Anasetti C, Martin PJ, Hansen JA, et al: A Phase I-II study evaluating the murine anti-IL-2 receptor antibody 2A3 for treatment of acute graft-versus-host disease. Transplantation 50(1):49-54, 1990.

115. Vey N, Blaise D, tiberghien P, et al: A pilot study of autologous bone marrow transplantation followed by recombinant interleukin-2 in malignant lymphomas. Leukemia & Lymphoma 21:(1-2)107-14, 1996

116. Attal M, Blaise D, Marit G, et al: Consolidation treatment of adult acute lymphoblastic leukemia: a prospective, randomized trial comparing allogeneic versus autologous bone marrow transplantation and testing the impact of recombinant interleukin-2 after autologous bone marrow transplantation. BGMT Group. Blood 86:(4)1619-28, 1995

117. Giralt SA, Kantarjian HM, Talpez M, et al: Effect of prior interferon alfa therapy on the outcome of allogeneic bone marrow transplantation for chronic myelogenous leukemia. J Clin Oncol 11:(6)1055-61, 1993

118. Pavord S, Simvakumaran M, Durrant S, Chapman C: The role of alpha interferon in the pathogenesis of GVHD [letter]. Bone Marrow Transplant 10:(5)477, 1992

119. Morton AJ, Gooley T, Hansen JA, et al: Impact of pre-transplant interferon-a on outcome of unrelated donor marrow transplants for chronic myeloid leukemia in first chronic phase. Blood 90(Suppl 1): Abstract 536, 1997

120. Brok HP, Heidt PJ, van der Meide PH, et al. Interferon-gamma prevents graft-versus-host disease after allogeneic bone marrow transplantation in mice. J Immunol 151:(11)6451-9, 1993

121. Mason DW, Dallman M, Barclay AN: Graft-versus-host disease induces expression of Ia antigen in rat epidermal cells and gut epithelium. Nature 293:(5828)150-1, 1981

122. Huber C, Niederwieser D: Role of cytokines and major histocompatibility complex antigens in graft-versus-host disease: in vitro studies using T-cell lines and keratinocytes or hemopoietic targets. Hamatolgie und Bluttransfusion 33:652-4, 1990

123. Mowat AM: Antibodies to IFN-gamma prevent immunologically mediated intestinal damage in murine graft-versus-host reaction. Immunology 68:(1)18-23, 1989

124. Allen RD, Staley TA, Sidman CL: Differential Cytokine Expression. Eur J Immunol 23:(2)333-7,

1993

125. Garlisi CG, Pennline KJ, Smith SR, et al. Cytokine gene expression in mice undergoing chronic graft-versus-host disease. Molecular Immunol 30:(7)669-77, 1993

126. De Wit D, Van Mechelen M, Zanin C, et al: Preferential activation of Th2 cells in chronic graft-versus-host reaction. Journal of Immunology 150:(2)361-6, 1993

127. Steeg PS, Moore RN, Oppenheim JL: Regulation of murine macrophage Ia-antigen expression by products of activated spleen cells. J Exp Med 152:(6)1734-44, 1980

128. Gifford GE, Lohmann-Matthes ML: Gamma interferon priming of mouse and human macrophages for induction of tumor necrosis factor production by bacterial lipopolysaccharide. J Natl Cancer Inst 78:(1)121-4, 1987

129. Pace JL, Russell SW: Activation of mouse macrophages for tumor cell killing. I. Quantitative analysis of interactions between lymphokine and lipopolysaccharide. Journal of Immunology 126:(5)1863-7, 1981

130. De Maeyer E, De Maeyer-Guignard J: Interferon-gamma. [Review] [37 refs]. Current Opinion in Immunology 4:(3)321-6, 1992

131. McBride WH, Economou JS, Nayersina R, Comora S, . ER: Influences of interleukins 2 and 4 on tumor necrosis factor production by murine mononuclear phagocytes. Cancer Research 50:(10)2949-52, 1990

132. Gerard C, Bruyns C, Marchant A, et al: Interleukin 10 reduces the release of tumor necrosis factor and prevents lethality in experimental endotoxemia. J Exp Med. 177:(2)547-50, 1993

133. Wong HL, Costa GL, Lotze MT, Wahl SM: Interleukin (IL) 4 differentially regulates monocyte IL-1 family gene expression and synthesis in vitro and in vivo. J Exp Med 177:(3)1993

134. Fiorentino DF, Zlotnik A, Vieira P, et al: IL-10 acts on the antigen-presenting cell to inhibit cytokine production by Th1 cells. J Immunol 146:(10)3444-51, 1991

135. Umlauf SW, Beverly B, Kang SM, et al: Molecular regulation of the IL-2 gene: rheostatic control of the immune system. [Review] [68 refs]. Immulogical Reviews 133:177-97, 1993

136. Heinzel FP, Sadick MD, Holaday BJ, et al: Reciprocal expression of interferon gamma or interleukin 4 during the resolution or progression of murine leishmaniasis. Evidence for expansion of distinct helper T cell subsets. J Exp Med 169:(1)59-72, 1989

137. Symington FW, Symington BE, Liu PY, et al. The Relationship of Serum IL-6 Levels to Acute Graft-Versus-Host Disease and Hepatorenal Disease after Human Bone Marrow Transplant. Transplantation 54:547-462, 1992

138. Rabinowitz J, Petros WP, Stuart AR, Peters WP: Characterization of endogenous cytokine concentrations after high-dose chemotherapy with autologous bone marrow support. Blood 81:(9)2452-9, 1993

139. Tosato G, Jones K, Breinig MK, et al. Interleukin-6 Production in Posttransplant Lymphoproliferative Disease. J Clin Invest 91:2806-2814, 1993

140. Uguccioni M, Meliconi R, Nesci S, Lucarelli G: Elevated interleukin-8 serum concentrations in beta-thalassemia and graft-versus-host disease. Blood 81:(9)2252-6, 1993

141. Rosnet O, Mattei MG, Marchetto S, Birnbaum D: Isolation and chromosomal localization of a novel FMS-like tyrosine kinase gene. Genomics 9:(2)308-5, 1991

142. Matthews W, Jordan CT, Wiegand GW, et al. A receptor tyrosine kinase specific to hematopoietic stem and progenitor cell-enriched populations. Cell 65:(7)1143-52, 1991

143. Lyman SD, James L, Vanden BT, et al. Molecular cloning of a ligand for the flt3/flk-2 tyrosine kinase receptor: a proliferative factor for primitive hematopoietic cells. Cell 75:(6)1157-67, 1993

144. Hannum C, Culpepper J, Campbell D, et al. Ligand for FLT3/FLK2 receptor tyrosine kinase regulates growth of haematopoietic stem cells and is encoded by variant RNAs. Nature 368:(6472)643-8, 1994

145. Winton EF, Bucur SZ, Bray RA, et al: The hematopoietic effects of recombinant human (rh) Flt3 ligand administered to non-human primates. Blood 86 (suppl 1):1681a, 1995

146. Juan TS, McNiece IK, Van G, et al: Chronic expression of murine flt3 ligand in mice results in increased circulating white blood cell levels and abnormal cellular infiltrates associated with splenic fibrosis. Blood 90:(1)76-84, 1997

147. Wodnar-Filipowicz A, Chklovskaia E, et al: Effect of flt3 ligand on in vitro growth and expansion of colony-forming bone marrow cells from patients with aplastic anemia. Experimental Hematology 25:(7)573-81, 1997

148. Ebihara Y, Tsuji K, Lyman SD, et al: Synergistic action of Flt3 and gp130 signalings in human hematopoiesis. Blood 90:(11)4363-8, 1997

149. Veiby OP, Borge OJ, Martensson A, et al: Bidirectional effect of interleukin-10 on early murine B-cell development: stimulation of flt3-ligand plus interleukin-7-dependent generation of CD19(-) ProB cells from uncommitted bone marrow progenitor cells and growth inhibition of CD19(+) ProB cells. Blood 90:(11)4231-31, 1997

150. Lemieux ME, Chappel SM, Miller CL, Eaves CJ: Differential ability of flt3-ligand, interleukin-11, and Steel factor to support the generation of B cell progenitors and myeloid cells from primitive murine fetal liver cells. Exp Hematol 25:(9)1997

151. Petzer AL, Hogge DE, Landsdorp PM, et al. Self-renewal of primitive human hematopoietic cells (long-term-culture-initiating cells) in vitro and their expansion in defined medium. Proc Natl Acad Sci USA 93:(4)1470-4, 1996

152. Esche C, Subbotin VM, Maliszewski C, Lotze MT, Shurin MR: FLT3 ligand administration inhibits tumor growth in murine melanoma and lymphoma. Cancer Research 58:(3)380-3, 1998

153. Alcorn MJ, Holyoake TL: Ex vivo expansion of haemopoietic progenitor cells. Blood Reviews 10:(3)167-76, 1996

154. Cervantes F, Pierson BA, McGlave PB, Verfaillie CM, Miller JS: Autologous activated natural killer cells suppress primitive chronic myelogenous leukemia progenitors in long-term culture. Blood 87:(6)2476-85, 1996

155. Silla LM, Whiteside TL, Ball ED: The role of natural killer cells in the treatment of chronic myeloid leukemia. J Hematother 4:(4)269-79, 1995

156. Baldwin NG, Rice CD, Tuttle TM, Bear HD, Hirsch JI, Merchant RE: Ex vivo expansion of tumor-draining lymph node cells using compounds which activate intracellular signal transduction. I. Characterization and in vivo anti-tumor activity of glioma-sensitized lymphocytes. J Neuro-Oncology 32:(1)19-28, 1997

157. van Lunzen J, Schmitz J, Dengler K, Kuhlmann C, Schmitz H, Dietrich M: Investigations on autologous T-cells for adoptive immunotherapy of AIDS. Advances in Experimental Medicine & Biology. 374:57-70, 1995

4. Improving on Nature by Re-Engineering Hematopoietic Growth Factors

Yiqing Feng, John McKearn

Introduction

The hematopoietic cytokines or growth factors belong to a superfamily of proteins that regulate a variety of physiological conditions. They function as regulatory mediators by interacting with specific receptors expressed on the surface of hematopoietic and inflammatory target cells. Binding and activation of the receptors triggers a cascade of intracellular events that eventually elaborates their biological effect. Cytokines often act on a number of different cell types, frequently in concert with one another. Thus, they can have a wide-range of complex, and sometimes overlapping biological functions. In addition to playing essential roles in the growth, differentiation, and maturation of the hematopoietic cells and their precursors, cytokines have effects on inflammation, immunomodulation, angiogenesis, and apoptosis (see ref. 1).

Although the advent of biotechnology has provided a means to manufacture large amounts of purified cytokines, the native proteins may have other limitations which prevent them from being used as effective therapeutic agents. One common limitation is the pleiotropic character of many cytokines, which can limit their utility as therapeutic agents because a compromise has to be made between the beneficial and detrimental activities. Another problem is that some recombinant forms of cytokines are unstable or are cleared so rapidly from circulation that their efficacy is limited. In addition, the solubility of cytokines can influence how well they are delivered, which will affect their therapeutic efficacy. Thus, the clinical utility of cytokines depends on a number of biological and physical properties which are critical for their pharmacological effects. Given that the therapeutic applications of hematopoietic cytokines may require a different set of attributes and activities than nature has provided, protein engineering offers a means to improve them for use in modern medicine.

The hematopoietic cytokines have little primary sequence homology but have a remarkably conserved core structural motif consisting of an anti-parallel four-helical bundle [2]. They are relatively small proteins with molecular weights usually in the range of 15-30 kDa. Compared with many protein families such as immunoglobulins and serine proteases, whose members have high levels of amino acid sequence and structural similarity, the active (receptor binding) sites on cytokines have only recently been elaborated. The lack of the knowledge regarding the active sites of cytokines and more importantly, the features which allow cytokines to achieve their pleiotropic functions with relatively small polypeptide chains, has presented an obstacle for the engineering efforts.

Our knowledge of the structure-function relationship of cytokines, along with our ability to modify proteins, have increased dramatically over the past decade. The pioneering studies on human growth hormone by Wells and colleagues (reviewed in ref. 3 and 4) revealed many of the molecular characteristics of cytokine-receptor interactions, as well as defined the methodology used to elucidate the intearctions in many other cytokine-receptor systems. These studies shed light on the receptor binding sites and provided a basis for focusing protein engineering efforts to improve the receptor binding properties of these molecules. The understanding of the *in vivo* network in which the cytokines function, however, is far less developed. This complex *in vivo* system, including synergistic or antagonistic cytokine partners, as well as positive or negative regulators of the cytokines, remains a major challenge. Despite these difficulties, significant progress has been made on improving cytokines for clinical use.

The objective of this review is to provide an overview of the recent progress in engineering hematopoietic cytokines and improving their therapeutic utilities, especially in treating myelosuppressive conditions induced by cancer chemotherapies.

Improving the Bioactivity of Cytokines by Mutagenesis

Hematopoietic growth factors have important potential as therapeutic agents because they regulate a wide variety of biological activities, including the growth and maturation of pluripotent stem cells to committed progenitor cells as well as development of specific lineages of effector cells. However, the activity profile of some cytokines, including side effects, may limit their clinic applications. Mutagenesis and protein engineering offer an opportunity to alter the biological activity profile of these cytokines.

The biological activity of interleukin-3 (IL-3), also called multi-CSF, is mediated through a cell surface receptor composed of two subunits (see ref. 5). The 70-kDa α-subunit is specific for IL-3, while the 130-kDa β-subunit is shared by the IL-3, IL-5, and GM-CSF receptors. IL-3 promotes the survival, proliferation, and development of multipotential hematopoietic stem cells and of committed progenitor cells of the granulocyte/macrophage, erythroid, eosinophil, megakaryocyte, mast cell, and basophilic lineages [6,7]. These properties make it an attractive candidate for the treatment of different states of bone marrow failure or hematologic malignancies, for mobilization and expansion of hematopoietic progenitor cells, and for support of engraftment following bone marrow transplantation. Clinical experience with rhIL-3 has indicated that many patients receiving rhIL-3 suffered from side effects such as fever, headache, neck rigidity, chills, rash, nausea, vomiting, and edema in a dose-dependent manner [8,9]. Dose-limiting toxicity, linked to the release of inflammatory mediators such as sulfidoleukotrienes [9] and histamine [10], seriously limits the use of rhIL-3 as a therapeutic agent.

The relationship of IL-3's structure to its function has been a subject of numerous studies (e.g. refs. 11-17). McKearn and coworkers [15] have undertaken a systematic mutagenesis study of hIL-3 to define residues critical for activity and to discover mutants with enhanced proliferative activity. Analysis of a series of truncation mutants established that the minimally active fragment consisted of residues 15-118 (with two-fold higher proliferation activity than that of full length hIL-3), whereas residues 15-117 had less than 1% of the potency of hIL-3 in the AML-193.1.3 cell proliferation

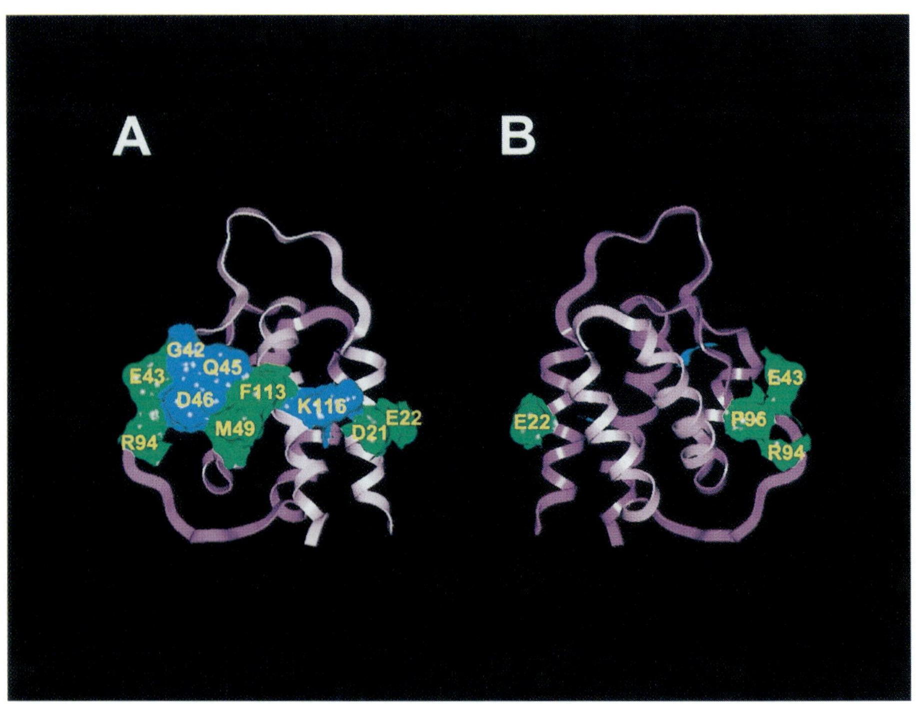

Figure 1. Ribbon diagram of the three-dimensional model of hIL-3$_{15-125}$ illustrating the putative hIL-3 receptor binding site. *Green* surface contours indicate residues where amino acid substitutions significantly impair cell proliferation activity and/or receptor binding affinity. *Blue* surface contours are for residues that gave greater than 10-fold increase in cell proliferation activity and/or receptor binding affinity upon substitution. *A*, view of the structure with helices A and D in front; *B*, the molecule in *A* rotated 180° so that helices B and C are in front (with permission from ref. 17).

assay. The fragment consisting residues 15 to 125 exhibited higher solubility than full length hIL-3 while retaining a 2- to 3-fold increase in activity. The increased solubility made the 15-125 fragment an ideal scaffold for mutagenesis studies because it permitted libraries of mutants to be efficiently secreted in *E.coli* in order to screen for activity. Libraries of random single-amino acid substitutions were constructed and tested at each of 105 positions in hIL-3 $_{15\text{-}125}$. The majority of positions in the hIL-3$_{15\text{-}125}$ sequence were found to tolerate a variety of amino acid substitutions without substantial loss of activity, while mutation at a small set of positions resulted in mutants with greater than a twenty-fold decrease in proliferation activity. After screening 770 single-point mutants, sixteen were confirmed upon purification to have 5- to 26-fold increased bioactivity in AML-193.1.3 cell line compared with hIL-3 [15]. Critical positions in the sequence were identified as those positions where substitution led to either significantly increased IL-3 activity or those that were surface-exposed but intolerant of substitution [17]. Although scattered in the primary sequence, when the critical positions from the mutagenesis studies were mapped onto the three-dimensional structure [18], they were found to form a continuous surface patch, which was proposed to be the binding site for the IL-3 receptor α-subunit [17] (Figure 1).

An iterative combinatorial mutagenesis strategy was employed to further optimize the biological profile of IL-3. The objective was to separate the multilineage proliferative activity from the proinflammatory activity in order to engineer an IL-3 receptor agonist with improved potency and therapeutic index (ref. 19 & unpublished data). The hIL-3$_{15\text{-}125}$ sequence was divided into four target regions. Substitutions at four to nine positions were made in each region separately, generating a total of 500 multiply substituted variants. The selection of positions to substitute was guided by the results of the previous single-point mutagenesis studies. Sites that gave rise to either enhanced IL-3 activity or maintained IL-3 activity [15] were given priority. The variants in which multiple substitutions were located in a single region exhibited up to 2.5-fold increased activity relative to hIL-3. Next, the most active multiple mutations from any two regions were combined to generate more extensively substituted variants. Combining substitutions from two regions resulted in highly active molecules exhibiting bioactivity as high as 12.5-fold that of hIL-3 in AML-193.1.3 cell proliferation assay. Subsequent combination of mutations from all four regions created hIL-3 variants with up to twenty-six amino acid substitutions evenly distributed throughout the sequence. While all the highly substituted molecules were at least as active as hIL-3, some of them achieved up to 24-fold higher potency than hIL-3 in AML-193.1.3 cell proliferation assay. The proinflammatory activity of these highly substituted hIL-3 variants was evaluated in cytokine-induced leukotriene release assay. While many variants exhibited proliferative activity that correlated with leukotriene release activity, several variants were found which displayed a separation of the two activities. These variants had 10- to 20-fold increases in proliferative activity relative to hIL-3, while their ability to stimulate leukotriene release was increased by only 2- to 4-fold relative to hIL-3. A potent and selectively enhanced IL-3 receptor agonist, daniplestim (SC-55494 or Synthokine), was the result of this combinatorial mutagenesis strategy [19].

Daniplestim is composed of Ala-hIL-3$_{15-125}$ with 26 mutations interspersed throughout the sequence [19]. In the AML-193.1.3 clonal cell line, daniplestim demonstrated 10-fold more potency than native rhIL-3 (Figure 2). The enhancement in hematopoietic activity was more pronounced in human CD34$^+$ bone marrow colony-forming assay, where daniplestim was 22-times more potent than rhIL-3 (Figure 3). In contrast to the hematopoietic activity, the daniplestim-induced sulfidoleukotriene synthesis and release from peripheral blood cells was increased by only 2-fold relative to native rhIL-3. Therefore, this engineered IL-3 receptor agonist is selectively biased towards the hematopoietic activity *in vitro*. The benefit of daniplestim *in vivo* was demonstrated in a non-human primate model of radiation-induced marrow aplasia [20]. In this model, daniplestim significantly reduced the duration of thrombocytopenia compared with albumin-treated controls. Daniplestim consistently lessened the depth of the nadir of the neutropenia, although it did not reduce its duration. More significantly, when daniplestim was co-administered with G-CSF in the irradiated rhesus model, it was more effective than G-CSF alone in reducing both the neutrophil and platelet nadirs [21]. Initial human clinical trials indicate that daniplestim when co-administered with G-CSF is well-tolerated and efficacious for mobilization of PBSC for autologous transplantation following chemotherapy [22].

Another example in which mutagenesis has been used to generate a hematopoietic growth factor with enhanced biological activity is nartograstim (Neu-up or KW-2228), a variant of human granulocyte colony-stimulating factor (hG-CSF). G-CSF specifically regulates the proliferation, differentiation, and maturation of hematopoietic cells of the neutrophilic lineage [5]. G-CSF has been developed to treat neutropenia as a result of cancer chemotherapy, bone marrow transplant, congenital defects, or infection. Untreated neutropenic conditions often lead to bacterial and fungal infections that require hospitalization and the use of antibiotics. Itoh and co-workers [23] engineered over 100 hG-CSF variants to identify novel G-CSF receptor agonists with superior biological activity and physicochemical properties. Although most of the variants with mutation or deletion at the internal and the C-terminal region of the molecule abolished activity, a few variants with mutations at the N-terminal region were found to be more potent than rhG-CSF. One of the best variants is nartograstim, which has five mutations in the N-terminal region of G-CSF and a 2- to 4-fold elevation in specific activity relative to native rhG-CSF in both cell proliferation [23] and human bone marrow progenitor colony-forming unit assays [24]. In normal mice, nartograstim showed improvement over rhG-CSF when administered in either single or multiple courses, especially at sub-optimal doses [24]. In addition, nartograstim was found to be significantly more stable than rhG-CSF [24]. The improvement in thermal stability and resistance to proteolysis resulting from just a few mutations is remarkable. Nartograstim retained about 70% of its activity after ten minutes at 56 °C in phosphate-buffered saline, while rhG-CSF completely lost activity under the same condition. In human plasma at 37 °C, nartograstim remained completely active for up to 50 hours, while rhG-CSF lost half of its activity after just ten hours due to proteolytic degradation.

The increased stability is not only observed *in vitro* but also *in vivo*. After a single intravenous injection in mice, the bioactive form of nartograstim was maintained at an elevated circulating level for at least an hour, whereas the concentration of rhG-CSF

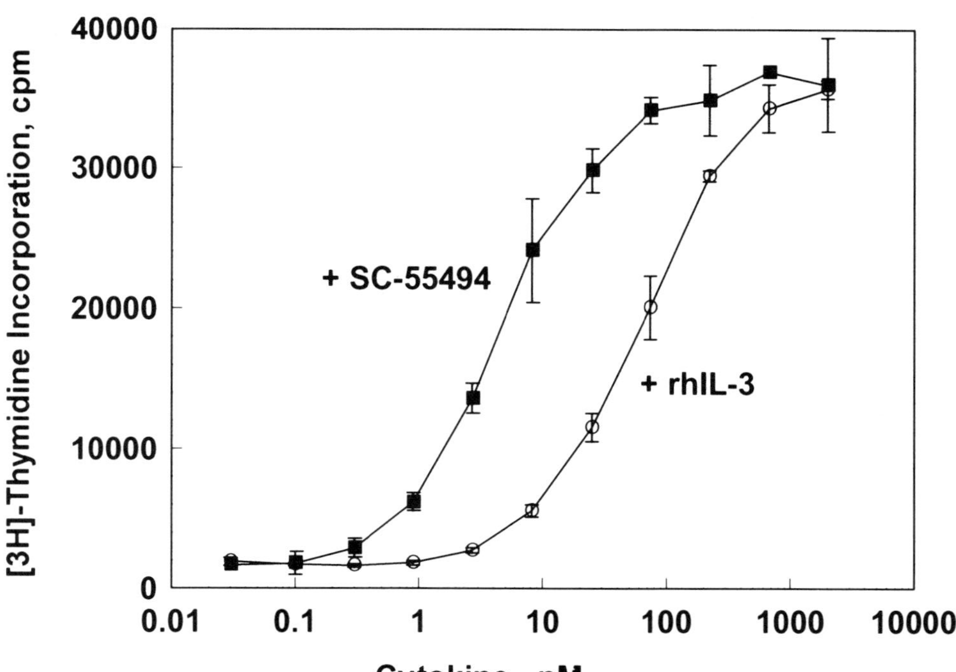

Figure 2. AML 193.1.3 clonal cell line growth assays for daniplestim (■) and rhIL-3 (O) (with permission from ref. 19).

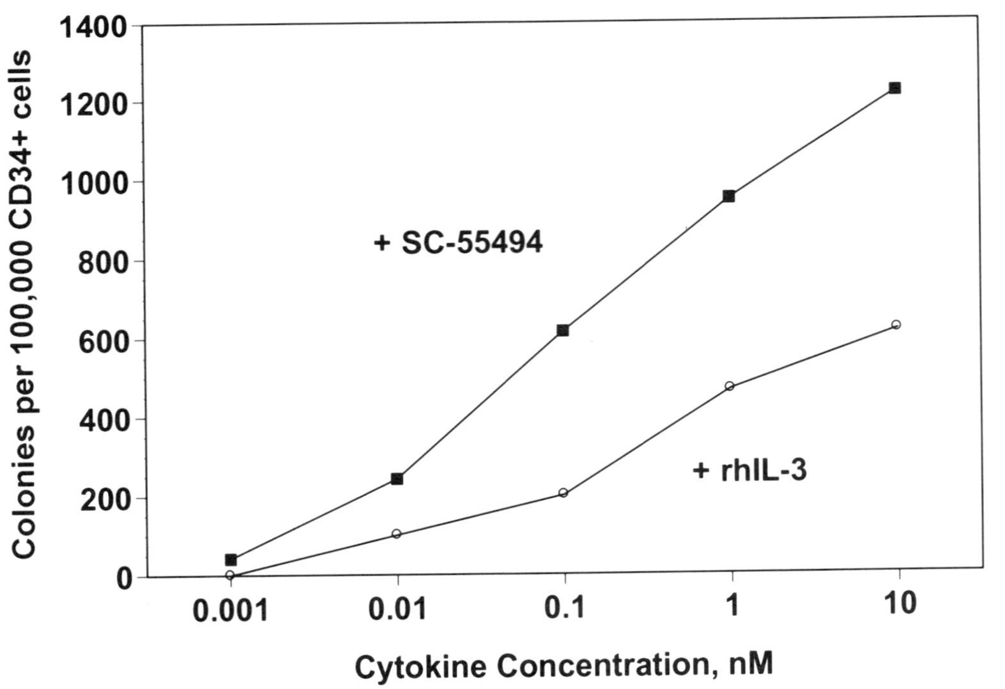

Figure 3. Methylcellulose hematopoietic colony-forming assay with normal human CD34[+] bone marrow cells. Number of CFUs per 100,000 CD34[+] cells was determined for both rhIL-3 (O) and daniplestim (■) (with permission from ref. 19).

decreased rapidly after just 5 minutes. The recently published crystal structure of nartograstim [25] revealed that although the overall structure is very similar to that of rhG-CSF [26, 27], there are additional interactions between the reengineered N-terminal region and the C-terminal sequence which result in reduced flexibility in the structure, especially in the long overhand loops which connect the helices and the terminal segments of the sequence. The improved properties of nartograstim were attributed to the conformational differences and the increased rigidity of the structure.

Improving the Pharmacokinetics of Cytokines by Post-translational or Post-production Modification

Although cytokines are expressed naturally at very low levels, advances in biotechnology in recent years have made it possible to obtain large quantities of active cytokines for therapeutic purposes. However, some cytokines are rapidly cleared from circulation after either intravenous or subcutaneous administration, limiting their clinical effectiveness. Post-translational or post-production modification has been found to offer an avenue to prolong the circulation time of proteins.

Naturally occurring G-CSF is a single polypeptide chain composed of either 174 or 177 amino acid residues depending on two alternative mRNA splice forms [28-30]. The insertion of three amino acids between residues 32 and 33 of the 174-residue G-CSF resulted in greatly diminished biological activity, so that only the 174-residue G-CSF has been pursued as a therapeutic agent. In contrast to many heavily glycosylated cytokines, natural hG-CSF contains only one O-linked carbohydrate chain at Thr-133[31].

Two forms of recombinant hG-CSF have been approved for clinical use in the U.S. and Europe. Filgrastim (Neupogen), an *E.coli*-derived hG-CSF, has an additional methionine at the amino-terminus and is non-glycosylated. Lenograstim (Neutrogen) is a glycosylated version of hG-CSF produced in Chinese hamster ovary (CHO) cells. In addition, the previously discussed multiple-substituted variant of G-CSF (nartograstim or KW-2228), also derived from *E.coli*, is available in Japan. Naturally occurring G-CSF and lenograstim differ in the structure of the sugar moiety [31]. The glycosylated and nonglycosylated forms of recombinant G-CSF show virtually identical conformation when assessed by circular dichroism, fluorescence [32], and NMR spectroscopies[33]. While the attachment of the sugar moiety has no effect on either receptor binding or activity in proliferation assays, it appears to increase the stability of the molecule against heat denaturation, pH change, aggregation, and proteolysis[34-36].

The difference in biological effect and pharmacokinetics among G-CSF produced from different sources has been extensively studied both *in vitro* and *in vivo* [28-45]. Although glycosylated G-CSF was shown to have an advantage in potency over the non-glycosylated form in human bone marrow neutrophil colony assays [38], in neutropenic and normal rats [42], and in normal human volunteers [44,45], both glycosylated and nonglycosylated G-CSF are rapidly cleared from the circulation, resulting in short-term pharmacological effects[46,39].

Covalent conjugation of polyethylene glycol (PEG) to G-CSF ("pegylation") has been shown to increase the half-life of G-CSF *in vivo* and therefore enhance the pharmacological effect of G-CSF [47-49]. Human G-CSF produced in *E.coli* (mw 19-kDa) was conjugated with PEG, resulting in PEG-rhG-CSF molecules with molecular weights ranging from 25- to 60-kDa. The *in vitro* activity of the PEG-rhG-CSF molecules was found to correlate negatively with the increasing molecular weight [48, 49](Table 1). For a conjugate of molecular weight 60-kDa, only 15% of the G-CSF activity was retained. When PEG-rhG-CSF of molecular weight 45-kDa or 60-kDa

Table 1. Comparison of Modified rHuG-CSFs.

Sample	MW (kDa)	activity *in vivo* (%)	activity *in vitro* (%)
rHuG-CSF	19	100	100
PEG (4,500)-rHuG-CSF	60	250	15
PEG (10,000)-rHuG-CSF	45	500	32

Activities are expressed using a value of 100% for intact rHuG-CSF. (Reproduced with permission from ref. 48)

was injected intravenously into mice, however, the *in vivo* response was significantly increased compared to unmodified G-CSF (Figure 4).

Another *in vivo* experiment in which a mixture of PEG-rhG-CSF with an average molecular weight of 45-kDa was injected into rats again showed a significant improvement in pharmacokinetics [47] (Table 2). The serum half-life of 1.8 h for rhG-CSF was increased to 7 h upon pegylation. In addition, pegylation was shown to significantly improve the storage stability of rhG-CSF [49].

Table 2. Pharmacokinetic parameters of rhG-CSF and PEG-rhG-CSF obtained after iv administration of 100 μg protein/kg to rats

Materials	AUC[a] (ng•h/ml)	CL (ml/h/kg)	$t_{1/2}$ (h)	MRT (h)
rhG-CSF	2,000	50.0	1.79[b]	1.65
PEG rhG-CSF[c]	16,195	6.2	7.05	10.8

[a] AUC, area under the serum concentration-time curve; CL, total body clearance; $t_{1/2}$, half-life; MRT, mean residence time.
[b] $t_{1/2}$ of rhG-CSF was determinded from the points between 2 and 8 h.
[c] The PEG rhG-CSF is rhG-CSF modified by activated PEG (10,000) and has an average mw of 45 kDa.
(Reproduced with permission from Ref.63)

Since the conformation of the modified G-CSF was shown to be unaltered by using biophysical methods such as circular dichroism (CD) and NMR spectroscopies [49], the decrease in *in vitro* activity could be attributed to PEG masking the receptor binding site [47, 48]. Activated PEG reacts only with amino groups, i.e., the ε-amino groups of

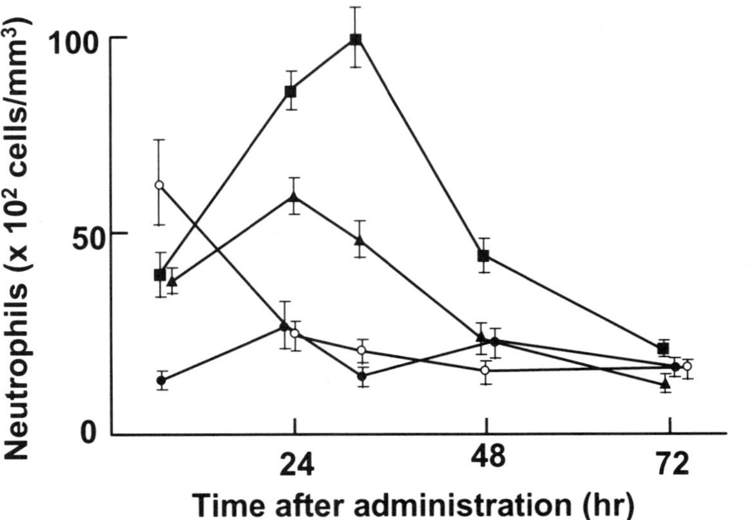

Figure 4. Time course of neutrophil counts in mice after injection of rHuG-CSF and PEG-rHuG-CSF. rHuG-CSF (O), PEG (4,500)-rHuG-CSF (60-kDa)(▲), PEG (10,000)-rHuG-CSF (45-kDa) (■) or vehicle (●) was injected intravenously to mice at a dose of 10 μg protein/kg. Each point is the mean of six animals with standard errors indicated by bars (with permission from ref. 48).

Lys and the N-terminal amino group. In rhG-CSF, there are five possible sites to which PEG can covalently link and all five are localized either in or near the first helix, a region which has been implicated as important for interacting with the receptor [50, 51]. The mechanism for the improved pharmacokinetics of PEG-rhG-CSF has been speculated to have two sources [47]. First, it may be the result of slower clearance rates by the kidney since glomerular filtration rate decreases with increasing molecular weight [52] and pegylation of rhG-CSF dramatically increases the molecular weight. It may also be explained by protection of proteolytic sites within rhG-CSF by the bulky PEG moieties, leading to slower degradation rates *in vivo*.

Recently, pegylation was applied to recombinant megakaryocyte growth and development factor (MGDF) to generate PEG-rMGDF [53]. MGDF is a fully active N-terminal domain of the newly discovered cytokine thrombopoietin (TPO) or c-mpl ligand [54-58]. This cytokine has a potent effect on megakaryocyte progenitor cell expansion and maturation which makes it a potential agent for treatment of thrombocytopenic disorders [59-61]. It has been shown that pegylation increased the *in vivo* potency of MGDF by increasing its circulating half-life [62].

A different approach can be used to improve pharmacokinetics and increase the biological response. This approach employs covalent attachment of albumin and has been applied to rhG-CSF [63]. Paige and coworkers linked the N-terminus of rhG-CSF to the unpaired cysteine residue in albumin (Cys-34) through a heterobifunctional PEG spacer, resulting in 1:1 albumin:rhG-CSF conjugate with a molecular weight over 80-kDa. The modified molecules were tested in rats and compared to both unmodified rhG-CSF and a non-covalent equal molar mixture of albumin and rhG-CSF. Table 3 shows that the modified rhG-CSF was eliminated more slowly from the circulation than either the unmodified rhG-CSF or the non-covalent mixture of albumin and rhG-CSF. The slower clearance rate of the modified molecules corresponds to enhanced efficacy *in vivo*.

Table 3. Pharmacokinetic Parameters in Rats After IV Dosage[a]

Drug	n	Dose (μg/kg)	MRT (min)	Vss (ml/kg)	CLp (ml/min/kg)
RSA-EM	4	477	1393 ± 34	194 ± 11	0.140 ± 0.011
HSA-EM	4	629	1003 ± 107	150 ± 16	0.151 ± 0.024
RSA-PEG-GLY	2	500	957 ± 2	214 ± 7	0.224 ± 0.007
HSA-PEG-GLY	3	480	1033 ± 7	298 ± 5	0.289 ± 0.007
RSA-PEG-GCSF	3	50	394 ± 28	67 ± 2	0.172 ± 0.013
HSA-PEG-GCSF	4	50	425 ± 12	60 ± 3	0.141 ± 0.005
rhG-CSF	8	50	90 ± 16	75 ± 13	0.839 ± 0.121
rhG-CSF + HSA	4	75	124 ± 9	66 ± 2	0.533 ± 0.025

[a] Data shown are mean ± SD. (Reproduced with permission from ref. 63)

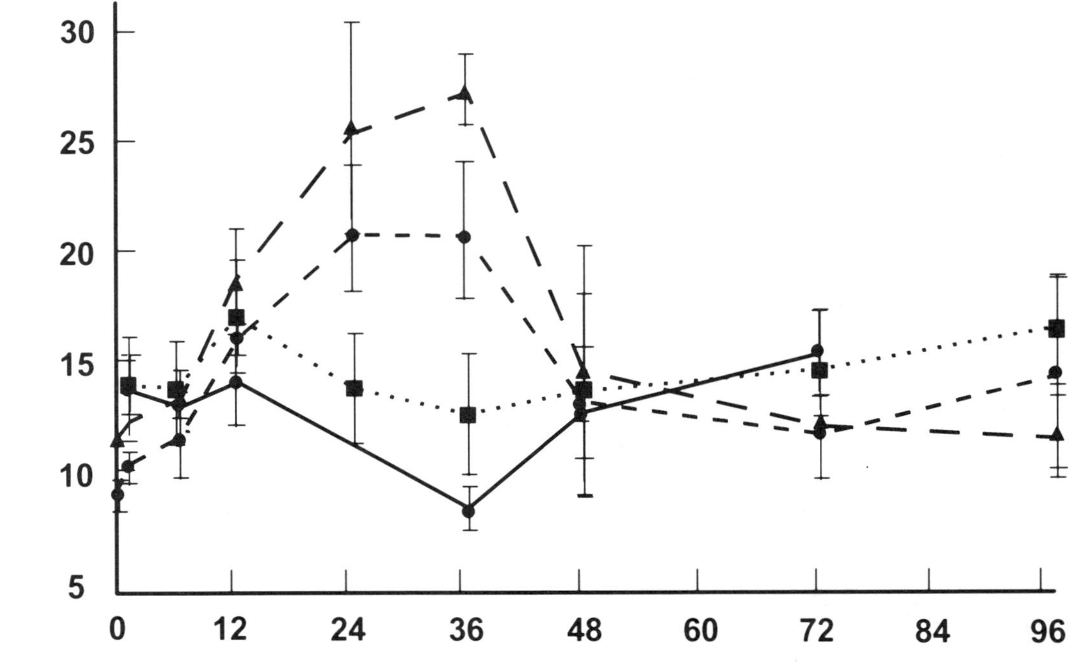

Figure 5. The WBC response in rats comparing a 50µg/kg dose of rhG-CSF (■), RSA-PEG-rhG-CSF (●), HSA-PEG-rhG-CSF (▲), and a 75 µg/kg dose of non-covalent mixture of rhG-CSF and HSA (◆). Data shown are ±SD of the mean (N≥3). (Reproduced with permission from ref.63).

The average WBC level of rats that received the modified G-CSF is higher than that of rats that received unmodified rhG-CSF or the non-covalent mixture (Figure 5). The duration of the WBC response was also increased upon the modification. Coupling of albumin appears to protect rhG-CSF against degradation in serum; the rate of degradation in rat serum was decreased 5-fold in comparison to rhG-CSF.

Erythropoietin (EPO) is another growth factor that has been engineered for improved pharmacokinetic properties. EPO, a primary regulator of erythropoiesis [64, 65], stimulates the proliferation and differentiation of erythroid progenitor cells by binding to a specific cell surface receptor [66]. EPO has been used in patients to treat a variety of anemias, including those that result from renal insufficiency (inadequate production of EPO in the kidney), or those induced by chemotherapy (such as in cancer and AIDS patients) (e. g. refs. 67& 68). Naturally occurring EPO is a heavily glycosylated protein with 40% of its mass being attributed to carbohydrates [69]. The role of carbohydrate in the biology and pharmacokinetics of EPO has been extensively studied. There are three N-linked carbohydrates at positions 24, 38, and 83 and one O-linked carbohydrate at position 126. Site-directed mutagenesis studies have shown that glycosylation at these sites is essential for the proper biosynthesis and secretion of EPO, and for its *in vivo* but not *in vitro* bioactivity [70-75], although there is a controversy over whether the O-linked carbohydrate chain is important for secretion [70, 72, 74]. In addition, the N-linked carbohydrates were found to prevent EPO from aggregating upon heating and are therefore essential for its stability [76].

The *in vivo* activity of EPO is not only dependent on the presence of carbohydrate, but also sensitive to the structure and composition of the carbohydrate chains. The N-linked carbohydrate chains in natural EPO are highly-branched as well as highly sialyated (see ref. 77). Kobata and coworkers [78] have shown that the *in vivo* activity of EPO correlated positively with the ratio of tetraantennary to biantennary oligosaccharides. The two CHO cell-derived EPO molecules, epoetin alfa (Epogen, Amgen; ref. 79) and epoetin beta (Marogen, Chugai-Upjohn; refs. 69, 80) demonstrated small differences in pharmacokinetics in a comparative clinical trial [81]. Epoetin beta administered intravenously showed a slightly greater volume of distribution (8-17%) and prolonged half-life (20%) compared with epoetin alfa, whereas epoetin beta administered subcutaneously exhibited a delayed drug absorption compared with epoetin alfa. These phenomena are presumably due to small differences in their heterogeneous populations of glycosylation [82]. Sialidase treatment to remove the terminal sialic acid from the oligosaccharide chains rendered the still heavily glycosylated EPO molecules inactive *in vivo* [83-87]. A further demonstration of the importance of terminal sialic acid is that recombinant EPO produced in tobacco cells, which lacks sialic acid residues in the N-linked oligosaccharides, or in Φ2 cells, which produce only limited sialylation of N-linked oligosaccharides, had no *in vivo* activity [88, 89]. Studies of partially or fully enzymatically desialyated hEPO revealed a linear relationship between the specific activity *in vivo* and the number of sialic acids[90] (Figure 6). The terminal salic acids are thought to provide protection against recognition by a hepatic asialoglycoprotein binding lectin [91, 92], thereby reducing the rate of elimination.

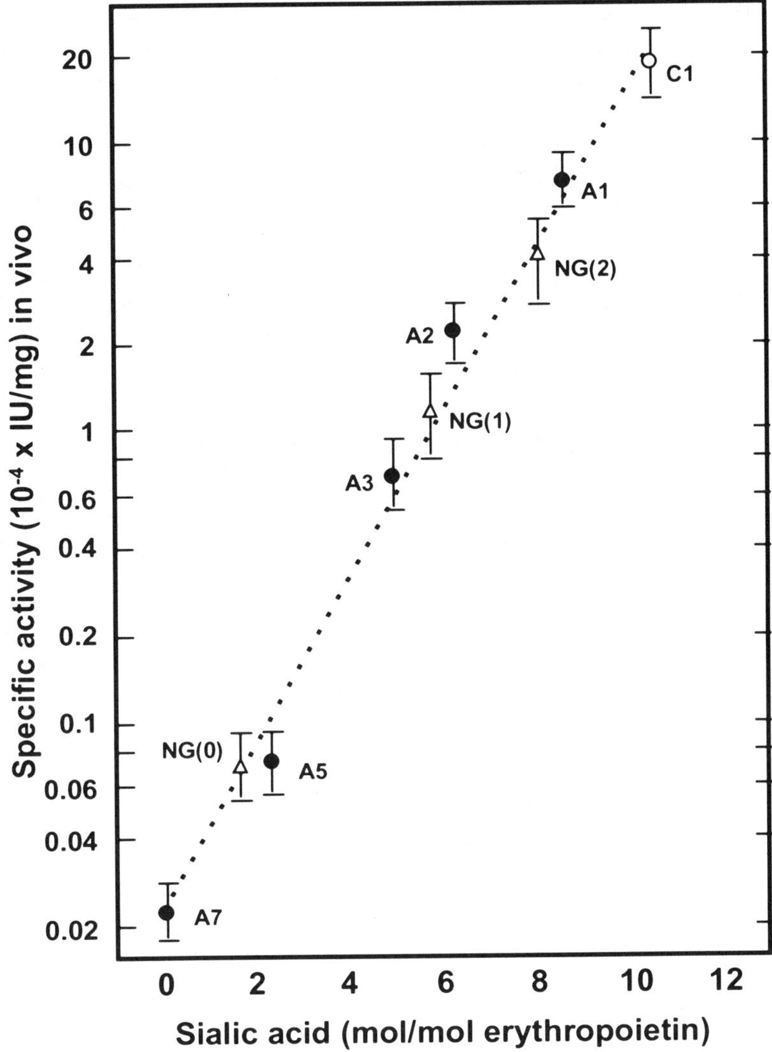

Figure 6. Relationship between the *in vivo* activity and the number of sialic acid residues. Samples of standard erythropoietin preparations were subcutaneously injected into five female Crj: CD-1(1CR) mice (seven weeks old) at 0.2 ml/mouse for three days. Blood was collected from the inferior vena cava on the next day, and was treated with stromatolyzing reagent after dilution. Residual reticulocytes were counted in an automatic micro cell counter. The activity was determined by the parallel-line method and the vertical bar indicated 95% confidence limits. (O) Intact erythropoietin (C1); (●) desialylated erythropoietins [A1, A2, A3, A5 (partially desialylated) and A7 (fully desialylated)]; (▲) de-*N*-glycosylated erythropoietins [NG(2), NG(1) and NG(0); number in parenthesis indicates the number of N-linked oligosaccharide chains] (with permission from ref. 90).

The above observations led to the hypothesis that further increases in the amount of carbohydrates which are rich in sialic acid may result in EPO molecules with improved pharmacokinetic and therapeutic profiles. Egrie and coworkers [93] tested this hypothesis by engineering an EPO mutant with two additional N-linked glycosylation sites. The new glycosylation sites were designed into the EPO sequence after a careful examination of the information concerning the EPO structure and the receptor binding site so that they would not interfere with either. The resulting novel erythropoiesis stimulating protein (NESP) has 52% carbohydrate by weight compared with 40% in natural hEPO or rhEPO. When tested in animal models, NESP exhibited a three-fold increase in serum half-life and a 3.6-fold enhanced potency compared to the less glycosylated rhEPO. The prolonged half-life observed in animals appears to also be present in humans according to a preliminary report [94]. These improvements hold promise for a less frequent dosing schedule and therefore a better quality of life for patients.

Improving Hematopoietic Efficacy using Chimeric Cytokines

Human hematopoiesis is a complex process that requires the intricate interplay of a large number of growth factors. These growth factors act at different stages of this process to produce mature, functional cells from stem cell progenitors in the bone marrow. It has frequently been found that combinations of many of the hematopoietic cytokines, especially mixtures of specific early-acting and late-acting factors, potentiate the activity of one another (see refs. 95, 96). Several attempts have been made to extend these observations by combining two cytokines into a single chain chimeric molecule [97-101].

Pixykine (PIXY321or milodistim) is a fusion protein in which GM-CSF and IL-3 are linked through a flexible peptide linker [97]. The high affinity heterodimeric receptors for each of these cytokines share a common subunit [102]. GM-CSF (sargramostim) is an effective stimulator of the production of cells of myeloid lineage [5] and has been used clinically for the relief of neutropenia[103]. IL-3 has a biological profile which overlaps but is nonetheless distinct from that of GM-CSF; IL-3 acts on earlier progenitors and supports multipotential progenitor cells as well as committed progenitors of the megakaryocytic, erythroid, and granulocytic lineages [6,7]. Co-administration of the two cytokines have a synergistic effect in aminal models [104-106]. It was thought that the combination of GM-CSF and IL-3 in a single polypeptide chain would create a single protein that could stimulate multiple hematopoietic lineages for treatment of both neutropenia and thrombocytopenia.

Pixykine exhibited superior *in vitro* activity in comparison to each growth factor, either alone or in combination. Receptor binding studies indicated that pixykine was capable of binding to GM-CSF receptor (GM-CSFR) and IL-3 receptor (IL-3R) on cells that express either receptor alone (JM-1 & HL-60) or both receptors (KG-1 & AML-193) [97]. For cells that express both receptors, the affinity of pixykine to IL-3R was about 10- to 20-fold greater when compared to cells expressing IL-3R alone. In AML-193 cell proliferation assays, pixykine again exhibited a ten-fold enhancement relative to the co-addition of GM-CSF and IL-3 (Figure 7). Synergy was demonstrated in human bone marrow colony-forming unit assays that examined the production of CFU-GEMM, BFU-E, and CFU-GM, where pixykine was shown to be 10- to 20-fold more potent than either growth factor alone or in combination. Pixykine was also found to promote CFU-MK and BFU-MK colony formation, thereby establishing its effect on human megakaryocytopoiesis [107]. Its ability to stimulate BFU-MK colony formation was equivalent to that of the combination of GM-CSF and IL-3. The effect of pixykine on CFU-MK, however, is less potent than GM-CSF plus IL-3. When tested in irradiated rhesus monkeys, pixykine accelerated the recovery of both neutrophils and platelets, an effect that neither cytokine alone was unable to achiev [108]. Synergy of pixykine in hemotopoiesis, however, has not been demonstrated beyond the *in vitro* studies. Clinical trials of pixykine have shown that it is well tolerated and efficacious, although its biological profile in humans is similar to that of IL-3 alone [109-111]. The less impressive results of pixykine in humans might be due to the inhibition of GM-CSF binding to GM-CSFR by IL-3 [112] and the fact that GM-CSFR and IL-3R share the same component [102].

The myelopoietins (MPO) represent a novel class of chimeric molecules that bind and activate both IL-3 and G-CSF receptors [101, 113-115]. The design of this class of engineered molecules was motivated by the observation that this combination of growth factors has greater hematopoietic activity over using either of them alone[21,22, 116-118]. MPO-1 is a chimera of a multiply substituted IL-3 variant and a variant of G-CSF. MPO-1 (SC-68420) binds to cells expressing either IL-3R or G-CSFR with affinities in the nanomolar range. It binds to the IL-3R on cells expressing both IL-3 and G-CSF receptors (AML-193.1.3) with a 7-fold higher affinity than to cells expressing only the IL-3 receptor (TF-1) [113]. Mechanistic studies have been carried out on a family of MPO molecules containing a library of IL-3 variants with various degrees of amino acid substitutions (ref. 115 & unpublished data), as well as a library of G-CSF receptor agonists. An ensemble of different sites in the G-CSF receptor agonist for connection to the IL-3R agonist domain has also been explored [114].

The IL-3 receptor binding property of the MPO molecules was found to be either similar or quite different compared to the single IL-3R agonist domains, depending on the specific IL-3 receptor agonist incorporated[115]. This suggests that each IL-3 receptor agonist interacts in a specific manner with the rest of the chimeric molecule. By comparison, the order of the agonist domains in the sequence and the linker had a smaller effect on the binding property. The effect of the relative orientation of the IL-3R and G-CSFR agonist domains was investigated using circularly permuted G-CSF (cp-GCSFs) sequences [114]. Circular permutation leads to domains in which the termini are in different locations on the surface of G-CSF, resulting in different spatial connections to the IL-3 receptor agonist moiety of MPO. The G-CSFR agonist activity of these MPO molecules was found to be similar to the activity of the isolated cpG-CSF domains in some cases, while in other cases significant differences were observed compared with the isolated cpG-CSF domains suggesting a connectivity effect. The ability to connect the cpG-CSF domain in a number of different ways provides a convenient means for modulating the relative activity of the constituent domains.

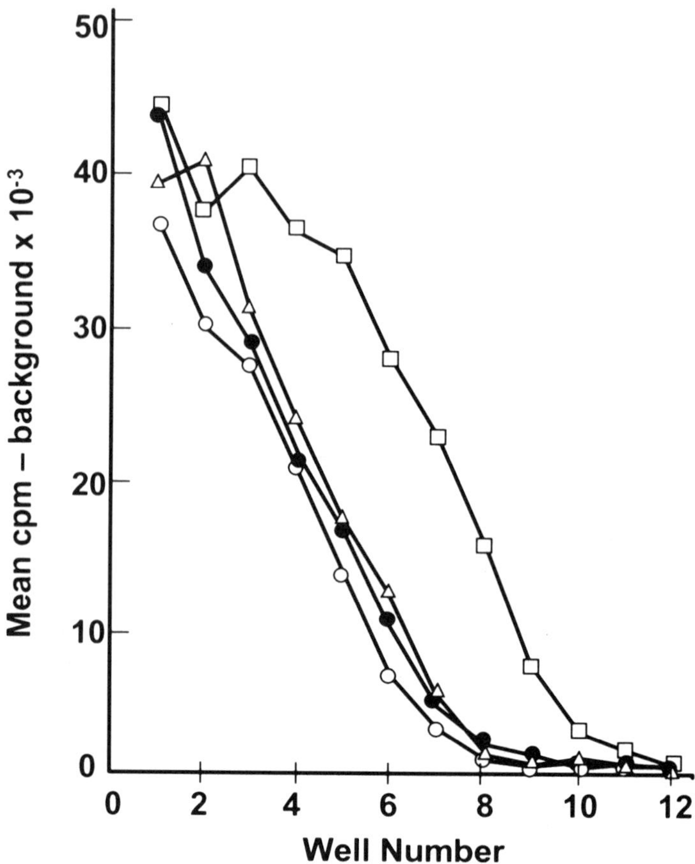

Figure 7. PIXY321 demonstrated an enhanced capacity to stimulate the proliferation of the AML-193 cell line. Data points are the mean of triplicate determination in one representative study. ●, Human IL-3; O, Human GM-CSF; □, PIXY321; ▲, human GM-CSF and IL-3 (with permission from ref. 97).

The dual receptor agonist property of MPO-1 provided an advantage in stimulating proliferation of cells expressing both receptors. While MPO-1 supported the proliferation of cells that express either the IL-3 receptor or G-CSF receptor alone, its potency increased about 5-fold in cells expressing both receptors [113]. The human bone marrow CD34[+] colony-forming unit assays revealed more dramatic improvement of MPO-1 over the combination of the component growth factors [113] (i.e., daniplestim with G-CSF; Figure 8). MPO-1 was significantly more potent in stimulating colony formationcompared with co-addition of the individual components, and the enhancement was more pronounced at concentrations that were sub-optimal for the combined single agonists. The growth of CFU-GM, CFU-G, CFU-M, BFU-E, and CFU-GEMM colonies in the presence of MPO-1, which was absent in the presence of only G-CSF, confirmed the multilineage nature of MPO-1. In contrast, the ability of MPO-1 to induce leukotriene release was reduced by 2- and 4-fold, respectively, in comparison to IL-3 and daniplestim. Thus MPO is a novel chimeric growth factor which not only has enhanced hematopoietic activity compared to the single growth factors but also preferentially targets certain populations of hematopoietic cells, presumably due to its dual receptor agonist nature.

The *in vivo* effect of MPO-1 was evaluated in non-human primates [119,120] as well as in humans [121]. The improved *in vitro* hematopoietic activity of MPO-1 appears to translate into enhanced *in vivo* activity. In normal and myelosuppressed rhesus monkeys [119, 120], MPO-1 efficiently mobilized CD34[+] stem and progenitor cells and more mature colony-forming cells, and significantly reduced the duration as well as the depth of nadirs of neutropenia and thrombocytopenia. For example, in the myelosuppression model, MPO-1 treatment using a BID dose schedule reduced the duration of the neutrophil nadir to 7.3 days from 14.8 days in the control animals, and the duration of thrombocytopenia to 2 days from 11.9 days. The depth of the neutrophil nadir was reduced to 390/μL (vs. 0/μL in the control) and the platelet nadir to 35,000/μL (vs. 5,000/μL in the control animals). The phase I/II study of MPO-1 [121] indicated that MPO-1 was well tolerated and was effective in PBSC mobilization of multilineage CD34[+] progenitors.

It should be pointed out that combining an early-acting with a late-acting cytokine does not guarantee enhanced activity. Fusion constructs of IL-3 and erythropoietin resulted in no enhancement of erythropoiesis over that observed with the co-addition of the individual cytokines [98]. Many factors including the complementary of the biological profiles, the signaling mechanism and distribution of the receptors, the length of the linker sequences, the order of the domains, and the linkage sites for connecting the domains all may contribute to the success of such chimeric molecules.

A different type of chimeric molecule was demonstrated to enhance the hematopoietic activity of interleukin-6 (IL-6) [122, 123]. Rather than combining two synergistic cytokines, this type of chimera combines a cytokine with a soluble form of its cognate receptor. IL-6 is a pleiotropic cytokine which acts on a variety of cells, leading to a number of effects on hematopoiesis, inflammation, immune response, neuron survival, and the growth of tumors [124-128]. IL-6 is a stimulator of thrombopoiesis especially in the presence of other growth factors such as IL-3[124,129, 130].

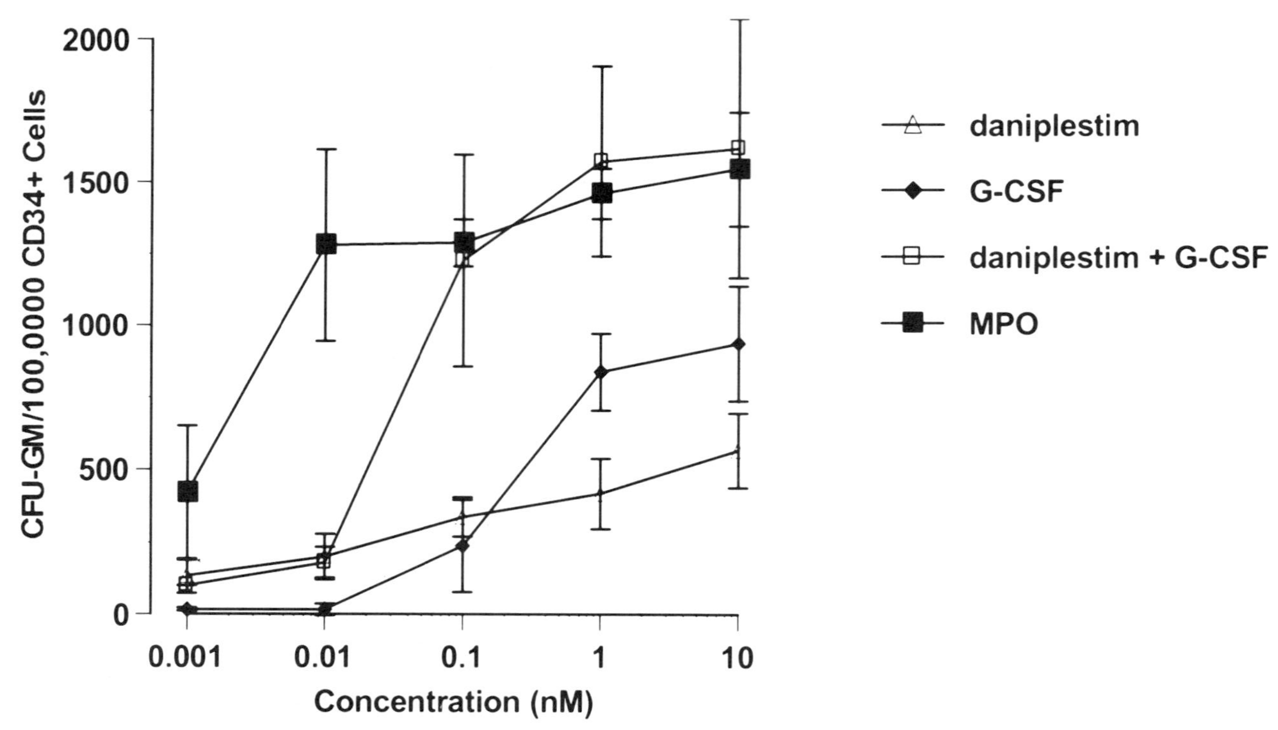

Figure 8. CFU activity of MPO-1 (■), daniplestim (▲), G-CSF (◆), or equimolar concentrations of G-CSF and daniplestim(□)

The use of IL-6 in combination with other cytokines is of potential benefit for ex vivo expansion of megakaryocytic progenitors [131]. The IL-6 receptor is composed of a ligand binding α-subunit (gp 80 or IL-6R) and a signal-transducing β-subunit [132] (gp130). Gp 130 is shared with the receptors for several other cytokines, including those for CNTF, IL-11 and LIF. High concentrations of the soluble form of the IL-6 specific receptor (sIL-6R) when combined with IL-6 were shown to stimulate human hematopoietic progenitor cells that express gp130 but not IL-6R [133]. Chimeras of sIL-6R and IL-6 were designed to promote the stability of the IL-6/sIL-6R complex. The stable pre-formed binary complex in turn was used to facilitate the formation of the IL-6/sIL-6R/gp130 ternary complex [122, 123], which is capable of signaling. The resulting chimeric molecule (H-IL-6) exhibited a 100- to 1000-fold higher potency than the combination of IL-6 and sIL-6R when assayed using a cell line that expresses only gp130 (Figure 9). The potency of H-IL-6 in a human CD34$^+$ colony-forming unit assay in the presence of SCF and IL-3 was significantly elevated compared with that of the co-addition of IL-6 and sIL-6R. The enhanced ability of the chimera to support the neuronal survival compared with the co-addition of IL-6 and sIL-6R was also observed in rat simpathetic neuron culture[134]. It has long been recognized that if subsets of desirable activities of pleiotropic cytokines can be enhanced, then they may have considerable therapeutic potential. These results suggest that cytokine and cytokine soluble receptor chimeras may be one way to achieve this goal.

Conclusions

In this review we have summarized recent data which demonstrates that certain experiments of nature or specific protein engineering technologies engender novel and sometimes desirable biological properties in hematopoietic cytokines. These properties include enhanced bioactivity or improved pharmacokinetics, or biological profiles that cannot be acheived by any single cytokine nature has provided. Our own experience using protein engineering to create a clinically useful therapeutic index for a family of IL-3 receptor agonists provided a structure-function database which has subsequently been expanded in our research program to include many of the key members of the hematopoietic cytokine superfamily. This experience also enabled us to create proteins with much greater hematopoietic activity and lower inflammatory activity. Extending this approach to a novel class of chimeric proteins further enabled the development of very high potency compounds with a number of distinct properties. Chimeric proteins which activate two different cell surface receptors display activities greater than any of their individual components (synergy). These activities include: increased biological potency, decreased inflammatory activity, greater protein stability, improved ease of protein manufacture and increases in circulating half-life *in vivo*. It should be emphasized that chimeras with enhanced activities are a unique subset of all fusion

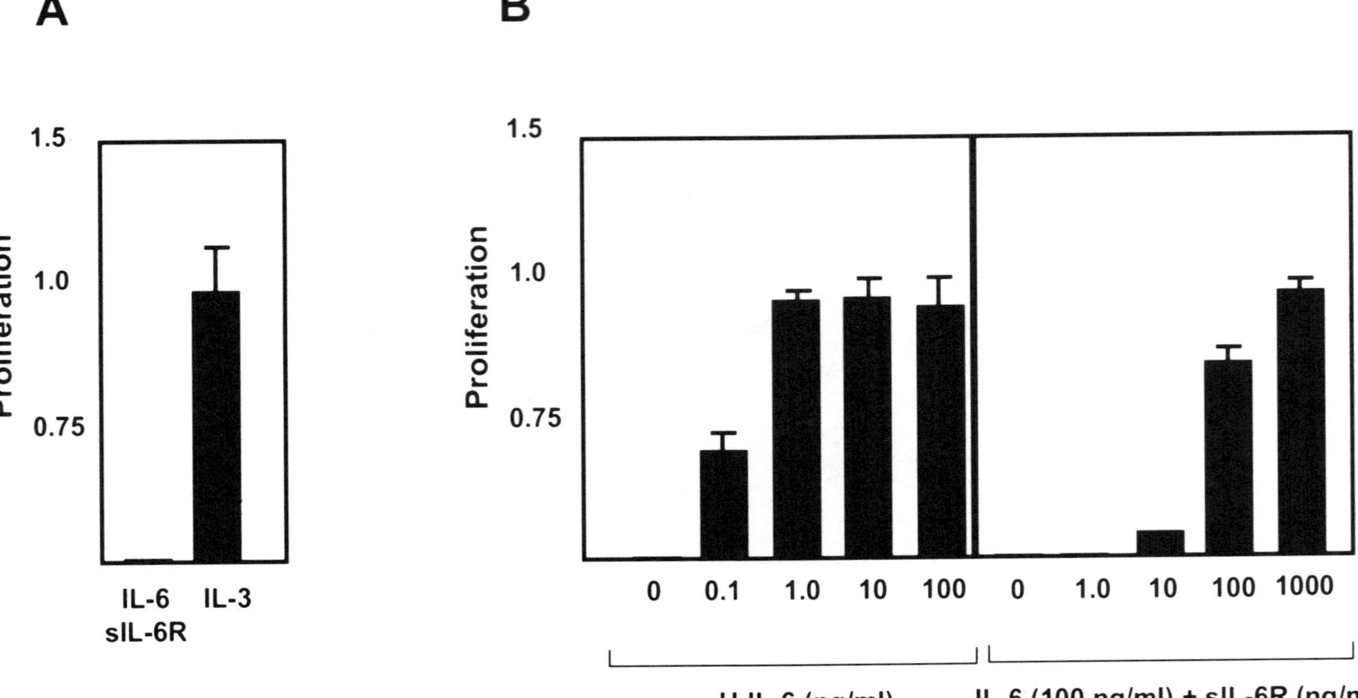

Figure 9. Proliferation of BAF/3 cells in response to H-IL-6 and IL-6/sIL-6R. BAF/3 cells (A) or BAF/3 cells stably transfected with human gp 130 cDNA (B) were stimulated with increasing amounts of H-IL-6 or increasing concentrations of sIL-6R in the presence of 100 ng/ml human IL-6. The mean of four experiments with positive standard deviation is shown. (Reprodued with permission from ref. 122).

proteins. Our on-going experience with large libraries of dual receptor chimeric proteins demonstrate that many chimeras exhibit properties that are superior to their components. Therefore, protein engineering approach allows the creation of unique, highly active and selective cytokines while providing critical new insights to understanding the receptor binding sites and other important properties of proteins belonging to the hematopoietic cytokine superfamily.

Acknowledgement

We thank Bob Forgey, Shari Burd, and Chuck Bogardus for assisting in the preparation of this manuscript, Dr. Keats Nelms, Dr. Joe Welply, Walter Smith, and Dr. Barbara Klein for critical reading of the manuscript.

References

1. Thomson AE: The cytokine handbook. (ed 2nd). New York, Academic Press, 1994
2. Sprang SR, Bazan JF: Cytokine structural taxonomy and mechanisms of receptor engagement. Curr. Opin. Struct. Biol. 3:815, 1993
3. Wells JA, de Vos AM: Hematopoietic receptor complexes. Annu. Rev. Biochem. 65:609, 1996
4. Wells JA: Binding in the growth hormone receptor complex. Proc. Natl. Acad. Sci. U. S. A. 93:1, 1996
5. Metcalf D, Nicola NA: The Hemopoietic Colony-Stimulating Factors. New York, Cambridge University Press, 1995
6. Schrader JW: The panspecific hemopoietin of activated T lymphocytes (interleukin-3). Annual Rev. Immunol. 4:205, 1986
7. Metcalf D: Control of granulocytes and macrophages: Molecular, cellular, and clinical aspects. Science 254:529, 1991
8. Biesma B, Willemse PH, Mulder NH, et al. Effects of interleukin-3 after chemotherapy for advanced ovarian cancer. Blood 80:1141, 1992
9. Denzlinger C, Walther J, Wilmanns W, Gerhartz HH: Interleukin-3 enhances the endogenous leukotriene production. Blood 81:2466, 1993
10. Mayer P, Valent P, Schmidt G, et al. The in vivo effects of recombinant human interleukin-3: demonstration of basophil differentiation factor, histamine-producing activity, and priming of GM-CSF-responsive progenitors in nonhuman primates. Blood 74:613, 1989
11. Dorssers LCJ, Mostert MC, Burger H, et al. Receptor and antibody interactions of human interleukin-3 characterized by mutational analysis. J. Biol. Chem. 266:21310, 1991
12. Kaushansky K, Shoemaker SG, Broudy VC, et al. Structure-function relationships of interleukin-3: an analysis based on the function and binding characteristics of a series of interspecies chimera of gibbon and murine interleukin-3. J. Clin. Invest. 90:1879, 1992
13. Lopez AF, Shannon MF, Barry S, et al. A human interleukin 3 analog with increased biological and binding activities. Proc. Natl. Acad. Sci. U. S. A. 89:11842, 1992
14. Barry SC, Bagley CJ, Phillips J, et al. Two contiguous residues in human interleukin-3, Asp21 and Glu22, selectively interact with the .alpha.- and .beta.-chains of its receptor and participate in function. J. Biol. Chem. 269:8488, 1994
15. Olins PO, Bauer SC, Braford-Goldberg S, et al. Saturation mutagenesis of human interleukin-3. J. Biol. Chem. 270:23754, 1995
16. Bagley CJ, Phillips J, Cambareri B, et al. A discontinuous eight-amino acid epitope in human interleukin-3 binds the .alpha.-chain of its receptor. J. Biol. Chem. 271:31922, 1996
17. Klein BK, Feng Y, McWherter CA, et al. The receptor binding site of human interleukin-3 defined by mutagenesis and molecular modeling. J. Biol. Chem. 272:22630, 1997
18. Feng Y, Klein BK, McWherter CA: Three-dimensional solution structure and backbone dynamics of a variant of human interleukin-3. J. Mol. Biol. 259:524, 1996
19. Thomas JW, Baum CM, Hood WF, et al. Potent interleukin 3 receptor agonist with selectively enhanced hematopoietic activity relative to recombinant human interleukin 3. Proc. Natl. Acad. Sci.

U. S. A. 92:3779, 1995

20. Farese AM, Herodin F, McKearn JP, et al. Acceleration of hematopoietic reconstitution with a synthetic cytokine (SC-55494) after radiation-induced bone marrow aplasia. Blood 87:581, 1996

21. MacVittie TJ, Farese AM, Herodin F, et al. Combination therapy for radiation-induced bone marrow aplasia in nonhuman primates using synthokine SC-55494 and recombinant human granulocyte colony-stimulating factor. Blood 87:4129, 1996

22. DiPersio JF, Abboud CN, Schuster MW, et al. Phase II study of mobilization of PBSC by administration of daniplestim (SC-55494) and G-CSF in patients with breast cancer or lymphoma. Proc. ASCO 16:87a, 1997

23. Kuga T, Komatsu Y, Yamasaki M, et al. Mutagenesis of human granulocyte colony stimulating factor. Biochemical and Biophysical Research Communications 159:103, 1989

24. Okabe M, Asano M, Kuga T, et al. In vitro and in vivo hematopoietic effect of mutant human granulocyte colony-stimulating factor. Blood 75:1788, 1990

25. Fujii I, Nagahara Y, Yamasaki M, et al. Structure of KW-2228, a tailored human granulocyte colony- stimulating factor with enhanced biological activity and stability. FEBS Lett. 410:131, 1997

26. Hill CP, Osslund TD, Eisenberg D: The structure of granulocyte-colony-stimulating factor and its relationship to other growth factors. Proc. Natl. Acad. Sci. U. S. A. 90:5167, 1993

27. Zink T, Ross A, Lüers K, et al. Structure and dynamics of the human granulocyte colony-stimulating factor determined by NMR spectroscopy. Loop mobility in a four-helix-bundle protein. Biochemistry 33: 8453, 1994

28. Souza LM, Boone TC, Gabrilove J, et al. Recombinant human granulocyte colony-stimulating factor: effects on normal and leukemic myeloid cells. Science 232:61, 1986

29. Nagata S, Tsuchiya M, Asano S, et al. Molecular cloning and expression of cDNA for human granulocyte colony-stimulating factor. Nature 319:415, 1986

30. Nagata S, Tsuchiya M, Asano S, et al. The chromosomal gene structure and two mRNAs for human granulocyte colony-stimulating factor. EMBO J. 5:575, 1986

31. Oheda M, Hase S, Ono M, Ikenaka T: Structures of the sugar chains of recombinant human granulocyte-colony-stimulating factor produced by Chinese hamster ovary cells. J. Biochem. (Tokyo) 103:544, 1988

32. Arakawa T, Prestrelski SJ, Narhi LO, et al. Cysteine 17 of recombinant human granulocyte-colony stimulating factor is partially solvent-exposed. J. Protein Chem. 12:525, 1993

33. Gervais V, Zerial A, Oschkinat H: NMR investigations of the role of the sugar moiety in glycosylated recombinant human granulocyte-colony-stimulating factor. Eur. J. Biochem. 247:386, 1997

34. Oheda M, Hasegawa M, Hattori K, et al. O-linked sugar chain of human granulocyte colony-stimulating factor protects it against polymerization and denaturation allowing it to retain its biological activity. J. Biol. Chem. 265:11432, 1990

35. Kishita M, Motojima M, Oh-eha M: Stability of granulocyte colony-stimulating factor (rHuG-CSF) in serum. Clin. Rep. 26:221, 1992

36. Mire-Sluis AR, Tivmamm HA, Gaines-Das R, Thorpe R: The role of glycosylation in the biological activity of granulocyte colony-stimulating factor. Exp. Haemat. A461, 1995

37. Cohen AM, Zsebo KM, Inoue H, et al. In vivo stimulation of granulopoiesis by recombinant human granulocyte colony-stimulating factor. Proc. Natl. Acad. Sci. U. S. A. 84:2484, 1987

38. Nissen C, Dalle Carbonare V, Moser Y: In vitro comparison of the biological potency of glycosylated versus nonglycosylated rG-CSF. Drug Invest. 7:346, 1994

39. Kuwabara T, Kobayashi S, Sugiyama Y: Pharmacokinetics and pharmacodynamics of a recombinant human granulocyte colony-stimulating factor. Drug Metab. Rev. 28:625, 1996

40. De Arriba F, Lozano ML, Ortuno F, et al. Prospective randomized study comparing the efficacy of bioequivalent doses of glycosylated and nonglycosylated rG-CSF for mobilizing peripheral blood progenitor cells. Br. J. Haematol. 96:418, 1997

41. Theocharis SE, Agapitos EB, Margeli AP, et al. Effect of two forms of granulocyte colony-stimulating factor on hepatic regeneration after 70% partial hepatectomy in rats. Clin. Sci. 92:315, 1997

42. Nohynek GJ, Plard JP, Wells MY, et al. Comparison of the potency of glycosylated and nonglycosylated recombinant human granulocyte colony-stimulating factors in neutropenic and nonneutropenic CD rats. Cancer Chemother. Pharmacol. 39:259, 1997

43. Tanaka H, Tanaka Y, Shinagawa K, et al. Three types of recombinant human granulocyte colony-stimulating factor have equivalent biological activities in monkeys. Cytokine 9:360, 1997

44.   Watts MJ, Addison I, Long SG, et al. Crossover study of the hematological effects and pharmacokinetics of glycosylated and non-glycosylated G-CSF in healthy volunteers. Br. J. Haematol. 98:474, 1997

45.   Hoglund M, Smedmyr B, Bengtsson M, et al. Mobilization of CD34[+] cells by glycosylated and nonglycosylated G-CSF in healthy volunteers - a comparative study. Eur. J. Haematol. 59:177, 1997

46.   Tanaka H, Okada Y, Kawagishi M, Tokiwa T: Pharmacokinetics and pharmacodynamics of recombinant human granulocyte-colony stimulating factor after intravenous and subcutaneous administration in the rat. J. Pharmacol. Exp. Ther. 251:1199, 1989

47.   Tanaka H, Satake-Ishikawa R, Ishikawa M, et al. Pharmacokinetics of recombinant human granulocyte colony-stimulating factor conjugated to polyethylene glycol in rats. Cancer Res. 51:3710, 1991

48.   Satake-Ishikawa R, Ishikawa M, Okada Y, et al. Chemical modification of recombinant human granulocyte colony-stimulating factor by polyethylene glycol increases its biological activity in vivo. Cell Struct. Funct. 17:157, 1992

49.   Yamasaki M, Asano M, Okabe M, et al. Modification of recombinant human granulocyte colony-stimulating factor (rhG-CSF) and its derivative ND 28 with polyethylene glycol. J. Biochem. (Tokyo) 115:814, 1994

50.   Reidhaar-Olson JF, De Souza-Hart JA, Selick HE: Identification of Residues Critical to the Activity of Human Granulocyte Colony-Stimulating Factor. Biochemistry 35:9034, 1996

51.   Young DC, Zhan H, Cheng Q-L, et al. Characterization of the receptor binding determinants of granulocyte colony stimulating factor. Protein Sci. 6:1228, 1997

52.   Guyton AC: Textbook of medical physiology. Philadelphia, W. B. Sanders Company, 1986

53.   Hokom MM, Lacey D, Kinstler OB, et al. Pegylated megakaryocyte growth and development factor abrogates the lethal thrombocytopenia associated with carboplatin and irradiation in mice. Blood 86:4486, 1995

54.   Lok S, Kaushansky K, Holly RD, et al. Cloning and expression of murine thrombopoietin cDNA and stimulation of platelet production in vivo. Nature 369:565, 1994

55.   de Sauvage FJ, Hass PE, Spencer SD, et al. Stimulation of megakaryocytopoiesis and thrombopoiesis by the c-Mpl ligand. Nature 369:533, 1994

56.   Kuter DJ, Beeler DL, Rosenberg RD: The purification of megapoietin: a physiological regulator of megakaryocyte growth and platelet production. Proc. Natl. Acad. Sci. U. S. A. 91:11104, 1994

57.   Hunt P, Li Y-S, Nichol JL, et al. Purification and biologic characterization of plasma-derived megakaryocyte growth and development factor. Blood 86:540, 1995

58.   Kato T, Ogami K, Shimada Y, et al. Purification and characterization of thrombopoietin. J. Biochem. (Tokyo) 118:229, 1995

59.   Sheridan WP, Choi E, Toombs CF, et al. Biology of thrombopoiesis and the role of Mpl ligand in the production and function of platelets. Platelets 8:319, 1997

60.   Archimbaud E: Clinical trials of pegylated recombinant human megakaryocyte growth and development factor (PEG-rHuMGDF). Haematol. Blood Transfus. 39:343, 1998

61.   Wendling F, Cohen-Solal K, Villeval J-L, et al. Mpl ligand or thrombopoietin: biological activities. Biotherapy (Dordrecht, Neth.) 10:269, 1998

62.   de Boer RH, Basser RL: Pegylated recombinant megakaryocyte growth and development factor. Drugs Future 22:987, 1997

63.   Paige AG, Whitcomb KL, Liu J, Kinstler O: Prolonged circulation of recombinant human granulocyte-colony stimulating factor by covalent linkage to albumin through a heterobifunctional polyethylene glycol. Pharm. Res. 12:1883, 1995

64.   Krantz SB: Erythropoietin. Blood 77:419, 1991

65.   Jelkmann W: Erythropoietin: structure, control of production, and function. Physiol. Rev. 72:449, 1992

66.   Spivak JL: The mechanism of action of erythropoietin. Int. J. Cell Cloning 4:139, 1986

67.   Peeters HRM, Jongen-Lavrencic M, Vreugdenhil G, Swaak AJG: Effect of recombinant human erythropoietin on anemia and disease activity in patients with rheumatoid arthritis and anemia of chronic disease: A randomized placebo controlled double blind 52 weeks clinical trial. Ann. Rheum. Dis. 55:739, 1996

68.   Ganser A, Karthaus M: Clinical use of hematopoietic growth factors. Curr. Opin. Oncol. 8:265, 1996

69.   Jacobs K, Shoemaker C, Rudersdorf R, et al. Isolation and characterization of genomic and cDNA clones of human erythropoietin. Nature 313:806, 1985

70.   Dube S, Fisher JW, Powell JS: Glycosylation at specific sites of erythropoietin is essential for

biosynthesis, secretion, and biological function. J. Biol. Chem. 263:17516, 1988
71. Yamaguchi K, Akai K, Kawanishi G, Ueda M, Masuda S, Sasaki R: Effects of site-directed removal of N-glycosylation sites in human erythropoietin on its production and biological properties. J. Biol. Chem. 266:20434, 1991
72. Wasley LC, Timony G, Murtha P, et al. The importance of N- and O-linked oligosaccharides for the biosynthesis and in vitro and in vivo biologic activities of erythropoietin. Blood 77:2624, 1991
73. Higuchi M, Oheda M, Kuboniwa H, et al. Role of sugar chains in the expression of the biological activity of human erythropoietin. J. Biol. Chem. 267:7703, 1992
74. Delorme E, Lorenzini T, Giffin J, et al. Role of glycosylation on the secretion and biological activity of erythropoietin. Biochemistry 31:9871, 1992
75. Kitagawa Y, Sano Y, Ueda M, et al. Glycosylation of erythropoietin is critical for apical secretion by Madin-Darby canine kidney cells. Exp. Cell Res. 213:449, 1994
76. Endo Y, Nagai H, Watanabe Y, Ochi K, Takagi T: Heat-induced aggregation of recombinant erythropoietin in the intact and deglycosylated states as monitored by gel permeation chromatography combined with a low-angle laser light scattering technique. J. Biochem. (Tokyo) 112:700, 1992
77. Takeuchi M, Kobata A: Structures and functional roles of the sugar chains of human erythropoietins. Glycobiology 1:337, 1991
78. Takeuchi M, Inoue N, Strickland TW, et al. Relationship between sugar chain structure and biological activity of recombinant human erythropoietin produced in Chinese hamster ovary cells. Proc. Natl. Acad. Sci. U. S. A. 86:7819, 1989
79. Lin FK, Suggs S, Lin CH, et al. Cloning and expression of the human erythropoietin gene. Proc. Natl. Acad. Sci. U. S. A. 82:7580, 1985
80. Recny MA, Scoble HA, Kim Y: Structural characterization of natural human urinary and recombinant DNA-derived erythropoietin. Identification of des-arginine 166 erythropoietin. J. Biol. Chem. 262:17156, 1987
81. Halstenson CE, Macres M, Katz SA, et al. Comparative pharmacokinetics and pharmacodynamics of epoetin alfa and epoetin beta. Clin. Pharmacol. Ther. (St. Louis) 50:702, 1991
82. Storring PL, Tiplady RJ, Das REG, et al. Epoetin alfa and beta differ in their erythropoietin isoform compositions and biological properties. Br. J. Haematol. 100:79, 1998
83. Lowy PH, Keighley G, Borook H: Inactivation of erythropoietin by neuraminidase and by mild substitution reactions. Nature 185:102, 1960
84. Winkert JW, Gordon AS: Enzymatic actions on the human urinary erythropoietic-stimulating factor. Biochim. Biophys. Acta 42:171, 1960
85. Dordal MS, Wang FF, Goldwasser E: The role of carbohydrate in erythropoietin action. Endocrinology 116:2293, 1985
86. Takeuchi M, Takasaki S, Shimada M, Kobata A: Role of sugar chains in the in vitro biological activity of human erythropoietin produced in recombinant Chinese hamster ovary cells. J. Biol. Chem. 265:12127, 1990
87. Tsuda E, Kawanishi G, Ueda M, et al. The role of carbohydrate in recombinant human erythropoietin. Eur. J. Biochem. 188:405, 1990
88. Matsumoto S, Ikura K, Ueda M, Sasaki R: Characterization of a human glycoprotein (erythropoietin) produced in cultured tobacco cells. Plant Mol. Biol. 27:1163, 1995
89. Goto M, Akai K, Murakami A, et al. Production of recombinant human erythropoietin in mammalian cells: host-cell dependency of the biological activity of the cloned glycoprotein. Bio/Technology 6:67, 1988
90. Imai N, Higuchi M, Kawamura A, et al. Physicochemical and biological characterization of asialoerythropoietin. Suppressive effects of sialic acid in the expression of biological activity of human erythropoietin in vitro. Eur. J. Biochem. 194:457, 1990
91. Fukuda M, Sasaki H, Fukuda MN: Structure and role of carbohydrate in human erythropoietin. Adv. Exp. Med. Biol. 271:53, 1989
92. Spivak JL, Hogans BB: The in vivo metabolism of recombinant human erythropoietin in the rat. Blood 73:90, 1989
93. Egrie JC, Dwyer E, Lykos M, et al. Novel erythropoiesis stimulating protein has a longer serum half-life and greater in vivo biological activity than recombinant human erythropoietin.1. Blood (Suppl. 1) 90:56a, 1997
94. Macdougall IC, Gray SJ, McEvoy O, et al. Comparison of the pharmacokinetics of Novel Erythropoiesis Stimulating Protein (NESP) and epoetin alfa (rhEPO) in dialysis Patients. American

Society of Nephrology annual meeting (Abs). , 1997

95. Moore MAS: The use of colony stimulating factors in combination. Curr. Opin. Biotechnol. 2:854, 1991

96. Lowry PA: Hematopoietic stem cell cytokine response. J. Cell. Biochem. 58:410, 1995

97. Curtis BM, Williams DE, Broxmeyer HE, et al. Enhanced hematopoietic activity of a human granulocyte/macrophage colony-stimulating factor-interleukin 3 fusion protein. Proc. Natl. Acad. Sci. U. S. A. 88:5809, 1991

98. Weich NS, Tullai J, Guido E, et al. Interleukin-3/erythropoietin fusion proteins: in vitro effects on hematopoietic cells. Exp. Hematol 21:647, 1993

99. Rock F, Everett M, Klein M: Overexpression and structure-function analysis of a bioengineered IL-2/IL-6 chimeric lymphokine. Protein Eng. 5:583, 1992

100. Zhao C, Tang P, Wang J, et al. Overexpression and characterization of recombinant human fusion protein IL-6/IL-2 (CH925). Stem Cells 12:339, 1994

101. McKearn JP, Hood WF, Monahan JB, et al. Myelopoietin - A multifunctional agonist of human IL-3 and G-CSF receptors. Blood (Suppl. 1) 86:259a, 1995

102. Kitamura T, Sato N, Arai K, Miyajima A: Expression cloning of the human IL-3 receptor cDNA reveals a shared β subunit for the human IL-3 and GM-CSF receptors. Cell 66:1165, 1991

103. Hill ADK, Naama HA, Calvano SE, Daly JM: The effect of granulocyte-macrophage colony-stimulating factor on myeloid cells and its clinical applications. J. Leukocyte Biol. 58:634, 1995

104. Broxmeyer HE, Williams DE, Hangoc G, et al. Synergistic myelopoietic actions in vivo after administration to mice of combinations of purified natural murine colony-stimulating factor 1, recombinant murine interleukin 3, and recombinant murine granulocyte/macrophage colony-stimulating factor. Proc. Natl. Acad. Sci. USA 84:3871, 1987

105. Donahue RE, Seehra J, Metzger M, et al. Human IL-3 and GM-CSF act synergistically in stimulating hematopoiesis in primates. Science 241:1820, 1988

106. Krumwieh D, Weinmann E, Seiler FR: Human recombinant derived IL-3 and GM-CSF in hematopoiesis of normal cynomolgus monkeys. Behring Inst. Mitt. 83:250, 1988

107. Bruno E, Briddell RA, Cooper RJ, Brandt JE, Hoffman R: Recombinant GM-CSF/IL-3 fusion protein: its effect on in vitro human megakaryocytopoiesis. Exp. Hematol 20:494, 1992

108. Williams DE, Dunn JT, Park LS, et al. A GM-CSF/IL-3 fusion protein promotes neutrophil and platelet recovery in sublethally irradiated rhesus monkeys. Biotechnology Therapeutics 4:17, 1993

109. Vadhan-Raj S, Broxmeyer HE, Andreeff M, et al. In vivo biologic effects of PIXY321, a synthetic hybrid protein of recombinant human granulocyte-macrophage colony-stimulating factor and interleukin-3 in cancer patients with normal hematopoiesis: a phase I study. Blood 86:2098, 1995

110. Ghielmini M, Pettengell R, Coutinho LH, et al. The effect of the GM-CSF/IL-3 fusion protein PIXY321 on bone marrow and circulating hemopoietic cells of previously untreated patients with cancer. Br. J. Haematol. 93:6, 1996

111. Bishop MR, Jackson JD, O'Kane-Murphy B, et al. Phase I trial of recombinant fusion protein PIXY321 for mobilization of peripheral-blood cells. J. Clin. Oncol. 14:2521, 1996

112. Taketazu F, Chiba S, Shibuya K, et al. IL-3 specifically inhibits GM-CSF binding to the high affinity receptor. J Cell Physiol 146:251, 1991.

113. Giri JG, Abegg A, Abrams M, et al. In vitro hematopoietic activity of myelopoietin, a chimeric dual agonist for IL-3 and G-CSF receptors. Blood submitted, 1998

114. McWherter CA, Feng Y, Busfluh LL, et al.: Circular permutation of the G-CSF receptor agonist domain of myelopoietin. Biochem, submitted 1998

115. Hood W, Feng Y, Monahan JB, et al.: Structure fucntion studies of bifunctional chimeric interleukin-3 and granulocyte-colony stimulating factor agonists binding to the interleukin-3 receptor. BBA submitted, 1998

116. Geissler K, Peschel C, Niederwieser D, et al. Potentiation of granulocyte colony-stimulating factor-induced mobilization of circulating progenitor cells by seven-day pretreatment witn interleukin-3. Blood 87:2732, 1996

117. Lemoli RM, Rosti G, Visani G, et al. Concomitant and sequential administration of recombinant human granulocyte colony-stimulating factor and recombinant human interleukin-3 to accelerate hematopoietic recovery after autologous bone marrow transplantation for malignant lymphoma. J. Clin. Oncology 14:3018, 1996

118. Huhn RD, Yurkow EJ, Tushinski R, et al. Recombinant human interleukin-3 (rhIL-3) enhances the mobilization of peripheral blood progenitor cells by recombinant human granulocyte colony-stimulating factor (rhG-CSF) in normal volunteers. Exper. Hematol. 24:839, 1996

119. MacVittie TJ, Farese AM, Davis TA, et al. Myelopoietin, a chimeric agonist of human IL-3 and G-CSF receptors mobilizes CD34$^+$ cells and hematopoietic clonegenic cells in normal nonhuman primates relative to daniplestim, G-CSF and daniplestim plus G-CSF. Blood submitted, 1998

120. MacVittie TJ, Farese AM, Lind LB, et al. Myelopoietin, an engineered chimeric IL-3 and G-CSF receptor agonist, stimulates multilineage hematopoietic recovery in a nonhuman primate model of radiation-induced myelosuppression. Exp Hematol submitted, 1998

121. DiPersio JF, Abboud CN, Winter JN, et al. Phase I/II study of mobilization of PBSC by SC-68420 in patients with breast cancer or lymphoma. Blood (Suppl. 1) :97a, 1997

122. Fischer M, Goldschmitt J, Peschel C, et al. A bioactive designer cytokine for human hematopoietic progenitor cell expansion. Nat. Biotechnol. 15:142, 1997

123. Chebath J, Fischer D, Kumar A, et al. Interleukin-6 receptor-interleukin-6 fusion proteins with enhanced interleukin-6 type pleiotropic activities. Eur. Cytokine Network 8:359, 1997

124. Ishibashi T, Kimura H, Uchida T, et al. Human interleukin 6 is a direct promoter of maturation of megakaryocytes in vitro. Proc. Natl. Acad. Sci. U. S. A. 86:5953, 1989

125. Carroll G, Bell M, Wang H, et al. Antagonism of the IL-6 cytokine subfamily. A potential strategy for more effective therapy in rheumatoid arthritis. Inflammation Res. 47:1, 1998

126. Gruol DL, Nelson TE: Physiological and pathological roles of interleukin-6 in the central nervous system. Mol. Neurobiol. 15:307, 1997

127. Greipp PR: Biology and treatment of myeloma. Curr. Opin. Oncol. 8:20, 1996

128. Revel M, Katz A, Eisenbach L, et al. Interleukin-6: Effects on tumor models in mice and on the cellular regulation of transcription factor IRF-1. Ann. N. Y. Acad. Sci. 762:342, 1995

129. Ishibashi T, Kimura H, Shikama Y, et al. Interleukin-6 is a potent thrombopoietic factor in vivo in mice. Blood 74:1241, 1989

130. Ikebuchi K, Wong GG, Clark SC, et al. Interleukin 6 enhancement of interleukin 3-dependent proliferation of multipotential hemopoietic progenitors. Proc. Natl. Acad. Sci. U. S. A. 84:9035, 1987

131. Kallen K-J, Meyer zum Buschenfelde K-H, Rose-John S: The therapeutic potential of interleukin-6 hyperagonists and antagonists. Expert Opin. Invest. Drugs 6:237, 1997

132. Kishimoto T, Akira S, Taga T: Interleukin-6 and its receptor: a paradigm for cytokines. Science 258:593, 1992

133. Sui X, Tsuji K, Tanaka R, et al. Gp130 and c-Kit signalings synergize for ex vivo expansion of human primitive hemopoietic progenitor cells. Proc. Natl. Acad. Sci. U. S. A. 92:2859, 1995

134. Marz P, Cheng J-G, Gadient RA, et al. Sympathetic neurons can produce and respond to interleukin 6. Proc. Natl. Acad. Sci. U. S. A. 95:3251, 1998

II

Management of Neutropenia and Neutropenic Fever

5. The Influence of Colony-Stimulating Factors on Neutrophil Production, Distribution, and Function

J. Milton Gaviria, W. Conrad Liles, David C. Dale

Introduction

The colony-stimulating factors (ie. interleukin 3, granulocyte-macrophage colony-stimulating factor, granulocyte colony-stimulating factor and monocyte/macrophage colony stimulating factor) are a group of glycoproteins that regulate the proliferation and differentiation of hematopoietic precursor cells [1-4]. In addition to their effects on hematopoiesis, colony-stimulating factors (CSFs) modulate the function of fully mature cells and therefore play an important role in regulating inflammatory responses vital to host defense. Here we review recent information that describes the biological activity of CSFs, particularly focusing on their modulation of neutrophil production, distribution, and function. The spectrum of biological activity of granulocyte colony-stimulating factor (G-CSF) and granulocyte-macrophage colony-stimulating factor (GM-CSF) is summarized in Table 1.

Differential effect of G-CSF and GM-CSF on neutrophil function.

In vitro marrow culture studies have furthered our understanding of the different effects of CSFs on hematopoietic proliferation and differentiation. For instance, when hematopoietic stem cells were cultured in the presence of 100 U/mL of IL-3, a 100-fold increase in cell number was seen within 7 days. Throughout this time course, more than 95% of the cells exhibited a primitive blast morphology. Very little spontaneous differentiation was observed, but when present, the maturing cells consisted of metamyelocytes [8,9]. When the IL-3 concentration was reduced to 1 U/mL, only limited proliferation was observed, but a greater proportion of mature cells was present following 7 days of culture, including some mature neutrophils. When cells were grown with GM-CSF only, little increase in cell number was seen after 7 days, but the cultures contained more mature neutrophils and macrophages. These data indicate that IL-3 supports the maintenance and proliferation of early cells, whereas GM-CSF acts predominantly as a differentiation factor [8].

Recent studies have shown that a combination of early acting factors affecting the kinetics of cell cycle-dormant primitive stem cells is necessary to stimulate the proliferation and differentiation of primitive hematopoietic stem/progenitor cells. Combinations of stem cell factor (SCF; c-kit ligand) or a ligand for type III receptor tyrosine kinase (flt3 RTK; FL) with IL-3 or GM-CSF showed a distinct synergistic effect on primitive stem cells [10,11]. Furthermore, the combination of three signals through the activation of gp130 (a signal-transducing receptor), c-kit, and IL-3 receptor (IL-3R) exerted a dramatic synergistic action on hematopoietic colony formation [12]. In the presence of these three signals, multipotential progenitors and committed cells could proliferate and differentiate to form colonies in the absence of terminally acting

Table 1. Effects of G-CSF and GM-CSF on Neutrophil Distribution and Function

	IN VITRO		IN VIVO	
	G-CSF	GM-CSF	G-CSF	GM-CSF
Adhesion	↑ [60, 61] n [57, 58]	↑ [57,58,62,63]	↑ [64,65,66, 67]	↑ [63]
Chemotaxis	↑ [68, 69] n [70] ↓ [72, 73]	↑ [69,74] ↓ [70-72, 75]	↑ [85] n [80-83] ↓ [39, 65-67, 76, 77]	n [71, 83, 84] ↓ [23, 78, 79]
CD11b/CD18	↑ [57, 58, 60, 70, 72]	↑ [57, 58, 62, 63, 70, 72, 87, 88]	↑ [64, 66, 84, 90, 91]	↑ [23, 57, 92]
L-selectin	↓ [57, 58, 70, 96, 97]	↓ [57, 58, 70]	↓ [57, 96 ,97]	↓ [57]
Phagocytosis	↑ [69, 77, 90, 102, 104]	↑ [69, 87, 90, 102, 103, 105]	↑ [66,77,85,90,107,108] n [82,106]	↑ [78]
FcgRI	↑ [109] n [69, 88, 110, 111]	↑ [69] n [88]	↑ [65,66,110,112,113]	n [23, 112]
FcgRII	↑ [109]		↑ [66]	n [23]
FcgRIII	↑ [88, 89]	n [88] ↓ [115]	n [66] ↓ [65,73,89,113,115]	n [23] ↓ [116]
CR 1	n [69]	↑ [69]	↑ [66,67]	
Respiratory Burst	↑ [60,70,72,117,118, 122,143] ↓ [136]	↑ [70,72,87,102,117, 119,120, 121,122]	↑ [38,66,67,91,124-126, 127,130-134] n [66] ↓ [137]	↑ [128-130, 132, 133, 135]
Microbicidal Activity	↑ [69,72,105,109, 142,143] n [140]	↑ [69,138,139] n [103,119]	↑ [140,144] n [136,145]	↑ [146]
ADCC	↑ [27,145,147,148]	↑ [27,147,148,149]	↑ [93,112]	↑ [150]
Degranulation	↑ [131]	↑ [101,102, 121,139, 151]	↑ [89,154]	↑ [154]
CD14	↑ [92]	↑ [92]	↑ [65,73,92,93,115]	n [92]
Apoptosis	↓ [165,166,168,176]	↓ [-165-170]	↓ [177,178]	↓ [178]

↑- increased; ↓ - decreased; n − no effect.

lineage-specific factors, such as G-CSF, erythropoietin, and thrombopoietin. Moreover, data from single-cell suspension cultures suggested that IL-3 support was important for survival and initial proliferation, whereas SCF was important for enhancement of progenitor cell proliferation [12,13].

Because of the known synergistic activities of hematopoietic growth factor combinations [14,15] and based on the assumption that normal hematopoiesis is regulated by such combinations, *in vitro* studies have been conducted to stimulate cell proliferation and simultaneously facilitate differentiation and maturation. *In vitro* expansion of progenitors and neutrophil precursors from enriched CD34[+] marrow cells has been achieved by the combination of IL-3, GM-CSF and G-CSF, which also increased the proportion of cells expressing the myeloid antigens CD13, CD15, CD11b and CD14 [13]. Addition of SCF to this mixture of factors further increased the production of progenitors and precursors and helped to maintain the cells at a less differentiated stage early in the cultures [13].

In vivo, human studies have shown that IL-3 is a powerful activator of the proliferation of all myelopoietic progenitors. The effect is dose dependent, and the various progenitors have different degrees of sensitivity; megakaryocyte progenitors appear to be the most sensitive, followed by erythroid and granulocyte/monocyte progenitors, orderly [16]. Furthermore, IL-3 acts as a primer for the action of other cytokines. Purified marrow progenitors obtained at the end of 7 days of IL-3 administration are more sensitive *in vitro* to the effect of optimal doses of G-CSF. This priming effect, also observed *in vivo* in the presence of physiological concentrations of G-CSF, could explain the modest increase in the proliferative activity of the morphologically recognizable granulocyte progenitors induced by IL-3 [17]. The same priming effect is seen with GM-CSF, which induces simultaneous stimulation of granulopoiesis, eosinophilopoiesis, and monocytopoiesis [18,19]. Clinical trials with IL-3 alone, however, have resulted in significant side effects with only very modest changes in blood cell counts [20-22]. Likewise, *in vivo* studies in healthy volunteers showed that GM-CSF at a dose of 250 mcg/m^2 causes neutrophilia mainly by accelerating delivery of neutrophils from the bone marrow to the blood and by decreasing migration from the blood to the tissues, with only a modest effect on neutrophil production and blood half-life [23]. Combinations of IL-3 and GM-CSF have been used in an attempt to better stimulate granulopoiesis. A study in cancer patients, showed a 3.2-fold amplification in neutrophil production, which required at least 2 extra divisions in the marrow [19]. The results were comparable with those of a previous trial using GM-CSF alone, but significant ineffective granulopoiesis developed in this earlier study [24]. These findings further suggest that IL-3 serves as a priming factor to increase the proliferative activity of precursors, while GM-CSF functions primarily as a differentiation factor. Similar results were seen in patients after bone marrow transplantation [25,26].

Like other growth factors , G-CSF stimulates cell proliferation and function by interacting with a specific cell surface receptor [27,28]. The G-CSF receptor is a 140-kDa homodimer, similar in structure to the receptors for erythropoietin and some interleukins. In contrast, other hematopoietic growth factor receptors are composed of two or three dissimilar components. Although G-CSF receptors may be found in other tissues, biologic functions are largely limited to hematopoietic cells. Experimental evidence indicates that G-CSF is necessary not only for the maintenance of normal neutrophil levels but also for the development of neutrophilia with infections.

Hammond et al. showed that dogs given repeated injections of human G-CSF produced antibodies that cross-reacted with recombinant canine G-CSF. Dogs with the anti-G-CSF antibodies developed sustained neutropenia that lasted until the antibodies had declined to undetectable levels, suggesting that G-CSF is necessary for the maintenance of a normal neutrophil count [29]. However, the bone marrow of these animals showed neutrophil development that appeared normal in its early stages, suggesting that other cytokines may support the earlier phases of neutrophil formation. Lieschke et al. reported the presence of chronic neutropenia (with levels 20%-30% of normal) in G-CSF knockout mice, with marrow histology similar to that of dogs with G-CSF deficiency [30]. The mice responded to G-CSF administration by developing normal blood neutrophil levels. It is noteworthy that dogs repeatedly injected with human GM-CSF and mice rendered deficient in GM-CSF by "gene knockout" experiments are not neutropenic [31,32].

Circulating G-CSF levels rise promptly as an acute-phase response to endotoxin injections and in various infectious diseases [33-35]. A dramatic example of this response was reported in a patient who self-injected 1 mg of *Salmonella minnesota* endotoxin and subsequently developed hypotension and sepsis syndrome. Twenty two hours later, the G-CSF level was 277 ng/mL, equivalent to the levels achieved after intravenous injection of approximately 25 mcg/kg recombinant G-CSF [36]. Cebon et al. examined the level of G-CSF, interleukin-6 (IL-6), GM-CSF, and monocyte/macrophage colony-stimulating factor (M-CSF) in normal subjects, febrile neutropenic patients, and bacteremic patients who were not neutropenic [37]. G-CSF, IL-6, and M-CSF levels were elevated with fever, but GM-CSF levels were not. In multiple regression analysis, the investigators showed that G-CSF levels correlated with fever, neutropenia, and pathogen type (higher levels in patients with gram-negative infections compared to those with gram-positive infections). Thus, a growing body of evidence suggests that G-CSF is necessary not only for the maintenance of normal neutrophil levels but also for the development of neutrophilia with infections.

Normally, neutrophil development requires approximately 6 days from the last stage of cell division, the myelocyte stage, before entry into the blood, as measured by *in vivo* labeling with ^{3}H-TdR [38]. Daily injection of G-CSF (30 mcg/day) to healthy young and elderly volunteers reduced this interval to approximately 4.5 days. A higher dose of G-CSF (300 mcg/day) further reduced the transit time to approximately 3 days and expanded the neutrophil mitotic pool, without significantly affecting blood neutrophil circulatory half-life or the distribution of blood neutrophils between the marginal and circulating pools [38,39]. A single injection of G-CSF (300 mcg) increased the blood neutrophil count about 4 fold [40]. Repeated administration of G-CSF over several days in hematologically healthy volunteers causes sustained neutrophilia [39-42]. Thus, daily subcutaneous G-CSF injection induces a progressive elevation of the base line count to a plateau, with superimposed acute increases in the count after each dose is given, which far exceeds the normal variation. On the basis of the observation that the percentage of circulating band neutrophils is increased, the acute neutrophilia after G-CSF administration is generally attributed to the release of maturing cells from bone marrow neutrophil reserves resulting from the dose-dependent shortening of the marrow transit time [38-40].

G-CSF also causes neutrophilia by stimulating proliferation of all stages of neutrophil development through the myelocyte stage [39,41,43]. Cells of the neutrophil lineage, including undifferentiated cells (CD34$^+$ CD33$^-$), have receptors for G-CSF and respond to this cytokine with increased proliferation [44]. G-CSF is also able to raise circulating CD34$^+$ hematopoietic progenitor cells in peripheral blood of healthy volunteers, cancer patients and severely ill patients with the acquired immunodeficiency syndrome (AIDS) [45]. Histologically, a prompt increase in the percentage of cells engaged in active DNA synthesis is present in marrow aspirate and biopsy samples [46]. Marrow cells exhibit features arising from both stimulated production and accelerated marrow release [38-40]. With aging, there seems to be no apparent difference in the hematopoietic-precursor response to factors that are regarded as early multilineage regulators (i.e., IL-3 and GM-CSF). In addition, bone marrow hematopoietic progenitors from healthy elderly subjects have reduced sensitivity, but similar absolute responsiveness to G-CSF compared to healthy young subjects [39,40,44,47,48].

M-CSF exerts its physiologic activity on cells committed to the monocyte/macrophage lineage, enhancing their replication, differentiation, and protein synthesis. Early clinical studies with M-CSF reported amelioration of neutropenia induced by conventional dose chemotherapy for solid tumors [49], and a more rapid neutrophil recovery in patients undergoing bone marrow transplantation (BMT) [50]. However, more recent clinical studies have been unable to demonstrate any effect of M-CSF on neutrophil recovery after BMT [51-53]. Current available data suggest that this growth factor has no significant activity on neutrophils [54].

Effects of Colony-Stimulating Factors on Neutrophil Distribution

Neutrophils leave the marrow storage compartment and enter the blood, and there is no evidence that they re-enter the marrow or recirculate once they leave the blood and enter the tissues[55]. The total blood neutrophil pool consists of all the neutrophils in the vascular spaces. A substantial percentage of these neutrophils do not circulate freely but adhere to the endothelium of blood vessels. These adherent cells constitute the marginated neutrophil pool, which accounts for approximately half of the total number of neutrophils [56]. The behavior of neutrophils in the blood appears to be controlled predominantly by two classes of membrane-bound adhesion proteins, L-selectin (LAM-1) and the β_2 integrin receptor CD11b/CD18, which regulate neutrophil rolling and transendothelial migration, respectively [57-59].

The mature neutrophil lacks IL-3 receptors and, thus, is not affected by IL-3. However, *in vitro* stimulation of peripheral blood neutrophils with either G-CSF or GM-CSF leads to rapid (maximal by 30 min) up-regulation of CD11b/CD18 and down-regulation of L-selectin (LAM-1) [57,58]. Early *in vitro* studies reported increased neutrophil adherence after treatment with G-CSF [60,61], but recent investigators have failed to detect an effect of G-CSF on neutrophil adherence [57,58]. In contrast, GM-CSF has consistently been shown to increase neutrophil adhesion to vascular endothelium [57,58,62,63]. In addition, GM-CSF is also able to down-regulate neutrophil L-selectin (LAM-1) expression [57]. When G-CSF was administered to healthy volunteers, neutrophils displayed enhanced expression of CD11b/CD18 and increased adhesion to E-selectin and ICAM-1 (CD54) [64]. G-CSF treatment of patients with cancer and severe neutropenia also resulted in an increased adherence of the induced neutrophils to plastic surfaces [65]. Yong et al. demonstrated that GM-CSF enhances neutrophil adherence to human endothelial monolayers *in vitro*, while G-CSF, despite producing a rise in CD11b expression of similar magnitude to that of GM-CSF, had no effect on neutrophil adherence [57]. G-CSF administered to healthy volunteers and patients with aplastic anemia caused increased neutrophil adhesion to nylon wool, which peaked on day 4 or 5 of treatment [64,66,67]. *In vivo,* although the time course and magnitude of the margination responses are similar for G-CSF and GM-CSF, the kinetics of margination differ. Following G-CSF, neutrophils marginate earlier with complete recovery of counts by 60 minutes, whereas at 2 hours after GM-CSF, peripheral cell counts were still at 50 percent of preinfusion levels [57].

Effects of Colony-Stimulating Factors on Neutrophil Function

<u>Neutrophil chemotaxis and tissue migration.</u> Chemotaxis refers to the directed migration of neutrophils along a concentration gradient of a particular stimulus, known as a chemotatic factor. G-CSF has been shown to serve as a chemotactic agent for neutrophils *in vitro* [68]. Checkerboard experiments performed using polycarbonate filters showed that maximal induction of migration occurred in the presence of a positive concentration gradient [68]. Bober et al. showed that pre-exposure of neutrophils to G-CSF or GM-CSF for 15 minutes stimulated the motility of the cells toward soluble stimuli such as formyl-methionyl-leucyl-phenylalanine (FMLP) [69]. However, other in vitro experiments have yielded contrasting results, including a dose-related inhibition of neutrophil chemotaxis after priming with GM-CSF [70-72]. Other studies have shown no effect or inhibition of chemotaxis after priming with G-CSF [70,72,73]. In general, the balance of data indicates that both G-CSF and GM-CSF enhance neutrophil chemotaxis *in vitro* at low concentrations and inhibit neutrophil motility at high concentrations [68,70,71,74,75]. This biphasic response presumably serves to attract and immobilize neutrophils at sites of inflammation. Chemokinesis, which refers to the random migration of neutrophils in response to a particular stimulus, is stimulated *in vitro* by both G-CSF [58,68] and GM-CSF [58].

In vivo experiments in healthy volunteers [65,66], patients with cancer [65,66], patients with aplastic anemia [67], and patients following bone marrow transplantation [76] have demonstrated decreased neutrophil chemotaxis after administration of G-CSF. In one study, chemotaxis toward FMLP was decreased after 2-3 d of treatment and returned to normal values 3-5 d after cessation of G-CSF therapy [65]. Furthermore, studies performed in our laboratory in healthy volunteers showed decreased neutrophil migration after administration of 300 mcg/d of G-CSF for 5 days, as demonstrated by the lack of proportional increase in neutrophil count in skin chambers and buccal neutrophils [39]. Similar results were observed after daily administration of GM-CSF (250 mcg/m^2) [23]. Other *in vivo* studies investigating neutrophil function in G-CSF-treated healthy volunteers and patients with cancer have shown decreased neutrophil migration into tissues [65,66,76,77]. During continuous intravenous infusion of GM-CSF, a markedly reduced neutrophil migration was found in a skin chamber assay [78,79]. However, other studies have not shown impairment of neutrophil migration *in vivo* after treatment with G-CSF [80-82] or GM-CSF [83,84]. Lieschke et al. evaluated the presence of neutrophils in the oral cavity in patients after bone marrow transplantation using a mouth rinse assay [80]. The percentage of neutrophils recovered from the oral cavity was not altered by G-CSF administration, suggesting that G-CSF did not impair tissue migration of primed neutrophils. In addition, another study demonstrated that G-CSF was able to improve abnormal neutrophil chemotaxis when given to patients with myelodysplastic syndrome [85]. Factors that might be responsible for the variable results on neutrophil chemotaxis and tissue migration include the use of different assays, different doses and routes of administration, and different intervals between administration of the growth factor and blood collection.

Integrins and selectins. The β_2 integrin subfamily of adhesion molecules play an important role in the regulation of neutrophil adhesion and migration into tissues [86]. Expression of CD11b, an α-subunit of the β_2 integrin subfamily, is up-regulated on neutrophils by G-CSF [57,58,60,70,72] and GM-CSF [57,58,62,63,70,72,87,88] *in vitro*. Up-regulation of CD11b has been observed following administration of G-CSF to healthy volunteers [64,66,89] and patients with malignancy[90,91]. Likewise, GM-CSF administered *in vivo* stimulated CD11b expression in healthy volunteers [23] and cancer patients[57,92]. Up-regulation of CD11b is a very early event after administration of G-CSF, with maximal expression levels seen approximately 1 hour after administration [90,91,93]. These changes in surface expression of adherence molecules may represent the mechanism underlying the acute but transient neutropenia observed following the administration of either G-CSF [41,94] or GM-CSF [23].

In vitro studies performed in healthy volunteers have shown that both G-CSF and GM-CSF down-regulate expression of L-selectin (LAM-1) on neutrophils [58,70]. Also, both colony stimulating factors have been reported to initially increase the affinity of L-selectin (LAM-1) for its ligand [95], then to decrease L-selectin (LAM-1) surface expression via shedding [57,95,96,97]. Serum concentrations of soluble L-selectin (sL-selectin) and sE-selectin were elevated after administration of G-CSF to healthy volunteers and patients with cancer [98]. sL-selectin retained functional activity and inhibited L-selectin-dependent leukocyte attachment to endothelial cells [99,100]. Conceivably, altered L-selectin expression may play a role in the regulation of the adhesive functions of primed neutrophils.

Phagocytosis. *In vitro*, GM-CSF [69,87,101-104] and G-CSF [69,101,105] stimulate phagocytic activity of normal neutrophils. The phagocytic activity of neutrophils stimulated with GM-CSF [78] and G-CSF [66,77,82,90,106,107] *in vivo* was enhanced or normal in most studies. G-CSF has been found to enhance the abnormal phagocytic activity of neutrophils in patients with myelodysplastic syndrome [85] and chronic graft-versus-host disease [108]. The enhancement of neutrophil phagocytosis by GM-CSF and G-CSF is related to increased expression of Fc receptors for IgG (FcγR) [known as the high-affinity receptor FcγRI (CD64) and the low-affinity receptors FcγRII (CD32) and FcγRIII (CD16)], and receptors for the C3b and C3bi complement fragments known as complement receptor 1 (CR1; CD35) and CR3 (CD11b/CD18) [74,109].

Immunoglobulin and complement receptors. Under natural conditions, expression of FcγRI (CD64) is restricted to monocytes in various stages of development and early precursors of the myelocyte lineage [110]. With maturation into band forms and polymorphonuclear cells, Fcγ RI (CD64) expression diminishes strongly. Studies have shown that GM-CSF and G-CSF have only a marginal effect *in vitro* on CD64 expression by mature neutrophils [69,88,110,111]. However, during G-CSF-induced *in vitro* myeloid differentiation, the CD64 receptor remains expressed during final maturation [110]. Sullivan et al. reported increased expression of FcγRI (CD64) after *in vitro* stimulation of mature neutrophils with G-CSF [109]. A strong induction of FcγRI (CD64) on mature neutrophils has been observed after administration of G-CSF to healthy volunteers [65,66,110] and patients with cancer [65,112,113], cyclic neutropenia [112] and AIDS [113]. Administration of GM-CSF to healthy volunteers failed to affect on expression of FcγRI (CD64) [23].

Mature neutrophils constitutively express low affinity receptors for multimeric IgG, [FcγRII (CD32) and FcγRIII (CD 16)] which mediate binding and lysis of cells coated with IgG, in a process known as antibody-dependent cellular cytotoxicity (ADCC), as well as binding and phagocytosis of immune complexes [114]. *In vitro*, G-CSF stimulates the expression of FcγRII (CD32) [109] and FcγRIII (CD16) [88,89], while expression of FcγRIII (CD16) is either decreased or unaltered by GM-CSF [88,115]. In studies conducted in healthy volunteers, administration of G-CSF increased neutrophil expression of FcγRII (CD32), whereas FcγRIII (CD16) expression did not differ from base line [66]. Others have found the expression of FcγRIII to be strongly decreased after G-CSF administration to healthy volunteers [65,89], patients following cancer chemotherapy [65,113], and patients with congenital neutropenias [73,115]. GM-CSF *in vivo* produced decreased neutrophil expression of FcγRIII (CD16) in one study [115] and no effect in expression of FcγRII (CD32) and FcγRIII (CD16) in another study [23].

The decreased expression of FcγRIII (CD16) after administration of G-CSF and GM-CSF may be related to either their respective actions on neutrophil precursors, favoring the release of partially immature granulocytes from the marrow, or shedding of the receptor. Kerst et al. found that levels of soluble FcγRIII (sFcγRIII; sCD16) were increased for as long as 10 days in healthy volunteers after a single dose of G-CSF [93]. Similar results have been published by others [113]. More research is needed to clarify the biological and clinical relevance of these changes on neutrophil function.

In vitro studies have shown that expression of CR1 (CD35) and CR3 (CD11b/CD18) is increased in GM-CSF-primed neutrophils. In contrast, G-CSF reportedly does not enhance expression of these cell-surface receptors [69]. Nevertheless, when neutrophil microbicidal activity against *S. aureus* was evaluated, no difference was seen between GM-CSF- or G-CSF-primed neutrophils. In a different set of studies, increased expression of CR1 (CD35) and CR3 (CD11b/CD18) was observed after G-CSF treatment of healthy volunteers and patients with cancer or aplastic anemia [66,67].

<u>Respiratory oxidative burst.</u> *In vitro* stimulation with G-CSF or GM-CSF fails to activate the respiratory burst of neutrophils in suspension, but induces a delayed but substantial respiratory burst in adherent neutrophils [117]. Although the maximal response to both CSFs is roughly equivalent, it is noteworthy that GM-CSF is the more potent stimulus when compared on the basis of weight [117]. After a short incubation time (15 min) with either GM-CSF or G-CSF, neutrophils demonstrate a marked enhancement in their ability to undergo a respiratory burst in response to FMLP or zymosan-activated serum [60,70,72,87,102,117-122]. Although both agents exert similar priming effects on neutrophils, their respective signal transduction pathways differ [123].

We have previously shown that *in vivo* administration of G-CSF [38,124,125,126] and GM-CSF [23] to healthy volunteers primed neutrophils for an enhanced production of reactive oxygen species (ROS). The neutrophil respiratory burst is increased after administration of GM-CSF and G-CSF to patients with cancer [66,91,127-130], myelodysplasia [131-133], aplastic anemia [67], diabetes [134] and after bone marrow transplantation [135]. Other studies, however, have failed to demonstrate this priming effect. Höglund et al. found that G-CSF *in vivo* did not stimulate the neutrophil respiratory burst in healthy volunteers [66]. Others have found a decreased production of ROS by neutrophils of patients with severe congenital neutropenia (SCN) after priming with G-CSF and stimulation with FMLP, but normal values after stimulation with the direct activator, phorbol myristate acetate (PMA) [136,137]. The balance of experimental evidence indicates that GM-CSF and G-CSF enhance the respiratory burst of normal and dysfunctional neutrophils both *in vitro* and *in vivo*.

<u>Microbicidal activity.</u> *In vitro*, G-CSF significantly enhanced the microbicidal activity of normal neutrophils and defective neutrophils from HIV-1-infected patients against *Staphylococcus aureus* [105,109], while GM-CSF stimulated the bactericidal activity of neutrophils obtained from patients following allogeneic bone marrow transplantation against *Staphylococcus aureus* [138]. Other *in vitro* studies showed that GM-CSF and G-CSF were able to correct the decreased neutrophil killing of *S. aureus* in patients with myelodysplasia [72] and in dexamethasone-suppressed neutrophils [69]. However, in other studies GM-CSF failed to augment bactericidal activity of neutrophils *in vitro* despite increasing phagocytic activity and stimulating production of ROS [103,119]. GM-CSF enhanced the fungicidal activity of normal neutrophils *in vitro* against blastospores of *Torulopsis glabrata* [139] and *Candida albicans* [69]. Conflicting results have been reported with G-CSF, however, which failed *in vitro* to enhance the fungicidal activity of neutrophils against *C. albicans* blastospores [69,140], despite its ability to augment the neutrophil respiratory burst in response to blastoconidia and pseudohyphae of the yeast [141]. In contrast, other *in* vitro studies conducted with neutrophils obtained from healthy volunteers showed that neutrophils stimulated with G-CSF had enhanced fungicidal activity against different Candida species [142] and *Aspergillus fumigatus* [143].

Administration of G-CSF to HIV-1-infected patients caused significant enhancement of neutrophil fungicidal activity against *C. albicans* and *C. neoformans* [140]. Furthermore, treatment with G-CSF enhanced neutrophil bactericidal activity in cancer patients [144]. However, in a group of patients with SCN [136] or hairy cell leukemia [145], treatment with G-CSF resulted in normal neutrophil bactericidal activity. Non-human primates treated with GM-CSF showed enhanced neutrophil bactericidal activity against *E. coli* [146].

<u>Antibody-dependent cellular cytotoxicity (ADCC).</u> Both G-CSF and GM-CSF are capable of stimulating neutrophil ADCC *in vitro* as well as *in vivo*. G-CSF has been shown to enhance *in vitro* neutrophil ADCC in healthy volunteers [27,147,148], HIV-infected patients [147] and hairy-cell-leukemia patients [145]. *In vitro*, GM-CSF also enhanced ADCC of neutrophils from healthy volunteers [27,102,147-149] and patients with chronic granulomatous disease (CGD) [147]. Furthermore, G-CSF stimulated *in vivo* ADCC when given to healthy volunteers [93] and cancer patients [112]. A similar effect was observed following administration of GM-CSF to HIV-infected patients [150].

<u>Degranulation.</u> *In vitro* assays have shown that GM-CSF primes neutrophils for an augmented release of constituents from both specific and azurophil granules in response to *C. albicans* [101], *Torulopsis glabrata* [139], Sephadex particles [151], opsonized inflammatory microcrystals [121] and FMLP [102]. *In vitro*, G-CSF is able to induce leukocyte alkaline phosphatase (LAP) mRNA [152] and to increase LAP activity in

126

neutrophils [153]. Furthermore, G-CSF has been shown to increase LAP activity in neutrophils from patients with myelodysplastic syndrome and chronic myelogenous leukemia (CML) [131]. G-CSF also induces *in vivo* activation of neutrophils, as demonstrated by the mobilization and release of secretory vesicles (LAP and CD11b), specific granules (lactoferrin, CD11b, and CD66b), and azurophil granules (elastase and α-1 antitripsin) [89]. Administration of GM-CSF or G-CSF, but not M-CSF, to patients recovering from autologous bone marrow transplantation primed neutrophils for enhanced neutrophil degranulation [154].

<u>Other receptor expression and function.</u> The receptor for lipopolysacharide (LPS) and LPS-binding protein (LBP) known as CD14 is expressed by neutrophils at low levels under natural conditions [155]. *In vitro*, both G-CSF and GM-CSF stimulated expression of CD14 antigen in mature neutrophils [92]. Increased surface expression of CD14 on neutrophils has been found after administration of G-CSF to healthy volunteers [65,92,93], patients post-chemotherapy [66] and patients with congenital neutropenias [73,115]. In contrast, GM-CSF failed to alter CD14 expression on neutrophils [92]. In addition, the level of soluble CD14 (sCD14) rose in plasma after healthy volunteers received G-CSF[93].

<u>Apoptosis.</u> Programmed cell death or apoptosis refers to the non-pathologic or physiological mode of cell death, which occurs via a characteristic sequence of events with morphologic features distinct from necrosis [156]. Because apoptosis induces the recognition and phagocytosis of senescent neutrophils by monocyte-derived macrophages and phagocytes, death via apoptosis results in the removal of intact neutrophils at tissue sites, presumably preventing the release of their toxic compounds into the tissues [157,158]. Apoptosis is now recognized to play a fundamental role in the regulation of the immune system and the inflammatory response [159,160]. As neutrophils proceed through apoptosis, functional activity declines. Apoptotic neutrophils lose FcγRIII (CD16) expression [161,162] and demonstrate a reduce ability to degranulate, generate respiratory burst, or undergo shape changes in response to external stimuli such as FMLP [163,164].

Recent evidence indicates that the functional life span of mature human neutrophils can be significantly extended *in vitro* by incubation with pro-inflammatory mediators, including G-CSF, GM-CSF, interferon-γ (IFN-γ), tumor necrosis factor-α (TNF-α), IL-1β, IL-2, endotoxic lipopolysaccharide (LPS) and complement factor 5a (C5a) [165-168], or adenosine triphosphate (ATP) and the diadenosine polyphosphates Ap$_3$A, Ap$_4$A, Ap$_5$A and Ap$_6$A [169-171], or dexamethasone[166]. *In vitro* studies have shown that the combination of GM-CSF together with ATP and diadenosine polyphosphates results in more pronounced protection from apoptosis than that of any of the components alone [169,170].

Niessen et al. showed that G-CSF delays spontaneous neutrophil apoptosis in part by activation of the vacuolar proton ATPase (v-ATPase) which plays a role in maintaining cellular pH balance. G-CSF may stimulate v-ATPase synthesis or its translocation to the plasma membrane [171]. Other laboratories, including ours, have studied another important mechanism involved in the regulation of spontaneous neutrophil apoptosis, the Fas (APO-1; CD95)/Fas-ligand (FasL) pathway, showing that neutrophils are highly susceptible to death through this system [166,172,173]. Although Fas is constitutively expressed on human neutrophils, monocytes and eosinophils, constitutive expression of cell surface FasL is relatively restricted to neutrophils [166,172-174]. As a result of constitutive co-expression of both Fas and FasL, neutrophils may be destined to undergo rapid cell death via the Fas apoptotic pathway. *In vitro* experiments have shown that G-CSF, GM-CSF, IFN-γ, TNF-α, or dexamethasone can suppress Fas-mediated neutrophil apoptosis and partly maintain neutrophil function [166,168,175].

Neutrophil apoptosis has been found to be accelerated in patients with advanced HIV infection (AIDS) [176]. The defect appears to be intrinsic and not related to serum factors. *In vitro* incubation of neutrophils from AIDS patients with G-CSF significantly delayed apoptosis [176]. *In vivo* administration of G-CSF to healthy volunteers and cancer patients increased subsequent neutrophil survival *ex vivo* by approximately 24 hours longer than that observed in controls which did not receive G-CSF [177]. Other studies examining neutrophil apoptosis in the acute respiratory distress syndrome (ARDS) have shown that the proportion of apoptotic neutrophils recovered from the lungs of patients with ARDS is low throughout the course of ARDS. In addition, the alveolar microenviroment of patients with established ARDS contains factors that prolong the survival of normal human neutrophils *in vitro*. G-CSF and GM-CSF appear to account for the majority of anti-apoptotic activity detected in the bronchoalveolar fluid from patients with ARDS [178].

Summary

Scientific data support the concept that IL-3 in combination with other early acting factors (SCF; c-kit ligand and flt3 RTK; FL) are required to stimulate the proliferation and differentiation of primitive hematopoietic stem/progenitor cells. GM-CSF, on the other hand, acts predominantly as a differentiation factor for granulocyte/monocyte progenitors. G-CSF has a more restricted activity, limited mainly to the granulocyte lineage, where it is necessary not only for the maintenance of normal neutrophil level but also for the development of neutrophilia with infections. In contrast, M-CSF exerts its activity on the comminted monocyte/macrophage cell lineage, with very little or no activity on the granulocyte cell lineage. Mature neutrophils lack IL-3 receptors and are, therefore, not affected by IL-3. In contrast, GM-CSF and G-CSF act on mature neutrophils modulating not only their distribution in blood and tissues but also their function.

References

1. Metcalf D. The granulocyte-macrophage colony-stimulating factors. Science 229: 16-22 , 1985.
2. Clark SC, Kamen R. The human hematopoietic colony-stimulating factors. Science 236: 1229-1237, 1987.
3. Demetri GD, Griffin JD. Granulocyte colony-stimulating factor and its receptor. Blood 78: 2791-2808, 1991.
4. Lieschke GJ, Burgess AW. Granulocyte colony-stimulating factor and granulocyte-macrophage colony-stimulating factor. N Engl J Med 327: 28-35, 1992.
5. Metcalf D. The molecular control of normal and leukemic granulocytes and macrophages. Proc R Soc London 230: 389-423, 1987.

6.	Spivak J, Smith RR, Ihle JN. Interleukin 3 promotes the *in vitro* proliferation of murine pluripotent hematopoietic stem cells. J Clin Invest 76: 1613-1621, 1985.

7.	Lord BI, Molineux G, Pojda Z, et al. Myeloid cell kinetics in mice treated with recombinant interleukin-3, granulocyte colony-stimulating factor (CSF), or granulocyte-macrophage CSF in vivo. Blood 77: 2154-2159, 1991.

8.	Heyworth CM, Dexter TM, Kan O, Whetton AD. The role of hemopoietic growth factors in self-renewal and differentiation of IL-3 dependent multipotential stem cells. Growth Factors 2: 197-211, 1990.

9.	Spooncer E, Heyworth CM, Dunn A, Dexter TM. Self renewal and differentiation of interleukin 3 dependent multipotent stem cells are modulated by stromal cells and serum factors. Differentiation 31: 111-118, 1986.

10.	Sonoda Y, Sakabe H, Ohmisono Y, et al. Synergistic actions of stem cell factor and other burst-promoting activities on proliferation of CD34+ highly purified blood progenitors expressing HLA-DR or different levels of c-kit protein. Blood 84: 4099-4106, 1994.

11.	Sonoda Y, Kimura T, Sakabe H, et al. Human flt3 ligand acts on myeloid as well as multipotential progenitors derived from purified CD34+ blood progenitors expressing different levels of c-kit protein. Eur J Haematol 58: 257-262, 1997.

12.	Kimura T, Sakabe H, Tanimukai S, et al. Simultaneous activation of signals through gp130, c-kit, and interleukin-3 receptor promotes a trilineage blood cell production in the absence of terminally acting lineage-specific factors. Blood 90: 4767-4778, 1997.

13.	Smith SL, Bender JG, Maples PB, et al. Expansion of neutrophil precursors and progenitors in suspension cultures of CD34⁺ cells enriched from human bone marrow. Exp Hematol 21: 870-877, 1993.

14.	Broxmeyer HE, Williams DE, Hangoc G, et al. Synergistic myelopoietic actions *in vivo* after administration to mice of combinations of purified natural murine colony stimulating factor 1, recombinant murine interleukin 3, and recombinant murine granulocyte/macrophage colony stimulating factor. Proc Natl Acad Sci USA 84: 3871-3875, 1987.

15.	Heyworth CM, Ponting ILO, Dexter TM. The response of hemopoietic cells to growth factors: developmental implications of synergistic interactions. J Cell Sci 91: 239-247, 1988.

16.	Aglietta M, Pasquino P, Sanavio F, et al. Granulocyte-macrophage colony-stimulating factor and interleukin 3: target cells and kinetics of response in vivo. Stem Cells 11(suppl 2): 83-87, 1993.

17.	Lemoli RM, Fortuna A, Fogli M, et al. Proliferative response of human marrow myeloid progenitor cells to in vivo treatment with granulocyte colony-stimulating factor alone and in combination with interleukin-3 after autologous bone marrow transplantation. Exp Hematol 23: 1520-1526, 1995.

18.	Aglietta M, Sanavio F, Stacchini A, et al. Interleukin 3 in vivo: kinetics of response of target cells. Blood 82: 2054-2061, 1993.

19.	Lord BI, Testa NG, Bretti S, et al. Haemopoietic progenitor and myeloid cell kinetics in humans treated with interleukin-3 and granulocyte/macrophage colony-stimulating factor in combination. Int J Cancer 59: 483-490, 1994.

20.	Ganser A, Ottmann OG, Seipelt G, et al. Effect of long term treatment with recombinant human interleukin-3 in patients with myelodisplastic syndromes. Leukemia 7: 696-701, 1993.

21.	Tepler I, Elias A, Kalish L, et al. Effect of recombinant human interleukin-3 on haematological recovery from chemotherapy-induced myelosuppression. Br J Haematol 87: 678-686, 1994.

22.	Scadden DT, Levine JD, Bresnahan J, et al. *In vivo* effects of interleukin 3 in HIV type 1-infected patients with cytopenia. AIDS Res Hum Retrov 11: 731-739, 1995.

23.	Dale DC, Liles WC, Llewellyn C, Price TH. Effects of granulocyte-macrophage colony-stimulating factor (GM-CSF) on neutrophil kinetics and function in normal human volunteers. Am J Hematol 57: 7-15, 1998.

24.	Lord BI, Gurney H, Chang J, et al. Haematopoietic cell kinetics in humans treated with rGM-CSF. Int J Cancer 50: 26-31, 1992.

25.	Crump M, Couture F, Kovacs M, et al. Interleukin-3 followed by GM-CSF for delayed engraftment after autologous bone marrow transplantation. Exp Hematol 21: 405-410, 1993.

26.	Albin N, Douay L, Fouillard L, et al. *In vivo* effects of GM-CSF and IL-3 on hematopoietic cell recovery in bone marrow and blood after autologous transplantation with mafosfamide-purged marrow in lymphoid malignancies. Bone Marrow Transplant 14: 253-259, 1994.

27.	Avalos BR, Gasson JC, Hedvat C, et al. Human granulocyte colony-stimulating factor: biologic activities and receptor characterization of hematopoietic cells and small cell lung cancer cell lines. Blood 75: 851-857, 1990.

28. D'Andrea AD. Cytokine receptors in congenital hematopoietic disease. N Engl J Med 330: 839-846, 1994.

29. Hammond WP, Csiba E, Canin A, et al. Chronic neutropenia: a new canine model induced by human G-CSF. J Clin Invest 87: 704-710, 1991.

30. Lieschke GJ, Grail D, Hodgson G. Mice lacking granulocyte colony-stimulating factor have chronic neutropenia, granulocyte and macrophage progenitor cell deficiency, and impaired neutrophil mobilization. Blood 84: 1737-1746, 1994.

31. Stanley E, Lieschke GJ, Grail D, et al. Granulocyte-macrophage colony-stimulating factor-deficient mice show no major perturbation of hematopoiesis but developed a characteristic pulmonary pathology. Proc Natl Acad Sci USA 91: 5592-5596, 1994.

32. Dranoff G, Crawford AD, Sadelain M, et al. Involvement of granulocyte-macrophage colony-stimulating factor in pulmonary homeostasis. Science 294: 713-716, 1994.

33. Cheers C, Haigh AM, Kelso A, et al. Production of colony-stimulating factors (CSFs) during infection: separate determinations of macrophage-, granulocyte-, and multi-CSFs. Infect Immun 56: 247-251, 1988.

34. Dale DC, Lau S, Nash R, et al. Effect of endotoxin on serum granulocyte and granulocyte-macrophage colony-stimulating factor levels in dogs. J Infect Dis 165: 689-694, 1992.

35. Kawakami M, Tsutsumi H, Kumakawa T, et al. Levels of serum granulocyte colony-stimulating factor in patients with infections. Blood 76: 1962-1974, 1990.

36. Taveira Da Silva AMT, Kaulbach HC, Chuidian FS, et al. Brief report: shock and multiple-organ dysfunction after self-administration of salmonella endotoxin. N Engl J Med 328: 1993 1457-1460.

37. Cebon J, Layton J, Maher D, Morstyn G. Endogenous haemopoietic growth factors in neutropenia and infection. Br J Haematol 86: 265-274, 1994.

38. Price TH, Chatta GS, Dale DC. The effect of recombinant granulocyte colony-stimulating factor (G-CSF) on neutrophil kinetics in normal human subjects. (abstract) Blood 80: 350a, 1992.

39. Price TH, Chatta GS, Dale DC. Effect of recombinant granulocyte colony-stimulating factor on neutrophil kinetics in normal young and elderly humans. Blood 88: 335-340, 1996.

40. Chatta GS, Price TH, Allen RC, Dale DC. Effects of in vivo recombinant methionyl human granulocyte colony-stimulating factor on the neutrophil response and peripheral blood colony-forming cells in healthy young and elderly adult volunteers. Blood 84: 2923-2929, 1994.

41. Morstyn G, Campbell L, Souza LM, et al. Effect of granulocyte colony-stimulating factor on neutropenia induced by cytotoxic chemotherapy. Lancet 1: 667-672, 1988.

42. Lieschke GJ, Burgess AW. Granulocyte colony-stimulating factor and granulocyte-macrophage colony-stimulating factor. N Engl J Med 327: 28-35, 99-106, 1992.

43. Linderman A, Herrmann F, Oster W, et al. Hematologic effects of recombinant human granulocyte colony-stimulating factor in patients with malignancy. Blood 74: 2633-2651, 1989.

44. Chatta GS, Andrews RG, Roger E, et al. Hematopoietic progenitors and aging: alterations in granulocyte precursors and responsiveness to recombinant human G-CSF, GM-CSF, and IL-3. J Gerontol 48: M207-212, 1993.

44. Nielsen SD, Dam-Larsen S, Nielsen C, et al. Recombinant human granulocyte colony-stimulating factor increases circulating CD34-positive cells in patients with AIDS. Ann Hematol 74: 215-220, 1997.

46. Lord BI, Bronchud MH, Owens S, et al. The kinetics of human granulopoiesis following treatment with granulocyte colony-stimulating factor in vivo. Proc Natl Acad Sci USA 86: 9499-9503, 1989.

47 Lipschitz D, Udupa K, Milton K, Thompson C. Effect of age on hematopoiesis in man. Blood 63: 502-509, 1984.

48. Timmafy M. A comparative study of bone marrow function in young and old individuals. Geront Clin 4: 13-18, 1962.

49. Motoyoshi K, Takaku F, Maekawa T, et al. Protective effect of partially purified human urinary colony-stimulating factor on granulocytopenia after antitumor chemotherapy. Exp Hematol 14: 1069-1075, 1986.

50. Masaoka T, Motoyoshi K, Takaku F, et al. Administration of human urinary colony-stimulating factor after bone marrow transplantation. Bone Marrow Transplant 3: 121-127, 1988.

51. Khwaja A, yong K, Jones HM, et al. The effect of macrophage colony-stimulating factor on haematopoietic recovery after autologous bone marrow transplantation. Br J Haematol 81: 288-295, 1992.

52 Laughlin MJ, Kirkpatrick G, Sabiston N, et al. Hematopoietic recovery following high-dose combined alkylating-agent chemotherapy and autologous bone marrow support in patients in phase-

I clinical trials of colony-stimulating factors: G-CSF, GM-CSF, IL-1, IL-2, M-CSF. Ann Hematol 67: 267-276, 1993.

53. Schuening FG, Neumunaitis J, Appelbaum FR, Storb R. Hematopoietic growth factors after allogeneic marrow transplantation in animal studies and clinical trials. Bone Marrow Transplant 14: S74-S77, 1994.

54. Nemunaitis J. A comparative review of colony-stimulating factors. Drugs 54: 709-729, 1997.

55. Zimmerman GA, Prescott SM, McIntyre TM. Endothelial cell interactions with granulocytes: Tethering and signaling molecules. Immunol Today 13: 93-98, 1992.

56. Athens JW, Raab SO, Haab OP, et al. Leukokinetic studies. III. The distribution of granulocytes in the blood of normal subjects. J Clin Invest 40: 159-167, 1961.

57. Yong KL, Linch DC. Differential effects of granulocyte and granulocyte-macrophage colony-stimulating factors (G- and GM-CSF) on neutrophil adhesion *in vitro* and *in vivo*. Eur J Haematol 49: 251-259, 1992.

58. Yong KL. Granulocyte colony-stimulating factor (G-CSF) increases neutrophil migration across vascular endothelium independent of an effect on adhesion: comparison with granulocyte-macrophage colony-stimulating factor (GM-CSF). Br J Haematol 94: 40-47, 1996.

59. Yong KL, Linch DC. GM-CSF differentially regulates neutrophil migration across IL-1 activated, and nonactivated, human endothelium. J Immunol 150: 2449-2456, 1993.

60. Yuo A, Kitagawa S, Ohsaka A, et al. Recombinant human granulocyte colony-stimulating factor as an activator of human granulocytes: potentiation of responses triggered by receptor-mediated agonists and stimulation of C3bi receptor expression and adherence. Blood 74: 2144-2149, 1989.

61. Okada Y, Kawagishi M, Kusaka M. Effect of recombinant human granulocyte colony-stimulating factor on human neutrophil adherence *in vitro*. Experientia 46: 1050-1053, 1990.

62. Devereux S, Bull HA, Campos-Costa D, et al. Granulocyte-macrophage colony-stimulating factor induced changes in cellular adhesion molecule expression and adhesion to endothelium: *in vitro* and *in vivo* studies in man. Br J Haematol 71: 323-330, 1989.

63. Yong KL, Rowles PM, Patterson KG, Linch DC. Granulocyte-macrophage colony-stimulating factor induces neutrophil adhesion to pulmonary vascular endothelium *in vivo*: role of β_2 integrins. Blood 80: 1565-1575, 1992.

64. Håkansson L, Höglund M, Jonsson U-B, et al. Effects of *in vivo* administration of G-CSF on neutrophil and eosinophil adhesion. Br J Haematol 98: 603-611, 1997.

65. Spiekermann K, Emmendoerffer A, Elsner J, et al. Altered surface marker expression and function of G-CSF induced neutrophils from test subjects and patients under chemotherapy. Br J Haematol 87: 31-38, 1994.

66. Höglund M, Håkansson L, Venge P. Effects of *in vivo* administration of G-CSF on neutrophil functions in healthy volunteers. Eur J Haematol 58: 195-202, 1997.

67. Yasui K, Tsuno T, Miyabayashi M, et al. Effects of high-dose granulocyte colony-stimulating factoron neutrophil functions. Br J Haematol 92: 571-573, 1996.

68. Wang JM, Chen ZG, Colella S, et al. Chemotactic activity of recombinant human granulocyte colony-stimulating factor. Blood 72: 1456-1460, 1988.

69 Bober LA, Grace MJ, Pugliese-Sivo C, et al. The effect of GM-CSF and G-CSF on human neutrophil function. Immunopharmacology 29: 111-119, 1995.

70. Wheeler JG, Huffine ME, Childress S, Sikes J. Comparison of colony stimulating factors on in vitro rat and human neutrophil function. Biol Neonate 66: 214-220, 1994.

71. Buescher ES, McIlheran SM, Vadhan-Raj S. Effects of in vivo administration of recombinant human granulocyte-macrophage colony-stimulating factor on human neutrophil chemotaxis and oxygen metabolism (letter). J Infect Dis 158: 1140-1142, 1988.

72. Boogaerts M, Meeus P, Verhoef G, et al. Differential effects of IL-3, GM-CSF and G-CSF on preleukemic granulocytes. (abstract) Blood 72: 110a, 1988.

73. Idenbach T, Roesler J, Elsner J, et al. *In vitro* functions of granulocyte colony-stimulating factor induced neutrophils. In: Freund M, Link H, Schmidt RE, Welte K (eds). Cytokines in Hemopoiesis, Oncology, and AIDS II. Springer. Berlin pp. 521-527, 1992.

74. Wang JM, Colella S, Allavena P, Mantovani A. Chemotactic activity of human recombinant granulocyte-macrophage colony-stimulating factor. Immunology 60: 439-444, 1987.

75. Weisbart RH, Golde DW. Physiology of granulocyte and macrophage colony-stimulating factors in host disease. Hematol Oncol Clin North Am 3: 401-409, 1989.

76. Turilli I, Bowers D, Aronson I, et al. G-CSF and neutrophil chemotaxis (letter). Br J Haematol 90: 232-233, 1995.

77. Bronchud MH, Potter MR, Morgenstern G, et al. In vitro and in vivo analysis of the effects of recombinant human granulocyte colony-stimulating factor in patients. Br J Cancer 58: 64-69, 1988.

78. Peters WP, Stuart A, Affronti ML, et al. Neutrophil migration is defective during recombinant human granulocyte-macrophage colony-stimulating factor infusion after autologous bone marrow transplantation in humans. Blood 72: 1310-1315, 1988.

79. Addison IE, Johnson B, Devereux S, et al. Granulocyte-macrophage colony-stimulating factor may inhibit neutrophil migration in vivo. Clin Exp Immunol 76: 149-153, 1989.

80. Lieschke GJ, Ramenghi U, O'Connor MP, et al. Studies of oral neutrophil levels in patients receiving G-CSF after autologous marrow transplantation. Br J Haematol 82: 589-595, 1992.

81. Hammond WP, Price TH, Souza LM, Dale DC. Treatment of cyclic neutropenia with granulocyte colony-stimulating factor. N Engl J Med 320: 1306-1311, 1989.

82. Bowski AA, Souza L, Kelly F, et al. Effects of human granulocyte colony-stimulating factor in a patient with idiopathic neutropenia. N Engl J Med 320: 38-42, 1989.

83. Toner GC, Jakubowski AA, Crown JP, et al. Colony-stimulating factors and neutrophil migration (letter). Ann Intern Med 110: 846-847, 1989.

84. Montgomery B, Bianco JA, Jacobsen A, Singer JW. Localization of transfused neutrophils to site of infection during treatment with recombinant human granulocyte-macrophage colony-stimulating factor and pentoxifylline (letter). Blood 78: 533-534, 1991.

85. Negrin RS, Haeuber DH, Nagler A, et al. Treatment of myelodysplastic syndromes with recombinant human granulocyte colony-stimulating factor. A phase I-II trial. Ann Intern Med 110: 976-984, 1989.

86. Carlos TM, Harlan JM. Leukocyte-endothelial adhesion molecules. Blood 84: 2068-2101, 1994.

87. Lopez AF, Williamson DJ, Gamble JR, et al. Recombinant human granulocyte-macrophage colony-stimulating factor stimulates in vitro mature human neutrophil and eosinophil function, surface receptor expression, and survival. J Clin Invest 78: 1220-1228, 1986.

88. Buckle AM, Hogg N. The effect of IFN-γ and colony-stimulating factors on the expression of neutrophil cell membrane receptors. J Immunol 143: 2295-2301, 1989.

89. Haas M, Kerst JM, Van der Schoot CE, et al. Granulocyte colony-stimulating factor administration to healthy volunteers: analysis of the immediate activating effects on circulating neutrophils. Blood 84: 3885-3894, 1994.

90. Katoh M, Shirai T, Shikoshi K, et al. Neutrophil kinetics shortly after initial administration of recombinant human granulocyte colony-stimulating factor: neutrophil alkaline phosphatase activity as an endogenous marker. Eur J Haematol 49: 19-24, 1992.

91. Ohsaka A, Kitagawa S, Sakamoto S, et al. *In vivo* activation of human neutrophil functions by administration of recombinant human granulocyte colony-stimulating factor in patients with malignant lymphoma. Blood, 74: 2743-2748, 1989.

92. Hansen PB, Kjaersgaard E, Johnsen HE, et al. Different membrane expression of CD11b and CD14 on blood neutrophils following *in vivo* administration of myeloid growth factors (published erratum appears in Br Haematol 1994 86: 240). Br J Haematol 85: 50-56, 1993.

93. Kerst JM, de Haas M, van der Schoot E, et al. Recombinant granulocyte colony-stimulating factor administration to healthy volunteers: induction of immunophenotypically and functionally altered neutrophils via an effect on myeloid progenitor cells. Blood 82: 3265-3272, 1993.

94. Demetri GD, Griffin JD. Granulocyte colony-stimulating factor and its receptor. Blood 78: 2791-2808, 1991.

95. Spertini O, Kansas GS, Munro JM, et al. Regulation of leukocyte migration by activation of the leukocyte adhesion molecule-1 (LAM-1) selectin. Nature 349: 691-694, 1991.

96. Liles WC, Rodger ER, Dale DC. Differential regulation of human neutrophil surface expression of CD14, CD11b, CD18, and L-selectin following the administration of G-CSF in vivo and in vitro (abstract). Clin Res 42:304A, 1994.

97. Ohsaka A, Saionji K, Sato N, et al. Granulocyte colony-stimulating factor down-regulates the surface expression of the human leukocyte adhesion molecule-1 on human neutrophils in vitro and in vivo. Br J Haematol 84: 574-580, 1993.

98. Ohsaka A, Saionji K, Igari J. Granulocyte colony-stimulating factor administration increases serum concentrations of soluble selectins. Br J Haematol 100: 66-69, 1998.

99. Schleiffenbaum B, Spertini O, Tedder TF. Soluble L-selectin is present in human plasma at high levels and retains functional activity. J Cell Biol 119: 229-238, 1992.

100. Spertini O, Callegari P, Cordey A-S, et al. High levels of the shed form of L-selectin are present

in patients with acute leukemia and inhibit blast cell adhesion to activated endothelium. Blood 84: 1249-1256, 1994.

101. Fabian I, Kletter Y, Mor S, et al. Activation of human eosinophil and neutrophil functions by haemopoietic growth factors: comparisons of IL-1, IL-3, IL-5 and GM-CSF. Br J Haematol 80: 137-143, 1992.

102. Burgess AW, Begley G, Johnson GR, et al. Purification and properties of bacterially synthesized human granulocyte-macrophage colony-stimulating factor. Blood 69: 43-51, 1987

103. Fleischman J, Golde DW, Weisbart RH, Gasson J. Granulocyte-macrophage colony-stimulating factor enhances phagocytosis of bacteria by human neutrophils. Blood 68: 708-711, 1986.

104. Richardson MD, Chung I. GM-CSF-modulated phagocytosis of *Trichosporon beigelii* by human neutrophils. J Med Microbiol 46: 321-325, 1997.

105. Roilides E, Walsh TJ, Pizzo P, Rubin M. Granulocyte colony-stimulating factor enhances the phagocytic and bactericidal activity of normal and defective human neutrophils. J Infect Dis 163: 579-583, 1991.

106. Katoh M, Takada M, Nakatani N, et al. Chemotaxis and phagocytosis of the neutrophils mobilized by granulocyte colony-stimulating factor in healthy donors for granulocyte transfusions. Am J Hematol 49: 96-97, 1995.

107. Lawry J, Smith MO, Lorigan PC. Monitoring neutrophil phagocytosis in lung cancer patients or normal stem cell donors, treated with G-CSF. Biochem Soc Trans 25: 197S, 1997.

108   Stoppa AM, Fossat C, Sainty D, et al. *In vivo* administration of recombinant granulocyte colony-stimulating factor corrects acquired neutrophil function deficiency associated with chronic graft-versus-host disease. Br J Haematol 83: 169-170, 1993.

109.   Sullivan GW, Gelrud AK, Carper HT, et al. Interaction of tumor necrosis factor-α and granulocyte colony-stimulating factor on neutrophil apoptosis, receptor expression, and bactericidal function. Proc Assoc Amer Phys 108: 455-466, 1996.

110. Kerst JM, Van de Winkel GJ, Evans AH, et al. Granulocyte colony-stimulating factor induces hFcgRI (CD64 antigen)- positive neutrophils via an effect on myeloid precursor cells. Blood 81: 1457-1464, 1993.

111. Buckle AM, Jayaram Y, Hogg N. Colony-stimulating factors and interferon-γ differentially affect cell surface molecules shared by monocytes and neutrophils. Clin Exp Immunol 81: 339-342, 1990.

112. Alerius T, Repp R, de Wit TPM, et al. Involvement of the high-affinity receptor for IgG (FcγRI CD64) in enhanced tumor cell cytotoxicity of neutrophils during granulocyte colony-stimulating factor therapy. Blood 82: 931-939, 1993.

113. Ersten MJ, de Jong S, Evers LM, et al. Addition of granulocyte colony-stimulating factor to chemotherapy in patients with AIDS-related lymphoma: effects on neutrophil Fcg receptor expression and soluble FcgRIII plasma levels. Br J Haematol 99: 537-541, 1997.

114. Ravetch JV, Kinet JP. Fc-receptors. Ann Rev Immunol 9: 457-492, 1991.

115. Elsner J, Roesler J, Emmendoerffer A, et al. Altered function and surface marker expression of neutrophils induced by rhG-CSF treatment in severe congenital neutropenia. Eur J Haematol 48: 10-19, 1992.

116. Maurer D, Fischer GF, Felzmann T, et al. Ratio of complement receptor over Fc-receptor III expression: a sensitive parameter to monitor granulocyte-macrophage colony-stimulating factor effects on neutrophils. Ann Hematol 62: 135-140, 1991.

117. Nathan CF. Respiratory burst in adherent human neutrophils: triggering by colony-stimulating factors CSF-GM and CSF-G. Blood 73: 301-306, 1989.

118. Kitagawa S, You A, Souza LM, et al. Recombinant human granulocyte colony-stimulating factor enhances superoxide release in human granulocytes stimulated by chemotactic peptide. Biochem Biophys Res Commun 144: 1143-1146, 1987.

119. Weisbart RH, Golde DW, Clark SC, et al. Human granulocyte-macrophage colony-stimulating factor is a neutrophil activator. Nature 314: 361-363, 1985.

120. Eisbart RH, Kwan L, Golde DW, Gasson JC. Human GM-CSF primes neutrophils for enhanced oxidative metabolism in response to the major physiological chemoattractants. Blood 69: 18-21, 1987.

121. Burt HM, Jackson JK. The priming action of tumor necrosis factor-alpha (TNF-α) and granulocyte-macrophage colony-stimulating factor (GM-CSF) on neutrophils activated by inflammatory microcrystals. Clin Exp Immunol 108: 432-437, 1997.

122. Meyer CN, Nielsen H. Priming of neutrophil and monocyte activation in human immunodeficiency

virus infection. APMIS 104: 640-646, 1996.

123. Balazovich KJ, Almeida HI, Boxer LA. Recombinant human G-CSF and GM-CSF prime human neutrophils for superoxide production through different signal transduction mechanisms. J Lab Clin Med 118: 576-584, 1991.

124. Liles WC, Rodger ER, Dale DC. *In vivo* administration of granulocyte colony-stimulating factor (G-CSF) to normal human subjects: priming of the respiratory burst and inhibition of apoptosis in neutrophils. (abstract) Blood 84: 24a, 1994.

125. Liles WC, Huang JE, van Burik J-A H, et al. Granulocyte colony-stimulating factor administered in vivo augments neutrophil-mediated activity against opportunistic fungal pathogens. J Infect Dis 175: 1012-1015, 1997.

126. Allen RC, Stevens PR, Price TH, et al. In vivo effects of recombinant human granulocyte colony-stimulating factor on neutrophil oxidative functions in normal human volunteers. J Infect Dis 175: 1184-1192, 1997.

127. Lindermann A, Herrmann F, Oster W, et al. Hematologic effects of recombinant human granulocyte colony-stimulating factor in patients with malignancy. Blood 74: 2644-2651, 1989.

128. Harazmi A, Nielsen H, Hovgaard D, et al. Modulation of neutrophil and monocyte function by recombinant human granulocyte-macrophage colony-stimulating factor in patients with lymphoma. Eur J Clin Invest 21: 219-224, 1991.

129. Kaplan SS, Basford RE, Wing EJ, Shadduck RK. The effect of recombinant human granulocyte-macrophage colony-stimulating factor on neutrophil activation in patients with refractory carcinoma. Blood 73: 636-638, 1989.

130. Wiltschke C, Krainer M, Nanut M, et al. *In vivo* administration of granulocyte-macrophage colony-stimulating factor and granulocyte colony-stimulating factor increases neutrophil oxidative burst activity. J Interf Cytok Res 15: 249-253, 1995.

131. Uo A, Kitagawa S, Okabe T, et al. Recombinant human granulocyte colony-stimulating factor repairs the abnormalities of neutrophils in patients with myelodysplastic syndromes and chronic myelogenous leukemia. Blood 70: 404-411, 1987.

132. Iki S, Yuo A, Yagisawa M, et al. Increased neutrophil respiratory burst in myeloproliferative disorders: selective enhancement of superoxide release triggered by receptor-mediated agonists and low responsiveness to in vitro cytokine stimulation. Exp Hematol 25: 26-33, 1997.

133. Zabernigg A, Hilbe W, Eisterer W, et al. Cytokine priming of the granulocyte respiratory burst in myelodysplastic syndromes. Leukemia Lymphoma 27: 137-143, 1997.

134. Sato N, Kashima K, Tanaka Y, et al. Effect of granulocyte colony-stimulating factor on generation of oxygen-derived free radicals and myeloperoxidase activity in neutrophils from poorly controlled NIDDM patients. Diabetes 46: 133-137, 1997.

135. Zimmerli W, Zarth A, Gratwohl A, et al. Granulocyte-macrophage colony-stimulating factor for granulocyte defects of bone marrow transplant patients. Lancet I: 494-497, 1989.

136. Roesler J, Emmendorffer A, Elsner J, et al. *In vitro* functions of neutrophils induced by treatment with rhG-CSF in severe congenital neutropenia. Eur J Haematol 46: 112-118, 1991.

137. Elsner J, Roesler J, Emmendoerffer A, et al. Abnormal regulation in the signal transduction in neutrophils from patients with severe congenital neutropenia: relation of impaired mobilization of cytosolic free calcium to altered chemotaxis, superoxide anion generation and F-actin content. Exp Hematol 21: 38-46, 1993.

138. Fabian I, Kletter Y, Bleiberg I, et al. Effect of exogenous recombinant human granulocyte and granulocyte-macrophage colony-stimulating factor on neutrophil function following allogeneic bone marrow transplantation. Exp Hematol 19: 868-873, 1991.

139. Kowanko IC, Ferrante A, Harvey DP, et al. Granulocyte-macrophage colony-stimulating factor augments neutrophil killing of *Torulopsis glabrata* and stimulates neutrophil respiratory burst and degranulation. Clin Exp Immunol 83: 225-230, 1991.

140. Vecchiarelli A, Monari C, Baldelli F, et al. Beneficial effect of recombinant human granulocyte colony-stimulating factor on fungicidal activity of polymorphonuclear leukocytes from patients with AIDS. J Infect Dis 171: 1448-1454, 1995.

141. Roilides E, Uhlig K, Venzon D, et al. Neutrophil respiratory burst in response to blastoconidia and pseudohyphae of *Candida albicans*. J Infect Dis 166: 668-673, 1992.

142. Roilides E, Holmes A, Blake C, et al. Effects of granulocyte colony-stimulating factor and interferon-γ on antifungal activity of human polymorphonuclear neutrophils against pseudohyphae of different medically important *Candida* species. J Leukoc Biol 57: 651-656, 1995.

143. Roilides E, Uhlig K, Venzon D, et al. Enhancement of oxidative response and damage caused by

human neutrophils to *Aspergillus fumigatus* hyphae by granulocyte colony-stimulating factor and gamma interferon. Infect Immun 61: 1185-1193, 1993.

144. Fossat C. Stoppa AM, Sainty D, et al. G-CSF *in vivo* improves neutrophil bactericidal activity against *Pseudomonas aeruginosa* in cancer patients. (abstract) Blood 76: 137a, 1990.

145. Glaspy JA, Baldwin JC, Robertson PA, et al. Therapy for neutropenia in hairy cell leukemia with recombinant human granulocyte colony-stimulating factor. Ann Intern Med 109: 789-795, 1988.

146. Mayer P, Lam C, Obenaus H, et al. Recombinant human GM-CSF induces leukocytosis and activates peripheral blood polymorphonuclear neutrophils in non-human primates. Blood 70: 206-213, 1987.

147. Baldwin GC, Fuller ND, Roberts RL, et al. Graanulocyte- and granulocyte-macrophage colony-stimulating factors enhance neutrophil cytotoxicity toward HIV-infected cells. Blood 74: 1673-1677, 1989.

148. Baldwin GC, Chung GY, Kaslander C, et al. Colony-stimulating factor enhancement of myeloid effector cell cytotoxicity towards neuroectodermal tumor cells. Br J Haematol 83: 545-553, 1993.

149. Metcalf D, Begley CG, Johnson GR, et al. Biologic properties *in vitro* of a recombinant human granulocyte-macrophage colony-stimulatimg factor. Blood 67: 37-45, 1986.

150. Baldwin GC, Gasson JC, Quan SG, et al. Granulocyte-macrophage colony-stimulating factor enhances the neutrophil function in acquired immunodeficiency syndrome patients. Proc Natl Acad Sci USA 1988 85: 2763-2766.

151. Carlson M, Peterson C, Venge P. The influence of IL-3, IL-5, and GM-CSF on normal human eosinophil and neutrophil C3b-induced degranulation. Allergy 48: 437-442, 1993.

152. Sato N, Mizukami H, Tani K, Asano S. Regulation of mRNA levels of alkaline phosphatase gene in neutrophilic granulocytes by granulocyte colony-stimulating factor and retinoic acid. Eur J Haematol 46: 107-111, 1991.

153. Sato N, Takatani O, Koeffler HP, et al. Modulation by retinoids and interferons of alkaline phosphatase activity in granulocytes induced by granulocyte colony-stimulating factor. Exp Hematol 17: 258-262, 1989.

154. Tsakona CP, Goldstone AH. Patterns of primary degranulation as indicated by the mean myeloperoxidase index (MPXI) during bacteremia in lymphoma transplants treated with growth factors. Clin Lab Haematol 14: 273-280, 1992.

155. Ziegler-Heitbrock HWL, Ulevitch RJ. CD14: cell surface receptor and differentiation marker. Immunol Today 14: 121-125, 1993.

156. Ellis RE, Yuan J, Horvitz HR. Mechanisms and functions of cell death. Annu Rev Cell Biol 7: 663-698, 1991.

157. Newman SL, Henson JE, Henson PM. Phagocytosis of senescent neutrophils by human monocyte-derived macrophages and rabbit inflammatory macrophages. J Exp Med 156: 430-442, 1982.

158. Savill JS, Wyllie AH, Henson JE, et al. Macrophage phagocytosis of aging neutrophils in inflammation: programmed cell death in the neutrophil leads to its recognition by macrophages. J Clin Invest 83: 865-875, 1989.

159. Cohen JJ. Programmed cell death in the immune system. Adv Immunol 50: 55-85, 1991.

160. Cohen JJ, Duke RC, Fadok VA, Sellins KS. Apoptosis and programmed cell death in immunity. Annu Rev Immunol 10: 267-293, 1992.

161. Dransfield I, Buckle A, Savill A, et al. Neutrophil apoptosis is associated with reduction in CD16 (FcγRIII) expression. J Immunol 153: 1254-1263, 1994.

162. Homburg CHE, de Haas M, Von dem Borne AEG, et al. Human neutrophils lose their surface FcgRIII and acquire annexin V binding sites during apoptosis in vitro. Blood 85: 532-540, 1995.

163. Dransfield I, Stocks SC, Haslett C. Regulation of cell adhesion molecule expression and function associated with neutrophil apoptosis. Blood 85: 3264-3273, 1995.

164. Whyte MKB, Meagher LC, MacDermot J, Haslett C. Impairment of function in aging neutrophils is associated with apoptosis. J Immunol 150: 5124-5134, 1993.

165. Colotta F, Re F, Polentarutti N, et al. Modulation of granulocyte survival and programmed cell death by cytokines and bacterial products. Blood 80: 2012-2020, 1992.

166. Liles WC, Kiener PA, Ledbetter JA, et al. Differential expression of Fas (CD95) and Fas ligand on normal human phagocytes: implications for the regulation of apoptosis in neutrophils. J Exp Med 184: 429-440, 1996.

167. Lee A, Whyte MKB, Haslett C. Inhibition of apoptosis and prolongation of neutrophil functional longevity by inflammatory mediators. J Leukoc Biol 54: 283-288, 1993.

168. Hu B, Yasui K. Effects of colony-stimulating factors (CSFs) on neutrophil apoptosis: possible roles

at inflammatory site. Int J Hematol 66: 179-188, 1997.

169. Gasmi L, McLennan AG, Edwards S. The diadenosine polyphosphates Ap_3A and Ap_4A and adenosine triphosphate interact with granulocyte-macrophage colony-stimulating factor to delay neutrophil apoptosis: implications for neutrophil:platelet interactions during inflammation. Blood 87: 3442-3449, 1996.

170. Gasmi L, McLennan AG, Edwards S. Neutrophil apoptosis is delayed by the diadenosine polyphosphates, Ap_5A and Ap_6A: synergism with granulocyte-macrophage colony-stimulating factor. Br J Haematol 95: 637-639, 1996.

171. Niessen H, Meisenholder GW, Li HL, et al. Granulocyte colony-stimulating factor upregulates the vacuolar proton ATPase in human neutrophils. Blood 90: 4598-4601, 1997.

172. Liles WC, Dale DC, Klebanoff SJ. Fas (APO-1 CD95) activation induces apoptosis in human phagocytes. (abstract) Blood 84: 371a, 1994.

173. Iwai K, Miyawaki T, Taakizawa T, et al. Differential expression of bcl-2 and susceptibility to anti-Fas-mediated cell death in peripheral blood lymphocytes, monocytes, and neutrophils. Blood 84: 1201-1208, 1994.

174. Matsumoto K, Schleimer RP, Saito H, et al. Induction of apoptosis in human eosinophils by anti-Fas antibody treatment in vitro. Blood 86: 1437-1443, 1995.

175. Liles WC, Dale DC, Klebanoff SJ. Glucocorticoids inhibit apoptosis of human neutrophils. Blood 86: 3181-3188, 1995.

176. Pitrak DL, Tsai HC, Mullane KM, et al. Accelerated neutrophil apoptosis in the acquired immunodeficiency syndrome. J Clin Invest 98: 2714-2719, 1996.

177. Adachi S, Kubota M, Lin YW, et al. *In vivo* administration of granulocyte colony-stimulating factor promotes neutrophil survival *in vitro*. Eur J Haematol 53: 129-134, 1994.

178. Matute-Bello G, Liles WC, Radella II F, et al. Neutrophil apoptosis in the acute respiratory distress syndrome. Am J Respir Crit Care Med 156: 1969-1977, 1997.

6. Evidence-Based Use of Hematopoietic Cytokines in Clinical Oncology

George D. Demetri

Introduction

The history of medicine is replete with examples which show how certain new technology and new therapeutics improve clinical outcomes. The introduction of hematopoietic cytokines into the clinical practice of oncology represents one of the more interesting recent examples of technologic innovation translating into clinical therapeutics. The corporate-sponsored research that tested these recombinant agents in humans set new standards for rapidly turning laboratory findings such as cloned human cytokine genes into useful therapeutic compounds such as recombinant human granulocyte colony-stimulating factor (G-CSF), recombinant human granulocyte-macrophage colony-stimulating factor (GM-CSF), and recombinant human erythropoietin (epoetin alfa, EPO). However, once G-CSF , GM-CSF, and EPO were commercially available for broad use by oncologists, it became clear that the optimal and appropriate use of these agents required more study and analysis. It is important also to note that hematopoietic cytokines are not unique in cancer medicine: many new cancer therapeutic agents are very expensive, and after initial regulatory approval, the field of oncology continually re-assesses the use of new agents. Often, for cytotoxic chemotherapies, this involves more broad use of a new agent outside of the initial tumor type for which the drug was approved (so-called "off label" use in practice). Such expansion of chemotherapy use can yield important new uses for a drug. For example, the novel cytotoxic agent gemcytabine, although initially approved by the United States Food and Drug Administration (USFDA) for palliative therapy of pancreatic carcinoma, also has important clinical activity in non-small cell lung cancer and other tumor types. This ongoing assessment of new therapeutic agents which often broadens the scope of use of drugs, has been more focused on limiting the scope of use for CSFs to those patients who stand to gain the most from these drugs. One key difference in CSF investigation compared to other drug development strategies is that CSFs were developed solely as agents of supportive care. If the supportive care were absolutely required in order to deliver the anticancer therapy, and if the anticancer therapy were of proven clinical value, then it would follow logically that the supportive care was a necessary part of the anticancer treatment overall. However, prior to the USFDA approval of G-CSF and GM-CSF in 1991, there had been lengthy prior experience in oncology of successful anticancer therapy without this supportive care methodology. Therefore, while the CSFs had measurable benefits that convinced the USFDA that these agents merited approval, critics quickly noted that these agents were not lifesaving breakthroughs. After all, it was argued, the cytotoxic anticancer therapies supported by CSFs had given to patients prior to 1991. This argument persists, and in this era of cost-consciousness, physician accountability, and evidence-based medicine, it is critical for physicians, oncology nurses, and managed care organizations to understand the costs, benefits, and controversies surrounding the appropriate utilization of hematopoietic cytokines in the supportive care of cancer patients. This review will summarize the clinical development of hematopoietic cytokines to mitigate the myelosuppressive toxicities of anticancer chemotherapy. From this background, oncology care providers and payers will need to formulate policies, which determine the "standard of care" in cytokine use. All too often, such decisions have been made without the input of patients and their own "willingness to pay" preferences, and this factor also needs to be taken into account.

The Starting Point: How Dangerous Is Myelosuppression in Oncology Practice?

The risks of myelosuppression were initially reported in the initial experiences of using myelotoxic chemotherapy to treat acute leukemias in the early 1960's. Bodey et al noted that the clinical risk of severe infectious complications was significantly related to the severity and length of severe neutropenia following antileukemic chemotherapy [1]. Other risks of myelosuppression were also noted in the 1960's, such as the increased risk of hemorrhagic complications in acute leukemia patients with severe and prolonged thrombocytopenia [2]. These life-threatening complications of severe and prolonged myelosuppression diminished the overall favorable impact of cytotoxic therapy for leukemia [3]. Interestingly, the model of leukemia treatment was subsequently extrapolated to the care of patients with solid tumors, although the approach to these malignancies is quite different. Oncologists rarely induce hematologic toxicities of the severity and prolonged duration that is commonly noted in the induction therapy of acute leukemia. Most cytotoxic regimens developed to treat solid tumors were developed to avoid significant hematologic toxicities. In the development of drugs to treat solid tumors, grade IV (severe) myelosuppression (even if uncomplicated by fever with neutropenia or bleeding) was judged as unacceptably severe toxicity, whereas grade IV myelosuppression is the goal in induction therapy of acute leukemia. Additionally, even if moderate to severe myelosuppression is induced in conventional solid tumor practice, (such as with the aggressive combination chemotherapy regimens used to treat testis cancer, sarcoma, or breast cancer), the duration of myelosuppression is generally only a few days at worst, compared to weeks in the case of acute leukemia therapy.

The truth is that myelosuppression is occasionally a limiting factor in the delivery of standard-dose chemotherapy for solid tumors – but only occasionally. The vast majority of patients can tolerate "standard" regimens in solid tumor oncology without the support of hematopoietic cytokines. Why then was the arrival of G-CSF and GM-CSF in 1991 greeted with such widespread enthusiasm and acceptance by oncologists? First, from the 1960's to the present day 1990's, the standard of care for management of fever with neutropenia has been inpatient hospitalization and administration of broad-spectrum empiric parenteral antibiotics. With modern antibiotics, deaths from such standard empiric treatment of fever with neutropenia have become very rare. Given the excellent outcomes with empiric antibiotics, many changes in management of fever with neutropenia have been promulgated. Most importantly, many providers are managing routine, uncomplicated fever with neutropenia with antibiotics in the outpatient setting, avoiding the costly and unpleasant hospitalization for the patient. This subject will be covered in more detail in a separate chapter in this book, and remains the subject of large national clinical trials randomizing empiric management between outpatient and inpatient care. Nonetheless, fever with neutropenia does still have a quality-of-life impact on a patient, since it interrupts the patient's normal life and requires immediate attention, often with time-consuming and expensive use of emergency department services. Avoidance of neutropenia is still, therefore, regarded as a desirable goal, especially in patients whose prior courses of therapy have been complicated by infectious problems.

It is also useful to put into context the 1991 introduction of G-CSF and GM-CSF into clinical oncology standard practice. The decade of the 1980's had been rather bleak from the standpoint of drug discovery and development of novel therapeutics. Unlike the 1990's, with the rich pipelines of investigational agents and promising new technologies, the focus of the 1980's was on maximizing the anticancer activity of "standard" cytotoxic agents through dose intensification. The use of bone marrow transplantation had made myeloablative therapy accessible to patients with leukemias, lymphomas, and solid tumors. However, bone marrow transplantation in the 1980's was limited to relatively few academic and research centers. The costs of bone marrow transplantation at that time were quite high due to the lengthy duration of hospitalization required to treat regimen-related toxicities, and the human costs in terms of mortality and morbidity were also considerable. With the impact of CSFs to minimize the myelotoxicity of chemotherapy drugs came renewed enthusiasm in dose escalation of cytotoxic drugs as the key strategy to overcome the generally suboptimal results seen with chemotherapy of solid tumors. These interrelated and connected threads (early enthusiasm for "breakthrough" recombinant DNA technology, optimistic faith in the worth of chemotherapy dose escalation) were key drivers which developed the current patterns of use for CSF support in clinical practice.

The Concept of Chemotherapy Dose/response: Is "More Toxic" Necessarily "More Effective"?

The concept that the anticancer activity of chemotherapy is directly related to the dose delivered is as old as cancer pharmacology itself. Given the nonspecific toxicities induced by most "standard" chemotherapy drugs, dose escalation is limited by a variety of factors. For many chemotherapy drugs, the adverse impact on the patient's hematopoietic function is the first dose-limiting factor. If myelosuppressive toxicities are overcome for certain drug classes (e.g. alkylating agents such as cyclophosphamide), several-fold increases in dose can be achieved before the next dose-limiting organ toxicity is noted (usually dose limiting toxicity to an epithelial system, such as mucositis or hemorrhagic cystitis). For other agents, such as anthracyclines, the ability to dose escalate significantly in the absence of myelotoxicity is more restricted, due to concerns of cardiotoxicity and severe epithelial toxicities such as palmar-plantar erythrodysesthesia (the "hand-foot syndrome" of palm and sole irritation, redness, and sloughing).

Solid tumor oncology is in a time of transition, with several new agents in clinical practice and more in development. At one time, it was taken as a truism that toxicity limited the effectiveness of cancer chemotherapy. Several well-publicized retrospective analyses promoted the theory that chemotherapy dose is a crucial determinant of chemotherapy activity [4-6]. Preclinical models strongly supported this view as well, although with all the obvious caveats about not being able to extrapolate from mouse or cell culture models to human physiology in actual patients. The field of dose-intensity analysis has captured the imagination of the more mathematically-minded oncologists, and several innovative schemes have been devised to analyze and explain data, as well as to predict clinical activity of dose-intensified chemotherapy. However, all models need verification, and without such verification the impact of faulty assumptions may render even the most elegant dose-intensity predictions not representative of clinical reality. An enormous number of small, nondefinitive trials have shown that dose escalation of chemotherapy with cytokine and/or stem cell support is feasible. However, in only a handful of well-conducted, prospective, randomized clinical trials has the importance of dose been tested and validated [e.g. 7]. Reasonably powerful data have been generated to support the use of very high-dose therapy with stem cell support in leukemia, relapsed intermediate to high-grade lymphomas, and multiple myeloma. For the vast majority of more common human solid tumors, dose escalation of chemotherapy to the degree requiring the support of hematopoietic cytokines has not yet been prospectively proven to be of worth [8-9].

Development of Hematopoietic Cytokines as Supportive Care for Clinical Oncology

The biology of hematopoietic cytokines indicated that recombinant molecules such as G-CSF, GM-CSF, or EPO might possess clinical activity, which could be developed to help cancer patients tolerate myelotoxic therapies [10-13]. Even the first dose-ranging clinical trials of hematopoietic cytokines with ability to stimulate leukocyte production (e.g. GM-CSF and G-CSF) confirmed that these molecules could increase circulating levels of white blood cells in a dose- and schedule-dependent manner [14 - 17]. Additionally, certain early studies in patients with marrow failure syndromes such as myelodysplasia suggested that these agents might stimulate leukocyte production even in the setting of impaired host hematopoiesis [18-20].

Besides the obvious clinical activity in stimulating host hematopoiesis *in vivo*, recombinant human cytokines such as G-CSF, GM-CSF, and EPO were remarkably well tolerated overall. The most common adverse effect noted with both GM-CSF and G-CSF is a mild to moderate ache in bones, particularly the low back and pelvis. The etiology of this "medullary bone pain" remains poorly understood, although it is routinely attributed to the rapid proliferation of marrow elements. The pain is clearly dose-related, with more severe pain noted at very high doses of these agents, and also worse with very vigorous marrow recovery to high levels of circulating neutrophils. Interestingly, no dose-limiting toxicities (other than bony pain) have been reported for G-CSF (Filgrastim) at any dose (highest clinical doses tested have been in the range of 115 μg/kg/day) [11-12]. In contrast, GM-CSF administration is associated more frequently with toxicities, and these adverse effects represent a more complex set of inflammatory processes, consistent with the more complex and multipotent biology of GM-CSF [12]. Certainly, there is a higher incidence of GM-CSF-related toxicities with higher doses of GM-CSF. Although, initial dose-ranging studies of GM-CSF showed biological effects at the lowest doses tested (< 5 μg/kg/day), administration of higher doses of GM-CSF (> 30 μg/kg/day) was associated with dose-limiting toxicities such as pleuropericarditis, thrombotic complications, and third-spacing of fluid [12, 15]. These toxicities may have limited relevance for routine clinical practice, however, since there is no clinical indication for such excessively high doses of GM-CSF and since clinical activity is noted at safer lower doses. These systemic toxicities of GM-CSF are also very consistent with the biology of this inflammatory mediator, which rarely reaches detectable levels in the circulation. This is in contrast to G-CSF, which is routinely detectable at high levels in the systemic circulation of patients recovering from myelosuppression or from infection. Such biological differences may be useful clues indicating the optimal use of these agents in different therapeutic indications.

<u>Definitive Randomized Studies of Hematopoietic Cytokines</u>. Initial clinical trials paved the way for rapid development of hematopoietic cytokines. With the goals of proving both "safety" and "efficacy" of these recombinant molecules, various biotechnology and pharmaceutical companies focused their strategic development plans on how best to demonstrate "efficacy". Prospective, placebo-controlled, randomized clinical trials still represent the gold standard for drug development in oncology, and the key strategic decisions in this field centered around choosing the proper clinical scenario and the most achievable endpoints. In the pilot dose-ranging studies of GM-CSF and G-CSF, the increased numbers of circulating leukocytes induced by these molecules were only a fascinating laboratory finding, without documented clinical benefits [11,12, 14-17]. Higher levels of circulating leukocytes were considered a "surrogate endpoint" for other, more meaningful clinical endpoints such as lower rates of infection, less days of parenteral antibiotics, or fewer toxic deaths from myelosuppressive chemotherapy. After dose-finding studies had been performed, the next generation of randomized trials aimed to prove that CSF-stimulated leukocyte production and EPO-enhanced erythropoiesis had clinically relevant beneficial impacts on endpoints other than a complete blood count.

To be able to show an impact on ameliorating myelosuppressive toxicities, such toxicities must be induced with high incidence. While this might seem common sense, it is quite a challenge in standard oncology practice, where most conventional chemotherapy regimens were developed in the pre-CSF era specifically to avoid unacceptably myelotoxicity. Most of the data, therefore, from randomized studies of hematopoietic cytokines, comes from unique populations of study patients who may not be representative of "routine" clinical oncology practice. GM-CSF was primarily developed using bone marrow transplant patients as the model. This degree of hematopoietic toxicity obviously would have only limited relevance for non-transplant patients. G-CSF was primarily developed using a severely myelotoxic combination chemotherapy regimen of cyclophosphamide, doxorubicin, and etoposide to treat patients with small-cell lung cancer. The definitive randomized studies of EPO accrued the broadest possible patient population, but selected patients who already were anemic at the time of study entry. This points out a difference in clinical development strategies as well as in potential clinical use of these agents. Most of the definitive clinical research studies of either G-CSF or GM-CSF were trying to prevent infectious complications of myelosuppressive therapy **before** any complications had ever occurred. This use of hematopoietic cytokines is defined as **"primary**

prophylaxis" of infectious complications, and represents the preventive use of these agents to decrease the risks of potential adverse clinical events (such as fever with neutropenia). In contrast, the development of EPO studied a **"therapeutic"** use of this agent, since all of the patients already had anemia [24]. The analogous clinical situation for leukocyte CSFs is the use of CSF as therapy (in addition to parenteral antibiotics) of empiric fever with neutropenia [25]. Another potential scenario for the use of hematopoietic cytokines includes **"secondary prophylaxis,"** which is the attempt to prevent **subsequent** recurrences of a treatment-associated complication after one episode had already occurred. For example, if a patient experiences an episode of fever with neutropenia during her third cycle of chemotherapy given without an adjunctive CSF, the preventive use of CSF during the subsequent fourth cycle of chemotherapy would typify "secondary prophylaxis." In a sense, the randomized studies of EPO could also be considered studies of "secondary prophylaxis". This has been the least-studied area of CSF use in rigorously designed randomized studies.

Randomized Studies of G-CSF or GM-CSF as Primary Prophylaxis. Both G-CSF [11,12, 21,22] and GM-CSF [12, 23] have been documented to improve certain clinical outcomes in prospective randomized clinical trials. However, it is important to note that these data from randomized trials may have limited relevance to the routine practice of clinical oncology. For example, for the vast majority of cancer patients treated with cytotoxic therapy, the incidence of severe myelotoxicity with infectious complications does not approach the 60% to 100% incidence noted in the pivotal trials of G-CSF or GM-CSF. Thus, the data may be directly applicable only to the small subset of patients treated with exceptionally myelotoxic regimens and with very high-dose treatments requiring autologous stem cell transplantation. If this limitation were to be overlooked, there might be a tendency to overuse CSF support as primary prophylaxis via an overenthusiastic extrapolation of the randomized data to less myelosuppressive clinical scenarios which would not ordinarily require CSF support. To avoid irresponsible and wasteful use of CSFs, then , it is important to recognize the clinical benefits and to target appropriate utilization to achieve these goals. G-CSF demonstrated the ability to decrease by half the duration of severe neutropenia following aggressive combination chemotherapy. Several measurable clinical benefits tracked along with this accelerated hematopoietic recovery, including a decreased rate of hospital admissions for febrile neutropenia, somewhat decreased duration of hospitalizations for toxicity management, and shortened duration of parenteral antibiotic administration. Although a relatively small trial with differences in survival, this trial was taken to show definitively that the increased levels of circulating neutrophils produced in response to exogenous dosing of recombinant human G-CSF are indeed fully functional effector cells. The limitations of the trials are also clear: these studies gave no indication at all as to the potential for G-CSF to support dose-intensified chemotherapy, and they gave no guidance as to which regimens would be appropriate for CSF support. Nonetheless, the initial USFDA approval of Filgrastim (G-CSF) in February 1991 was remarkably broad in scope, approving the use of G-CSF as an adjunct to myelosuppressive chemotherapies of all types in the treatment plan for virtually any non-myeloid malignancy.

In contrast to the testing of G-CSF with aggressive, but nonetheless standard dose chemotherapy, most of the initial registration data for GM-CSF were generated in the setting of extremely high-dose chemotherapy or chemoradiotherapy with autologous bone marrow transplantation (ABMT). Patients treated with GM-CSF exhibited significantly more rapid leukocyte recovery following ABMT than those who had received placebo. This translated into a more rapid discharge from hospital (on the order of one week earlier than the placebo group) and a lower requirement for parenteral antibiotics in the group receiving adjunctive GM-CSF. Fewer documented infections and fewer fungal infections were noted in the group receiving adjunctive GM-CSF. This study, in addition to much pilot data, led to the USFDA approval of the Sargramostim version of GM-CSF in February 1991. However, based upon the limitations of the pivotal data which applied uniquely to ABMT, the initial U.S. approval was far more limited than the one granted nearly simultaneously for G-CSF, approving GM-CSF only as supportive care for patients with non-myeloid malignancies undergoing ABMT. This lack of approval for the more generalized scenario of "myelosuppressive chemotherapy" without stem cell infusion (just when the USFDA was cracking down on off-label promotion of drugs in cancer medicine) was one early difference in the acceptance of these cytokines by clinical oncologists. This clearly was one variable among many that fostered the market dominance of G-CSF today to accelerate leukocyte recovery post-chemotherapy.

<u>Randomized Studies of EPO in Cancer Patients.</u> As noted earlier, EPO was tested in cancer patients who were already anemic, not in those "at risk" to develop anemia [24]. This more targeted approach in the initial registration strategy also was far less targeted in another dimension: the first randomized trials did not specify any one tumor type or single chemotherapy regimen. Instead, broad entry criteria allowed accrual of anemic cancer patients who reflected the variety of diseases seen in any clinical oncologist's practice. While this is a strength of the initial studies, it is also a weakness: this heterogeneous pool of patients had many co-variables which could muddy the interpretation of data and limited the ability to discern what important effects were due to EPO and what may have been observed by chance alone in this varied group of patients. EPO was shown to diminish the severity of anemia, to modestly decrease the need for red blood cell transfusions, and to improve certain indices associated with patient-reported quality of life [24]. Further nonrandomized community-practice based studies have expanded and confirmed these initial observations [26,27]. These data will be discussed in greater detail elsewhere in this volume.

How to use G-CSF, GM-CSF, and EPO Outside of Clinical Research: Implications for Practice

While the recombinant versions of human G-CSF, GM-CSF, and EPO are impressive examples of technology assessment, development, and commercialization, these molecules present novel and pressing problems for the practice of oncology. These agents do not "treat cancer" *per se*: they are simply mechanisms to improve the supportive care of patients receiving myelotoxic chemotherapy. The budgetary impact of these agents created an immediate need to determine appropriate utilization: these agents used irresponsibly could waste billions of health care dollars. On the other hand, these molecules used responsibly could clearly benefit cancer patients in significant ways. The challenge was for oncology professionals to decide based on data how best to use these new tools of supportive care. In an effort to address these thorny issues head-on, the American Society of Clinical Oncology (ASCO) embarked upon its first-ever venture into the development of evidence-based clinical practice guidelines. An *ad hoc* expert panel was convened to dissect the research literature on hematopoietic cytokines and to make reasonable judgements about appropriate guidelines for use. These guidelines have been published [28] and updated regularly [29]. To disseminate the information, the guidelines are even available on-line at the Internet Web Site of ASCO (www.asco.org). Rather than repeat these in detail, it would be better to seek out the primary source guidelines for full information. However, in brief, the guidelines were formulated to answer specific questions in practice and to focus efforts on where additional clinical research data might help to guide practice. For example, sample questions regarding optimal use of CSFs included the following:

• **Which Cancer Patients Should Receive Hematopoietic Cytokines as Supportive Care?** The optimal strategy for use of hematopoietic cytokines remains open to discussion. Certainly, one should scoff at the routine use of CSFs as primary prophylaxis in <u>all</u> patients with non-myeloid malignancies treated with any myelosuppressive chemotherapy. Although this broad definition would technically be covered under the USFDA-approved indication for G-CSF, such universal use would clearly represent wasteful and inappropriate use of an expensive agent. The vast majority of cancer patients do not receive chemotherapy that is sufficiently myelosuppressive to induce a high risk for clinical complications. For example, the vast majority of patients receiving adjuvant CMF (cyclophosphamide, methotrexate, 5-fluorouracil) or 5-FU/leucovorin chemotherapy for breast or colon cancer, respectively, do not experience clinically relevant infectious complications. For such patients, the routine use of CSF support as "primary prophylaxis" would likely be overtreatment. On the other hand, in selected high-risk patients, the judicious use of CSF support might truly be appropriate and clinically beneficial. The efficacy of CSF support in high-risk populations (e.g. the very elderly, patients with severe co-morbid disease, etc.) requires further study, but was judged appropriate by the ASCO Guidelines Committee. It is also important to note that there remains a large element of clinical judgement even with evidence-based medical guidelines. How much risk of infectious complications is "sufficient" to justify use of CSF support? For economic reasons, this risk level has been set at approximately 40% [30]. However, there may be risk-averse patients for whom a willingness-to-pay analysis might show that a 25% risk would be sufficient to use CSF support. More data are clearly needed to set these levels more accurately. However, since many commonly-used chemotherapy regimens have <10% chance of inducing severe toxicities, it has been acceptable to use primary prophylaxis in relatively few clinical scenarios outside of clinical research trials (e.g. curative-intent aggressive chemotherapy).

• **Should One Use Secondary Prophylaxis with CSF Support or Dose Reduction?** Secondary prophylaxis represents one reasonable strategy for limiting irresponsible CSF use, since the patient population would be selected on the basis of clinical parameters (i.e. prior poor tolerance of chemotherapy) and would represent a more restricted subset than a universally-applied "primary prophylaxis" approach. Many skeptics are quick to note that chemotherapy was given safely for many years without CSF support simply by reducing doses if unacceptable toxicities had been induced. Many lines of evidence, though, support the notion of minimal "dose thresholds" to achieve optimal anticancer effects from chemotherapy [e.g. 7]. Thus, dose reduction may interfere with the oncologist's ability to induce durable remissions or obtain the most benefits from adjuvant chemotherapy. Given the evidence supporting dose thresholds in diseases such as breast cancer, it is unlikely that significant dose reductions would ever be viewed as superior to dose maintenance with CSF support. Nonetheless, for purely palliative care, it is still reasonable to question the universal use of CSF support for secondary prophylaxis, and for research to objectively demonstrate the benefits of such CSF support.

- **Should CSF Support be used to Intensify Chemotherapy Dosing Beyond Conventional Levels?** Nearly all clinical trials have demonstrated an increased ability of patients to tolerate higher "dose intensities" of chemotherapy with equivalent toxicities if adjunctive CSF support is utilized. This can be achieved by increasing the chemotherapy doses administered ("dose intensification"), increasing the frequency of chemotherapy administration ("schedule-based intensification"), or both ("dose-dense administration"). This leads to the obvious question: how clinically significant are such increases in dose or schedule intensity? Do patients really do better by measurable and quantifiable criteria if they are treated intensively than if they receive the same drugs in a somewhat less intensive manner? The controversy surrounding dose intensity has generated fervor of a near-religious fanaticism. However, data tends to quiet unsubstantiated beliefs, and the next few years should bring maturation of many randomized clinical trials to test these hypotheses. As noted above, most data support the hypothesis that a certain threshold of chemotherapy dose must be attained to achieve optimal clinical anticancer efficacy. This is supported, for example, by the large randomized study performed by the Cancer and Leukemia Group B in patients with early breast cancer [7]. Several thoughtful reviews have come to the conclusions of the ASCO Guidelines Committee: dose- or schedule-based intensification of chemotherapy should be undertaken only in the context of clinical research trials [8,9]. Additional well-designed trials are required to prove that important clinical outcomes are improved by the administration of higher-than-standard doses of chemotherapy. This is particularly important in this era of new therapeutics (e.g. navelbine, gemcytabine) which are significantly less myelotoxic than the older cytotoxic agents of the 1980's.

- **What is the Optimal Dose and Schedule of CSF Administration?** G-CSF, GM-CSF, and EPO, like many biotherapeutic agents, present interesting problems which diverge from the traditional path of cytotoxic drug development in oncology. For example, these agents are highly active over a wide dose range. There may not be significantly increased clinical efficacy at higher doses, and a reasonably bioactive dose may not be synonymous with the maximal tolerated dose. More research is required to define more specifically the CSF dose/response curve and the relevance of CSF schedule of administration to clinical outcome. Early pilot studies which evaluated differences between CSF doses or schedules were terribly underpowered to detect differences due to the inclusion of very small numbers of patients in different dosing cohorts [31-33]. Clinically important questions remain regarding the schedule of CSF administration, such as whether the initiation of CSF dosing can be delayed a few days in a chemotherapy cycle or whether the CSF can be stopped earlier in the cycle. Although these issues may seem trivial, the answers would have an enormous impact upon CSF use in routine practice and will be relevant to analyses of cost-effectiveness.

● Is the Therapeutic Use of CSFs Indicated in any Patients? As defined earlier, the "therapeutic use" of hematopoietic cytokines represents the administration of these agents to treat some active problem, not to prevent problems at risk of developing. The "therapeutic" use of G-CSF alongside empiric antibiotics for patients with febrile neutropenia is widely used in the routine practice of oncology although there are relatively few objective research data to justify the use in that setting. In the modern era of routine, broad-spectrum parenteral antibiotics, mortality from febrile neutropenia is quite rare. Most studies have shown that the therapeutic use of G-CSF can modestly decrease the time to recovery from severe neutropenia by approximately 1 day [25]. However, this improvement in hematologic recovery does not consistently lead to a significant decrease in the lengths of hospital stays in this patient population. Further research will be required to decide whether the costs of "therapeutic" CSF administration as adjuncts to standard antibiotics in the setting of acute infectious complications from chemotherapy justify this application. Prospective randomized data have shown that there is no indication whatsoever for the "therapeutic" use of G-CSF in patients with uncomplicated (afebrile) neutropenia [34].

● Should CSFs be used to Support the Cytotoxic Therapy of Patients with Leukemia? Although much concern has been raised about the potentially dangerous effects of CSFs to stimulate the proliferation of myeloid leukemia cells, randomized trials have not shown this to be clinically relevant [35-37]. This will be discussed in more detailed in a later chapter in this volume. However, the use of CSFs to support the intensive myelotoxic chemotherapy of leukemia has been one of the first "label expansions" for these agents based on the strength of more recent clinical trial data.

● How to Combine Hematopoietic Cytokines active on other cell lineages besides leukocytes? This is an area of intensive investigation. Currently, the only other USFDA approved hematopoietic cytokines are recombinant human EPO and the thrombopoietic cytokine Interleukin-11 (IL-11). Given the difficulty in identifying patients who should receive G-CSF to support levels of leukocytes, it is clear that the task is magnified significantly when other hematologic cell lineages are taken into account. For EPO and IL-11, the task is made more difficult because transfusion of blood components (red blood cells and platelets, respectively) represents a standard "substitute service" for the cytokine support. For EPO, the potential to improve patient-assessed quality of life is a novel therapeutic goal [26,27]. Most oncologists are still wary of trying to guide practice from quality of life research, and the use of EPO has not been addressed in the ASCO Clinical Practice Guidelines. This will clearly be an area in rapid evolution over the next several years.

Summary – Responsible Utilization of Hematopoietic Cytokines in Clinical Oncology

This is an era of enormous promise in cancer medicine. New technologies are being translated into useful therapeutics with striking speed. The development of hematopoietic cytokines offers lessons from success. There is no question that these agents can stimulate host hematopoiesis, and that this stimulation of blood cell production can have clinically beneficial consequences. However, because of the costs involved, the appropriate use of hematopoietic cytokines remains a subject of intense discussion, controversy, and investigation. Much of the utility of the leukocyte-stimulating agents (G-CSF and GM-CSF) is tied to the delivery of highly myelosuppressive chemotherapy. If a patient is at high risk from a severely myelosuppressive regimen, these agents certainly have a proven track record of diminishing the risks and accelerating the expected hematologic recovery as primary prophylaxis. As will be discussed elsewhere in this volume, for very-high-dose stem cell-supported therapies, all would agree that the hematopoietic stimulation offered by G-CSF or GM-CSF is not only effective but also cost-effective. For less myelotoxic scenarios involving conventional chemotherapy, however, it may be most prudent to hold CSF support for the more selected subset of patients with significant co-morbidity or for those who have previously suffered a clinical complication of therapy ("secondary prophylaxis"). This strategy may well decrease the costs of CSF use in general while maximizing the benefits to selected and appropriate patients. Dose intensification requiring CSF support remains an area of clinical investigation. Until such trials provide proof that clinical outcomes are improved by dose-intensified chemotherapy, less toxic chemotherapy should remain the standard of care outside of a research setting. Decisions regarding the use of EPO are far more complicated, since improvements in patient-reported quality of life may be difficult to model across broad patient and cultural groups. The field of hematopoietic supportive care is changing constantly, and clinicians need to stay current with the research literature to make rational prescribing decisions. Patients will best be served by an evidence-based decision-making process which takes into account medical appropriateness, the effectiveness of these agents, as well as the complexity and variety of situations encountered by medical oncologists and hematologists in clinical practice.

References

1. Bodey GP, Buckley M, Sathe YS,Freireich E: Quantitative relationship between circulating leukocytes and infections in patients with acute leukemia. Ann Intern Med 64: 328-340, 1966
2. Gaydos LA, Freireich EJ, Mantel N, et al: The quantitative relation between platelet count and hemorrhage in patients with acute leukemia. N Engl J Med 266: 905, 1962
3. Hersh EM, Bodey GP, Niles BA,Freireich EJ: Causes of death in acute leukemia - a ten year study of 414 patients from 1954-1963. JAMA 193: 99, 1965
4. Frei III E,Canellos GP: Dose: a critical factor in cancer chemotherapy. Am J Medicine 69: 585-594, 1980
5. Henderson I, DF H,Gelman R: Dose-response in the treatment of breast cancer: a critical review. J Clin Oncol 6: 1501-1515, 1988
6. Hryniuk W,Bush H: The importance of dose intensity in chemotherapy of metastatic breast cancer.

J Clin Oncol 2: 1281-1288, 1984

7. Wood WC, Budman DR, Korzun AH, et al. Dose and dose intensity of adjuvant chemotherapy fo stage II, node-positive breast carcinoma. N Engl J Med 330: 1253-1257, 1994.

8. Siu LL and Tannock IF: Chemotherapy dose escalation: Case Unprõven (editorial). J Clin Oncol 15: 2765-2768, 1997

9. Savarese DMF, Hsieh CC, Stewart FM: Clinical Impact of Chemotherapy Dose Escalation in Patients With Hematologic Malignancies and Solid Tumors. J Clin Oncol 15:2981-2995, 1997.

10. Moore MAS: Clinical implications of positive and negative hematopoietic stem cell regulators. Blood 78: 1-19, 1991

11. Demetri GD,Griffin JD: Granulocyte colony-stimulating factor and its receptor. Blood 78: 2791-2808, 1991

12. Lieschke GJ,Burgess AW: Granulocyte colony-stimulating factor and granulocyte-macrophage colony-stimulating factor (parts I and II). New Engl J Med 327: 28-35, 99-106, 1992

13. Metcalf D: Hematopoietic Regulators: Redundancy or Subtlety? Blood 82: 3515-3523, 1993

14. Groopman JE, Mitsuyasu RT, DeLeo MJ, et al: Effect of recombinant human granulocyte-macrophage colony-stimulating factor on myelopoiesis in the acquired immunodeficiency syndrome. N Engl J Med 317: 593-8, 1987

15. Antman K, Griffin J, Elias A, et al: Effect of recombinant human granulocyte-macrophage colony-stimulating factor on chemotherapy-induced myelosuppression. N Engl J Med 319: 593-598, 1988

16. Gabrilove JL, Jakubowski A, Fain K, et al: Phase I study of granulocyte colony-stimulating factor in patients with transitional cell carcinoma of the urothelium._. J Clin Invest 82: 1454-61, 1988

17. Morstyn G, Campbell L, Souza LM, et al: Effect of granulocyte colony stimulating factor on neutropenia induced by cytotoxic chemotherapy. Lancet 1: 667-72, 1988

18. Vadhan-Raj S, Keating M, LeMaistre A, et al: Effects of recombinant human granulocyte-macrophage colony-stimulating factor in patients with myelodysplastic syndromes. N Engl J Med 317: 1545-1552, 1987

19. Vadhan-Raj S, Buescher S, Broxmeyer HE, et al: Stimulation of myelopoiesis in patients with aplastic anemia by recombinant human granulocyte-macrophage colony-stimulating factor. N Engl J Med 319: 1628-34, 1988

20. Negrin RS, Haeuber DH, Nagler A, et al: Treatment of myelodysplastic syndromes with recombinant human granulocyte colony-stimulating factor. A phase I-II trial. Ann Intern Med 110: 976-84, 1989

21. Crawford J, Ozer H, Stoller R, et al: Reduction by granulocyte colony-stimulating factor of fever and neutropenia induced by chemotherapy in patients with small-cell lung cancer. N Engl J Med 325: 164-170, 1991

22. Trillet-Lenoir V, Green J, Manegold C, et al: Recombinant granulocyte colony stimulating factor reduces the infectious complications of cytotoxic chemotherapy. Eur J Cancer 29A: 319-324, 1993

23. Nemunaitis J, Rabinowe SN, Singer JW, et al: Recombinant granulocyte-macrophage colony-stimulating factor after autologous bone marrow transplantation for lymphopid cancer. N Engl J Med 324: 1773-1778, 1991

24. Abels R: Erythropoietin for anaemia in cancer patients. Eur J Cancer 29A: S2-S8, 1993 (suppl 2)

25. Maher D, Green M, Bishop J, et al: Filgrastim in patients with chemotherapy-induced febrile neutropenia. A double-blind, placebo-controlled trial. Ann Intern Med 121: 492-501, 1994.

26. Glaspy J, Bukowski R, Steinberg D, et al: Impact of therapy with epoetin alfa on clinical outcomes in patients with nonmyeloid malignancies during cancer chemotherapy in community oncology practice. J Clin Oncol 15:1218-1234, 1997

27. Demetri GD, Kris M, Wade J, et al: Quality-of-Life Benefit in Chemotherapy Patients Treated with Epoetin Alfa is Independent of Disease Response or Tumor Type: Results From a Prospective Community Oncology Study. J Clin Oncol (1998, in press)

28. ASCO Ad Hoc Committee on Hematopoietic Growth Factors: American Society of Clinical Oncology Recommendations for the Use of Hematopoietic Colony-Stimulating Factors: Evidence-Based, Practice Guidelines. J Clin Oncol 12:2471-2508, 1994.

29. ASCO Ad Hoc Committee on Hematopoietic Growth Factors: Update of Recommendations for the Use of Hematopoietic Colony-Stimulating Factors: Evidence-Based, Clinical Practice Guidelines J Clin Oncol 16: 1957-1960, 1996.

30. Lyman GH, Lyman CG, Sanderson RA,Balducci L: Decision analysis of hematopoietic growth factor use in patients receiving cancer chemotherapy. J Natl Cancer Inst USA 85: 488-493, 1993

31. Morstyn G, Campbell L, Lieschke G, et al: Treatment of chemotherapy-induced neutropenia by subcutaneously administered granulocyte colony-stimulating factor with optimization of dose and

duration of therapy. J Clin Oncol   7: 1554-62, 1989

32. Gianni A, Bregni M, Siena S, et al: Recombinant human granulocyte-macrophage colony-stimulating factor reduces hematologic toxicity and widens clinical applicability of high-dose cyclophosphamide treatment in breast cancer and non-Hodgkin's lymphoma. J Clin Oncol 8: 768-778, 1990

33. Neidhart JA, Mangalik A, Stidley CA, et al: Dosing regimen of granulocyte-macrophage colony-stimulating factor to support dose-intensive chemotherapy. J Clin Oncol 10: 1460-1469, 1992

34. Hartmann LC, Tschetter LK, Habermann TM, et al: Granulocyte colony-stimulating factor in severe chemotherapy-induced afebrile neutropenia. N Engl J Med 336:1776-1780, 1997

35. Rowe JM, Anderson JW, Mazza JJ, et al. A randomized placebo-controlled Phase III study of granulocyte-macrophage colony-stimulating factor in adult patients (> 55 to 70 years of age) with acute myelogenous leukemia: a study of the Eastern Cooperative Oncology Group (E1490). Blood 86:457-462, 1995.

36. Stone RM, Berg DT, George SL, et al. Granulocyte-macrophage colony-stimulating factor after initial chemotherapy for elderly patients with primary acute myelogenous leukemia. N Engl J Med 332:1671-1677, 1995.

37. Dombret H, Chastang C, Fenaux P, et al. A controlled study of recombinant human granulocyte colony-stimulating factor in elderly patients after treatment for acute myelogenous leukemia. N Engl J Med 332:1678-1683, 1995.

7. Economic, Public Health, and Policy Implications of Hematopoietic Growth Factors, High-dose Chemotherapy, and Stem Cell Rescue

Charles L. Bennett, Tammy J. Stinson

Introduction

The use of hematopoietic growth factors (HGF) and high dose therapy with stem cell transplant (SCT) are two relatively new weapons in the battle against cancer that have gained widespread acceptance among oncologists in the United States and abroad. HGFs, granulocyte colony-stimulating factor (G-CSF) and granulocyte-macrophage colony-stimulating factor (GM-CSF), have been shown to reduce the time to hematopoietic recovery following myelosuppressive chemotherapy and SCT for both solid tumors and hematopoietic malignancies. These new technologies have improved patient outcomes, but are also relatively costly. Their development has resulted in a myriad of economic, public health, and policy concerns related to costs, regulation, legislation, and access to care.

In an era of health care reform, cost-effectiveness of medical therapies are under intense scrutiny by policy makers, insurers, and patients.[1-7] It is no longer true that a therapy will be accepted if it can provide some benefit over therapies without taking into consideration the costs of the therapies. Medical technologies must not only produce improvements in survival and/or quality of life, but they must also do so at a cost that is considered affordable. In other words, medical therapies such as HGFs and SCT must prove to be both effective and cost-effective.

As physicians and health policy makers, we must be able to evaluate the cost-effectiveness of medical therapies. To address these questions, it is important to analyze the following determinants: costs; benefits; cost-effectiveness; cost-reduction methods; and health care decision making, comparing alternatives in therapies based on cost-effectiveness. In this chapter, we will outline some of the basic principles used by researchers to evaluate the costs of medical technologies. Then we will discuss the current literature on costs and cost-effectiveness of HGFs and HGFs for SCT.

Some Basic Principles of Cost and Cost-Effectiveness Analyses

<u>Types of Costs</u>. The costs of therapy are generally divided into direct, medical indirect and indirect costs. Direct costs reflect medical care given during the episode of illness and include physician fees, hospital charges, medications, blood products, etc.[8] Medical indirect costs include out of pocket costs borne by the patient and their family during the treatment and recovery period, such as travel to and from the hospital or clinic, lodging, food, domestic help required while the patient is recovering (baby-sitting, house cleaning, yard work), and insurance deductibles. The final category are indirect costs borne by society, such as the loss of productivity from the patient and

their care giver. Many of the studies discussed in this chapter concentrate on direct costs, which are the costs from the perspective of the third party payer. This information is the easiest to measure with the best developed methodologies. Studies that report information that include indirect costs include the perspective of the patient and/or society. These type of analyses have become important as more oncology treatment moves to the outpatient setting.

Types of Analyses. There are different methodologies for given situations in cost analyses. The two most commonly published are "cost minimization" and "cost effectiveness". A cost minimization analysis measures the incremental cost difference between two agents or procedures that have essentially the same effectiveness. In this type of analysis the focus is on differences in drug administration costs and costs associated with treatment and diagnosis of adverse events. Many studies published on the cost of HGFs are of this type, as conclusive evidence of improvement in survival has not been demonstrated. A cost effectiveness analysis divides the incremental cost difference by the incremental survival difference. The incremental cost of the experimental treatment is reported in units of "cost per life year gained" ($/LYG). The LYG data may be "quality adjusted" in order to account for differences in quality of life between treatment arms. This is accomplished by evaluating "utilities". This methodology measures the quality of life for a patient with a particular health state and quantitates it, by attaching a value from 0 to 1 for the quality of life for a year spent in a given health state (1 being perfect health and 0 being death). This value is then multiplied by the years of survival to determine the "quality adjusted life years" (QALY). This type of analysis is typically conducted for a new therapy that has been proven to provide a significant survival advantage in comparison to standard therapy.

Costs Associated with the Treatment of Neutropenia

Patients with neutropenia require specialized care to prevent infectious complications. A number of specific resource areas related to this care are investigated in analyses of the costs. Most studies demonstrating a benefit to the use of HGFs report shorter hospitalization times for patients receiving cancer therapy in conjunction with G-CSF or GM-CSF. Since the cost of hospitalization for these patients often requires intensive care facilities at a room rate of $700-$1400 per day, shortened hospitalization times can lead to significantly lower costs.[9] Also of interest in these economic studies are pharmaceutical costs. This includes the cost of the HGF and its administration costs, the costs of antibiotics or antifungals to treat infection, and the cost of intravenous fluids and drugs to treat adverse events. A third type of resource investigated is diagnostic services, such as laboratory tests and radiologic examinations to diagnose and monitor neutropenia or infection. In the transplant setting the use of blood products, red blood cell or platelet transfusions, are also noted in cost analyses. Each of these types of resources are monitored in cost studies of HGFs and when shown to be decreased in the G-CSF or GM-CSF arm of the study can lead to lower overall costs. But the cost of HGFs can be high, as high as $400 per day plus administration costs, and outweigh savings seen in other areas of supportive care if they are not significant enough.[9]

The Use of Clinical Trial Data

The use of data from phase III clinical trials offers several advantages to an economic analysis.[10] Patients are accrued from multiple sites, randomized to treatment arms and treated on highly-defined protocols which provide well-balanced comparative groups with limited confounding factors. Clinical data, which often coincides or correlates to resource utilization data, are collected prospectively and thoroughly on specifically designed case report forms or treatment flow sheets. Clinical endpoints are evaluated at a centralized statistical facility by personnel with strong epidemiologic backgrounds. Portions of the information from clinical statistical reports (e.g., hospital days, days of fever) can also be useful in calculating costs of treatment.[10]

While there are advantages to utilizing these data, the clinical trial setting is an artificial environment that may not reflect routine clinical practice. Depending upon the study, the population may not be generalizable due to strict inclusion criteria; patients generally have better outcomes and survival than nontrial patients whether they receive control or treatment due to trial eligibility (often times only patients with good a prognosis are included, i.e. early stage disease or those with limiting confounding disease); a disproportionate number of physicians who participate are from academic institutions with potentially greater access to high tech facilities and highly-trained, multidisciplinary staff; patients are monitored more closely for adverse events and compliance as part of a highly defined protocol, and similarly, the staff may manage these patients with extra caution because of the new trial drug than they may once treatment is established; costs to treat toxicity are higher until physicians have enough experience with side effects to treat them efficiently; new agents are expensive until they become routinely used or added to formularies where they can be purchased in bulk.[11]

Cost Analyses of Hematopoietic Growth Factors

It has been well established that HGFs shorten the recovery time of patients prone to neutropenia from myelosuppressive therapy and those undergoing high dose therapy and SCT. Consequences of shortened recovery times have included shorter hospitalizations, fewer documented infections and a decreased use of supportive agents, such as antibiotics. Yet the high cost of these agents has led to the conclusion that their use is most cost-effective when the expected risk of neutropenic fever is >40%. [12,13] This has led to several investigations as to which clinical applications show reductions in resource use that lead to lower overall costs of care. Specific examples in particular clinical settings are discussed in the following.

Growth Factors for Myelosuppressive Chemotherapy in Pediatric Oncology

The costs of HGF use for the prophylaxis of neutropenia associated with chemotherapy in pediatric oncology has been analyzed by a number of investigators. One report in the literature found a cost savings for G-CSF use in the pediatric setting . Riikonen, et al, demonstrated a $1,033 savings per chemotherapy cycle for 16 pediatric cancer patients (mainly hematologic malignancies).[14] While two other reports have found that the costs of G-CSF use break even, i.e. the cost of G-CSF offsets any benefits from lower resource use. Pui, et al, reported shorter hospital stays and fewer documented infections in pediatric patients with acute lymphoblastic leukemia who received G-CSF during induction versus those who received placebo. [15] Despite these clinical improvements the median costs of supportive care were similar, $8,678 for the G-CSF arm and $8,616 for the placebo arm. Pajeau et al, in a study of the costs of G-CSF for prevention of neutropenia during induction and maintenance therapy for T-cell leukemia and advanced lymphoblastic lymphoma determined a cost difference of $34,190 for G-CSF versus $28,653 for no G-CSF from a Pediatric Oncology Group clinical trial.[16] There was no overall costs savings from the use of G-CSF despite the fewer days of hospitalization and lesser use of antibiotics in the G-CSF arm. Clearly the use of growth factors, while seeming to provide some clinical benefit for pediatric lymphoma and leukemia, requires further investigation and optimization.

Growth Factors for Elderly Patients Treated for Hematologic Malignancies

Because considerable morbidity and mortality and large medical costs are associated with chemotherapy for older patients with acute myeloid leukemia (AML) and non-Hodgkin's lymphoma (NHL), studies have investigated the economic impact of the prophylactic use of HGFs on the total costs of treatment for these patients. A study by Bennett, et al based on an Eastern Cooperative Oncology Group trial comparing GM-CSF to placebo administered to elderly patients receiving intensive induction chemotherapy for AML determined a cost savings of $12,513 per patient.[17] Savings primarily resulted from lower intensive care room, laboratory and radiology costs. In cost-effectiveness study by Woronoff-Lemsi, et al a savings of $9,122 per life year gained was estimated, based on 5 year survival, for the use of GM-CSF compared to placebo for patients >55 –70 years old.[18] In a study of the costs of G-CSF use for elderly patients receiving chemotherapy for NHL, Zagonel et al determined that the total costs of therapy for the G-CSF arm were $13,300 compared to $8,440 for the placebo arm. In this instance the cost of the G-CSF displaced the savings seen due to lower hospitalization and antibiotic therapy costs.[19] The use of HGFs for elderly patients receiving intensive chemotherapy for hematologic malignancies has been well supported clinically, but appears economically to be best indicated for patients with AML.

Growth Factors for Treatment of Therapy-Induced Febrile Neutropenia

Studies investigating the use of HGFs as treatment for patients with chemotherapy-induced febrile neutropenia have shown a reduction in neutrophil recovery, but no reduction in the length of time with fever. Studies have also considered how these outcomes affect costs. Uyl-de Groot, et al found that the total costs of treatment of febrile neutropenia with GM-CSF for patients with hematologic and non-hematologic malignancies were more expensive than placebo, $5,177 versus $4178, respectively.[20] Whereas in a study by Mayordomo, et al, considering both G-CSF or GM-CSF in comparison to standard antibiotic treatment, the use of HGFs resulted in 2 less days hospitalized for neutropenic complications and a cost savings of $1300-1400.[21] In the pediatric setting, Mitchell, et al determined a 20% reduction in treatment costs, mainly due to reductions in hospital stay, for 112 pediatric patients (both hematologic and solid malignancies) receiving G-CSF as treatment for febrile neutropenia.[22] The use of HGFs in established febrile neutropenia has not proven to be as effective as treatment started immediately following chemotherapy and is indicated by the American Society of Clinical Oncology guidelines only for high risk patients.[13] While there appears to be some economic benefit in these few studies, it is generally agreed that starting at-risk patients on HGF therapy 24 hours after completion of chemotherapy is a more cost-effective strategy.

Growth Factors Following Autologous Stem Cell Transplant

HGFs have been shown to reduce the time to hematopoietic recovery for patients receiving high dose therapy and autologous bone marrow transplantation (ABMT), helping to avert serious and/or life threatening infections. Three published studies have investigated the costs and outcomes of HGFs in this setting. Gulati and Bennett analyzed the resource use and costs of 24 Hodgkin's disease patients randomized to receive GM-CSF versus placebo following high dose therapy and autologous bone marrow transplant.[23] The group receiving GM-CSF had significantly lower total in-hospital charges (post bone marrow infusion), $39,800 versus $62,000 for placebo. Cost savings were due lower hospital room, antibiotic, blood product, laboratory and physical therapy costs. A study by Luce et al considered in-hospital costs plus the costs of follow-up treatment to 100 days post-transplant for leukemia and lymphoma patients who received GM-CSF or placebo following high dose therapy and autologous bone marrow transplantation.[24] The total costs (from bone marrow infusion to 100 days post transplant), including any readmissions was $70,300 for the GM-CSF patients versus $82,500 for placebo patients. The savings from GM-CSF use were significantly lower during the hospitalization period, but were not statistically significantly different overall. A third study, a French multi-site study by Souetre et al, measured the cost of G-CSF versus usual care from the time of transplant through 100 days post-SCT for patients with lymphomas.[25] The total cost of treatment was $43,341 with G-CSF versus $44,656 without. The most significant savings were seen in costs for the hospital room and laboratory tests, as well as for post-ABMT hospitalization. As judged from these studies, there is significant cost savings to be gained from the use of HGFs following autologous bone marrow transplant for hematologic disease. But, technology changes rapidly in the field of stem cell transplantation. The benefits of shorter neutrophil recovery and hospitalization gained by HGF use has been quickly surpassed by the use of HGF-stimulated peripheral blood progenitor cells (PBPC), as discussed in the next paragraph.

Growth Factors for Mobilization of Peripheral Blood Progenitor Cells

The use of PBPCs for transplant has clinical and economic advantages over ABMT. During harvest, anesthesia and operating room costs and potential complications are avoided, but often time multiple leukophereses are required to obtain enough cells for transplant. Following transplant, platelet recovery and hospitalization are reduced. Four studies have been published that describe in detail the costs of HGF-stimulated PBPC transplant in comparison to ABMT. Chao et al compared G-CSF mobilized PBPCT to ABMT with post transplant G-CSF and showed a significant difference in total costs in favor of PBPCT (approximate 45% decrease).[26] The majority of the savings were due to cost differences in platelet transfusions and hospital stay. Faucher et al conducted a study in patients with non-Hodgkins lymphoma, Hodgkin's disease or breast cancer comparing the two transplant regimens analyzing costs through 30 days post transplant.[27] PBPCT patients had shorter hospital stays and no readmissions during follow-up. The total cost were $24,140 for the BMT group compared to $19,770 for the PBPCT group, over a 15% cost difference. Uyl de Groot et al conducted a similar study including patients with breast cancer, Hodgkin's disease, non-Hodgkin's lymphoma, germ cell tumors, neuro or medulloblastoma.[28] There was a 7 day difference in hospital stay between the ABMT and PBPCT patients and a reduced use of blood products and G-CSF post transplant. The harvest costs were slightly higher in the PBPCT group, but overall costs were reduced from $32,433 for BMT to $21809 for PBPCT. Savings resulted from decreased hospital stay and lower medication and blood product costs. The most recent study confirming these findings was conducted by Smith et al, comparing PBPCT to ABMT for relapsed Hodgkin's disease and non-Hodgkin's lymphoma.[29] Patients in the PBPCT arm had shorter hospitalization stays and fewer platelet transfusions. The total costs of PBPCT were 23% lower than for ABMT, $45,792 versus $59,314.

Public Health and Policy Implications

The cost of treating cancer in the US has become very high, estimated at $60 billion in 1996.[30] Policy makers and care providers agree that these costs must be contained. Managed care impacts on cancer treatment, cutting costs of care for many patients. The government has renewed interest in legislation regarding reimbursement for Medicare treatment (50-60% of cancer treatment in this country is paid by Medicare).[31] With the increased importance of cost in medicine, pharmaceuticals for supportive care have more of a challenge gaining reimbursement. Strongly favorable conclusions in cost-effectiveness analyses will become increasingly important, while at the same time the scientific quality of these studies will also be more rigorously scrutinized. To date, many of the published studies have been retrospective in nature and compared HGFs to placebo or no treatment. Studies of clinical trials with economics as a prospectively determined endpoint are needed, so that data collection and sample size considerations of the cost component of the study could be incorporated into the research design. Also of importance would be studies that compare HGFs to the next best alternative, which is prophylactic antibiotics (under certain circumstances).

As managed care and Medicare exert more restrictions on providers of cancer care, reimbursement becomes an issue in treatment choices. Currently Medicare patients are limited in the use of HGFs in the outpatient setting, as only those doses administered in the doctors office are reimbursed, resulting in inconvenience to patients and physicians. There is also the potential for disruption in the dosing schedule during the weekend days when the physician's office is not open. A second dilemma currently being worked-out between legislators and oncology representatives is that of reimbursement for outpatient chemotherapy. To date, physicians have been reimbursed for these drugs based on the Average Wholesale Price (AWP). Physicians actually negotiate the price they pay for these drugs with the pharmaceutical companies and often pay significantly less, using the surplus to pay for costs associated with the highly-skilled nurses, assistants and equipment required to administer these therapies. Legislation is currently under review to lower the reimbursement to 95% of the AWP, significantly cutting into what oncologists agree is their already under-funded operating budgets.

Also of importance to policy makers and oncologists when regarding the costs of HGFs is the issue of long-term care. As cure rates rise and survivors live longer, it is important to consider the increased costs of treatment of therapy-related, long-term adverse events and second cancers, as well as the increased productivity and lowered costs incurred by prevention or alleviation of these events. A study of AML patients cured of their disease for three years or longer, showed 74% of patients under 50 years of age working full time. The odds ratio of developing a secondary cancer was 1.70 for all patients, and 1.05 for those under 40 years of age.[32] This represents a significant gain to the public of treating cancer efficiently with limited adverse events. The National Cancer Institute has recently made the investigation of long-term cancer survivors a research focus. The economics of this issue, particularly from a societal perspective, will be a key aspect of this research.

Conclusions

With the substantial current use, and potentially expanding use of growth factors in oncology and their high costs, growth factors have the ability to increase health care costs and pharmacy budgets. But at the same time there is the potential for reduced costs in other areas of cancer treatment, such as hospitalization, antibiotics and blood products, particularly in stem cell transplant, that may reduce the overall costs of treatment in certain clinical settings. The economic assessment of these costs is of essential importance to assure that this valuable technology is utilized optimally. The high costs of cancer care in the US, and the influx of managed care into cancer care have made economic analyses increasingly important in justifying costly new technologies such as HGFs. Issues before policy makers and oncologists when considering the appropriateness of these agents include the quality of cost-effectiveness research available, reimbursement policies and the effects of long-term survivorship.

References

1. McVie JC. Counting costs of care. J Clin Oncol 6: 1529- 1531, 1988.
2. Eisenberg JA. Clinical economics. Ag guide to the economic analysis of clinical practice. JAMA 262: 2879- 2886, 1989.
3. Drummond M, Stoddart G, LaBelle R et al. Health economics: an introduction for clinicians. Ann Intern Med 107: 88- 92, 1987.
4. Smith TJ, Desch CE, Hillner BE. Analysis of economic issues. In High dose cancer therapy: Pharmacology, Hematopoietins, and stem cells. (Antman K, Armitage JO eds). Philadelphia: Williams and Wilkins, 1992.
5. Goddard M, Hutton J. Economic evaluation of trends in cancer therapy: Marginal or average costs.

Int J of Tech Assessment in Health Care. 7: 594- 603, 1991.

6. Wodisnky HB. The costs of caring for cancer patients. J of Palliative Care 8: 24- 27, 1992.

7. Robinson R. Economic evaluation and health care: Costs and cost-minimization analyses. BMJ 307: 726- 728, 1993.

8. Hodgson TA, Meiners MR. Cost-of-illness methodology: a guide to current practices and procedures. Milbank Mem Fund Q 60: 429- 462, 1982.

9. Weber RJ. Pharmacoeconomic issues in the use of GM-CSF for bone marrow transplantation or chemotherapy-induced neutropenia. Clin Ther 15:180-91, 1993.

10. Bennett CL, Westerman IL. Economic Analysis During Phase III Clinical Trials: Who, What, When, Where and Why? Oncol 9(11):1-7, 1995.

11. Fayers PM, Hand DJ. Generalisation from Phase III Clinical Trials: Survival, Quality of Life, and Health Economics. Lancet 350:1025-27, 1997.

12. Lyman GH, Lyman CG, Sanderson RA, et al. Decision analysis of hematopoietic growth factor use in patients receiving cancer chemotherapy. J Natl Cancer Inst 85:488-93, 1993.

13. American Society of Clinical Oncology recommendations for the use of hematopoietic colony-stimulating factors: Evidence based, clinical practice guidelines. J Clin Oncol 12: 2471-2508, 1994.

14. Riikonen P, Rahiala J, Salonvaara M, et al. Prophylactic administration of granulocyte colony-stimulating factor after conventional chemotherapy in children with cancer. Stem Cells 13:289-94, 1995.

15. Pui CH, Boyett JM, Hughes WT, et al. Human granulocyte colony stimulating factor after induction chemotherapy in children with acute lymphoblastic leukemia. N Engl J Med 336:1781-87, 1997.

16. Pajeau TS, Lane D, Bennett CL, et al. Economic Analysis of G-CSF use with Intensive Treatment for Pediatric Lymphoma and T-Cell Leukemia. Blood 90(10) Suppl. 1:316-I.

17. Bennett CL, Golub RM, Waters TM, et al. Economic analyses of phase III cooperative cancer group clinical trials: Are they feasible? Cancer Invest 15:227-36, 1997.

18. Woronoff-Lemsi MC, Demoly P, Arveux P, Ifrah N, Tellier Z, Harousseau JL, Cahn JY, Witz F. Cost-effectiveness analysis of GOELEM SA3, a randomized placebo-controlled protocol of GM-CSF for elderly patients with acute myeloid leukemia. Blood 90(10) Supplement 1:72a, 1997.

19. Zagonel V, Babare R, Merola MC, et al. Cost-benefit of granulocyte colony stimulating factor administration in older patients with non-Hodgkin's lymphoma treated with combination chemotherapy. Ann Oncol 5:127-132, 1994.

20. Uyl-de Groot CA, Vellenga E, de Vries EG, et al. Treatment costs and quality of life with granulocyte-macrophage colony stimulating factor in patients with antineoplastic therapy-related febrile neutropenia. Pharmacoecon 12:351-60, 1997.

21. Mayordomo JI, Rivera F, Diaz-Puente MT, et al. Improving treatment of chemotherapy-induced neutropenic fever by administration of colony-stimulating factors. J Natl Cancer Inst 87:803-08, 1995.

22. Mitchell PLR, Morland B, Stevens MCG, et al. Granuloycyte colony-stimulating factor in established febrile neutropenia: a randomized study of pediatric patients. J Clin Oncol 15(3):1163-70, 1997.

23. Gulati SC, Bennett CL. Granulocyte-macrophage colony-stimulating factor as adjunct therapy in relapsed Hodgkin's disease. Ann Intern Med 116:177-82, 1992.

24. Luce BR, Singer JW, Weschler JM, et al. Recombinant human granulocyte-macrophage colony-stimulating factor after autologous bone marrow transplantation for lymphoid cancer. Pharmacoecon 6:42-48, 1994.

25. Souetre E, Qing W, Penelaud PF. Economic analysis of the use of recombinant human granulocyte colony stimulating factor in autologous bone marrow transplantation. Eur J Cancer 32A:1162-65, 1996.

26. Chao NJ, Schriber JR, Grimes K, et al. Granulocyte colony stimulating factor mobilized peripheral blood progenitor cells accelerate granulocyte and platelet recovery after high-dose chemotherapy. Blood 81:2031, 1993.

27. Faucher C, le Corroller AG, Blaise D, et al. Comparison of G-CSF primed peripheral blood progenitor cells and bone marrow autotransplantation: clinical assessment and cost-effectiveness. Bone Marrow Transplant 14:895-901, 1994.

28. Uyl-de Groot CA, Richel DJ, Rutten FFH. Peripheral blood progenitor cell transplantation mobilized by G-CSF: A less costly alternative to autologous bone marrow transplantation. Eur J Cancer 30A:1631-35, 1994.

29. Smith TJ, Hillner BE, Schmitz N, et al. Economic analysis of a randomized clinical trial to compare filgrastim-mobilized peripheral blood progenitor cell transplantation and autologous bone marrow

transplantation in patients with Hodgkin's and non-Hodgkin's lymphoma. J Clin Oncol 15:5-10, 1997.

30. Rundle RL. Salick pioneers selling cancer care to HMOs. The Wall Street Journal, Monday August 12:B1-B2, 1996.

31. Mortenson LE. Health care policies affecting the treatment of patients with cancer and cancer research. Cancer 74:2204-07, 1994.

32. De Lima M, Strom SS, Keating M, et al. Implications of potential cure in AML: Development of subsequent cancer and return to work. Blood 90:4719-24, 1997.

8. Outpatient Management of Neutropenic Fever: Antibiotics, Growth Factors or Both?

Edward B Rubenstein, Linda S. Elting,
Charlotte C. Sun, Kenneth V.I. Rolston

Introduction

The association of neutropenia and infection in patients with cancer receiving myelosuppressive chemotherapy was established over three decades ago by Bodey et al., who demonstrated that the risk of infection began to increase as the neutrophil count fell below 1000/mm^3 and was greatest at levels below 100/mm^3 (Figure 1) [1]

Figure 1. Episodes of severe infection related to number of circulating neutrophils

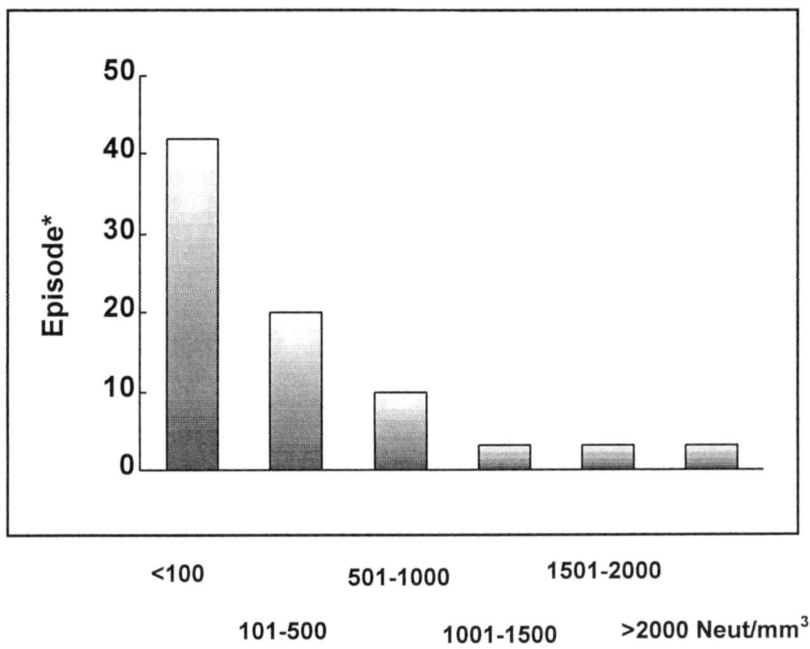

Number of severe infections per 1000 days without severe infection

Infection continues to be a leading cause of morbidity and mortality in patients with febrile neutropenic episodes [2]. However, patients with fever and neutropenia are not a homogenous group; that is, not all such patients have the same risk of developing serious complications or of dying during a febrile episode. This chapter will review the theoretical framework which underpins the concept of risk assessment in patients with febrile neutropenic episodes, summarize the clinical trials which evaluate the management of low risk febrile neutropenic patients, and critically examine whether white cell growth factors are of incremental benefit beyond antibiotics for treatment of febrile neutropenic patients outside the hospital setting.

Risk Assessment in Febrile Neutropenic Patients

Risk assessment implies evaluating certain patient, disease or treatment factors that influence the outcome or course of a patient's illness [3]. Although it has been recognized for some time that risk varies substantially in subsets of febrile neutropenic patients, our ability to predict risk early during the course of a febrile episode has been limited. Before proceeding with a risk assessment strategy there must be an explicit understanding of how risk is defined. In the setting of outpatient management of febrile neutropenic episodes, risk is implicitly understood to be risk of developing major medical complications or of dying during the course of treatment of the febrile event. Patients with a high risk of these "bad" outcomes should be initially managed in the hospital setting so that early intervention can improve these potentially bad outcomes.

Talcott and colleagues were the first to develop a formal statistically-based clinical prediction rule that defined risk groups among febrile neutropenic patients. In a retrospective study of 261 patients at the Dana Farber Cancer Institute, they derived a model which identified outcomes of patients with febrile neutropenia [4]. They subsequently validated this model in a prospective study of 444 cancer patients with fever and neutropenia [5]. The model identified the patients' risk of developing serious medical complications or of dying during their hospitalization for febrile neutropenia using clinical information available on the first day of their febrile episode. Talcott's model categorized patients into 4 risk-groups.

Group 1 consisted of patients who were hospitalized when they developed their febrile neutropenic episodes. These were patients with hematologic disorders and those who had undergone bone marrow transplantation. Group 1 patients had substantial morbidity and an overall mortality rate of 13%. Group 2 included outpatients with concurrent comorbidity (hypotension, altered mentation, respiratory failure, uncontrolled bleeding, dehydration, hypercalcemia, cord compression, etc.) who independently required inpatient management. Serious complications occurred in approximately 40% of these patients and the overall mortality in this group was 12%. Group 3 consisted of patients who developed fever and neutropenia as outpatients, had no concurrent comorbidity, but had progressive, uncontrolled cancer. Serious complications occurred in 25% of these patients and 18% died. Patients in Group 4 were clinically stable outpatients who did not have progressive disease. These patients rarely developed serious complications (3%) and in the combined derivation and validation set had no mortality. Table 1 shows the summary data from these 2 studies. Talcott and his colleagues concluded from these 2 studies that perhaps Group 4 patients could be treated with a less intensive approach than the usual standard of care, which has been inpatient intravenous antibiotic therapy for the entire duration of the febrile episode.

Table 1. Clinical outcomes of patients with fever and neutropenia*

	No. Patients	No. Complications (%)	No. Deaths (%)	
Group I	369	85 (23)	48 (13)	
Group II	65	15 (23)	8 (12)	
Group III	55	11 (20)	8 (15)	
Group IV	<u>216</u>	<u>2 (1)</u>	<u>0 (0)</u>	p<0.0001
TOTAL	705	113 (16)	64 (9)	

I - inpatients at the time neutropenia and fever occur; II - outpatients with concurrent
III - outpatients with progressive uncontrolled cancer; IV - clinically stable outpatients
*Modified after Talcott et al. (ref. #4)

Based upon their risk assessment model, Talcott and associates performed a pilot study of early discharge after initial hospitalization for 48 hours, followed by home intravenous antibiotic therapy in low-risk (Group 4) febrile neutropenic patients[6]. They excluded Group 4 patients who had significant infections (bacteremia, pneumonia, urinary tract infection) or were older than 65 years of age. Eligible patients received standard intravenous antibiotics in the hospital. The initial regimens used were either mezlocillin plus gentamicin, or ceftazidime as a single agent. Modifications were made as needed by the patients' primary physicians. After two days of in-hospital observation, stable patients were enrolled in the early discharge phase of the study. After discharge, patients were evaluated daily at home by a nurse who examined them for new signs and symptoms of infection and for the development of adverse effects. Patients were readmitted at the discretion of treating physicians, or when a complication occurred. Patients who remained on the study underwent standardized laboratory evaluations, and were examined in the clinic by a physician 2 to 4 days after discharge, and weekly thereafter. The mean duration of neutropenia among the 30 patients treated in this manner was 6 days (however, 5 patients had neutropenia of 13-36 days duration). Only 5 (18%) had clinically documented infections and the rest had FUO. Patients were treated at home for a median of 3.5 days (range 1-24 days). The response rate to the initial regimen was only 53%. Four developed serious medical complications (hypotension, acute renal failure, disseminated fungal infection, coagulase-negative staphylococcal bacteremia) and required prolonged hospitalization after readmission. Five were readmitted for persistent fever, and 5 received additional antibiotics at home.

Although no patients died, the high rate of readmission (30%) and frequent modifications of the initial antibiotic regimen suggest that important prognistic factors may have been omitted from Talcott's clinical prediction rule. In particularly, talcott's rule did not account for one of the most important factors in the outcome of febrile neutropenic episodes, namely, duration of neutropenia. The duration of neutropenia, or (perhaps more accurately) the rate at which the granulocyte count returns, is of overriding importance in determining the complexity of a patient's clinical course following the onset of fever [1, 7-10]. This factor was not included in the model because it is not known until the episode is resolved. A clinical prediction rule of risk for a febrile neutropenic episode must be available early in the course of the episode, preferably in the first 6-24 hours after the onset of fever. Table 2 shows the relationship between the duration of neutropenia and outcomes of febrile episodes

Table 2. Risk groups and medical complications of patients with neutropenia lasting 7 days or less

Patient Group	Neutropenia <7 Days No. Pts. With Complications	%	Neutropenia >7 Days No. Pts. With Complications	%	p
Group I	19/83	23	75/185	41	.006
Group II	9/33	27	5/10	50	.25
Group III	1/15	7	5/14	36	.08
Group IV	2/69	3	3/35	9	.33
All patients (100%)	31/200	16	88/244	36	<0.00001

From Talcott et al.(ref.#5)

in Talcott's validation study [5]. For each subgroup, duration of neutropenia is either statistically significant or shows a trend towards significance (and is only limited in statistical significance by small numbers in the sample sizes). The rate of complications is three-fold higher in Group 4 patients with neutropenia >7 days compared to Group 4 patients with duration of neutropenia < 7 days. In many prospective clinical trials duration of neutropenia and recovery of neutrophil count influences the response to antibiotics and outcome of patients during their febrile episode [7-10,11,12]. The importance of duration of neutropenia as a determinant of outcome in febrile neutropenic events is further highlighted by the following study conducted at the National Cancer Institute.

In 1984, Rubin et al. examined the influence of the duration of neutropenia on outcomes of febrile neutropenic episodes in patients who had fever of undetermined origin (FUO) [13]. Patients with <7 days of neutropenia had response rates to initial antimicrobial therapy of 95%, compared to only 32% in patients with >14 days of neutropenia (p<0.001). These results demonstrated that the duration of neutropenia strongly influenced the requirement for modifications to the initial antibiotic regimen (Table 3). Patients with short durations of neutropenia (defined in this study as < 7 days) also became afebrile much more quickly (2 days vs. 5 days) compared to the group with neutropenia > 14 days (p<0.001).

A large number of prospective, randomized trials of empiric antibiotic therapy in febrile neutropenic patients have also demonstrated significantly better response rates in patients with documented infections in whom recovery from neutropenia occurs, as compared to those with persistent neutropenia [7-12, 14-16]. At greatest risk are patients with hematologic malignancies and recipients of bone marrow transplantation because the duration of severe neutropenia often exceeds 2 weeks in such patients. In contrast, most patients with solid tumors, except those undergoing dose-intensive chemotherapy, have neutropenia lasting less than 7-10 days and are at much lower risk. The depth of neutropenia has also been shown to correlate with an increased frequency of infectious complications, with more bacteremias and pneumonias occurring at an absolute neutrophil count (ANC) <100/mm^3 as reported in the early studies of Bodey et al. [1, 17]. It is important to note that the studies of Bodey [1], Talcott [4-6] and Rubin [13]

Table 3. Outcome of Patients with FUO

	Low Risk Neutropenia <7 Days	Neutropenia 7-14 days	High Risk Neutropenia >14 days
No. episodes	331	166	93
Time to afebrile (days)			
median	2	4	5
range	1-7	1-14	1-30
Recurrent fever (%)	2 (0.6)	7 (4)	35 (38)
Outcome:			
Success without modification (%)	315 (95)	131 (79)	30 (32)
Success with modification (%)	14 (4)	32 (19)	60 (65)
Death (%)	2 (1)	3 (2)	3 (3)

Adapted from Rubin et al (ref. #13).

were conducted before the routine use of myeloid growth factors; therefore, it is not known how modulation of risk factors such as depth and duration of neutropenia by the use of cytokines would have influenced important outcomes such as response rates to antibiotics and survival from serious infections in these reports.

Various other factors increase the risk of developing infection and/or serious complications during a febrile episode. These include severe mucositis [18] induced by intensive chemotherapeutic regimens and damage to the skin by vascular access devices or bone marrow aspiration/biopsies [19]. These impairments in host defenses may serve as important portals of infection for a variety of pathogenic and opportunistic organisms.

Outpatient Antibiotic Therapy for Febrile Neutropenic Patients

Some clinical trials have demonstrated the efficacy of outpatient antibiotic therapy in febrile patients with neutropenia without using risk-adjusted eligibility criteria. In a multicenter trial, 68 episodes of fever and neutropenia in patients with lymphoma were treated with a regimen consisting of oral pefloxacin (400 mg BID) and amoxicillin/clavulanate (500/125 mg TID). These were patients in whom the expected duration of neutropenia was less than 7 days [20]. Patients self-administered these drugs upon development of fever without prior examination by a physician and without initial laboratory evaluation. Patients were expected to contact the study center principal investigator if they were still febrile or otherwise symptomatic after 72 hours of antibiotic therapy. This approach was successful in 59 episodes (87%). Among the 9 failures, 8 responded to hospital-based therapy. One patient with methicillin-susceptible *Staphylococcus aureus* bacteremia died despite therapy with vancomycin plus amikacin. The average duration of neutropenia in these patients was 5 days. This study demonstrated that broad-spectrum, oral antibiotic therapy in patients with relatively short-lived neutropenia was associated with a high response rate and such therapy could be given in an ambulatory/home setting. However the lack of a physical examination and baseline laboratory evaluation along with cultures makes it impossible to accurately perform a prospective risk assessment. The infection-related death may have been preventable if baseline blood cultures were available for directing early modifications of the empiric antibiotic regimen.

In a similar study, Malik and colleagues studied the efficacy of self-administered oral ofloxacin (400 mg BID) for the treatment of low-risk febrile neutropenic patients with nonhematologic malignancies and an expected duration of neutropenia of <1 week [21]. These were patients who either lived too far away from the oncology center or were unable to afford hospital-based therapy. As in the previously described French study, patients instituted oral antibiotics prior to initial contact with a physician. Of the 111 episodes treated on this study, 83% responded to oral ofloxacin outside the hospital environment. Of the 19 patients who did not respond to ofloxacin, two died before they could reach a hospital, and one died in the hospital after prolonged neutropenia and fever. This study provided further evidence that patients with anticipated short duration neutropenia could be managed with oral antibiotics in an outpatient setting. It also adds evidence that patients who live too far from the cancer center are at risk of dying during febrile neutropenic episodes. One of the criteria for successful outpatient management strategies should be to ensure that patients have rapid access to care. It also raises an ethical consideration. Should patients receive myelosuppressive chemotherapy and not have access to the appropriate medical infrastructure for management of expected complications such as febrile neutropenia?

Two prospective randomized clinical trials have been conducted at the University of Texas M. D. Anderson Cancer Center utilizing a different approach. The hypothesis that low-risk febrile neutropenic patients with cancer could be identified and safely and effectively treated in the ambulatory setting was tested in a randomized clinical trial which was initiated more than a decade ago. In what can be considered a pilot study using clinical trials methodology, low-risk febrile neutropenic patients were explicitly defined prior to study. Eligibility criteria for outpatient therapy included: fever which developed outside the hospital setting, patients without comorbidity that otherwise required hospitalization (e.g. hypotension acidosis/respiratory distress, severe electrolyte abnormalities), and patients with normal liver and renal function.

Psychosocial criteria for eligibility for outpatient therapy also included a history of compliance with medical therapy, telephone in the local residence (which had to be within a 30 mile radius of the cancer center), and a willing caregiver to assist with following the treatment protocol.

Patients underwent a standardized evaluation to determine the focus of infection, complete blood and laboratory evaluations, appropriate cultures, and a chest x-ray. Eligible patients were randomized to oral therapy with ciprofloxacin 750 mg plus clindamycin 600 mg every 8 hours or intravenous antibiotics consisting of aztreonam 2 gm plus clindamycin 600 mg every 8 hours.

Patients received their first dose of antibiotics in the emergency center, were observed for 4-6 hours, and discharged to home. Patients randomized to the intravenous regimen were met at home by a nurse from a local home infusion therapy company who connected the patients pre-existing central venous catheter to computerized infusion pumps each containing a 24 hour supply of antibiotic programmed to deliver the appropriate dose every 8 hours. All patients returned to the clinic to see one of two physician investigators (K.R. or E.B.R.) on the next day for evaluation of response to therapy and toxicity. All patients were seen daily either at home by the home infusion therapy nurse (who also performed standardized assessments of the patients on oral antibiotics), or in the clinic by one of the physician investigators.

Eighty-three episodes were evaluated in this trial; 40 on the oral regimen and 43 on the intravenous regimen [22]. Twenty-six percent of patients had hematologic malignancies and 93% were moderately or severely neutropenic (<500 neutrophils/mm^3) when enrolled on the study. Thirty-nine percent had documented infections, of which 88% were microbiologically documented, including bacteremias, urinary tract infections, and other skin/soft tissue infections. If otherwise eligible, patients above 65 years of age were not excluded. Response rates for both regimens were much higher than those obtained in the pilot study by Talcott et al. (Table 4). The

Table 4. Response rate to outpatient antibiotics for treatment of low risk febrile neutropenic episodes

	P.O. Ciprofloxacin plus clindamycin		I.V. Aztreonam plus clindamycin		
Type of episode	Episode	Response	Episode	Response	P value
Documented Infection	16	81%	16	94%	0.60
Fever of undetermined origin	24	92%	27	96%	0.60
Total	40	88%	43	95%	0.25

From Rubenstein et al (ref. #22).

intravenous regimen was associated with a response rate of 95%, and the oral regimen with a response rate of 88% (p = 0.19), giving a combined response rate of 92% for outpatient antibiotic therapy. The oral regimen was associated with unexpected renal toxicity. Combining safety and efficacy, the intravenous regimen was superior. Of the 83 episodes, only 6 required admission to the hospital, 3 for management of renal toxicity and 3 for treatment of persistent fever. There were no infection- related complications such as septic shock and no infection-related deaths among patients on this trial. Only 6 patients in this trial received growth factors (GM-CSF) as part of their prior chemotherapy regimen and there was no apparent difference in safety, efficacy or outcome in the patients who received GM-CSF compared to those who did not receive growth factors.

The high response rates seen with both initial regimens (similar to the rate of low risk patients with FUO reported by Rubin et al. in Table 3) and the low rate of admission (7%) suggested that this model of eligibility for outpatient management accurately defined a low-risk population.

These results were reproduced using the same eligibility criteria in another clinical trial [23]. The intravenous regimen was retained but the oral regimen was changed to ciprofloxacin 500 mg plus amoxacillin/clavulanate 500 mg every 8 hours. Using a similar study design, 179 patients were randomized to either outpatient intravenous antibiotics (91 patients), or outpatient oral antibiotic therapy (88 patients). The median age of the patients in each group was 46 years and the majority had solid tumors, primarily sarcoma and breast cancer. At the time of study entry, 89% of the patients on the intravenous regimen had a neutrophil count <500 per mm^3 compared to 86% for the oral regimen. In this study 40% of the patients were on growth factors at the time of their febrile episode, mostly G-CSF, and there was no improvement in outcome associated with its use.

For all episodes, the intravenous regimen had an 87% response rate compared to 90% for the oral regimen (p > 0.05). There was no major toxicity associated with either regimen and no patients developed septic shock or died from their infections. The duration of therapy was between 6-7 days for both the I.V. and P.O. regimens and the overall duration of neutropenia was <7 days for the majority of patients. Subgroup analysis suggested a trend toward a slightly higher response rate in the patients randomized to the oral regimen who were already on growth factors compared to those who did not receive cytokines. Combined analysis of data from both clinical trials shows that these low risk patients had a bimodal duration of neutropenia. Approximately 85% of the patients had a duration of neutropenia < 7 days; the rest had more prolonged neutropenia with rare patients experiencing neutropenia >2 weeks. There were no statistically significant differences in the response rates, complication rates, or hospitalization rates between these 2 groups, although the numbers of patients evaluated in these studies with prolonged neutropenia were limited. Patients with acute leukemia had a lower response rate to both oral and intravenous antibiotics compared to patients with solid tumors and are no longer considered low risk in our institution. Recently the National Comprehensive Cancer Network (NCCN) developed guidelines for the treatment of febrile neutropenic cancer patients and also excluded patients with acute leukemia from the low risk strata (James Wade, personal communication).

Early Discharge Strategies

In a study at the NCI, febrile neutropenic patients who became afebrile within 72 hours after administration of parenteral antibiotic monotherapy (either ceftazidime or imipenem/cilastatin) were randomized to either continue I.V. antibiotics or to complete their course with oral ciprofloxacin [24]. Patients who were persistently neutropenic and had either FUO or a documented infection were eligible if they were able to take medicine by mouth, had no evidence of organ failure and were hemodynamically stable. Patients who had recovered their granulocyte counts to >500/mm^3 and were to complete a 10-14 day course of therapy for a documented infection were also included.

About half the patients had solid tumors and the mean duration of neutropenia following the 72 hour evaluation period was 10 days in both groups (range 1-37 days).

Of 27 evaluable episodes that were randomized to continue parenteral antibiotics, 24 (89%) were successfully treated without modifications, and 22 of 29 patient episodes (76%) in the oral treatment group completed therapy outside of the hospital without modification. Seven patients who had been discharged on ciprofloxacin required readmission to the hospital for recurrent fever, approximately 3 days after discharge. Six of the seven readmitted patients had no identified source for recurrent fever and one had a culture negative pharyngitis. All patients responded to the reinstitution of their original parenteral antibiotic therapy, with no major complications or deaths.

The high rate of recurrent fever (24%) in the oral ciprofloxacin group may be related to the prolonged duration of neutropenia in this group since selection was not based on expected continued duration of neutropenia. Another possibility is that occult Gram-positive infections accounted for recurrent fever, since ciprofloxacin has weak activity against these organisms, particularly the streptococci.

Recently, another group has explored a similar strategy in febrile neutropenic children who had defervesced on parenteral antibiotics after 72 hours [25]. Patients who had negative blood cultures, were hemodynamically stable and who remained granulocytopenic were treated with the oral combination of cefixime (8mg/kg/day as a single daily dose and cloxacillin (100 mg/kg/day in four divided doses). Of 23 patients treated, the first 12 were observed on oral therapy in the hospital and the remaining 11 patients were followed as outpatients until resolution of granulocytopenia. Median time from switch to oral therapy until recovery of the absolute neutrophil count was 3 days (range 1-10 days). Three patients (13%) had recurrent fever, with negative cultures, and all survived with inpatient treatment.

Bash et al. permitted a change to oral therapy and discharge in 30 persistently neutropenic children with localized infections who had defervesced on initial intravenous antibiotics, as long as they showed signs of impending marrow recovery, e.g. increasing neutrophil, leukocyte and/or platelet counts [26]. Five (16%) of these children required readmission for recurrent fever, but all were stable and responded to the reinstitution of intravenous antibiotics.

These studies suggest that there is a role for the strategy of switching from an initial course of intravenously administered inpatient-based antibiotics to an oral regimen in selected febrile neutropenic patients. Although it has been shown that low risk patients can be safely managed with initial outpatient oral therapy, sequential intravenous-to-oral therapy may be more acceptable for some patients and physicians. Several days of hospital-based therapy provides an opportunity to observe patients and identify those who are at "low risk" for subsequent complications. It also allows for intravenous therapy during the critical period following onset of fever, when some patients may have nausea or mucositis that limits oral intake, or have rapid hemodynamic changes associated with dehydration or sepsis. Early discharge, after this initial observation period and prior to recovery of the absolute neutrophil count, would still decrease the costs and risks associated with a more prolonged hospitalization.

Role of Growth Factors in Established Febrile Neutropenia

Most studies of colony stimulating factors have examined questions of dose intensity[27], evaluated the impact of shortening the duration of neutropenia associated with chemotherapy [28] or studied the prevention of febrile neutropenic events[29,30]. Nevertheless a few studies are available which have been designed to study the added benefit of growth factors in addition to antibiotics in the treatment of febrile neutropenic episodes.

Mayordomo et al. compared the effect of adding granulocyte colony-stimulating factor (G-CSF) or granulocyte-macrophage colony-stimulating factor (GM-CSF) to standard antibiotic therapy in cancer patients with fever and chemotherapy-induced neutropenia [31]. This study involved 121 patients; 39 patients were randomized to the G-CSF arm; 39 to the GM-CSF arm; and 43 to antibiotics alone. The initial empiric antibiotic regimen consisted of ceftazidime 2 gms I.V. every 8 hours plus amikacin 500 mg I.V. every 12 hours. Patients who had documented sites of infection were treated as follows: vancomycin was added for catheter-related infection; for dental, intra-abdominal infections or aspiration pneumonia, imipenem was substituted for ceftazidime. Treatment was initiated within 8 hours of onset of neutropenic fever. Antibiotics were modified if patients had significant positive cultures and remained febrile, new infectious sites were noted after admission, and patients remained persistently febrile. Vancomycin was added if patients had persistent fever and neutropenia for 72 hours; if fever persisted > 7 days then amphotericin B was added. CSF treatment or placebo was stopped as soon as the ANC was > 1000/mm^3 for 2 consecutive days. Antibiotics were discontinued when the patient remained afebrile and had an ANC of >1000 per mm^3 for 2 consecutive days. Patients remained on antibiotics for a minimum of 5 days according to a pre-established policy and patients were not discharged until antibiotics were discontinued.

The primary endpoint was length of hospital stay (LOS), including median hospital stay and risk of prolonged hospitalization. Other endpoints included duration of grade IV neutropenia (<500/mm^3), duration of fever, and cost of therapy (hospitalization, antibiotics due to persistent febrile neutropenia) and the percentage of patients who needed modification of therapy for any reason including toxicity.

Patients with non-leukemic malignancies, [primarily solid tumors including non-Hodgkin's lymphoma (25); breast cancer (23); lung cancer (21) patients; ovarian cancer (15), were treated in a medical oncology ward and their vital signs were monitored every 8 hours; physical exam and CBC were performed every 24 hours; complete blood and urine chemistries (plus cultures, if febrile, every 48 hours). Other tests were conducted as clinically indicated.

Not surprisingly, the mean duration of grade IV neutropenia was significantly shorter in patients who received either CSF (2 days, range 1-6) than in patients on placebo (3 days, range 1-16) (p<.001). The mean duration of neutropenia < 1000/mm^3 was also significantly shorter for patients receiving CSFs compared to placebo. There was no significant difference in the duration of neutropenia < 100/mm^3, with the median number of days for both CSFs (0 days) versus 1 day for patients on antibiotics alone. Both growth factors decreased the proportion of patients with prolonged neutropenia

(ANC of < 1000/mm^3 for > 10 days) compared to the patients who received antibiotics alone (0% vs. 21%) (p<.05).

Duration of fever was not significantly different in the 3 arms of the study. The number of patients who required a change in antibiotics was also not significantly different in 3 groups. Median hospital stay was shorter in patients receiving CSFs compared to placebo, however the data is difficult to interpret given the existence of policies which dictated preexisting standards for continued hospitalization. For patients receiving antibiotics plus G-CSF the median LOS was 5 days (range 5-14), for the antibiotics plus GM-CSF group LOS was 5 days (range 5-10) and for the group receiving antibiotics alone it LOS was 7 days (range 5-34). There were 8 deaths: 4 infection-related and 4 due to tumor progression. All deaths occurred in patients with severe neutropenia and positive blood cultures. CSF-related toxicity was reported as mild.

The authors did not perform a formal cost-effectiveness analysis using accepted methodology since only normative data was used. They only included the assigned cost of hospital days ($500 per day), the cost of G-CSF ($320 per 300 micrograms), the cost of GM-CSF (assumed to be the same as G-CSF) and the cost of antibiotics. No toxicity costs were included.

Although the duration of neutropenia end points were shorter in the groups that received CSFs, there is little, if any, evidence this led to clinical benefit. The shorter duration of hospitalization was simply a function of a protocol policy that required patients to be on antibiotics for 2 consecutive days after their neutrophil count recovered. There is no evidence that this is necessary. Our policy is to discontinue antibiotics when the patient is afebrile for 4 consecutive days regardless of what is happening with the neutrophil count as long as the patient is showing other signs of clinical improvement and has an adequate duration of therapy based upon his/her site of infection [9, 10, 22].

In another study that examined the effects of myeloid growth factors along with antibiotics on outcomes of febrile neutropenic episodes, Maher et al. conducted a multicentered double-blinded randomized clinical trial involving 218 patients over 4 years [32]. Patients with fever, chemotherapy-induced neutropenia and a variety of malignancies (both solid tumor and hematologic) were randomized to receive antibiotics including piperacillin and tobramycin along with G-CSF or antibiotics alone. Patients remained on study until 4 consecutive afebrile days passed and ANC > 500/mm^3 , or until 28 days had passed.

The primary endpoint of the study was the effect of G-CSF on the number of febrile days and days of neutropenia associated with infection treated with antibiotics. Also studied were duration of neutropenia (time to ANC > 500/mm^3 and time to ANC > 1000/mm^3). Other endpoints of interest included time to resolution of fever and development of late fever. Prospectively defined secondary endpoints included LOS and modification of the initial antibiotic regimen.

Of 216 evaluable patients, 109 received G-CSF and 107 received placebo. Seventeen of the G-CSF and 14 of placebo group were removed prior to study completion but were included in the intent-to-treat analysis. Out of these 31 patients, 11 died, 5 were treatment failures, 8 had persistent fever thought to not be caused by infection, 4 patients requested to be removed from the study and 3 were taken off study for unreported technical reasons.

G-CSF significantly reduced the median number of days of neutropenia (ANC<500/mm^3) from 4 to 3 (placebo versus G-CSF respectively) and from 5 to 3 (ANC<1000/mm^3). The median number of days with fever were the same but fewer patients receiving G-CSF had prolonged fever. There was no difference in time to fever resolution , although time to resolution of febrile neutropenia was lower in the group who received G-CSF. No significant differences in LOS were observed, although the trend indicated lower mean days for the G-CSF group. The number of days of treatment and total dose of antibiotics were almost identical in the 2 groups. G-CSF was given for a median of 7 days. There was also no difference in the 2 groups in the number of treatment days, total dose of piperacillin and tobramycin and no difference in use of other I.V. antibiotics.

In subgroup analyses, G-CSF decreased the number of days of neutropenia and accelerated neutrophil recovery regardless of baseline neutrophil count. Statistically significant differences occurred in patients who had moderate and severe neutropenia at baseline. G-CSF resulted in reduction of time to resolution of fever only in patients with baseline ANC <100/mm.^{3} In patients with lymphoma, G-CSF was associated with fewer days of neutropenia, however the number of days of fever and days in the hospital were similar in the 2 groups for this subset of patients. G-CSF did reduce the number of days of fever and hospitalization in patients with solid tumors but this was not statistically significant. In subsets of patients with microbiologically or clinically documented infections, G-CSF reduced the median number of days of neutropenia from 5 to 4 days, (ANC<1000/mm^3). However, no difference was observed in time to fever resolution. In patients with FUO, no statistically significant reduction in number of fever days was observed.

This study was conducted when the standard of care was to assume that all patients had the same risk for outcomes during their febrile episode and inpatient management was the only accepted strategy. Once again a policy that required patients to remain in the hospital until neutropenia resolved most likely accounts for the effect seen with G-CSF on the length of stay endpoint. Time to fever resolution in patients with documented infections was not different suggesting no benefit with G-CSF compared to antibiotics alone. The one subgroup that might benefit is the patient population with expected prolonged duration of neutropenia, a group previously discussed as non-low risk.

Avilés et al. conducted a prospective clinical trial of 119 patients with microbiologically proven infections and severe granulocytopenia after intensive chemotherapy to investigate the effectiveness and toxicity of G-CSF [33]. All patients were treated with amikacin 7.5 mg/kg I.V. every 12 hours and ceftazidime 2 gm I.V. every 8 hours. Patients were randomized to receive antibiotics or antibiotics plus G-CSF. Patients with hematologic malignancies (lymphoma, myeloma or Hodgkin's disease which was previously untreated) treated with intensive chemotherapy during induction phase who had fever, radiographic and microbiological evidence of bacterial infection, and granulocyte count <100/mm^3 in 2 consecutive measurements at 12 hour intervals were enrolled. Patients were eligible for analysis if they had microbiologically documented infection and received the antimicrobial agent and/or G-CSF for a minimum of 3 days.

Response to therapy was classified as improvement (resolution of fever >15 days after cessation of treatment with overall clinical improvement and elimination of infecting organism with no change to antibiotic regimen); failure (persistence of fever or infecting organism > 3 days, requiring modification of antibiotic therapy); or non-evaluable (either infection was unlikely, the patient had a non-bacterial infection or there was a protocol violation). Superinfection rates were also documented as secondary endpoints.

The response rate for bacteremias in the control group patients was 53%, while patients in the G-CSF group had a response rate of 80%. The addition of G-CSF significantly improved granulocyte recovery and G-CSF patients had fewer febrile days and days in the hospital than patients on antibiotics alone. Fifty-two percent of Gram-negative bacterial infections treated with antibiotics alone improved compared to 81% in G-CSF patients (p<0.01). There were no significant differences in response rates for patients with Gram-positive infections. Patients randomized to receive antibiotics alone demonstrated an increased incidence of superinfections (20% vs. 6%) compared to patients who received G-CSF. A total of 20 patients died during the infectious episodes (15 on antibiotics alone, 5 in the G-CSF group). Eleven patients died during the initial episode of infection due to multiorgan failure.

This study is of interest because on first glance it appears to show a major benefit associated with the use of G-CSF in addition to antibiotics for the treatment of documented infections in patients with hematologic diseases who are undergoing intensive induction chemotherapy. The results, however, raise concerns about the similarities of the treatment groups. The overall mortality rate of 25% in the group who received antibiotics without G-CSF is exceptionally high, raising questions about the comorbid conditions or severity of illness of this population at the time of randomization. Furthermore, the median time to defervescence was 11.4 days in this group compared to 6.0 days in the group who received G-CSF, suggesting that there were more complex or tissue-based infections in the group who received antibiotics alone. The data does not allow for separation of pneumonias from urinary tract infections which could explain the overall differences in response and mortality if there were more patients in the antibiotic alone arm who had pneumonia and bacteremia. Pneumonia with bacteremia is a condition with a well-recognized lower response rate to antibiotics that in some studies is associated with mortality rates as high as 40% [34]. In addition, this study does not report responses with the modified regimens, raising questions about the analysis. Nevertheless, if confirmed by other studies, this clinical trial suggests that for serious documented infections in neutropenic patients with hematologic tumors (a non-low risk subset), G-CSF adds benefit above that of antibiotics alone.

Mitchell et al. conducted a double-blind study in which pediatric patients with febrile neutropenia were randomized to receive either G-CSF or placebo in addition to antibiotics [35]. Eligibility criteria included patients < 18 years of age; fever or clinical evidence of sepsis such as rigors or septic shock; and neutropenia (ANC < 500/mm^3). Each patient could be randomized for up to 4 independent febrile events. Patients were randomized to receive either G-CSF or placebo which began within 24 hours of antibiotic therapy.

The primary endpoint was hospital length of stay, defined as from the point of randomization to discharge upon completion of treatment for febrile neutropenia. Febrile neutropenia with FUO was considered resolved when patients were afebrile > 72 hours and ANC > 200/mm^3 in a clinically stable patient. Patients with positive blood cultures were treated for > 7 days with inpatient I.V. antibiotics. Other endpoints included duration of I.V. antibiotic usage, time to afebrile and time to recovery of neutrophil count (ANC of 200/mm^3 and 500/mm^3).

There were 186 febrile episodes (94 G-CSF and 92 placebo) in 112 patients. The median duration of hospital stay was reduced from 7 days to 5 days for patients on placebo compared to G-CSF patients (p=0.04). Febrile neutropenia was successfully treated in all patients, with no readmissions for recurrent sepsis and no deaths. Recurrence of fever occurred in 14% of G-CSF patients and 13% of placebo patients. G-CSF patients had a median of 3 days for recovery of ANC >500/mm^3 while patients receiving antibiotics alone experienced a median of 5 days to recovery of ANC (p=0.02). G-CSF patients required a median of 5 days of antibiotic therapy compared to 6 days for placebo patients (p=.02). However, there was no difference in proportion of patients requiring change to second line antibiotics or amphotericin therapy.

Hospital LOS was the main cost outcome for treatment of febrile neutropenia. Costs were reduced by 29% (a reduction of 2 days) for G-CSF treated patients. Median costs of patients on placebo were $5046 per patient admission as compared to $3604 per G-CSF treated patient admission (p=0.04). Antimicrobial agents were reduced in cost by 27% in patients on G-CSF (p=0.04). Overall costs were reduced by 20% per patient admission, from a median cost of $5169 per patient admission for those in the placebo group to $4147 per patient admission for those in the G-CSF group. Patients with acute lymphocytic leukemia (ALL) who received G-CSF had significantly shorter hospital stays, from a median of 7 days to 5 days (p ≤ .01). Costs were reduced for treatment of febrile neutropenia mainly due to decreased length of hospital stay.

It is difficult to interpret studies like the one summarized above when so many factors influence the length of hospital stay. Antibiotic regimens may be similar in terms of their initial and modified response rates but not in the *speed* with which they induce response rates [36]. In the study reported by Mitchell et al., the antibiotic regimen was set by local policies and could have been gentamicin plus pipracillin plus flucloxacillin or imipenem-cilastatin plus gentamicin. Preliminary reports suggest that patients respond more quickly to carbapenem-based regimens [36]. Time to defervescence can also be influenced the presence or absence of tissue based or complex infections as well as the degree of underlying mucositis [34]. Arbitrary rules such as waiting for the ANC to reach 200/mm^3 may also create additional time in the hospital when there is little evidence to suggest that it is necessary despite its widespread acceptance. Studies that call for early modifications in antibiotic regimens before 72-96 hours may also create delays in response since it is well recognized that some febrile neutropenic patients may not become afebrile until 5 days after starting antibiotics [13]; changing regimens too soon may cause even further delays.

Other studies in non-low risk patients include Annaisie et al.'s trial of antibiotics with or without GM-CSF for patients with fever and anticipated prolonged neutropenia[37]. This was a randomized prospective study to see if GM-CSF would improve response rates to antibiotic therapy and shorten the duration of neutropenia.

Patients were randomized to ticarcillin/clavulanate plus netilmicin (TN) or TN plus GM-CSF. Risk factors such as age, underlying cancer, indwelling central venous catheters, type and site of infection were recorded and evaluated. Patients were monitored for clinical improvement, duration of neutropenia, and toxicity. Patients responding to therapy were treated for a minimum of 7 days or 4 days after resolution of all signs/symptoms of infection, whichever was longer. GM-CSF was begun at 3μg/kg/day, as a 4 hr I.V. infusion.

The primary endpoints were response on day 4 of the presenting febrile episode to the initial regimen and time to neutrophil recovery ($> 1000/mm^3$). Secondary endpoints included: response on day 8, at end of therapy, and at 6 weeks after completion of therapy; incidence and type of side effects; rate and type of superinfection; and mortality. Prospective subgroup analyses included: response according to diagnosis (FUO, documented infection); response according to underlying disease (acute leukemia versus others); response according to organism; response according to neutrophil count and trend; time to defervescence; time to recovery of WBCs (other than neutrophils) and platelets and leukemic progression.

The addition of GM-CSF to antibiotics improved outcome of all febrile episodes in 100 evaluable episodes in 92 patients at day 4 of therapy (p=0.03) and for patients with leukemia (p=0.04), but not for the intent-to-treat population (p>0.05). In documented infections, 96% of 24 episodes responded to TN-GM-CSF, whereas 79% of 33 episodes responded to TN alone (p=0.12). Treatment with TN-GM-CSF was associated with improved outcome over treatment of TN in patients with organ infections (100% vs. 59%, p=0.03) but this subgroup had small numbers of observations. Both arms had similar rates of response for Gram positive and Gram negative infections.

Response to therapy was evaluated in relation to patients' initial neutrophil counts and changes in counts during therapy. In patients with severe neutropenia, response rates were higher among patients on GM-CSF (p=0.06). Outcome was poorer in patients whose neutrophil count did not increase, especially in patients who had severe neutropenia at the beginning of treatment. Most failures occurred in this group of patients. Shorter duration of neutropenia was found in patients who responded to treatment of their fever (median 7 days) than those who did not respond (median 16 days) (p=0.02).

More TN-GM-CSF patients recovered from severe neutropenia, allowing the next cycle of chemotherapy to be given on time(p=0.02). No significant difference was found in median time to increase in neutrophils to $>500/mm^3$ or to increase in other WBCs or in platelets ($>50,000/\mu L$). Leukemic progression was not increased due to GM-CSF.

Eleven evaluable episodes did not respond after 4 days of therapy (2 TN-GM-CSF and 9 TN). Of these, 4 responded to administration of amphotericin B (1 with TN-GM-CSF and 3TN), 1 responded to change in antibiotics after development of drug-related skin rash (TN-GM-CSF), 2 responded to addition of vancomycin (TN) and the remaining 4 (TN) failed to respond to all modifications to therapy due to persistent neutropenia. Median duration of fever was similar in both groups (4 days) and median duration of antibiotic therapy was also similar (p=0.11). There were no significant differences in the median duration of therapy in subgroups of patients with leukemia (p=0.16). No superinfections developed in the TN-GM-CSF group whereas 3 superinfections occurred in the TN group.

Evaluation at 6 weeks after end of therapy showed no significant reduction of subsequent infections between the 2 groups (21 infections after 50 febrile episodes for TN-GM-CSF (42%) vs. 14 infections after 50 febrile episodes for TN patients (28%), p=0.14). Hospital LOS was similar for the 2 groups (9 days TN-GM-CSF vs. 10 days TN) (p=0.19) and side effects were more common in patients who received GM-CSF.

This study failed to show that GM-CSF in addition to antibiotics shortened the overall duration of neutropenia, decreased the superinfection rate, or reduced the mortality rate associated with febrile neutropenic episodes for the entire population. Subgroup analyses did demonstrate benefit which emphasizes the need to prospectively identify these higher risk populations and design clinical trials of sufficient power to address questions of cost-effectiveness. In the setting of febrile neutropenic episodes it has been suggested that cytokines be reserved for patients who are at high risk for septic complications [38]. It will be important to develop these risk models and test their validity for predicting outcomes prior to embarking on clinical trials of growth factors to test their benefit.

Summary and Conclusions

Most of the studies conducted in low-risk patients have not explored the question of whether or not growth factors add benefit above and beyond that of antibiotics. Other studies have clearly shown benefit when growth factors are used in non low-risk settings such as high-dose chemotherapy and stem cell support as reported by Gilbert et al [39]. In this setting, shortening the duration of neutropenia facilitated an outpatient management strategy for a group of patients who otherwise required hospitalization.

It is unlikely that growth factors will prove to be cost-effective if used routinely in an attempt to prevent febrile neutropenic episodes in low-risk patients who are expected to have short durations of neutropenia. Lyman has shown that prophylactic growth factor administration is cost-effective if there is an expected high incidence of febrile neutropenia (>40%) for a prescribed chemotherapy regimen [40]; however, this decision analytic model assumed that all patients would be hospitalized for treatment of their episode and receive intravenous antibiotics a standard of care that is no longer practiced or necessary.

Although in some settings, growth factors can reduce the occurrence of fever during neutropenia, there is currently no proof that they decrease mortality from infection, improve response rates to antibiotics, or improve overall survival. As previously discussed, the notion that myeloid growth factors are cost-effective along with antibiotics for the treatment of febrile neutropenic episodes compared to antibiotics alone because they are associated with fewer days of hospitalization is poorly justified.

The proper approach is to perform a risk assessment at the time of the onset of febrile neutropenia. Low-risk patients (using an accepted model or strategy that has been clinically tested, reproduced, and generalized) should receive their initial treatment in the outpatient setting with oral or intravenous antibiotics (Table 5).

Recently the Multinational Association for Supportive Care in Cancer (MASCC) completed a study which may improve upon our ability to accurately identify patients risk for outcome at the onset of their febrile neutropenic episode. Preliminary data from MASCC's infectious disease study section suggests that a new model is predictive of a subset of low-risk febrile neutropenic patients. The MASCC model incorporates the following variables: clinically stable outpatient, serum creatinine <2mg/dl, no dehydration, normal CXR at presentation and patients with solid tumors or lymphoma [41].

Table 5. Low risk criteria for outpatient management of febrile neutropenic episodes

I. Solid Tumors	*Psychosocial Eligibility*
II. No comorbidity	▸ Live within 30 mile radius
III. Normal liver/renal function	▸ Willing caregiver
IV. No allergy to planned antibiotics	▸ Telephone in residence
V. History of compliance	
VI. No uncontrolled nausea/vomiting (if oral therapy is planned)	

With initial responses to antibiotics in the range of 85-95% and ultimate response rates of >99%, there is little to be gained by the addition of costly agents such as growth factors. It is most likely that growth factors will be useful in non-low-risk patients who have tissue-based or complex infections. These patients are traditionally hospitalized for management with broad spectrum intravenous antibiotics and can be targeted for specific strategies using cytokines and antibiotics to improve response rates. In addition, these strategies will hopefully lower mortality and decrease inpatient resource utilization. As always, well-designed studies in the appropriate, prospectively identified at-risk population are needed.

References

1. Bodey GP, Buckley M, Sathe YS, Freireich EJ. Quantitative relationships between circulating leukocytes and infections in patients with actue leukemia. Ann Intern Med 64:328-339, 1966.

2. Meunier F. "Infections in patients with acute leukemia and lymphoma." In *Principles and Practice of Infectious Diseases*, GL Mandell, RG Douglas Jr., JE Bennett, eds. New York: Churchill Livingstone, 1990.

3. Iezzoni, Lisa , ed. *Risk Adjustment For Measuring Health Care Outcomes*. Ann Arbor, Michigan: Health Administration Press, 1994.

4. Talcott JA, Finberg R, Mayer RJ, Goldman L. The medical course of cancer patients with fever and neutropenia. Arch Intern Med 148:2561-8, 1988

5. Talcott JA, Siegel RD, Finberg R, Goldman L. Risk assessment in cancer patients with fever and neutropenia: a prospective, two-center validation of a prediction rule. J Clin Oncol 10:316-22., 1992

6. Talcott JA, Whalen A, Clark J, et al. Home antibiotic therapy for low-risk cancer patients with fever and neutropenia: a pilot study of 30 patients based on a validated prediction rule. J Clin Oncol

12:107-114, 1994

7. Pizzo PA, Hawthorn JW, Hiemenz J, et al. A randomized trial comparing ceftazidime alone with combination antibiotic therapy in cancer patients with fever and neutropenia. New Engl J Med 315:552-558, 1986

8. Winston DJ, Ho WG, Brucker DA, et al. Controlled trials of double beta-lactam therapy with cefoperazone plus piperacillin in febrile granulocytopenic patients. Am J Med 85(Suppl):21-30, 1988

9. Bodey GP, Fainstein V, Elting LS, et al. Beta-lactam regimens for the febrile neutropenic patient. Cancer 65:9-16, 1990

10. Rolston KV, Berkey P, Bodey GP, et al. A comparison of imipenem to ceftazidime with or without amikacin as empiric therapy in febrile neutropenic patients. Arch Intern Med 152:283-91, 1992

11. Pizzo PA, Robichaud KJ, Gill FA, Witebsky FG. Empiric antibiotic and antifungal therapy for cancer patients with prolonged fever and granulocytopenia. Am J Med 72:101-11, 1982

12. Schimpff S, Satterlee W, Young VM, Serpick A. Empiric therapy with carbenicillin and gentamicin for febrile patients with cancer and granulocytopenia. New Engl J Med 284:1061-1065, 1971

13. Rubin M, Hathorn JW, Pizzo PA. Controversies in the management of febrile neutropenic cancer patients. Cancer Invest 6:167-184, 1988

14. DePauw BE, Dereskinski SC, Feld R, et al. Ceftazidime compared with piperacillin and tobramycin for the empiric treatment of fever in neutropenic patients with cancer: a multicenter randomized trial. Ann Intern Med 120:834-44, 1994.

15. Anaissie E, Fainstein V, Bodey GP, et al. Randomized trial of beta-lactam regimens in febrile neutropenic cancer patients. Am J Med 84:581-589, 1988.

16. Pizzo PA, Robichaud KJ, Gill FA, et al. Duration of empiric antibiotic therapy in granulocytopenic patients with cancer. Am J Med 1979 67:194-200.

17. Bodey GP. Overview of the problem of infections in the immunocompromised host. Am J Med 79 (suppl):56-61, 1985.

18. Rolston KVI, Bodey GP. "Infections in patients with cancer." In *Cancer Medicine*, JF Holland, E Frei, RC Bast, DW Kufe, DL Morton, RR Weichselbaum, eds. Philadelphia, PA: Lea & Febiger, 1993.

19. Schimpff SC. "Infections in cancer patients - diagnosis, prevention, and treatment." In *Principals and Practice of Infectious Diseases*, GL Mandell, JE Bennett, R Dolin, eds. New York: Churchill Livingstone, 1995.

20. Gardembas-Pain M, Desablens B, Sensebe L, et al. Home treatment of febrile neutropenia: an empirical oral antibiotic regimen. Ann Onc 2:485-7, 1991.

21. Malik IA, Khan WA, Aziz Z, Karim M. Self-administered antibiotic therapy for chemotherapy-induced, low-risk febrile neutropenia in patients with nonhematologic neoplasms. Clin Infect Dis 19:522-527, 1994.

22. Rubenstein EB, Rolston K, Benjamin RS, et al. Outpatient treatment of febrile episodes in low-risk neutropenic patients with cancer. Cancer 71(11):3640-3646, 1993 .

23. Rolston KVI, Rubenstein EB, Elting L, et al. Ambulatory management of febrile episodes in low-risk neutropenic patients (abstract 2235). In Programs and Abstracts of the 35th Interscience Conference of Antimicrobial Agents and Chemotherapy 1995, San Francisco, CA, p. 333.

24. Rolston KVI, Rubenstein EB, Freifeld A. Early empiric antibiotic therapy for febrile neutropenia patients at low risk. Infectious Disease Clinics of North America 10(2):223 - 237, 1996.

25. Lau RC, King SM, Richardson SE. Early discharge of pediatric febrile neutropenic cancer patients by substitution of oral for intravenous antibiotics. Pediatric Hem Oncol 11:417-21, 1994.

26. Bash RO, Katz JA, Cash JV, et al. Safety and cost effectiveness of early discharge of relatively low risk children with cancer hospitalized for fever and neutropenia (F/N). In Proceedings American Society Clinical Oncoly 11:381 (abstract), 1992.

27. Pettengell R, Gurney H, Radford JA, et al. Granulocyte colony-stimulating factor to prevent dose-limiting neutropenia in non-Hodgkin's lymphoma: a randomized controlled trial. Blood 80(6):1430-1436, 1992.

28. Gerhartz HH, Stern AC, Wolf-Hornung B, et al. Intervention treatment of established neutropenia with human recombinant granulocyte-macrophage colony-stimulating factor (rhGM-CSF) in patients undergoing cancer chemotherapy. Leukemia Research 17(2):175-185, 1993.

29. Trillet-Lenoir V, Green J, Manegold C, et al. Recombinant granulocyte colony stimulating factor reduces the infectious complications of cytotoxic chemotherapy. Eur J Cancer 29A(3):319-324, 1993.

30. Crawford J, Ozer H, Stoller R, et al. Reduction by granulocyte colony-stimulating factor of fever and neutropenia induced by chemotherapy in patients with small-cell lung cancer. Clin Infect Dis 18(Suppl 2):S189-96, 1994.

31. Mayordomo JI et al. Improving treatment of chemotherapy-induced neutropenic fever by administration of colony-stimulating factors. J Natl Cancer Inst 87:803-808, 1995.

32. Maher DW et al. Filgrastim in patients with chemotherapy-induced febrile neutropenia: a double-blind, placebo-controlled trial. Ann Intern Med 1994 121:492-501, 1995.

33. Avilés A, Guzmán R, García EL, et al. Results of a randomized trial of granulocyte colony-stimulating factor in patients with infection and severe granulocytopenia. Anti-Cancer Drugs 7:392-397, 1996.

34. Elting LS, Rubenstein EB, Rolston KVI, Bodey GP. Outcomes of bacteremia in neutropenic cancer patients: observations from two decades of epidemiologic and clinical trials. Clin Infect Dis 25(2):247-259, 1997.

35. Mitchell PLR, Morland B, Stevens MCG, et al. Granulocyte colony-stimulating factor in established febrile neutropenia: a randomized study of pediatric patients. J Clin Oncol 15(3):1163-1170, 1997.

36. Elting LS, Rubenstein EB, Rolston K, Bodey GP. Correlation between antibiotic regimen and duration of fever in gram negative bacteremias (GNB). 7th International Symposium Supportive Care in Cancer 1995 September 20-23 Luxembourg.

37. Anaissie EJ, Vartivarian S, Bodey GP, et al. Randomized comparison between antibiotics alone and antibiotics plus granulocyte-macrophage colony-stimulating factor (*Escherichia coli*-derived) in cancer patients with fever and neutropenia. Am J Med 100:17-23, 1996.

38. American Society of Clinical Oncology. American Society of Clinical Oncology recommendations for the use of hematopoietic colony-stimulating factors: evidence-based, clinical practice guidelines. J Clin Oncol 12:2471-2508, 1994.

39. Gilbert C, Meisenberg B, Vredenburgh J, et al. Sequential prophylactic oral and empiric once-daily parenteral antibiotics for neutropenia and fever after high-dose chemotherapy and autologous bone marrow support. J Clin Conol 12:1005-1011, 1994.

40. Lyman GH, Lyman CG, Sanderson RA, Balducci L. Decision analysis of hematopoietic growth factor use in patients receiving cancer chemotherapy. J Natl Cancer Inst 85:488-493, 1993.

41. J. Klastersky for MASCC. Prognostic factors for outcome in cancer patients with febrile neutropenia: a multinational survey from the infection committee of the Multinational Association for Supportive Care in Cancer. In Program Proceedings American Society Clinical Oncology Vol 17:419A (abstract # 1617) May 16-19; Los Angeles, CA, 1998.

9. The Use of Hematopoietic Growth Factors for Recruitment of Leukocytes for Transfusion

David B. Jendiroba, Benjamin Lichtiger,
Emil J Freireich

Introduction

Neutropenia and its related opportunistic infections have always been a concern, particularly in patients undergoing chemotherapy. Neutropenic infection is a leading cause of morbidity and mortality in patients who undergo chemotherapy. Improvement in antibiotic therapies as well as increased use of hematopoietic growth factors provide wider margins of safety for the use of higher doses of chemotherapy, with some regimens approaching marrow transplantation ablative potency. While the supportive use of growth factors and improved antibiotics have advanced cancer treatment, they have not, even in combination, provided enough support to counterbalance deeper peaks of neutropenia and prolonged nadirs caused by the more aggressive chemotherapy strategies. As a consequence, fewer cycles of chemotherapy, nowadays, induce longer periods of marrow aplasia with consequently longer recovery periods.

One procedure employed to overcome this problem is to provide adequate amounts of allogeneic functional granulocytes to granulocytopenic patients, until absolute neutrophil counts have recovered at the expense of their own marrow reserves.

Historical overview

The first systemic studies of granulocyte transfusions were done in the early and mid 1960s[1,2]. It had been established that one of the most important predictors for the success of granulocyte transfusion was the dose of transfused granulocytes; doses lower than 10^{10} granulocytes per square meter of body surface area of the recipient did not promote significant increments in the peripheral blood and failed to cause the cessation of febrile episodes. Doses in the order of 10^{11} granulocytes per square meter, however, did promote increments of ≥ 4.000 cells/μl, lasting 2 to 4 days before returning to the baseline values seen before transfusion. Transfusion did result in clinical benefit. Thereafter, collecting adequate numbers of fully functional granulocytes for transfusion has become a major goal.

Since its initial use, the collection of granulocytes evolved step by step. The first in a series of major breakthroughs was the development of a prototype continuous blood cell separator that could process larger volumes of blood [3]. Subsequently, red blood cells (RBC) sedimenting agents were used to increase the efficiency of the collection procedure by maximizing granulocyte separation. Corticosteroids were the next elements used to increase white blood cells (WBC) counts, but their effect was found to be short-lived. They improve collection parameters by mobilizing the marginal leukocyte compartment, but they do not stimulate bone marrow progenitor cells.

With the advent of growth factors such as granulocyte-colony stimulating factor (G-CSF) and granulocyte macrophage-colony stimulating factor (GM-CSF), which are potent marrow committed progenitor cell stimulators, granulocyte transfusion has increased its therapeutic importance.[4]

The advantage of hematopoietic growth factors

Hematopoietic growth factors such as G-CSF and GM-CSF were first used to decrease the leukocyte nadir as well as to induce faster recovery from leukopenia induced by myeloablative chemotherapeutic regimens[5,6]. Based on their capacity to stimulate both stem cells and committed progenitor cells, these growth factors were subsequently applied to harvest higher numbers of stem cells from either the peripheral blood or from the bone marrow of eligible bone marrow transplant donors. The advantages of those growth factors in particular were enough to initiate their use to stimulate leukocytes in normal volunteers for transfusion.

Increased numbers of transfused leukocytes. Both G-CSF and GM-CSF have been shown to increase considerably the leukocyte counts of normal volunteers above their baseline. In a recent study done, we have demonstrated that values of white blood cell counts assessed before the apheresis procedure - also known as "WBC pre-counts" - are very strong predictors of leukocyte yields, for a given volume of blood processed. Higher numbers of circulating leukocytes before apheresis means, therefore, better chances for collecting higher yields, with more beneficial effects of the transfusion to the neutropenic patients.

Collection of young myeloid cells. Well-known concerns in leukocyte transfusions are the amount and duration of the increments achieved after each treatment. Three factors at least have been recognized as predictors of increment values and their duration - recipient alloimmunization, amount of cells transfused, and percentage of immature granulocytes in the white cell concentrates. Taking these factors into account, it has been previously described that G-CSF and GM-CSF not only increase the amount of circulating mature leukocytes, but also increase the number of young cells released to the peripheral blood of stimulated donors. The positive effect of this action to the patient relies on the fact that immature transfused cells will produce a "depot" effect in the circulation, only migrating to the infected tissues after more complete maturation. Younger transfused myeloid cells extend, therefore, the kinetics of granulocyte migration, improving increment levels over time and assuring longer periods between transfusions.

Increase in stem cell numbers. Levin *et al* observed in the early studies with granulocyte transfusions that cells collected from chronic myelogenous leukemia (CML) donors and transfused to children with refractory opportunistic infections would promote a long lasting increment, sometimes as long as 72 hours, which was inconsistent with the normal kinetics of circulating white cells; a few recipients were noted to engraft temporarily after the leukocyte transfusions, documented by clones of Philadelphia positive cells present in their marrows[7]. This suggested that early progenitor cells or perhaps stem cells present in the peripheral blood of CML donors were responsible for the transient engraftment in the recipients. Likewise, hematopoietic progenitor cells (HPC), which are known to be stimulated by hematopoietic growth factors, seem to play a crucial role for the success of granulocyte transfusions.

Therefore, G-CSF and GM-CSF through their ability to mobilize large numbers of leukocytes that range from the fully mature to most undifferentiated progenitor cells

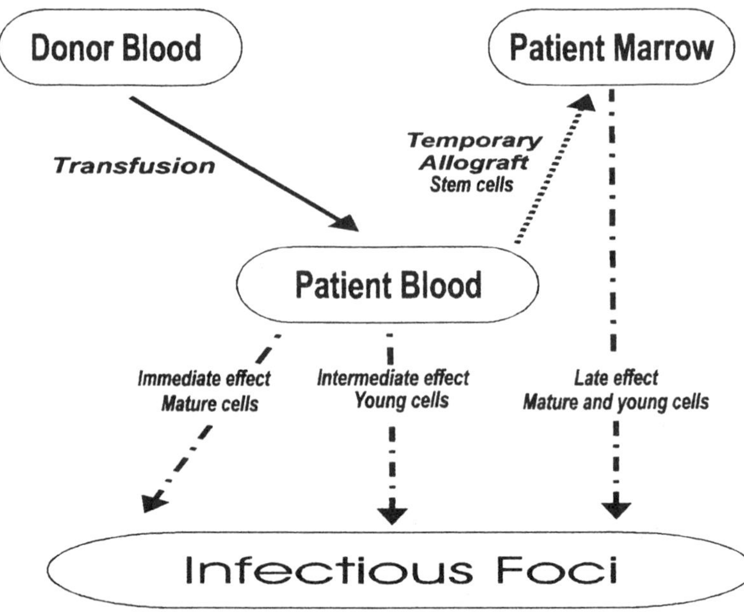

Figure 1. Beneficial effects of hematopoietic growth factors to the patient with neutropenia and infection. Bone marrow stimulation with G-CSF and GM-CSF may provide adequate support of effector cells through the release of leukocytes at varying differentiation levels, which will leave the peripheral blood of the recipient to the infectious foci progressively, as maturation occurs.

can provide not only adequate numbers of cells for transfusion, but also a whole array of functional cells that will function in a progressive chronologic time to provide a continuous anti infectious action against opportunistic infections (Figure 1).

<u>Improved leukocyte function</u>. In a recent review article, Spiekermann *et al* have described the effects that G-CSF and GM-CSF exert on the neutrophil population[8]. Spiekermann's studies reported that, among the many features analyzed, G-CSF and GM-CSF caused a significant increase in adherence, phagocytosis, killing, antibody-dependent cellular cytotoxicity and production of reactive oxygen species, for both *in vitro* and *in vivo* tests. However, chemotaxis was decreased for both *in vitro* and *in vivo*, for G-CSF and GM-CSF stimulated neutrophils. It has been suggested that GM-CSF, in addition to the features described above, also enhances the function of the immune system as a whole, since it also increases the function of monocytes/macrophages and lymphocytes[9-13]. As a whole, both growth factors enhance

the immune response of the host to infections, since the cytokine network activity that takes place among those cells during the inflammatory response is increased.

Enhanced cell viability: Besides stimulating production and function of leukocytes, G-CSF and GM-CSF have also been shown to increase leukocyte viability *in vitro* and *in vivo*[14-17]. It has been postulated that both G-CSF and GM-CSF promote such effect by inhibiting apoptosis; however, the implicated mechanisms may not solely rely on apoptosis inhibition and should, therefore, be further investigated.

Decrease in threshold sensitivity for synergistic action with other cytokines. Another important consideration regarding G-CSF and GM-CSF stimulated leukocytes is the ability of these growth factors to "prime" neutrophils. Priming is a very different biological event from activation. Neutrophil priming is characterized mainly by reinitiation of transcriptional events and translation of pre-existing or newly formed mRNA, so that cells become well supplied to perform their characteristic functions of chemotaxis, phagocytosis and killing. Neutrophils, under these circumstances, present with increased expression of surface receptors that will enhance their ability to interact with the surrounding environment, enabling them to become "active" upon specific stimuli. They will also have a boost in their enzymatic apparatus as well as considerable augmentation of oxygen reactive species production. As a consequence of such pre-mounted defensive state, once triggered by the appropriate stimuli, the primed neutrophil will perform its function faster and more efficiently, leaving fewer chances for the challenge to succeed.

In summary, both G-CSF and GM-CSF are potentially very promising agents for mobilization of leukocytes for collection. Their pharmacological action upon early and committed progenitor cells assure increased numbers of both mature and young leukocytes, which will assure prolonged coverage of the neutropenic patient's nadir. By promoting leukocyte enhanced functionality as well as longer viability, these growth factors replenish the pool of the immune network necessary for an elaborated adaptive response against opportunistic infections. It remains to be determined, however, the optimal schedules which will yield the most benefits from these hematopoietic factors.

G-CSF versus GM-CSF for mobilization of leukocytes

The effects of growth factors on collection parameters of normal individuals are far better known for G-CSF than for GM-CSF. While several studies have addressed the use of G-CSF for the recruitment of leukocytes for transfusion[18-26], as of yet, only one study, to our knowledge, has reported the effects of GM-CSF stimulation on normal volunteers[27].

Overall, the studies utilizing G-CSF have been able to mobilize yields of leukocytes which range from 3 to 7×10^{10}, an approximate 2 to 5-fold increase compared to corticosteroid stimulation or with no stimulation at all. Most mobilization schedules have used 5µg/kg/day of G-CSF given by subcutaneous infection. Acute side effects related to the administration of G-CSF have been reported to be mild and short-lasting, consisting of myalgia, arthralgia, bone pain and fever, which usually vanish without medication, when administration has stopped.

One important consideration for growth factor mobilized leukocytes is the optimization of schedules. Because the long-term side effects of G-CSF and GM-CSF have not been well established, and because cost of procedure is an issue becoming increasingly important in the current days, safer and cost-effective schedules, i.e., schedules that utilize smaller doses of growth factors to mobilize the same numbers of fully functional leukocytes would be desirable, but remain to be designed.

With that purpose, we have evaluated and compared 554 collection procedures from 194 normal donors who were stimulated according to one of four different mobilization schedules. A summary of the most important collection parameters pertaining to each of the four schedules is shown on Table 1.

Table 1. Features of the four mobilization schedules

Schedule	G-CSF 5μg/kg qd	G-CSF 5μg/kg qod	GM-CSF 5μg/kg qod	PDN[*] 60 mg po
Donors	77	59	31	27
Collections	221	179	90	64
Collections per donor	2.9	3.0	2.9	2.4
Mean liters of blood processed	7.0	7.5	8.4	6.0
Mean WBC pre-counts $x10^3/\mu l$	34.2	29.3	14.4	20.7
% monocytes in the bag concentrates	9.2	6.0	9.3	5.6
Monocyte yields $x10^9$	6.0	4.2	3.5	1.7
Mean ANC yields $x10^9$	42.3	46.2	22.2	28.7

[*]**Prednisone**

When granulocytes were stimulated with G-CSF according to both the qd and qod schedules, similar progressive and sustained increases in WBC pre-counts were seen during consecutive collection days in the order of 145% and 160% for G-CSF qd and G-CSF qod, respectively. The G-CSF qd donors showed a 5-fold increase from their baseline levels , while the G-CSF qod donors showed a 4-fold increase. GM-CSF stimulated donors showed a 2-fold increase in WBC pre-counts as compared to baseline levels, and did not increase progressively over the days of collection.

Granulocytes stimulated with prednisone (PDN) produced only a small and transient increase in WBC pre-count values between the first and the second day of collection. A minute decline was observed on the third day; a much larger decline was seen on the fourth day. The PDN donors showed a 2.7 fold increase in their WBC pre-counts from their baseline level. No PDN donors carried out apheresis until the fifth day of collection.

The difference in WBC pre-count values between the PDN schedule and the two G-CSF schedules is statistically significant. WBC pre-count values for the different mobilization schedules have been depicted in Figure 2.

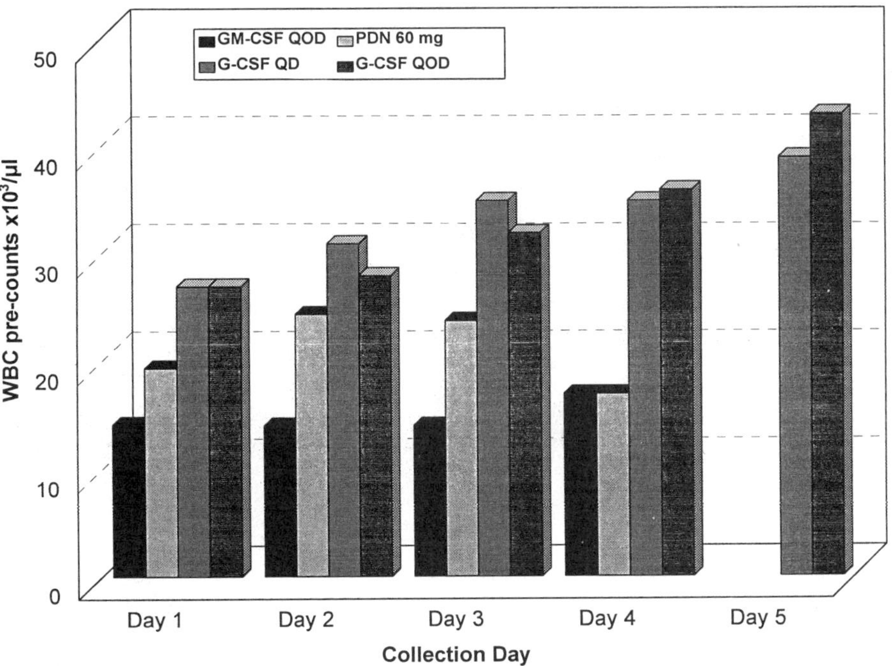

Figure 2. Mean WBC pre-counts for each mobilization schedule over the collection days.

Conclusion

Granulocyte transfusions have the potential to become a crucially important approach for overcoming neutropenia-related opportunistic infections. Its success rate in raising the number of circulating neutrophils in the recipient is directly proportional to the dose of functional cells transfused to the patient. To maximize granulocyte transfusion success rate and reduce procedural risks, cell collection must be monitored according to at least three apheresis parameters that directly influence the amount of cells collected - WBC pre-count values, the volume of blood processed, and the efficacy of the leukapheresis procedure. G-CSF and GM-CSF significantly increase WBC pre-counts in normal volunteers, with few side effects. Investigation of more effective schedules will provide higher numbers of functional leucocytes with smaller doses of the growth factors, and will therefore, minimize cost of the procedure and decrease long-term side effect risks for the donors. These important issues must be considered in any contemporary study design. Further study is needed to determine the effect of granulocyte transfusions on infection.

Acknowledgments

The authors are in debt to Lorraine A. Joyce and Nancy Kroning for assistance with the manuscript, and to the medical technologists of the M. D. Anderson Blood Bank, for data handling.

References

1. Freireich EJ, Morse EE, Bronson W, Carbone PP. Transfusion of granulocytes from donors with chronic myelocytic leukemia to leukopenic patients. Proceedings of the IX Congress of The International Society of Hematology 1:549-57, 1962

2. Morse EE, Freireich EJ, Carbone PP, et al. The transfusion of leukocytes from donors with chronic myelocytic leukemia to patients with leukopenia. Transfusion 6:183-92, 1966

3. Freireich EJ, Judson G, Levin RH. Separation and collection of leukocytes. Cancer Research 25:1516-20, 1965

4. Freireich EJ. White cell transfusions born again. Leukemia & Lymphoma 11:161-5, 1993

5. Chanock S, Freifeld A. The use of cytokines in fever and neutropenia. International Journal of Pediatric Hematology/Oncology 2:173, 1995

6. Chanock SJ, Gorlin JB. Granulocyte transfusions. Time for a second look. Infect Dis Clin N Am 10:327-43, 1996

7. Levin RH, Whang J, Tijo JH, et al. Persistent mitosis of transfused homologous leukocytes in children receiving antileukemic therapy. Science 142:1305-1, 1963

8. Spiekermann K, Roesler J, Emmendoerffer A, et al. Functional features of neutrophils induced by G-CSF and GM-CSF treatment: differential effects and clinical implications. Leukemia 11, 1997

9. Perkins RC, Vadhan-Raj S, Scheule RK, et al. Effects of continuous high dose rhGM-CSF infusion on human monocyte activity. Am J Hematol 43:279-85, 1993

10. Lydaki E, Bolonaki E, Stiakaki E, et al. Efficacy of recombinant human granulocyte colony-stimulating factor and recombinant human granulocyte-macrophage colony-stimulating factor in neutropenic children with malignancies. Ped Hematol Oncol 12:551-8, 1995

11. Steger GG, Kaboo R, deKernion JB, et al. The effects of granulocyte-macrophage colony-stimulating factor on tumour-infiltrating lymphocytes from renal cell carcinoma. Br J Cancer 72:101-7, 1995

12. Kowanko IC, Ferrante A, Harvey DP, Carman KL. Granulocyte-macrophage colony-stimulating factor augments neutrophil killing of Torulopsis glabrata and stimulates neutrophil respiratory burst and degranulation. Clin Exp Immunol 83:225-30, 1991

13. Lechner AJ, Lamprech KE, Potthoff LH, et al Recombinant GM-CSF reduces lung injury and mortality during neutropenic Candida sepsis. Am J Physiol 266:L561-8, 1994

14. Adachi S, Kubota M, Lin YW, et al. In vivo administration of granulocyte colony-stimulating factor promotes neutrophil survival in vitro. European Journal of Haematology 53:129-34, 1994

15. Colotta F, Re F, Polentarutti N, et al. Modulation of granulocyte survival and programmed cell death by cytokines and bacterial products. Blood 80:2012-20, 1992

16. Colotta F, Re F, Mantovani A. Granulocyte transfusions from granulocyte colony-stimulating factor-

treated donors: also a question of cell survival? [letter]. Blood 82:2258, 1993

17. Cohen DM, Bhalla SC, Anaissie EJ, et al. Effects of in vitro and in vivo cytokine treatment, leucapheresis and irradiation on the function of human neutrophils: implications for white blood cell transfusion therapy. Clinical & Laboratory Haematology 19:39-47, 1997

18. Hester JP, Rondon G, Huh YO, et al. Principles of bone marrow processing and progenitor cell/mononuclear cell concentrate collection in a continuous flow blood cell separation system. J Hematother 4:299-306, 1995

19. Jendiroba DB, Lichtiger B, Anaissie E, et al. Evaluation and comparison of three mobilization methods for the collection of granulocytes. Transfusion 38:722-728, 1998.

20. Dignani MC, Anaissie EJ, Hester JP, et al. Treatment of neutropenia-related fungal infections with granulocyte colony-stimulating factor-elicited white blood cell transfusions: a pilot study. Leukemia 11:1621-30, 1997

21. Sica S, Di Mario A, Salutari P, et al. Chemotherapy and recombinant human granulocyte colony-stimulating factor primed donor leukocyte infusion for treatment of relapse after allogeneic bone marrow transplantation. Bone Marrow Transplant 16:483-5, 1995

22. Sica S, Rutella S, Di Mario A, et al. rhG-Csf in healthy donors: mobilization of peripheral hemopoietic progenitors and effect on peripheral blood leukocytes. J Hematother 5:391-7, 1996

23. Katoh M, Takada M, Nakatani N, et al. Chemotaxis and phagocytosis of the neutrophils mobilized by granulocyte colony-stimulating factor in healthy donors for granulocyte transfusions [letter]. Am J Hematol 49:96-7, 1995

24. Caspar CB, Seger RA, Burger J, Gmur J. Effective stimulation of donors for granulocyte transfusions with recombinant methionyl granulocyte colony-stimulating factor. Blood 81:2866-71, 1993

25. Liles WC, Huang JE, Llewellyn C, et al. A comparative trial of granulocyte-colony stimulating factor and dexamethasone, separately and in combination, for the mobilization of neutrophils in the peripheral blood of normal volunteers. Transfusion 37:182-87, 1997.

26. Bhatia S, McCullough J, Perry EH, et al. Granulocyte transfusions: efficacy in treating fungal infections in neutropenic patients following bone marrow transplantation. Transfusion 34:226-32, 1994

27. Fritsch G, Fischmeister G, Haas OA, et al. Peripheral blood hematopoietic progenitor cells of cytokine-stimulated healthy donors as an alternative for allogeneic transplantation [letter]. Blood 83:3420-1,1994

III

Management of Anemia

10. Pathophysiology of the Anemia of Malignancy

John W. Adamson

Introduction

Anemia is common in patients with malignancy and there are many contributors to the anemia, as shown in Table 1. By far and away the most common form of anemia seen in patients with cancer or hematologic malignancies results from the underproduction of red cells - a hypoproliferative anemia.

Table 1. Mechanisms contributing to cancer-associated anemia

1. Anemia of chronic disease (inflammation).
2. Myelosuppressive effects of chemotherapy
   - Suppression of erythropoietin production
   - Direct suppression of marrow function
3. Blood loss
4. Nutritional deficiency (ies)
5. Hemolysis
   - Drug-induced
   - Microangiopathic
   - Autoimmune

Hypoproliferative anemias are characterized by a low reticulocyte (production) index and the absence of erythroid marrow hyperplasia despite significant, persistent anemia (hematocrit <30%, hemoglobin <10g/dL). The mechanisms which lead to a hypoproliferative anemia include: impaired erythropoietin (EPO) production, an impaired response of the erythroid marrow to EPO and mild iron deficiency, which itself impairs erythroid proliferation.

Generally, the chronic anemia associated with cancer is characterized by an inadequate production of EPO for a given hemoglobin and hematocrit[1] as well as an inadequate response of the erythroid marrow to endogenous EPO. In addition, there is impaired release of iron from iron storage sites so that, in chronic conditions, there is evidence of inadequate iron delivery to the developing erythroid marrow and, consequently, evidence of iron-deficient erythropoiesis. Finally, as with virtually all hypoproliferative anemias, there is a mild shortening of red cell survival. This constellation of findings is called the *anemia of chronic disease* (ACD)[2-4].

Anemia as a Consequence of Cancer

The importance of anemia in the cancer patient has only been moderately well characterized. Typical studies have used red cell transfusion needs as an indicator of significant anemia. However, given the fact that recent studies have demonstrated how important maintaining an adequate hemoglobin level is to the quality of life of cancer patients, the levels that have been accepted previously as appropriate for hemoglobin/hematocrit are being reconsidered. As an example, a frequently cited study of Skillings et al. indicated that in patients with malignancy only about 19%, overall, received blood transfusions for anemia[5]. However, of patients in that study with leukemia, 78% required red cell transfusions. In patients with solid tumors, those with lung cancer had the highest frequency of transfusion. Of interest, patients with lung cancer were transfused at a relatively high hemoglobin level; this was attributed to their generally older age as well as the higher likelihood of concurrent pulmonary disease. Finally, there was a clear and stepwise correlation between the number of patients transfused when segregated by baseline hemoglobin level prior to chemotherapy. In this study, all 8 patients whose baseline hemoglobin was less than 8.0 g/dL required transfusion, while only 8% of the patients whose hemoglobin was ≥ 12 g/dL required transfusion.

These results can be compared to the transfusion requirements of patients in the large US-based multicenter trial of EPO treatment for patients with anemia of cancer[6,7]. In that study, 28% of more than 300 patients required transfusions over the 1-2 months prior to entering the study. In the first month of the study, before the full effect of EPO therapy was seen, the percent of patients requiring transfusions rose to 44% in the group receiving cisplatin-based chemotherapy and remained at 26% in those patients receiving non-cisplatin-based chemotherapy. Studies have shown that platinum-based drugs, in and of themselves, reduce EPO production by the kidney in a manner which correlates with drug-induced renal tubular dysfunction[8].

Regulation of Normal Red Cell Production

To understand the mechanisms which result in anemia in cancer patients, it is useful to review the physiology of normal red cell production. The day-to-day production of red blood cells is under the control of the hormone, EPO. The major source of EPO production in adult mammals is the kidney - specifically, peritubular capillary lining (interstitial) cells of the proximal tubule. Using sensitive molecular probes, several groups have localized EPO mRNA to these cells[9,10].

While the preponderance of evidence implicates such interstitial cells in EPO production, other investigators have failed to confirm this, reporting that it is the renal tubular cells, themselves, that produce EPO[11].

Koury et al. have demonstrated a very interesting response of the mouse kidney to anemic hypoxia[12]. Using semiquantitative means, they calculated the number of renal cells/cm^2 of tissue section which were positive by in situ hybridization for the presence of EPO mRNA. They found that with progressively severe anemia, the strength of signal per cell did not change. Rather, as the hematocrit fell, the number of cells which were positive for EPO mRNA rose in a log-linear fashion, suggesting that the response to increasing hypoxia was the recruitment of additional EPO-producing cells. The corollary to this is the fact that some low number of renal interstitial cells displayed apparent constitutive production of EPO.

During fetal development, the liver is the major source of EPO production and retains the ability to produce EPO under extreme hypoxia or anemia, even into post-natal life. Koury et al. used molecular probes to localize EPO production principally to hepatocytes[13]. In contrast to the kidney, the increased hepatic production of EPO appears to result from increased EPO production per cell.

The mechanisms by which renal tissue recognizes hypoxia are unclear; however a heme protein has been postulated to be central to the process[14]. This heme protein will react with metals, including cobalt, to increase EPO production by Hep2B cells, a hepatoma cell line which responds in culture to hypoxia[15].

The kidney is substantially more sensitive to changes in oxygen delivery than is the liver and, consequently, hepatic production of EPO changes relatively little over the range of most hemoglobin concentrations seen with chronic anemia.

EPO is a glycoprotein of 30.4 kD molecular size[16]. It is heavily glycosylated (approximately 60%) and, once released, circulates in the plasma with a half-life in man of 4.9 ($\pm$1.7) hours[17,18]. In the bone marrow, EPO binds to specific receptors on erythroid cells[19]. While EPO receptors are found on cells in the brain, endothelial cells and trophoblastic cells, the function of EPO receptors in these nonerythroid tissues is unknown.

The cellular physiology of erythropoiesis has been well defined by using a variety of in vitro assays for progenitor cells capable of extensive proliferation. These assays have provided a picture of the hierarchy of progenitor cells of a number of lineages. Among erythroid progenitors, the assays have defined the growth factors necessary for proliferation and maturation of the various stages.

The earliest recognizable erythroid progenitor cell is characterized by its ability to generate large complex colonies (consisting of thousands of cells and multiple subcolonies) in semi-solid medium. The appearance of these colonies resembles a "burst" - hence, the name burst-forming unit-erythroid (BFU-E) was given to the cell that gives rise to such colonies[20]. The number of BFU-E in the marrow is independent of changes in circulating levels of EPO[21]. For in vitro growth, the initial cell divisions of the BFU-E depend on earlier-acting hematopoietic growth factors such as interleukin-3 (IL-3) or stem cell factor (SCF). However, EPO is required for the full maturation and hemoglobinization of the cells in the burst.

BFU-E express relatively few EPO receptors[22]. As the BFU-E divides, it gives rise to more differentiated erythroid progenitor cells - erythroid colony-forming cells (CFU-E). CFU-E give rise to colonies containing smaller numbers of cells (8-200) and it is the CFU-E population whose numbers in vivo depend upon the endogenous levels of EPO[21,23]. CFU-E also have the most EPO receptors per cell of any cell in hematopoiesis[22]. Neither BFU-E nor CFU-E are identifiable morphologically. The CFU-E probably precedes the first recognizable erythroblast by 1-2 cell divisions. As erythroblasts mature into reticulocytes and then adult red cells, the number of EPO receptors declines accordingly. As will be discussed, the intrinsic responsiveness of these various progenitor cell compartments to EPO or other growth factors isn't altered in patients with cancer-associated anemia, but the responsiveness of these cells to EPO can be altered substantially by a variety of inflammatory cytokines associated with malignancy and other chronic infectious or inflammatory states.

Iron Metabolism

Normal erythropoiesis depends upon the availability of critical vitamins, nutrients and, most especially, iron. Iron is a necessary element in the synthesis of hemoglobin, and an adequate supply of iron to the erythroid marrow is required for normal red cell production[24].

The pathway of iron metabolism in man is highly conserved with elemental iron needs in an adult male on the order of 1 mg per day. A schematic of the pathways of iron trafficking in man is shown in Figure 1.

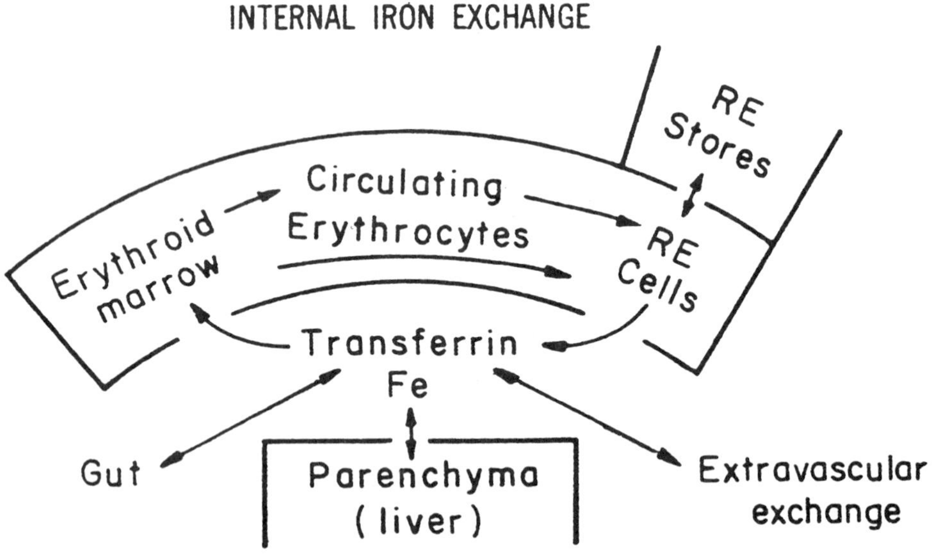

Figure 1: The pathways of internal iron trafficking in man. From The Red Cell Manual; R.S. Hillman and C.A. Finch, F.A. Davis, 1974, with permission.

Iron enters the body in three ways. Under normal circumstances, iron enters by being absorbed from dietary foodstuffs, and the amount of iron absorbed is regulated by body iron needs, the amount of iron in the diet, and the activity of the erythroid marrow. If the individual has reduced iron stores, the amount of iron absorbed is increased, and if the diet is rich in iron, the absolute amount of iron absorbed is also increased. Finally, through mechanisms which are not well understood, iron absorption is increased in the face of an increased erythroid marrow – irrespective of the amount of storage iron present in the body. The other means by which iron can enter the body are through red cell transfusions and parenteral iron administration.

Once absorbed, iron is transported through the circulation bound to its transport protein, transferrin. Each transferrin molecule can hold two iron atoms[24]. The iron-carrying transferrin interacts with specific transferrin receptors on the surface of erythroid progenitor cells. After binding to its receptor, the transferrin-iron-transferrin receptor complex is internalized, at which point the iron is separated from the transferrin molecule in an acidic endosome. At this point, the iron is either utilized for hemoglobin synthesis or complexed with apoferritin, an iron storage protein, to form ferritin, one of the normal storage forms of iron[24]. As red cells are released from the marrow, they take with them the iron in the form of hemoglobin. The hemoglobin iron in circulating red cells represents the largest "pool" of iron in the body - approximately 2-3 gm - and the iron remains in the pool for the lifespan of the red cell - normally 120 days. At the end of the red cell life cycle, senescent red cells are taken up by the cells of the reticuloendothelial system (RES), the hemoglobin is broken down, and iron is released either to be placed into storage or, for the most part, recycled to the surface of the RE cell where the iron is made available once again to circulate bound to transferrin.

This is an efficiently regulated pathway and is designed to preserve iron homeostasis. Typically, only 1 mg of iron is lost from the body per day in the form of cells desquamating from the intestinal track or the skin. Iron losses in females of childbearing age are approximately 2-3 mg per day, averaged over a month's time, due to menstrual blood loss[24].

The changes in red cell production which are associated with malignancy include changes in iron metabolism which are brought about by inflammatory cytokines released either by malignant cells or in response to the presence of malignant cells.

Changes in Red Cell Production Associated with Malignancy

The commonest features of malignancy-associated anemia are the features of ACD. The characteristics of ACD are: lower than expected circulating EPO levels in response to the anemia, alterations in iron metabolism, and a blunted erythroid progenitor cell response to EPO - all resulting in a hypoproliferative anemia.

The key to understanding mechanisms surrounding these changes with ACD lies in the alterations in the production of several inflammatory cytokines. These include interleukin-1 (IL-1), tumor necrosis factor alpha (TNFα) and the interferons (IFN).

These cytokines are produced by monocytes, resident macrophages, T-lymphocytes, bone marrow stromal cells and a variety of other tissues. They are only some of the cytokines involved in the complex networks of response to inflammation and tissue injury that are found in man. The presence in increased concentrations of these cytokines can have a profound effect on erythropoiesis.

EPO production

A useful system for the study of the regulation of EPO production has been hepatoma cell lines, such as Hep2G or Hep3B, which, when exposed to hypoxia, increase EPO production through transcriptional and translational mechanisms[15]. Using such a system, Faquin and co-workers showed that when Hep3B cells were exposed to hypoxia in the presence of IL-1, the expected increase in EPO mRNA expression and the release of bioactive EPO into the culture medium were blunted[25]. Similar findings were observed with TNFα. This was not a toxic effect on the cells since the Hep3B cells responded to a combination of IL-1 and IL-6 by increasing EPO mRNA levels. The degree of suppression of EPO mRNA was dependent on the concentration of IL-1 added to the culture. This group not only demonstrated cytokine concentration-dependent suppression of EPO mRNA accumulation but also provided a hierarchy of the effects of various cytokines with IL-1 β being more suppressive than IL-1 α and TNF α. Jelkmann et al. provided supportive results by demonstrating that IL-1 reduced EPO production by perfused rat kidneys[26].

One of the hallmarks of malignancy-associated anemia is the reduction in endogenous EPO levels with respect to the degree of anemia[1]. As shown in Figure 2,

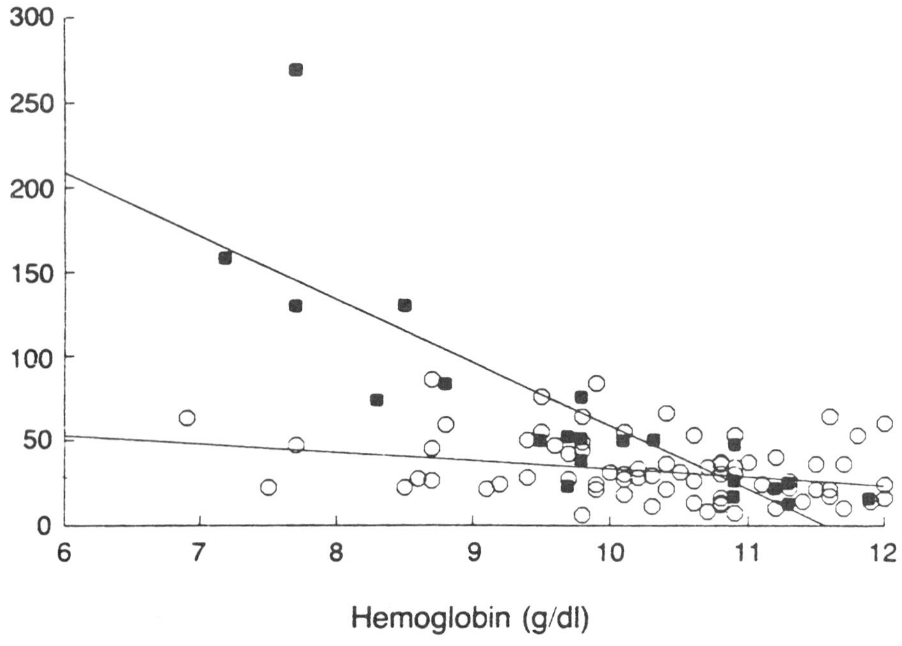

Figure 2: **The relationship between hemoglobin concentration and serum immunoreactive Epo concentration in 74 anemic cancer patients (open circles) and 24 patients with iron deficiency anemia (closed squares). From C.B. Miller, et al. (ref. 1), with permission.**

the expected inverse correlation between endogenous EPO levels, as measured by a sensitive radioimmunoassay, was lost in over 70 adult patients with malignancies of various kinds, including hematologic malignancies. In contrast, patients with uncomplicated iron deficiency anemia showed an increase in circulating levels of EPO which was inversely correlated with the decline in hemoglobin.

These laboratory and clinical studies have led to the current belief that EPO production is blunted in adult patients with malignancy by the increased production of inflammatory cytokines which interfere with hypoxia-induced upregulation of EPO gene expression. A recent report, however, suggests that an impaired response to endogenous EPO rather than impaired EPO production may characterize cancer-related anemia in children[27].

Erythroid marrow response to EPO

A great deal has been learned about the effect of various inflammatory cytokines on the response of the erythroid marrow to EPO. These studies have been conducted both in vitro and in vivo and have clearly identified a number of interacting mechanisms which likely contribute to the hypoproliferative nature of the ACD.

Some of the earliest studies employed bone marrow cells aspirated from anemic patients with infectious diseases such as tuberculosis or histoplasmosis. When bone marrow adherent cells were separated from non-adherent cells, and the non-adherent cells placed into semi-solid medium with EPO, there was a marked increase in the number of erythroid colonies (from CFU-E) observed when compared to cultures of unfractionated bone marrow cells[28]. When these same adherent cells (most likely macrophages) were added back to the culture of the non-adherent cells, erythroid colony growth was suppressed in a cell dose-dependent manner. Of significance, when adherent cells were separated from the marrow of nonanemic patients who had inflammatory/malignant disease, there was no increase in erythroid colony growth, and when the adherent cells were recombined in culture with the non-adherent cells, no suppression of colony growth was found.

Findings similar to these were reported by Roodman et al[29]. These investigators found that the removal of adherent cells from total bone marrow resulted in increased erythroid colony formation if the marrow source was a patient with anemia and chronic inflammatory disease or malignancy. Unlike the studies of Zanjani et al., however, there was no allogeneic inhibitory effect seen when the adherent cells from anemic patients were placed into co-culture with non-adherent cells from non-anemic subjects. Also, medium conditioned by adherent cells from anemic patients was inconsistent in its ability to suppress normal erythroid colony formation. Nevertheless, this set the stage for the identification of the soluble factors which were released by monocytes/macrophages under these conditions.

Two lines of investigation have provided insights into the process. First, in vitro studies conducted by Broxmeyer et al.[30] and Means et al. have demonstrated the complexity of the factors at work[4]. In early studies, the latter group showed that the addition of various cytokines to cultures of either human or murine bone marrow cells resulted in a concentration-dependent suppression of erythroid colony formation[31-34]. The most sensitive progenitor cells under these conditions were CFU-E as opposed to BFU-E. That this was not a toxic effect of certain cytokines on the progenitor cells was demonstrated by the restoration of full erythroid colony growth by the addition of high concentrations of EPO to the cultures.

Similarly, Johnson et al. demonstrated that the in vivo administration of IL-1 to mice resulted in a selective suppression of CFU-E numbers in bone marrow and spleen[35]. Again, this suppression could be overcome by the nearly simultaneous administration of EPO to the animals. Of interest, 48 hours after IL-1 administration, there was a   marked increase in the numbers of splenic and marrow BFU-E, granulocyte/macrophage colony forming cells (GM-CFC), G-CFC and megakaryocytic (Meg)-CFC.

Roodman and co-workers made similar observations in mice chronically exposed to TNF[36]. In these studies, nude mice were injected with Chinese hamster ovary cells which had been transfected with the human TNF gene. These cells produced high levels of TNF constitutively. In these animals, there was a profound suppression of the numbers of marrow and splenic BFU-E and CFU-E. In contrast, marrow and splenic GM-CFC and mixed-cell CFC were not affected.

Means et al. have provided an even more refined definition of the cytokine networks which may be involved in ACD[4]. Through a series of experiments beginning with unfractionated human marrow cells, this group showed that for IL-1 to suppress erythroid colony formation, accessory cells had to be present, and it was the accessory cells which released γINF in response to IL-1. This suppression of in vitro erythropoiesis was reversible by the addition of high concentrations of EPO to the culture system. In contrast, TNF was shown to suppress in vitro erythropoiesis by stimulating the release of β IFN from marrow stromal cells. This suppressive effect could not be overcome by exogenous EPO. Similarly, α IFN was shown not to suppress erythropoiesis directly but, rather, to stimulate the release of an as yet to be defined molecule from a subset of T-lymphocytes[37]. This effect also was not reversible by Epo.

These findings, taken together, demonstrated a specific cytokine-mediated suppression of erythropoiesis which was reversible by Epo in some instances, but not all. As these studies are examined retrospectively, it becomes clear why the doses of recombinant human EPO required to correct the anemia of malignancy are higher than the EPO doses required to correct the anemia of chronic renal failure. These findings also may explain why a subset of patients with malignancy-associated anemia did not respond to the doses of recombinant human EPO that were employed in the initial clinical trials[6,7].

Iron metabolism

The same cytokines which have an effect on EPO production and the erythroid marrow response to EPO also are believed to affect iron metabolism. Figure 3 shows schematically how at least some of the cytokines interact. Characteristic of the ACD is a reduction in the serum iron level, a modest reduction in the total iron-binding capacity (transferrin level) and a low to low-normal percent transferrin saturation (15-20%). In severe and chronic cases of ACD, the persistently low percent transferrin saturation results in impaired iron delivery to the developing erythroid marrow[2,24]. This, in turn, leads to the production of microcytic red cells and increased eythrocyte zinc protoporphyrin levels. These features of iron deficient red cells may be seen despite the presence of normal or increased bone marrow iron stores as demonstrated by direct examination of the marrow or an increased plasma ferritin level. This constellation of changes in iron metabolism appears to be mediated primarily by impaired release of iron from storage sites for binding to transferrin and, subsequently, delivery to the erythroid marrow. Again, although the precise molecular mechanisms are not known, the elevated levels of inflammatory cytokines seen in many patients with malignancy are likely to mediate these changes in iron metabolism[38].

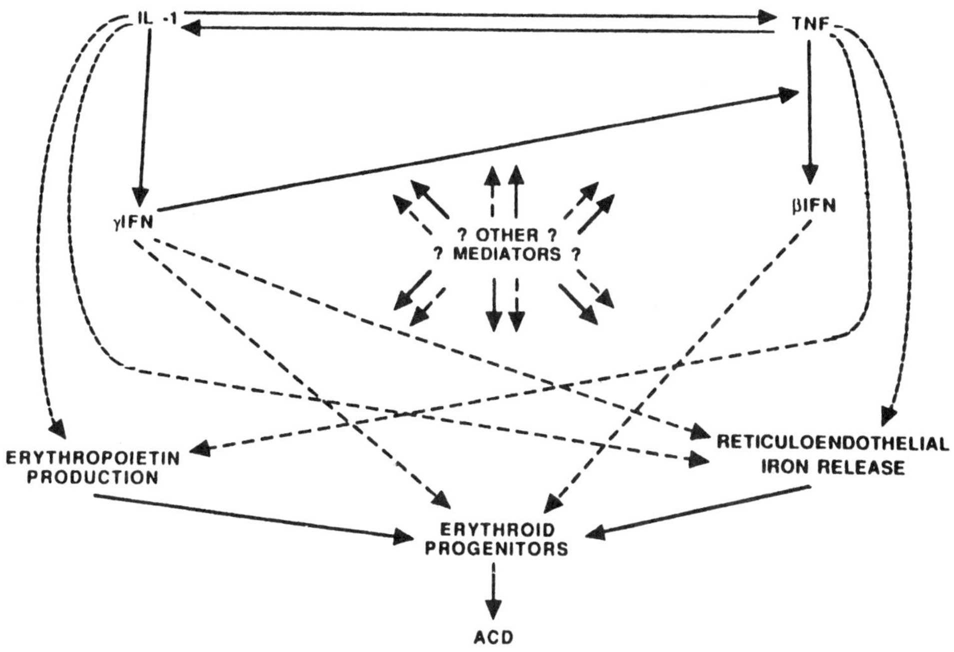

Figure 3: A schematic diagram of both the positive (solid lines) and negative (dotted lines) effects of various inflammatory cytokines which influence erythropoiesis in the ACD. From R. Means and S. Krantz, Blood 1992;80:1639-1647, with permission.

Two kinds of studies have clearly implicated the RES in this process. First, if radiolabeled heat-damaged red cells are injected into a normal individual, the red cells are rapidly removed from circulation by the RES. In the RES, the iron is recovered from the hemoglobin of the ingested red cell and then shuttled back to the cell surface to be made available for transferrin binding. This is a very efficient process and the radioiron reappears within minutes in the circulation bound to transferrin [24]. This same experiment, carried out in patients with chronic inflammation, results in a much lower "reutilization" of the labeled iron. However, if the RES is bypassed by giving radiolabeled iron already bound to transferrin, the iron is rapidly removed from the circulation by the erythroid marrow and efficiently (>90%) incorporated into the hemoglobin of newly formed red cells[24].

With long-standing ACD, many of the laboratory findings mimic true iron deficiency anemia - one of the confusing differentials in distinguishing iron deficiency from ACD. This distinction is clinically relevant since iron deficiency, itself, results in a hypoproliferative anemia and a blunted response to EPO stimulation. The relative or functional iron deficiency seen with malignancy has promoted studies of the potential value of supplemental intravenous iron administration along with recombinant human EPO in correcting cancer-associated anemia.

Summary

The increased knowledge of the pathophysiology of the anemia associated with cancer has resulted in a more focused and enlightened approach to anemia management. Given the fact that anemia is one of the most important contributors to the impaired quality of life of cancer patients, it is important that this knowledge be applied to rational therapy.

References

1. Miller CB, Jones RJ, Piantadosi S, et al. Decreased erythropoietin response in patients with the anemia of cancer. N Engl J Med 322:1689-1692, 1990.
2. Lee GR. The anemia of chronic disease. Semin Hematol 1983 20:61-80.
3. Cash JM, Sears DA. The spectrum of disease associated with the anemia of chronic disease: a study of 90 cases. Am J Med 87:638-644, 1990.
4. Means RT. Pathogenesis of the anemia of chronic disease: A cytokine mediated anemia. Stem Cells 13:32-37, 1995.
5. Skillings JR, Sridhar FG, Wong C, Paddock L. The frequency of red cell transfusion for anemia in patients receiving chemotherapy. Am J Clin Oncol 16:22-25, 1993.
6. Abels RI. Use of recombinant human erythropoietin in the treatment of anemia in patients who have cancer. Semin Oncol 19:29-35, 1992.
7. Henry DH, Abels RI. Recombinant human erythropoietin in the treatment of cancer and chemotherapy-induced anemia: Results of double-blind and open-label follow-up studies. Semin Oncol 21:21-28, 1994.
8. Wood PA, Hrushesky WJM. Cisplatin-associated anemia: An erythropoietin deficiency syndrome. J Clin Invest 95:1650-1659, 1995.
9. LaCombe C, Da Silva JL, Bruneval P, et al. Peritubular cells are the site of erythropoietin synthesis in the murine hypoxic kidney. J Clin Invest 81:620-623, 1988.
10. Koury ST, Bondurant MC, Koury MJ. Localization of erythrpoietin synthesizing cells in murine kidneys by in situ hybridization. Blood 71:524-527, 1988.
11. Maxwell AP, Lappin TRJ, Johnston CF, et al. Erythropoietin production in kidney tubular cells. Br J Haematol 74:535-539, 1990.
12. Koury ST, Koury MJ, Bondurant MC, et al. Quantitation of erythropoietin-producing cells in kidneys of mice by in situ hybridization: Correlation with hematocrit, renal erythropoietin mRNA, and serum erythropoietin concentration. Blood 74:645-651, 1989.
13. Koury ST, Bondurant MC, Koury MJ, et al. Localization of cells producing erythropoietin in murine liver by in situ hybridization. Blood 77:2497-2503, 1991.
14. Goldberg MA, Dunning SP, Bunn HF. Regulation of the erythropoietin gene: Evidence that the oxygen sensor is a heme protein. Science 242:1412-1414, 1988.
15. Goldberg, MA, Glass GA, Cunningham JM, Bunn HF. The regulated expression of erythropoietin by two human hepatoma cell lines. Proc Natl Acad Sci USA 84:7972-7976, 1987.
16. Davis JM, Arakawa T, Strickland TW, Yphantis DA. Characterization of recombinant human erythropoietin produced in Chinese hamster ovary cells. Biochemistry 26:2633-2638, 1987.
17. Cotes PM, Pippard MJ, Reid CDL, Winearls CG, et al. Characterization of the anaemia of chronic renal failure and the mode of its correction by a preparation of human erythropoietin (r-HuEPO). An investigation of the pharmacokinetics of intravenous erythropoietin and its effects on erythrokinetics. Q J Med New Ser 70:113-137, 1989.
18. Egrie, JC, Eschbach JW, McGuire T. Adamson JW. Pharmacokinetics of recombinant human erythropoietin (r-HuEPO) administered to hemodialysis (HD) patients. Kidney Int 33:Abstract 152,

1988.

19. Jones SS, D'Andrea AD, Haines L, Wong GG. Human erythropoietin receptor: cloning, expression and biological characterization. Blood 76:31-35, 1990.

20. Axelrad AA, McLeod DL, Shreeve MM, et al. Properties of cells that produce erythrocytic colonies in vitro. In: Robinson WA, ed. Hemopoiesis in Culture. Washington, D.C.: Second International Workshop, 1973:226-234 DHEW publication no. 74-205.

21. Adamson JW, Torok-Storb B, Lin N. Analysis of erythropoiesis by erythroid colony formation in culture. Blood Cells 4:89-103, 1978.

22. Sawada K-J, Krantz SB, Dai C-H, et al. Purification of human blood burst-forming units-erythroid and demonstration of the evolution of erythropoietin receptors. J Cell Physiol 142:219-230, 1990.

23. Iscove NN. The role of erythropoietin in regulation of population size and cell cycling of early and late erythroid precursors in mouse bone marrow. Cell Tissue Kinet 10:323-334, 1977.

24. Bothwell TH, Charlton RW, Cook JD, Finch, CA. Iron metabolism in man. Oxford: Blackwell Scientific Publications, :pp.576, 1979.

25. Faquin WC, Schneider TJ, Goldberg MA. Effect of inflammatory cytokines on hypoxia-induced erythropoietin production. Blood 79:1987-1994, 1992.

26. Jelkmann W, Pagel H, Wolff M, et al. Monokines inhibiting erythropoietin production in human hepatoma cultures and in isolated perfused rat kidneys. Life Sci 50:301-308, 1991.

27. Corazza F, Beguin Y, Bergmann P, et al. Anemia in children with cancer is associated with decreased erythropoietic activity and not with inadequate erythropoietin production. Blood 92:1793-1798, 1998.

28. Zanjani, ED, McGlave PB, Davies SF, et al. In vitro suppression of erythropoiesis by bone marrow adherent cells from some patients with fungal infection. Br J Haematol 50:479-490, 1982.

29. Roodman, GD, Horadam VW, Wright TL. Inhibition of erythroid colony formation by autologous bone marrow adherent cells from patients with the anemia of chronic disease. Blood 62:406-412, 1983.

30. Broxmeyer HE, Williams DE, Lu L, et al. The suppressive influences of tumor necrosis factors on bone marrow hematopoietic progenitor cells from normal donors and patients with leukemia: synergism of tumor necrosis factor and interferon-γ. J Immunol 136:4487-4495, 1986.

31. Means RT, Dessyrpis EN, Krantz SB. Inhibition of human colony-forming units erythroid by tumor necrosis factor requires accessory cells. J Clin Invest 86:538-541, 1990.

32. Means RT, Dessypris EN, Krantz SB. Inhibition of human erythroid colony-forming units by interleukin-1 is mediated by gamma interferon. J Cell Physiol 150:59-64, 1992.

33. Means, RT, Krantz SB. Inhibition of human erythroid colony-forming units by tumor necrosis factor requires beta interferon. J Clin Invest 91:416-419, 1993.

34. Means RT, Krantz SB, Luna J, et al. Inhibition of murine erythroid colony formation in vitro by gamma interferon and correction by interferon inhibitor. Blood 83:911-915, 1994.

35. Johnson CS, Keckler DJ, Topper MI, et al. In vivo hematopoietic effects of recombinant interleukin-1α in Mice: Stimulation of granulocytic, monocytic, megakaryoctyic, and early erythroid progenitors, suppression of late-stage erythropoiesis, and reversal of erythroid suppression with erythropoietin. Blood 73:678-683, 1989.

36. Johnson RA, Waddelow TA, Caro J, et al. Chronic exposure to tumor necrosis factor in vivo preferentially inhibits erythropoiesis in nude mice. Blood 74:130-138, 1989.

37. Means RT, Krantz SB. Inhibition of human erythroid colony-forming units by interferons alpha and beta: differing mechanisms despite shared receptor. Exp Hematol 1996 24:204-208.

38. Balkwill F, Burke F. Talbot D, et al. Evidence for tumor necrosis factor/cachectin production in cancer. Lancet 2:1229-1232, 1987.

11. The Use of Recombinant Erythropoietin in the Treatment and Prevention of Cancer and Chemotherapy-related Anemia

Jerry L. Spivak

Introduction

At the beginning of the twentieth century, Landsteiner's observations made blood transfusion a possibility [1] while at the century's end, recombinant DNA technology has provided the opportunity to obtain many of the benefits of blood transfusion without transfusing blood [2]. Although inventory concerns have always made blood conservation a priority of Transfusion Medicine specialists, after the introduction of the lethal retrovirus HIV into the blood supply, blood conservation became a major public health issue. While the development of sensitive molecular tests and more rigorous donor screening have greatly improved the safety of blood, [3] in addition to the public perception of risk, legitimate reasons still persist for concern about the non-infectious hazards of blood transfusion. These include immediate or delayed hemolytic reactions, alloimmunization, iron overload, volume overload, graft-versus-host disease, immunosuppression and suppression of marrow function. In addition, the issues of cost and inconvenience must always be considered. In the anemic patient, the various risks of blood transfusion whether immediate, remote or inevitable, need to be balanced against its positive effect with respect to improved tissue oxygenation, an effect which, unfortunately, is difficult to quantitate. To balance the risk-benefit equation, it has become standard practice in anemic, chronically transfused patients to limit the extent to which the red cell volume is restored. However, if anemic patients with end stage renal disease can serve as model, a decade of hormone replacement using recombinant human erythropoietin has made it abundantly clear that chronic anemia (hemoglobin level <10 gm%) has a deleterious effect on quality of life not only with respect to cardiovascular capacity but also cognitive function and psychological well being [4]. Since recombinant erythropoietin therapy carries with it none of the risks of blood transfusion, its application to the correction of anemia in patients with normal renal function was a logical progression. This chapter reviews the use of recombinant human erythropoietin for the correction or prevention of anemia in patients with solid tumors in the presence or absence of chemotherapy or irradiation.

The Anemia of Cancer

Although it has been long appreciated that anemia is a complication of cancer [5,6], studies of its epidemiology and pathophysiology have lagged in contrast to the anemia associated with end stage renal disease [7]. This may have been due in part to a lack of available remedies both for the correction of anemia and the treatment of cancer, as well as to the differences in life span of patients with cancer as opposed to those with end stage renal disease maintained by chronic hemodialysis, and also in part to the multifarious nature of the anemia associated with malignancy. (Table 1) Indeed, as little as 25 years ago, a prominent oncologist remarked with respect to research concerning the anemia associated with cancer, "I have not seen and do not anticipate

---

Table 1.   Causes of Anemia in Cancer Patients

- Blood loss
- Hemolysis
- Nutritional deficiencies
- Hemodilution
- Hypersplension
- Chemotherapy and radiotherapy
- Myelofibrosis

- Marrow necrosis
- Myelodysplasia
- Marrow involvement with tumor
- Infection
- Inflammation
- Renal failure

---

any remarkable new data in this field. Hematologists who are interested, have gone into other areas, but medical oncologists have not developed a keen interest. Surgeons need only know what the deficit is and to correct it by transfusion. This is not a pessimistic report, but instead, a statement of the current status of what is known, what has been done and what can be done."[8] Yet, powerful clues were available that pharmacologic correction of the anemia associated with cancer was possible [9,10], and with the development of more intensive chemotherapy regimens as well as the clinical availability of recombinant human erythropoietin, the anemia associated with cancer has come under greater scrutiny.

The exact extent to which anemia is a complication of cancer and its severity are not well documented but although the epidemiologic evidence is still incomplete, the incidence appears substantial. For example, at one tertiary center, 32% of patients referred with solid tumors were anemic [11], while at a radiation therapy clinic, 53% of referred patients were anemic [12]. In another survey of two cancer centers, 18% of patients required transfusions for anemia not associated with bleeding, and transfusions were most frequent in patients with lung cancer [13]. In a group of patients undergoing cyclic chemotherapy for ovarian cancer, 46% became severely anemic (hematocrit <25%) [14], while for another similarly treated group, anemia occurred in 67% . Anemia was also observed to complicate combined radiation and chemotherapy in 54% of a cohort of patients with nasopharyngeal carcinoma [16]. Interestingly, the use of GM-CSF appeared to be associated with the induction of significant anemia in advanced breast cancer patients treated with CEF [17], and in another study 40% of patients with non-small cell lung cancer undergoing chemotherapy required blood transfusions [18]. In a retrospective study of blood usage among cancer patients at a tertiary referral center, 219 patients required transfusions (mean of 3.7 units per patient) and 8.7% had some type of transfusion reaction [19]. A cost analysis indicated an expenditure of $552 per unit transfused in this center in the uncomplicated situation.

Anemia, however, has implications beyond cost, inconvenience and transfusion-associated risks. (Table 2) For example, in one survey, anemic cancer patients were more likely to have advanced disease and a shorter survival [12]. Anemic cancer patients were also more likely to require transfusions following chemotherapy then their nonanemic counterparts [13]. Anemia also appears to have an adverse effect on the local relapse rate after radiotherapy [20]. Whether the anemia was merely a reflection of the aggressive nature of the underlying tumor, or had an adverse effect on the efficacy of the radiotherapy is still matter of controversy [21,22]. A similar controversy exists with respect to the immunosuppressive effects of blood transfusion on tumor progression as well as susceptibility to infection. While there is little solid evidence for the

---

Table 2. **Consequences of Anemia in Cancer Patients**

- Imparied tissue oxygenation
- Impaired organ function
- Impaired quality of life
- Inability to make autologous blood donations

- Increased probability of blood transfusion after chemotherapy
- Increased iron absorption (with certain forms of anemia)
- Increased susceptibility to thrombo-cytopenic bleeding

---

former[23,24,25,26,27], more exists to support the latter [23,28,29]. Whether anemia contributes to cancer fatigue is an issue currently under investigation [30]. These issues taken together with the public perception of blood transfusion risks have fostered substantial interest in the use of recombinant human erythropoietin for the pharmacologic correction of the anemia associated with cancer and its therapy.

Erythropoietin

The fundamental premise for the use of recombinant erythropoietin is that this protein can provide many of the benefits of blood transfusion without transfusing blood. This premise is based on the principal physiologic role of erythropoietin which is to couple red cell production with long term tissue oxygen requirements. Erythropoietin's effects are essentially restricted to the promotion of the proliferation of early erythroid progenitor cells, which are largely dormant until triggered into cell cycle by the hormone, [31] and suppression of premature cell death in later erythroid progenitor cells, which are largely in cell cycle independent and, therefore, do not require erythropoietin for DNA synthesis[32]. Indeed, if programmed cell death is abrogated by overexpression of Bclx, erythroid progenitor cells can terminally differentiate in the absence of erythropoietin [33].

Erythropoietin is one of the few hematopoietic growth factors which behaves like a hormone - thrombopoietin being the other well-documented example [34]. Like thrombopoietin, the circulating level of erythropoietin reflects the mass and proliferative behavior of its target cells [35]. However, unlike thrombopoietin, erythropoietin production is not controlled by its metabolism, but, rather by the level of tissue oxygenation in the kidneys and, to a lesser extent, the liver. Hypoxia is the only known physiologic stimulus for erythropoietin production and controls both the rate of erythropoietin gene transcription and the stability of its mRNA [36]. Since erythropoietin behaves like a hormone, its plasma level provides useful information about its production as well as about tissue oxygenation in uncomplicated situations [37].

That is to say, there is an inverse log-linear correction between the plasma erythropoietin level and tissue oxygenation as assessed by the hemoglobin or hematocrit However, there appears to be a definite threshold with respect to this relationship since there was not a linear correlation between plasma erythropoietin and hemoglobin within the normal range of the hemoglobin level and plasma erythropoietin increased outside the normal range only when the hemoglobin fell below 10.5 gm% [38]. This is not meant to imply that lesser degrees of anemia do not produce an increase in erythropoietin synthesis and an increase in the plasma erythropoietin level. Rather, since the range of normal for plasma erythropoietin is so wide (4-26 mU/ml), unless a patient's normal base line level is known, an increase in plasma erythropoietin will not become apparent until its level rises outside the normal range and this only occurs below a hemoglobin of 10.5 gm%. It is also worth noting in this regard that erythrocytosis causes feed back inhibition of erythropoietin production, if not by improving tissue oxygenation, then by hyperviscosity [39]. This mechanism may also responsible for suppressing erythropoietin production when there is hyperviscosity due to macroglobulinemia or other forms of dysproteinemia [40].

The availability of recombinant erythropoietin provided the opportunity to develop a sensitive and specific immunoassay for erythropoietin which is normally present in the plasma in only picomolar quantities. Since erythropoietin functions like hormone, assay of plasma erythropoietin should serve to define those clinical situations in which there is erythropoietin deficiency or excess. Indeed, the most interesting observation from a survey of plasma erythropoietin levels in a variety of disease states was the number of situations in which erythropoietin production was depressed, in addition to the expected deficiency associated with chronic renal insufficiency [37] (Table 3). Of

---

Table 3.   **Clinical Situations in Which Erythropoietin Production is Impaired**

● Renal disease	● Neoplasia
● Hyperviscosity	● Cancer Chemotherapy*
● Inflammation	● Surgery
● Infection	● Bone marrow transplantation

* An initial elevation of plasma erythropoietin may occur due to marrow suppression but subsequently production can be depressed for many weeks.

---

great interest was the finding that not only were erythropoietin levels depressed in anemic cancer patients but that the inverse correlation between the hemoglobin or hematocrit level and plasma erythropoietin was lost as well [41]. This is similar to the situation in patients with end stage renal disease. It was also observed that recent chemotherapy was associated with depression of plasma erythropoietin. Most importantly, anemic cancer patients with an inappropriately low plasma erythropoietin level for their degree of anemia did not lack the ability to produce erythropoietin. On the contrary, given a sufficient hypoxic stimulus, their ability to produce erythropoietin was unimpaired [41]. A similar behavior has also been observed in patients with end stage renal disease [42]. Thus, it appeared that in these anemic cancer patients as well as those with renal disease, the hypoxic threshold for erythropoietin production was increased.

The mechanism for the low plasma levels of erythropoietin in anemic cancer patients is not fully understood. It is generally held, based on in vitro studies using erythropoietin-producing hepatoma cells or isolated kidney preparations, that suppression of erythropoietin production is due to elaboration of inflammatory cytokines such as IL-1, IL-6 and interferon [43,44]. It is also worth noting that in some patients, the erythropoietin deficit may be more apparent than real owing to plasma volume expansion [11]. While erythropoietin production is depressed in anemic cancer patients relative to their degree of anemia, it is not totally diminished [41]. This implies an element of end organ resistance to the ambient levels of endogenous erythropoietin. Once again the mechanisms involved are not completely understood. As indicated in Table 1, in some patients the anemia represents a dilutional phenomenon but this is not true for others [11]. Based on both in vivo and in vitro studies, it has been postulated that the same inflammatory cytokines, γinterferon and IL-1, which can suppress erythropoietin production in vitro, impair the proliferation of erythroid progenitor cells as well [45]. Tumor cells themselves may also release inhibitors of erythropoiesis [46] and stromal cell proliferation [47]. Importantly, the inhibitory effects of these inflammatory cytokines could be overcome by elevation of plasma erythropoietin, either exogenously or endogenously [48]. Erythroid progenitor cells harvested from the bone marrow of anemic cancer patients were normally responsive to erythropoietin in vitro, but even in the absence of chemotherapy their numbers were generally only similar to those present in normal bone marrow suggesting some depression of erythropoiesis in these anemic patients [49]. This is in keeping with the impairment of erythropoietin production observed in this situation. Chemotherapy in lung cancer patients has been also observed to reduce the number of erythroid colony-forming cells out of proportion to the number of myeloid colony forming cells, although a reduction in erythroid colony-forming cells was observed initially in the absence of chemotherapy [50]. This is of particular interest in view of the higher transfusion requirements of anemic patients with lung cancer[13].

Chemotherapy and Erythropoiesis

As mentioned above, recent chemotherapy is associated with impairment of erythropoietin production [41] and also appears to have a significant effect on hematopoietic progenitor cell proliferation as well. This latter effect must be taken in to consideration when anticipating the use of recombinant erythropoietin in patients undergoing chemotherapy. Although investigations in this area are incomplete, it is clear that many chemotherapeutic agents as well as irradiation damage the erythron apart from direct toxic or immunologic effects on mature erythrocytes. For example, actinomycin D selectively inhibits erythropoiesis and azathioprine can cause red cell aplasia [51]. There is controversy with respect to cisplatin with in vitro studies suggesting a direct toxic effect on erythroid progenitor cells [52,53] and in vivo studies suggesting that erythroid progenitor cells remain responsive to erythropoietin during cisplatin therapy [54,55].

Some chemotherapeutic agents such as 5-FU, cyclophosphamide and doxorubicin cause a transient reduction in erythropoietic activity and erythroid progenitor cell number which rebound within two weeks [56.] Others, such as irradiation or the nitrosourea carmustine are associated with an immediate depression of erythropoiesis followed by recovery and then a secondary depression [56,57]. Repeated courses of chemotherapy appear to deplete the peripheral blood stem cell pool more than the marrow stem cell pool and this depletion, which may persist for several years, is more marked for myeloid then erythroid progenitor cells [56]. While the correlation between progenitor cell pools and peripheral blood counts is inexact, it is clear that erythropoietin therapy may be less useful when there is only transient marrow suppression by chemotherapeutic agents than when such suppression is prolonged. Certainly, timing should also be an critical factor at least with single cell-cycle active drugs. For example, acute elevation of plasma erythropoietin following exposure to chemotherapy before there has been any change in the hemoglobin level represents depopulation or suppression of the erythroid progenitor cell pool [55,58,59,60,61]. Thus, administration of recombinant erythropoietin may be less effective during this time interval than before it or at a suitable interval after drug exposure. The influence of timing may, of course, be less important when noncycle-active drugs are employed. Indeed, kinetic experiments performed over two decades ago indicated that reduction in the hematopoietic stem cell pool need not be associated with impaired responsiveness on a sustained basis to exogenous erythropoietin [10]. The important lessons to be gained from these experiments are: 1) that repetitive doses of erythropoietin were necessary and 2) that the timing of erythropoietin administration was important. This is in keeping with the known physiology of erythropoietin, (Table 4) viz, that it is both a mitogen and a survival factor [31,32]. The initial dose of the hormone serves to trigger dormant erythroid progenitor

Table 4.   **Erythropoietin Physiology and Functions**

Major Functions	EPO Production	EPO Plasma Level
Viability factor	Constitutive	Constant
Mitogen	Inducible	Variable

cells into all cycle while subsequent doses permit the developing erythroid progenitor cells to survive during the time acquired for terminal differentiation and the use of other growth factors. This suggests that an initial high dose of erythropoietin followed by smaller doses may be the most appropriate therapeutic approach.

The Clinical Application of Recombinant Human Erythropoietin for Anemic in Cancer Patients

To date, the effect of recombinant human erythropoietin on cancer-associated anemia in the absence or presence of chemotherapy has been reported for over 4000 patients[50,62-94, 115]. This provides a data base sufficient to judge the safety and efficacy of the hormone in specifically defined situations and also to identify the direction for future clinical trials. It is of interest to note that the results from carefully selected conditions and exclusionary rules of the initial randomized, placebo-controlled [66] trials which do not usually recapitulate the realities of the clinic, have been broadly confirmed with very similar results obtained under routine practice conditions [93, 115].

Safety

Recombinant human erythropoietin has had a remarkable safety record in anemic cancer patients, which is in keeping with the experience in other cohorts of anemic patients with normal renal function and in contrast to the initial experience in anemic patients with end stage renal disease [95]. This is not surprising since not only are patients with end stage renal disease subject to cardiovascular complications, but the pharmacodynamics of erythropoietin therapy were not yet understood when it was first introduced. Furthermore, the intravenous administration of many growth factors is associated with systemic reactions such as flushing, bone pain and headache, which are not usually observed when the same agents are given subcutaneously. Thus, in every published report to date concerning erythropoietin administration in anemic cancer patients, side effects have been negligible with the highest incidence involving local skin reactions such as burning at the injection site, rash or pruritus. These reactions most likely relate to the excipient employed which has been reformulated to reduce injection site discomfort. Allergic reactions to the hormone are also rare as is the development of erythropoietin antibodies. To date, the description of these has been limited to patients with pure red cell aplasia [96].

Since erythropoietin is a hematopoietic growth factor, the possibility that the hormone could stimulate tumor cell proliferation has received scrutiny. Indeed, erythropoietin receptors have been identified in one myeloma cell line [97]. However, to date, neither in vitro studies nor clinical trials have given any indication that erythropoietin promotes tumor cell proliferation [98].

Exacerbation of preexisting hypertension or de novo hypertension were observed to occur with a high frequency in anemic hemodialysis patients [95], and anemic cancer patients are not immune to this side effect of recombinant erythropoietin therapy which is not a direct effect of the hormone [99]. Although the incidence of hypertension is very low compared to the hemodialysis population, it is worthwhile monitoring the blood pressure during the initial four to six weeks of therapy and this should be mandatory in patients with preexisting hypertension. In this latter group, as well as those patients with an elevated serum creatine, initiating therapy at lower dose of erythropoietin may also be judicious.

The most serious potential side effect of erythropoietin is vascular thrombosis and this is purely a function of the degree of expansion of the red cell mass. In this regard, it is essential to recognize that erythropoietin-driven erythrocytosis whether the stimulus is endogenous or exogenous, is associated with a reduction in plasma volume [100]. This is in contrast to the situation in polycythemia vera, where not only does the increase in red cell mass occur slowly, but there is simultaneous expansion of the plasma volume. Plasma volume contraction is probably also involved in erythropoietin-associated hypertension. Given the documented propensity of cancer patients to thrombosis, it is important to be vigilant that inappropriate expansion of the red cell mass does not occur when recombinant erythropoietin is employed.

Although there has been substantial interest concerning the effect of recombinant erythropoietin on platelet production, particularly as it relates to the potential for thrombosis, this interest is misguided. Erythropoietin has no effect on platelet production except possibly to the extent to which it induces iron deficiency and even in this instance, no example of erythropoietin-associated thrombocytosis has ever been reported. Indeed, transgenic mice which overexpress erythropoietin have erythrocytosis but not thrombocytosis or leukocytosis for that matter [101]. As a corollary, erythropoietin therapy does not result in thrombocytopenia or leukopenia. Furthermore, thrombocytosis has never been proven to cause major vessel thrombosis[102].

Extramedullary hematopoiesis as evidenced by circulating erythroblasts and myelocytes is not uncommon in cancer patients. To date, however, the development of splenomegaly associated with recombinant erythropoietin therapy has not been described in anemic cancer patients although this complication has been observed in patients with myeloproliferative disorders or myelodysplasia [82].

Efficacy

A number of randomized, double-blind, placebo-controlled studies have established that recombinant human erythropoietin can ameliorate the anemia associated with cancer and its therapy and alleviate transfusion requirements in transfusion-dependent patients[66,76,81,86]. The frequency of response varied amongst the reported clinical trials, but comparison of their results is frustrated by the use of different erythropoietin-dosing regimens, timing and routes of administration as well as the hybrid nature of most study populations with respect to tumor type and stage and variation in the use and type of anti- tumor therapy.

The mean overall response rate to recombinant erythropoietin in anemic cancer patients based on hemoglobin elevation alone was $63 \pm 15\%$ (N=17 studies). This figure represents results from both blinded and open label studies, involving patients with various types of hematologic malignancies as well as those with various types of solid tumors both on and off chemotherapy as well as a variety of erythropoietin regimens administered by different routes. In many series, the results for hematologic malignancies have been combined with those of solid tumors and for both often many different tumor types were studied under the same protocol making it impossible to dissect out the results for specific malignancies. However, even when the data could be dissected out, the overall mean response rate was not significantly different for solid tumors than for hematologic malignancies, with the exception that in the absence of chemotherapy, the response to erythropoietin may be poorer in patients with hematologic malignancies [80,85]. With respect to solid tumors, in one series anemic patients with squamous cell lung carcinoma responded better than those with adenocarcinoma and both responded better than anemic patients with breast cancer [80]. However, in another series, patients with breast cancer uniformly responded to recombinant erythropoietin [91]. In this latter series however, the patients were less anemic and were also receiving G-CSF simultaneously. Another large study has indicated tthat response to epoietin-α can occur independent of tumor type or response to chemotherapy [115].

Overall, there are currently insufficient data to make prognostic judgments with respect to responsiveness based on tumor type. Indeed, it may be that tumor stage is more important since failure to respond to recombinant-erythropoietin is a poor prognostic sign with respect to survival [103]. Given the realities of the clinic versus the artificiality of clinical trial protocols, the best current estimate of the success of recombinant erythropoietin therapy can probably be derived from the recent large open label community outpatient clinical trial in patients with solid tumors receiving chemotherapy, where the response rate was 54% [93], a rate similar to that of a previous smaller open label trial [80].

Another gauge of success and perhaps an even more important one from the perspective of cost and complications is reduction of transfusion usage or dependency. On average, a 50% reduction in red cell transfusions has been achieved with recombinant erythropoietin therapy but the range was broad, extending from no difference versus placebo to total independence. This in part reflects differences in patient status and transfusion practice as well as the conditions of the particular clinic trial [13]. Furthermore, since erythropoietin therapy takes 4 - 8 weeks to elevate the hemoglobin level, in many instances transfusions will not be avoidable.

Perioperative Erythropoietin Therapy

A different aspect of this same issue relates to the avoidance of transfusions associated with cancer surgery. A large prospective study established that anemic patients, many of whom had cancer, and required elective surgery were not only likely to have an inappropriately low plasma erythropoietin level preoperatively, but in spite of increasing anemia postoperatively, the plasma erythropoietin level remained depressed for up to 5 days [104]. Given these observations and the fact that the patient's own blood is the safest blood, it was logical to determine whether recombinant human erythropoietin could enhance autologous blood donation or by itself alleviate perioperative transfusion requirements. To date, 5 studies have examined this issue [78,86,88, 89,105]. In 4, the subjects were patients with gastric or colorectal cancer and in one, patients with head and neck cancer receiving preoperative chemotherapy [89]. Although not all were randomized double blind trials with the result that there were inequalities, for example, with respect to iron stores in the treatment and control populations, the net results were the same. Recombinant erythropoietin stimulated erythropoiesis, enabled anemia patients to donate up to 2 units for autologous use, and reduced homologous blood exposure. However, blood usage was not reduced. Indeed, those patients receiving erythropoietin who made autologous donations were more likely to be transfused than control patients (100% vs 36%) even through their preoperative hematocrit was higher than, average surgical blood loss the same, and the transfusion trigger was the same as the control [98]. This is not a cost-effective use of resources.

In the absence of autologous blood donation recombinant erythropoietin failed to eliminate or even reduce homologous blood exposure in spite of adequate doses of the hormone over what should have been a sufficient time interval [86,88,89,105]. This is not surprising since operative blood loss is independent of erythropoietin therapy as is age and the most important factors associated with transfusion needs were age, operative blood loss and a hemoglobin less than 11.5% [105]. Interestingly, these are the same factors associated with transfusion dependency in studies involving surgical patients with non-malignant disorders [106]. It is, of course, possible that, in contrast to patients without cancer, a longer duration of erythropoietin treatment was required. However, delaying cancer surgery does not have the same consequences as delaying a hip replacement. Taking everything together, since there is no proof that homologous blood transfusion promotes tumor metastases [23,27,29], based on these studies the perioperative use of recombinant erythropoietin to avoid homologous blood exposure cannot be justified on the basis of either cost or efficacy.

Erythropoietin Dosage and Route of Administration

Sufficient data has been accumulated to reach some conclusions about the route of administration and dosage of recombinant erythropoietin which are most effective. Studies in anemic hemodialysis patients established that subcutaneous administration of the hormone was not only equivalent to or even more effective than intravenous administration but also more convenient in an outpatient setting since self administration was possible. With a new excipient and more concentrated hormone preparations, subcutaneous administration is also more acceptable to patients. The standard three times weekly administration regimen has no physiologic or pharmacologic basis but merely reflects the frequency at which the initial study population, anemic patients with end stage renal disease, were dialyzed. A variety of administration regimens have been employed in anemic cancer patients without any significant differences in response rates and it appears that the cumulative weekly dose is more important than the frequency with which it is administered. Recent studies in orthopedic surgery patients have indicated that a single large weekly dose of hormone is as effective as multiple daily doses [107]. This is presumably because subcutaneous administration of the hormone provides a depot-like effect and with higher doses a higher blood level can be sustained for a longer interval. This is not unphysiologic since during hypoxia endogenous erythropoietin production does not appear to fluctuate but rather increase to a new steady state. Whether such a regimen would be effective in anemic cancer patients in whom marrow function is depressed remains to be determined.

With respect to the dose of recombinant erythropoietin, it has also been established that 300 U/kg three times weekly is not better than 150 U/kg. [50,65,108] On average 30,000-35,000 U per week should be an effective dose in the majority of patients regardless of whether it is administered in daily increments or in fewer divided doses. Smaller doses may also be effective but take much longer to increase the hematocrit [94]. It has generally been the practice to escalate the dose of erythropoietin if an effect has not been achieved after 4 to 6 weeks of therapy. However, one study suggested that it was equally efficacious to maintain the same dose for a longer time interval [108]. Finally, once a response has been obtained it appears to be durable, particularly in chemotherapy-treated patients [108].

Predicting a Response to Recombinant Erythropoietin

Given the fact that a substantial portion of anemic cancer patients do not respond to recombinant erythropoietin, a number of investigators have sought to develop predictive algorithms to avoid the unnecessary use of an expensive resource. Plasma erythropoietin is usually low relative to the degree of anemia in cancer patients and the plasma erythropoietin level has proved to correlate with hormone-responsiveness but the strength of this correlation appeared to vary with tumor type being better with myeloma then solid tumor [74,82,84,85,103]. When the level was greater than 400 mU/ml, in the absence of chemotherapy, a response was unlikely. [85]. In patients not undergoing chemotherapy, failure to achieve an increase in hemoglobin of at least 0.5 gm after 2 weeks of therapy together with an erythropoietin level of 100 mU/ml or greater had a positive predictive power of >90%. As an alternative, a serum ferritin of 400 ng/ml or greater after 2 weeks of therapy had a predictive power of 88% [103]. A similar conclusion at least with respect to hemoglobin was reached in patients with hematologic malignancies, most of whom were receiving chemotherapy [84] while in a larger study with both chemotherapy and nonchemotherapy-treated patients, a hemoglobin increment of >1gm after 4 weeks of therapy was thought to be a better predictor of responsiveness than a 0.5 gm increase after 2 weeks [109]. In this latter study, a reticulocyte count at 4 weeks of >40,000/ml was equivalent to the 1gm hemoglobin increment and together they had even a better predictive ability. Overall, however, the hemoglobin increment had greater strength than the reticulocyte count. Other factors associated with a response to recombinant erythropoietin have included a platelet count greater than 100,000 /ml [84,85], and low serum levels of TNF and IL-1 [90]. With respect to transfusion requirements, patients not requiring transfusions at the start of erythropoietin therapy will very likely not require them [93]. Given the expense of recombinant erythropoietin during chemotherapy more studies of these predictive algorithms and the other factors cited in specific patient populations undergoing standardized treatment regimens are clearly warranted.

Iron Therapy

Table 5 lists the factors' known to influence the efficacy of recombinant erythropoietin therapy in anemic cancer patients. Most are self explanatory, but iron deficiency

---

Table 5.   Factors influencing the efficacy of rErythropoietin in Anemic Cancer Patients

- Dose of recombinant erythropoietin
- Performance status
- Type of tumor (including histologic classification)
- Plasma erythropoietin level (>400 mU/ml)
- Duration of prior chemotherapy
- Type of chemotherapy or irradiation
- Iron deficiency
- Occult bleeding or hemolysis
- Splenomegaly
- Infection
- Surgery

---

deserves a comment. The initial experience with recombinant erythropoietin in anemic hemodialysis patients emphasized the importance not only of adequate body iron stores but also the provision of supplemental iron to sustain an erythropoietic response to the hormone. However, extrapolating these concerns to anemic patients with normal renal function is inappropriate. Hemodialysis patients are unique with respect to the magnitude of their ongoing iron-losses while normal iron-replete individuals provided with supplemental oral iron can tolerate weekly phlebotomies of 500 ml without developing significant anemia [110]. Thus, as long as the serum ferritin is greater than 100ng/ml, body can stores are sufficient for a response to recombinant erythropoietin and supplemental iron is not mandatory [111].

Quality of Life

In previous studies, involving anemic hemodialysis patients and anemic HIV-infected patients, recombinant erythropoietin therapy was demonstrated to significantly improve quality of life.[4,112]. These observations are important since in these patients as well as in anemic cancer patients, recombinant erythropoietin therapy would not be expected to have any impact on the underlying disease or patient survival. Five major studies have addressed the effect of recombinant erythropoietin therapy on quality of life in anemic cancer patients. Only one was a randomized double-blind, placebo-controlled multigroup study [66]; another was merely a randomized study [94], and the other three were open label nonrandomized studies [93,113, 115]. Dosing and administration of erythropoietin were comparable in all five studies as was the composition of the patient populations except for the randomized trial which was limited to patients with gastrointestinal malignancies [94]. In this latter study, the response rate with respect to hemoglobin increment (73%) was better than in the other studies (range 30-58%), with patients receiving chemotherapy performing better than those not receiving it. Overall, in each study a response to erythropoietin was associated with an improvement in quality of life. In one study, no change in Karnofsky score was observed in erythropoietin responders as compared with the nonresponders unless there was an increase in hemoglobin of at least 2 gm% [93]. In another, WHO performance status did increase in responders [113]. Although only overall quality of life was assessed in the one placebo-controlled study, the others addressed the issues of physical activity, energy, and psychosocial well-being, all of which were improved in those patients who responded to recombinant erythropoietin with a rise in hemoglobin. Indeed, even a small increment was associated with improvement [93, 115].

Dissecting out the contribution of a response to recombinant erythropoietin to improved quality of life from that of a tumor response to concomitant chemotherapy was a difficult issue with the consensus that both contributed to improvements in quality of life. Interestingly, the beneficial effects on life of epoietin-α-induced increases in hemoglobin levels appear to be independent of the tumor response to chemotherapy [115]. No improvement was seen in patients who failed to respond to either type of therapy, while improvement was seen in those who responded to either erythropoietin or chemotherapy. However, the degree of improvement was greatest when a response was observed to both[93,94.]. Since the hemoglobin levels in responders were always greater than the target hemoglobin level for transfusion therapy, one conclusion which could be drawn from these studies was that modest anemia (hemoglobin=9.0 gm%) is indeed associated with a reduced quality of life. This supports the findings in anemic patients with end stage renal disease treated with recombinant erythropoietin. The five studies cited above are encouraging in their consistency. Other appropriately designed, randomized, double-blind, placebo-controlled clinical trials are in progress to further validate these benefits.

Cost Considerations

Recombinant erythropoietin is an expensive pharmaceutical($0.01/U) and since it does not change the natural history of cancer or prolong patient survival, justification of its use must rely on other considerations. As discussed above, quality of life is one such consideration but, unfortunately, a subjective one for which quantification of benefits remains a challenge. Avoidance of blood transfusion is another important consideration given its potential risks. However, because of the limited life expectancy of many cancer patients, these risks have less meaning in terms of overall cost, while the safety of the blood supply has improved to the extent that risk of contracting HIV infection approximates that of experiencing a fatal hemolytic transfusion reaction [3]. The public perception of risk is, of course, a separate issue and additionally, although there is no proof that transfusions promote tumor spread, there is a very real association with susceptibility to infection [28]. Transfusions are also expensive and inconvenient. Therefore, if the cost of recombinant erythropoietin is equivalent or even reasonably close to that of blood transfusion, its use can be justified on the grounds of safety, convenience and risk reduction. At $0.01 /U and a requirement of 30,000 U/week, the cost of a week's supply of recombinant erythropoietin is $300.00. Thus, the cost of 4 weeks of erythropoietin therapy is close to that of 2 units of packed red cells @ $552/unit [19]. However, if the efficacy of erythropoietin therapy is such that at least 6 patients need to be treated to ensure a reduction in transfusion requirements in one of them [50], then cost becomes a major issue and justification for using the hormone rests solely on improvement in quality of life and also specific situations such as concomitant renal failure, alloimmunization, severe IgA deficiency, possession of a rare blood group or religious objection to blood transfusion. For example, in a recent study using recombinant erythropoietin to prevent anemia in lung cancer patients undergoing chemotherapy, 116 units of red cells were required in the control group ($64,032@ $552/unit)[50] and 54 units ($29808.@ $552/unit) in the erythropoietin-treated group. The cost of recombinant erythropoietin the latter group was $69,600.00. Thus, erythropoietin therapy while preventing the use of homologous blood in only 20% of treated patients added $35,376 or approximately $3000.00 per patient treated, to the cost of therapy. Of course, the value of therapies includes issues beyond costs, so that measurable improvements in quality of life become important for justifying costs of treatment.

Conclusions

Anemia is a complication of cancer and its therapy, but the exact frequency with which anemia occurs and the extent to which it is clinically significant are not well defined. There are many causes for cancer-associated anemia; some are trivial or easily remedied, others are correctable only by blood transfusion. Bone marrow suppression and the associated disruption of the erythropoietin-hemoglobin feed back loop, the mechanisms for which are not completely understood, were once in the latter category even though erythrooid progenitor cells in these situations were normally responsive to erythropoietin in vivo, while with significant tissue hypoxia anemic cancer patients could synthesize erythropoietin as well as normal individuals. Since erythropoietin production is not totally suppressed in cancer patients, the implication is that one mechanism for anemia was humoral inhibition of the erythropoietin-erythroid progenitor cell interaction. With the development of recombinant human erythropoietin, it was possible to overcome this inhibition with pharmacologic concentrations of the hormone. This was a welcome therapeutic advance given the cost, inconvenience and potential risks of blood transfusion and the debilitating effects of anemia. Unfortunately, however, not all anemic cancer patients respond to recombinant erythropoietin therapy and even when a response is obtained, blood transfusions cannot always be avoided. Considering the recent improvements with respect to the safety of blood, the most compelling argument for the use of recombinant erythropoietin in anemic cancer patients pertains to its effect on quality of life. This, of course, must be balanced against the cost of this therapy. In an effort to improve cost-effectiveness, algorithms have been devised to determine which patients will respond to the hormone, but these have not yet been tested prospectively in a controlled fashion. An alternative approach would be to define those chemotherapy regimens which predispose to symptomatic anemia. Unfortunately, this type of prospective data is not available either.

At present, the only approved use of recombinant erythropoietin in patients with nonmyeloid malignancies is as therapy of anemia associated with chemotherapy. This, however, ignores the potential use of the hormone in symptomatic or transfusion-dependent anemic cancer patients in whom chemotherapy might otherwise not be required or might be contraindicated, as well as in patients with azotemia, severely alloimmunized patients, those with rare blood groups or those with theologic objections to blood transfusion. Studies to date do confirm data from other patient populations that the perioperative use of recombinant erythropoietin is not likely to avoid exposure to homologous blood. Whether this would be true if the hormone were used in conjunction with normovolemic hemodilution remains to be determined. At this juncture, even though recombinant erythropoietin has been approved for use in anemic cancer patients, we do not yet know how to use it in the most efficient manner. Indeed, the real benefits of this remarkable hormone with respect to cost and efficacy will not be realized without further rigorously controlled clinical trials directed at defining those cancer patients who will most likely benefit from treatment with it and the situations when it would most benefit patients. For example, a risk model similar to that for identifying patients requiring platelet transfusions due to chemotherapy-induced thrompocytopenia has been developed and would be a useful contribution [114]. Finally, since a recent study suggests that physicians may not be employing recombinant erythropoietin properly [93], sustained cooperation between pharmaceutical companies and practitioners will be required to achieve these goals.

Acknowledgements

The assistance of Chester Young in the preparation of this chapter is acknowledged with gratitude.

References

1. Landsteiner K. Uber agglutination-sercheinungen normalen menschlichen. Blutes. Wien Klin Wochenschr 14:1132, 1901.
2. Lin F-K, Suggs S, Lin C, et al. Cloning and expression of the human erythropoietin gene. P.N.A.S. 82:7580, 1985.
3. Klein H G. New insights into the management of anemia in the surgical patient. Am. J. Med., 101(suppl.2A):12S, 1996.
4 . Evans RW, Rader B., Manninen D. L., and the Cooperative Multicenter EPO Clinical Trial Group. The quality of life of hemodialysis recipients treated with recombinant human erythropoietin. JAMA. 263:825, 1990.
5. Hyman GA. Anemia in malignant neoplastic disease. J Chron Dis. 16:645, 1963.
6. Zucker S. Anemia in cancer. Cancer Investigation. 3:249, 1985.
7. Adamson JW, Eschbach J, Finch CA. The kidney and erythropoiesis. Am J Med 4:725, 1968.
8. Berlin NI. Anemia of cancer. Annals NY Acad Sci. 230:209, 1974.
9. Kennedy J, Gilbertsen AS. Increased erythropoiesis induced by androgenic-hormone therapy. N. Engl. J. Med. 256:719, 1957.
10. Reissmann KR, Udupa KB. Effect of erythropoietin on proliferation of erythropoietin-responsive cells. Cell Tissue Kinet. 5:481, 1972.
11. Berlin NI, Hyde GM, Parsons RJ, Lawrence JH. The blood volume in cancer. Cancer 8:796, 1955.
12. Reed WR, Hussey DH, DeGowin RL. Implications of anemia of chronic disorders in patients anticipating radio-therapy. Amer. J. Med. Sci. 308:9, 1994.
13. Skillings JR, Sridhar FG, Wong C, Paddock L. The frequency of red cell transfusion for anemia in patients receiving chemotherapy. Am J Clin Oncol. 16:22, 1993.
14. Kuzur ME, Greco FA. Cisplatin-induced anemia. N. Engl. J. Med. 303:110, 1980.
15. Martoni A, Panetta A, Angelelli B, Melotti B, et al., A phase II study of carboplatin and cyclophosphamide in advanced ovarian carcinoma. J. Chemother. 5:47, 1993.
16. Al-Sarraf M, Pajak TF, Cooper JS, Mohiuddin M, et al., Chemo-radiotherapy in patients with locally advanced nasopharyngeal carcinoma: A Radiation Therapy Oncology Group study. J. Clin. Oncol. 8:1342, 1990.
17. Ardizzoni A, Venturini M, Sertoli MR, Giannessi PG, et al. Granulocyte-macrophage colony-stimulating factor (GM-CSF) allows acceleration and dose intensityincrease of CEF chemotherapy: a randomised study in patients with advanced breast cancer. Brit. J. Cancer 69:385, 1995.
18. Hesketh PJ, Cooley TP, Finkel HE, et. Al. Treatment of advanced non-small cell lung cancer with cisplatin, 5-fluorouracil, and mitomycin c. Cancer 62:1466, 1988.
19. Mohandas K, Aledort L. Transfusion requirements, risks, and costs for patients with malignancy. Transfusion 35:427, 1995.
20. Fein DA, Lee WR, Hanlon AL, et al. Pretreatment hemoglobin level influences local control and survival of T1-T2 squamous cell carcinomas of the glottic larynx. J. Clin Oncol. 13:2077, 1995.
21. Bush RS. The significance of anemia in clinical radiation therapy J. Rad. Oncol. Biol. Phys. 12:2047, 1986.
22. Poskitt TR. Radiation therapy and the role of red blood cell transfusion Cancer Invest. 5:231, 1987.
23. Williamson L. Annotation: Homologous blood transfusion: the risks and alternatives Brit. J. Haematol. 88:451, 1988.
24. Ness PM, Walsh PC, Zahurak M, et al. Prostate cancer recurrence in radical surgery patients receiving autologous or homologous. blood. Transfusion 32:31, 1992.
25. Busch ORC, Hop WCJ, Hoynck van Papendrecht MAW, et al. Blood transfusions and prognosis in colorectal cancer. N. Engl. J. Med. 32:1372, 1993.
26. Houbiers JGA, Brand A, van de Watering LMG, Hermans J, et al. Randomised controlled trial comparing transfusion of leucocyte-depleted or buffy-coat-depleted blood in surgery for colorectal cancer. Lancet. 344:573, 1994.
27. Donohue JH, Williams S, Cha S, Windschitl HE, et al. Perioperative blood transfusions do not affect disease recurrence of patients undergoing curative resection of colorectal carcinoma: A Mayo/North Central Cancer Treatment Group study. J. Clin. Oncol. 13:1671, 1995.
28. Heiss MM, Mempel W, Jauch K-W, et al. Beneficial effect of autologous blood transfusion on

infectious complications after colorectal cancer surgery. Lancet 342:1328, 1993.

29. Vamvakas EC. Transfusion-associated cancer recurrence and postopewrative infection: meta-analysis of randomized, controlled clinical trials. Transfusion 36:175, 1996.

30. Cella D. The functional assessment of cancer therapy-anemia (FACT-An) scale: A new tool for the assessment of outcomes in cancer anemia and fatigue. Sem. Hematol. 34:13, 1997.

31. Spivak JL, Pham T, Isaacs M. Erythropoietin is both a mitogen and a survival factor. Blood 77:1228, 1991.

32. Koury MJ, Bondurant MD. Erythropoietin retards DNA breakdown and prevents programmed death in erythroid progenitor cells. Science 248:378, 1990.

33. Silva M, Grillot, Benito A, et al. Erythropoietin can promote erythroid progenitor cell survival by repressing apoptosis through Bcl-x_L and Bcl-2. Blood 88:1576, 1996.

34. Gurney AL, Carver-Moore K, de Sauvage FJ, Moore MW. Thrombocytopenia in c-mpl-deficient mice. Science 265:1445, 1994.

35. Cazzola M, Guarnone R, Cerani P, et all. Red blood cell precursor mass as an independent determinant of serum erythropoietin level. Blood 91:2139, 1998.

36. Golberg MA, Gaut C C, Bunn HF. Erythropoietin mRNA levels are governed by both the rate of gene transcription and post transcriptional events Blood 77:271, 1991.

37. Spivak JL. Serum erythropoietin in health and disease Int. J. Cell Cloning 8: (Suppl 1):211, 1991.

38. Spivak JL, Hogans BB, et al. Clinical evaluation of radioimmunoassay for serum erythropoietin using reagents derived from recombinant erythropoietin [abstract].Blood 77:143, 1987.

39. Kilbridge TM, Fried W, Heller P. The mechanism by which plethora suppresses erythropoiesis. Blood 33:104, 1969.

40. Singh A, Eckardt KU, Zimmermann A, et al. Increased plasma viscosity as a reason for inappropriate erythropoietin formation. J. Clin. Invest. 91:251. 1993.

41. Miller CB, Jones RJ, Piantadosi S, et al. Decreased erythropoietin response in patients with the anemia of cancer. N. Engl. J. Med. 322:1689, 1990.

42. Chandra M, Clemons, GK, McVicar MI. Relation of serum erythropoietin levels to renal excretory function: Evidence for lowered set point for erythropoietin production in chronic renal failure. J. Pediatr. 113:1015, 1988.

43. Jelkmann W, Pagel H, Wolff M, et al. Monokines inhibiting erythropoietin production in human hepatoma cultures and in isolated perfused rat kidneys. Life Sci. 50:301, 1991.

44. Faquin WC, Schneider TJ, Goldberg MA. Effect of inflammatory cytokines on hypoxia-induced erythropoietin production. Blood 79:1987, 1992.

45. Means RT Jr, Krantz SB. Progress in understanding the pathogenesis of the anemia of chronic disease. Blood 80:1639, 1992

46. Zucker S, Lysik RM, DiStefano JF. Cancer cell inhibition of erythropoiesis. J. Lab & Clin. Med. 96:770, 1980.

47. DeGowin RL, Gibson DP, Knapp SA. Tumor bearing impairs hemopoietic recovery and survival after irradiation. Exp. Hematol. 11: 305, 1983.

48. DeGowin RL, Gibson DP. Erythropoietin and the anemia of mice bearing extramedullary tumor. J. Lab. Clin. Med. 94:303, 1979.

49. Dainiak N, Kulkarni V, Howard D, et. al. Mechanisms of abnormal erythropoiesis in malignancy. Cancer 51:101, 1983.

50. De Campos E, Radford J, Steward W, et al. Clinical and in vitro effects of recombinant human erythropoietin in patients receiving intensive chemotherapy for small-cell lung cancer. J. Clin. Oncol. 13:1623, 1995.

51. Doll DC, Weiss RB. Chemotherapeutic agents and the erythron Cancer Treat. Rev. 10:185, 1983.

52. Rothmann SA, Paul P, Weick JK, et al. Effect of cis-diamminodichloroplatinum on erythropoietin production and hematopoietic progenitor cells. Int. J. Cell Cloning 3:415, 1985.

53. Gebbia V, Valenza R, Rausa L. The *in vitro* effect of recombinant erythropoietin on cisdiamminedichloroplatinum - induced inhibition of murine erythroid stem cells. Anticancer Res. 10:1779, 1990.

54. Wood PA, Hrushesky WJM. Cisplatin-associated anemia: An erythropoietin deficiency syndrome. J. Clin. Invest. 95:1650, 1995.

55. Matsumoto, T., Endoh, K., Kamisango, K., et al. Effect of recombinant human erythropoietin on anticancer drug-induced anaemia. Brit. J. Haematol. 75:463, 1990.

56. Schreml W, Lohrmann H-P, Anger B. Stem cell defects after cytoreductive therapy in man. Exp. Hematol. 13:31, 1985.

57. Levin J, Andrews JR, Berlin NI. The effects of total body irradiation on some aspects of human iron metabolism. 1960

58. Schapira L, Antin JH, Ransil BJ, et. al. Serum erythropoietin levels in patients receiving intensive chemotherapy and radiotherapy Blood 76:2354, 1990.

59. Cerruti A, Castello G, Balleari E, et al. Serum erythropoietin increase in patients receiving adjuvant therapy with 5-fluorouacil and leucovorin. Exp. Hematol. 22:1261, 1994.

60. Oster W, Herrmann F, Cicco A, et. al. Erythropoietin prevents chemotherapy-induced anemia: Case report. Blut 60:88, 1990.

61. Birgegard G, Wide L, Simonsson B. Marked erythropoietin increase before fall in Hb after treatment with cytostatic drugs suggests mechanism other than anaemia for stimulation. Brit. J. Haemotol.: 72:462, 1989.

62. Piroso E, Erslev AJ, Caro J. Inappropriate increase in erythropoietin titres during chemotherapy. Am J. Hematol 32:248, 1989.

63. Oster W, Herrman F, Gamm, H, et al. Erythropoietin for the treatment of anemia of malignancy associate with neoplastic bone marrow infiltration. J. Clin. Oncol. 8:956, 1990.

64. Ludwig H, Fritz E, Kotzmann H, et al. Erythropoietin treatment of anemia associated with multiple myeloma. N. Engl. J. Med. 322:1693, 1990.

65. Platanias C, Miller CB, Mick R, et al. Treatment of chemotherapy-induced anemia with recombinant human erythropoietin in cancer patients. J. Clin Oncol. 9:2021, 1991.

66. Abels RI, Larholt KM, Krantz KD, Bryant E C. Recombinant Human Erythropoietin (r-HuEPO) for the treatment of the anemia of cancer. in Murphy, M. J., Jr., Ed. Blood Cell Growth Factors. Alpha Med Press p.122, 1991

67. Miller CB, Platanias LC, Mills SR., et al. Phase I-II trial of erythropoietin in the treatment of cisplatin-associated anemia. J. Nat. Cancer Inst. 84:98, 1988.

68. Ponchio L, Beguin Y, Farina G, et al. Evaluation of erythroid marrow response to recombinant human erythropoietin in patients with cancer anaemia. Haematol. 77:494, 1992.

69. James RD, Wilkinson PM, Belli F, et. al. Recombinant human erythropoietin in patients with ovarian carcinoma and anaemia secondary to cisplatin and carboplatin chemotherapy: Preliminary results. Acta Haematol. 87:12, 1992.

70. Vijayakumar S, Roach M III, Wara Wm, Chan SK, et. al. Effect of subcutaneous recombinant human erythropoietin in cancer patients receiving radiotherapy: Preliminary results of a randomized, open-labeled, phase II trial. Int. J. Radiation Oncol. Biol. Phys. 26:721, 1993.

71. Lavey RS, Dempsey WH. Erythropoietin increases hemoglobin in cancer patients during radiation therapy. Int. J. Rad. Oncol. Biol. Phys. 27:1147, 1993.

72. Markman M, Reichman B, Hakes T, et al. The use of recombinant human erythropoietin to prevent carbolplatin-induced anemia. Gynec. Oncol. 49:172, 1992.

73. Tsukuda M, Mochimatsu I, Nagahara T, Kokatsu T, et. al. Clinical application ofrecombinant human erythropoietin for treatments in patients with head and neck cancer. Cancer Immunol Immun. 36:52, 1992.

74. Barlogie B, Beck T. Recombinant human erythropoietin and the anemia of multiple myeloma. Stem Cells 11:88, 1993.

75. Cascinu S, Fedeli A, Fedeli S, Luzi, et. al. Cisplatin-associated anemia treated with subcutaneous erythropoietin. A pilot study. Br. J. Cancer 67:156, 1993.

76. Cascinu S, Fedeli A, Del Ferro E, et al. Recombinant human erythropoietin treatment in cisplatin-associated anemia: A randomized double-bllind trial with placebo. J. Clin Oncol. 12:1058, 1994.

77. Dusenbery KE, McGuire WA, Holt PJ, et al., Erythropoietin increases hemoglobin during radiation therapy for cervical cancer. Int. J. Rad. Oncol. Biol. Phys. 29:1079, 1994.

78. Braga M, Gianotti L, Vignalio A, et. al. Evaluation of recombinant human erythropoietin to facilitate autologous blood donation before surgery in anaemic patients with cancer of the gastrointestinal tract. Br. J. Surg. 82:1637, 1995.

79. Garton JP, Gertz MA, Witzig TE, et. al. Epoetin alfa for the treatment of the anemia of multiple myeloma. Arch Intern Med. 155:2069, 1995.

80. Ludwig H, Sundal E, Pecherstorfer M, et. al. Recombinant human erythropoietin for the correction of cancer associated anemia with and without concomitant cytotoxic chemotherapy. Cancer 76:2319, 1995.

81. Wurnig C, Windhager R, Schwameis E, Kotz R, et. al. Prevention of chemotherapy-induced anemia by the use of erythropoietin in patients with primary malignant bone tumors (a double-blind, randomized, phase III study). Transfusion 36:155, 1996.

82. Kasper C, Terhaar A, Fosså A, Welt A, et. al. Recombinant human erythropoietin in the treatment of cancer-related anaemia. Eur J Haematol. 58:251, 1997.

83. Mittleman M, Zeidman A, Fradin Z, et al. Recombinant human erythropoietin in the treatment of multiple myeloma-associated anemia. Acta Haematol 98:204, 1997.

84. Cazzola M, Messinger D, Battistel V, Bron D, et. al. Recombinant human erythropoietin in the anemia associated with multiple myeloma or non-Hodgkin's lymphoma: Dose finding and identification of predictors of response. Blood 86:4446, 1995.

85. Österborg A, Boogaerts MA, Cimino R, et. al. Recombinant human erythropoietin in transfusion-dependent anemic patients with multiple myeloma and non-Hodgkin's lymphoma - a randomized multicenter study. Blood 87:2675, 1996.

86. Heiss MM, Tarabichi A, Delanoff C, et. al. Perisurgical erythropoietin application in anemic patients with colorectal cancer: A double-blind randomized study. Surgery 119:523, 1996.

87. Chiou TJ, Chim YS, Wei CH, et. al. The effect of subcutaneous r-HuEPO in cancer patients receivng chemotherapy with anemia: a preliminary report. Chinese Medical 60:129, 1997.

88. Braga M, Gianotti L, Gentilini O, Di Carlo V. Erythropoietic response induced by recombinant human erythropoietin in anemic cancer patients candidate to major abdominal surgery. Hepato-Gastro. 44:685, 1997.

89. Dunphy FR, Dunleavy TL, Harrison BR, et. al. Erythropoietin reduces anemia and transfusions after chemotherapy with paclitaxel and carboplatin. Cancer 79: 1623, 1997.

90. Falcone MP, D'Arena A, Scalzulli G, et al. Clinical results of recombinant erythropoietin in transfusion-dependent patients with refractory multiple myeloma: role of cytokines and monitoring of erythropoiesis. E. J. Haematol 58:314, 1997.

91. Del Mastro L, Venturini M, Lionetto R, et al. Randomized phase III trial evaluating the role of erythropoietin in the prevention of chemotherapy induced anemia. J. Clin. Oncol. 15:2715, 1997.

92. Pawlicki M, Jassem J, Bosze P, Lotan C, et al. A multicenter study of recombinant human erythropoietin (epoetin alpha) in the management of anemia in cancer patients receiving chemotherapy. Anti-Cancer Drugs 8:949, 1997.

93. Glaspy J, Bukowski R, Steinberg T, et. al. Impact of therapy with epoetin alfa on clinical outcomes in patients with non-myeloid malignancies during cancer chemotherapy in community oncology practice. J. Clin. Oncol. 15:1218, 1997.

94. Glimelius B, Linné T, Hoffman K, Larsson L, et. al. Epoetin beta in the treatment of anemia in patients with advanced gastrointestinal cancer. J. Clin. Oncol. 16:434, 1998

95. Eschback JW, Abdulhadi MD, Browne JK, et. al. Recombinant human erythropoietin in anemic patients with end-stage renal disease. Results of a phase III multicenter clinical trial. Ann Intern Med. 111:992, 1989.

96. Casadevall N, Dupuy E, Molho-Sabatier P, et. al. Autoantibodies against erythropoietin in a patient with pure red-cell aplasia. N. Engl. J. Med. 334:660, 1996.

97. Okuno Y, Takahashi T, Suzuki A, Ichiba S, et al. Expression of the erythropoietin receptor on a human myeloma cell line. Biochem. Biophys. Res. Comm. 170: 1128, 1990.

98. Berdel WE, Oberberg D, Thiel E. Studies on the role of recombinant human erythropoietin in the growth regulation of human nonhematopoietic tumor cells in vitro. Hematol. 63:5, 1991.

99. McMahon FG, Vargas R, Ryan M, et. al. Pharmacokinetcs and effects of recombinant human erythropoietin after intravenous and subcutaneous injections in healthy volunteers. Blood. 76:1718, 1990.

100. Spivak JL. The clinical physiology of erythropoietin. Sem. Hematol. 30:2, 1993.

101. Semenza GL, Traystman MD, Gearhart JD, et al. Polycythemia in transgenic mice expressing the human erythropoietin gene. P.N.A.S. 86:2301, 1989.

102. Kessler CM, Klein HG. Untreated thrombocythemia in chronic myeloproliferative disorders Brit. J. Haematol. 50:157, 1982.

103. Ludwig H, Fritz E, Leitgeb C, et. al. Prediction of response to erythropoietin treatment in chronic anemia of cancer. Blood 84:1056, 1994.

104. Clemens J, Spivak JL. Serum immunoreactive erythropoietin during the perioperative period. Surgery 115:510, 1994

105. Kettelhack C, Hönes C, Messinger D, Schlag, P. M. Randomized multicentre trial of the influence of recombinant human erythropoietin on intraoperative and postoperative transfusion need in anaemic patients undergoing right hemicolectomy for carcinoma. Br. J. Surgery 85:63, 1998.

106. Sowale O, Warnke H, Scigalla P, Sowade B, et al. Avoidance of allogeneic bloodtransfusions by treatment with epoetin beta (recombinant human erythropoietin) in patients undergoing open-heart

surgery. Blood 89:411, 1997.

107. Goldberg MA, McCutchen JW, Jove M, et al. A safety and efficacy comparison study of two dosing regimens of epoetin alfa in patiants undergoing major orthopedic surgery. Amer. J. Orthopedics 544, 1996

108. Henry DH, Abels RI. Recombinant human erythropoietin in the treatment of cancer and chemotherapy-induced anemia: results of double-blind and open-label follow-up studies. Sem. Oncol. 21:21-28, 1994.

109. Henry D, Abels R, Larholt K. Prediction of response to recombinant human erythropoieitn (r-HuEPO/Epoetin-α) therapy in cancer patients. Blood. 85:1676, 1995.

110. Coleman DH, Stevens AR Jr, Dodge HT., Finch CA. Rate of blood regeneration after blood loss. Arch Int. Med 92:341, 1953.

111. Brugnara C, Colella GM, Cremins J, Langley RC Jr, et.al. Effects of subcutaneous recombinant human erythropoietin in normal subjects: development of decreased reticulocyte hemoglobin content and iron-deficient erythropoiesis. J. Lab. Clin. Med. 123:660, 1994.

112. Glaspy JA., Chap L. The clinical aplication of recombinant erythropoietin in the HIV-infected patient. Hematol./Oncol Clin. N.A. 8:945, 1994.

113. Leitgeb C, Pecherstorfer M, Fritz E, Ludwib H. Quality of life in chronic anemia of cancer during treatment with recombinant human erythropoietin.Cancer 73:2535, 1994.

114. Blay JY, Le Cesne A, Mermet C, Maugard C. A risk model for thrombocytopenia requiring platelet transfusion after cytotoxic chemotherapy. Blood. 92:405, 1998.

115. Demetri GD, Kris M, Wade J, et al. Quality of life benefit in chemtherapy patients treated with epoietin-α B independent of disease response or tumor type. J Clin Oncol 16:3412-3425, 1998.

IV

Management of Thrombocytopenia

12.   Regulation of Human Megakaryocytopoiesis

Ronald Hoffman, Michael W. Long

Introduction

Megakaryocytopoiesis is a complex biological process involving a series of cellular events that begins with the pluripotent hematopoietic stem cell and ultimately results in the biogenesis of platelets[1]. A hierarchy of MK progenitor cells, the progeny of which eventually proliferate and mature into MKs, has been defined[1-3].

A wide variety of regulatory signals act in concert to direct platelet production[1,4]. Cells comprising the MK lineage include: primitive, actively proliferating progenitor cells, post-mitotic MKs still capable of undergoing endoreduplication, and more differentiated MKs undergoing terminal maturation. This developmental process is regulated by a complex network of interacting stem cells, stromal cells, growth factors, and extracellular matrix proteins[1-8]. This process ultimately, results in the daily production of approximately 2×10^{11} platelets[8].

Although the exact makeup of the MK microenvironment is still unknown, many of its important elements have been defined. The cellular components are the parenchymal cells (i.e., cells committed to MK lineage) and the neighboring stromal cells such as fibroblasts, endothelial cells, and macrophages. These stromal cells produce both membrane-associated and soluble cytokines (growth factors) as well as extracellular molecules important to MK function. Among these growth factors, at least three interleukins (IL-3, IL-6, and IL-11) as well as stem cell factor (SCF), GM-CSF, thrombopoietin (TPO), and possibly, erythropoietin (EPO), stimulate both *in vivo* and *in vitro* MK development[1]. The final component of megakaryocytic microenvironment is the extracellular matrix (ECM). Once referred to as basement membrane, ECM is no longer thought to be an inert structural scaffold. Instead, it is a dynamic, complex cellular substrate, whose components stimulate cells to proliferate, differentiate, or migrate[9]. Recent studies demonstrate that, like other lineages, MKs have unique developmental requirements which are modulated by interactions with specific ECM molecules[5-7,10,11].

Megakaryocytopoiesis occurs within a number of locations throughout the body. Clearly, the primary site of MK development (and hence platelet production) is the bone marrow. However, it is known that MK precursors and some mature MKs circulate, which suggests that capillary beds might filter (trap) such cells[12,13]. If the surrounding microenvironment is appropriate, then MKs may develop in such extramedullary tissue. This is true for both the spleen and lungs, each of which contain MKs and produce platelets[14,15]. However, their contribution to total thrombocytopoiesis is likely on the order of only 7-15%[8,15].

Human MK Progenitor Cells

Various classes of hematopoietic progenitor cells have been identified by the use of *in vitro* clonal assay systems (Table 1) [3]. The kinetics of appearance of these various

Table 1. Characteristics of Human Megakaryocyte Progenitor Cells

Characteristics	HPPC-MK	BFU-MK	CFU-MK
Cells/colony	300-1000	108.6 ± 4.4	11.6 ± 1.2
Foci/colony	1.0 ± 0.0	2.3 ± 0.4	1.2 ± 0.1
Phenotype	CD34CDW109$^+$	CD34$^+$HLA-DR$^-$ ckit$^+$CD45RA	CD34$^+$ HLA-DR$^+$ ckit$^+$CD45RA$^-$ (CD41$^+$Mpl)†
Tissue source	Fetal bone marrow ? ? ?	Fetal bone marrow Adult Bone Marrow Cord blood Peripheral blood	Fetal bone marrow Adult Bone Marrow Cord blood Peripheral blood
Optimal time of appearance(days)	(21)	(16)21*	(7)12*

The number in parentheses indicates the time of appearance of fetal MK progenitor cells.
*Time of appearance of adult MK progenitor cell.
†A subpopulation of differentiated CFU-MK capable of forming small pure MK colonies in vitro are CD41+ and express the thrombopoietin receptor, Mpl

classes of colonies is consistent with a sequential developmental relationship between these various MK progenitor subpopulations [3]. The more primitive hematopoietic progenitor cells have a greater capacity for proliferation than their more differentiated counterparts and require longer periods of incubation *in vitro* for the appearance of their descendent colonies. A hierarchy of MK progenitor cells has been established based upon studies of *in vitro* megakaryocytopoiesis (Table 1) [3]. The most primitive lineage-restricted MK progenitor cell, referred to as MK-high proliferative potential-colony forming cell (MK-HPP-CFC) was first described in the murine system [16]. These progenitor cells exhibit a much higher degree of proliferation than other previously identified MK progenitor cells and require a longer incubation period to form macroscopic colonies *in vitro* [17]. Jackson et al have described, also in the mouse, a similar primitive lineage-restricted MK progenitor cell and termed it the HPP-CFU-MK [18]. The colonies derived from these cells *in vitro* form large unifocal aggregates when cultured from either bone marrow preparations obtained from animals pretreated with 5-fluorouracil or from lineage-negative bone marrow cells [18].

An extremely rare type of human MK progenitor cell that resembles the murine HPP-CFU-MK has been cloned from fetal bone marrow (FBM) CD34$^+$ cells in the presence of a combination of cytokines. Massive unifocal pure MK colonies are derived from these primitive progenitors which contain ≥ 300 cells (300-100), which form after 21 days of incubation (Table 1) [12]. These colonies represent the progeny of a unique type of lineage-restricted MK progenitor cell, termed the high proliferative potential cell-MK (HPPC-MK) (Fig. 1). Because of its extensive proliferative capacity, this progenitor cell appears to be the human equivalent of the murine MK

HPP-CFCs. It is possible that this very primitive MK progenitor cell in humans is unique to FBM, although the inability to assay these progenitors from adult bone marrow may merely reflect their extremely low frequency or the absence of a critical growth factor required for their proliferation *in vitro*. Although the phenotype of these primitive MK progenitor cells has not been entirely defined, recent studies have shown that a CD34$^+$CDw109$^+$ subpopulation of FBM is enriched for HPPC-MK [19]. The CDw109 antigen has been previously shown to be expressed by primitive human fetal hematopoietic stem cells [20].

The burst forming unit-MK (BFU-MK) is the most primitive progenitor cell committed to the MK lineage that can be presently assayed from adult marrow, peripheral blood and cord blood [3,17,21]. The more differentiated colony forming unit-MK (CFU-MK) can easily be distinguished from the BFU-MK by a variety of characteristics [17,21] (Table 1).

The HPPC-MK, BFU-MK, and CFU-MK are lineage-restricted progenitor cells which give rise to colonies exclusively composed of Mks [3]. Semisolid assays of human marrow to which are added combinations of hematopoietic growth factors also contain colonies composed of a variety of lineages including a minority population of Mks [3,22,23]. These mixed lineage progenitor cells, CFU-erythrocyte MK (CFU-EM), CFU-macrophage MK (CFU-MM), CFU-granulocyte erythrocyte macrophage MK (CFU-GEMM) likely represent oligopotent progenitor cells which are intermediate between pluripotent hematopoietic stem cells and unipotent hematopoietic progenitor cells [22]. The physiological significance of these mixed lineage progenitor cells which retain their ability to differentiate along the MK lineage remains unknown, although a hierarchy of these multipotential MK progenitor cells appears to exist.

Multiple lineages present within colonies derived from such multipotent progenitor cells are mitotically affected by such early acting cytokines as SCF and IL-3. Specific lineage within such colonies are driven toward terminal differentiation by lineage-specific signals (EPO and TPO) [19,24,27]. Debili and co-workers[23] utilized clonogenic assays and single cell cultures to further characterize a bipotent erythro-megakaryocytic progenitor cell (BFU-E/MK) in human adult bone marrow capable of producing only erythroid and megakaryocytic cells. CD34$^+$ bone marrow cells were subfractionated according to expression of the CD38 antigen [23]. The bipotent BFU-E/MK progenitor as well as a large fraction of pure MK progenitors were found in the CD34$^+$CD38$^\pm$ or in the CD34$^+$CD38$^-$ cell fractions but not in a CD34$^+$CD38$^+$ cell population [23]. The single cell origin of bipotent BFU-E/MK colonies was demonstrated in single cell cultures of CD34$^+$CD38^{low} cells[23]. After 12 days of incubation, 30% of the clones in individual wells contained glycophorin A$^+$ cells (erythroblasts) and some CD41$^+$cells (MKs) without the presence of CD14 cells (granulocytes) and CD15$^+$ cells (Macrophages). However, by day 20, clones containing erythroblasts and MKs were rare (5%) [23]. These findings support the existence of a compartment of bipotent progenitor cells with a differentiation program limited to two lineages (erythroid and megakaryocytic) which are dependent on the presence of EPO for the detection of their potential to differentiate along the erythroid pathway. These BFU-E/MK derived colonies are quite different from CFU-GEMM derived colonies which are composed of larger numbers of erythroblasts and require longer periods of incubation *in vitro* to appear (12 days versus > 18-20 days) [23]. The contribution of such mixed lineage progenitors to MK production has remained unknown. Papayannopoulou et al , however, have presented data which indicates that erythroid and MK cells can be generated from either bipotent (BFU-E/MK) or unilineage progenitors and that both EPO and TPO can affect both pure and bipotent progenitor cells [28]. These studies suggest that some fraction of marrow MKs ultimately originate not only from CFU-MK but also from BFU-E/MK.

The phenotypes of the classes of various MK progenitor cells are summarized in Table 1. All of the MK progenitors identified to date are CD34$^+$ [17,23,29]. CD34 expression diminishes as MK differentiation proceeds, yet a population of polyploid transitional immature MK still express CD34 [29]. The majority of BFU-MK and CFU-MK are CD45RA$^-$. A small number of CFU-MK with a limited proliferative capacity are CD34$^+$ CD41$^+$; this cell population likely represents the direct ancestor of the CD34$^+$CD41$^+$ polyploid transitional immature MK[29] . These CD34 CD41 cell populations that form small MK colonies *in vitro* express the TPO receptor (Mpl$^+$) [25]. The bipotent BFU-E/MK in adult marrow has also been shown to be CD34$^+$CD45RA$^-$CD41$^+$Mpl$^+$ [23,28].

A subpopulation of human MKs have also been shown to express the CD4 antigen [30-32]. CD4 is a 55Kd transmembrane glycoprotein originally identified as a differentiation antigen on T-cells that has recently been shown to be present on other hematopoietic lineages including monocytes, eosinophils and human and murine hematopoietic progenitor cells. The functional significance of CD4 expression by MKs remains unknown. Recently, Dolzhansky and co-workers examined the developmental changes in the expression of CD4 and CD34 on cells of the MK lineage [31]. They reported that MK cells are over-represented in the CD34$^+$ progenitor population and that CD4 expression occurs during relatively early stages of human MK maturation, when the MKs are still CD34$^+$ [31]. The loss of CD4 seems to be coincidental with the onset of endomitotic DNA replication and is associated with a loss of the ability of these cells to undergo normal mitotic division and form colonies *in vitro* [31]. Since CD4 is a receptor for the entry of HIV-1 into T-cells and monocytes, the presence of CD4 on immature transitional CD34$^+$CD41$^+$CD4$^+$ polyploid MKs makes this cell a potential target for HIV-1 infection.

The restriction of CD4 to more differentiated MK has been challenged by two other groups [30,32]. Both Louache et al and Zauli et al have detected a large fraction of CD34$^+$ cells (50%) which weakly stain with antiCD4 antibodies and include erythroid, granulocytic and MK progenitors [30,32]. This CD4 molecule present on the CD34$^+$CD4^{low} cells was reported to be capable of binding HIV-1 [32]. Resolution of this controversy concerning CD4 expression during MK differentiation may provide further insight into the pathobiology of HIV-1 induced thrombocytopenia.

Immature MKs (Promegakaryoblasts)

Promegakaryoblasts (ProMKBs) are transitional cells intermediate between the proliferating progenitor cells and the post-mitotic, mature Mks [33,34]. Morphologically, these immature cells are not readily observed *in vitro* or in bone marrow specimens, but can be identified by their expression of MK/platelet-specific markers such as platelet peroxidase, platelet glycoprotein IIb/IIIa, von Willebrand's factor (vWF) etc.

ProMKBs are restricted (or lacking) in proliferative potential [35,36]. They, thus, are the developmental stage at which MKs cease to proliferate but, rather, continue to acquire an increased DNA content. As such, they are endomitotic (a mechanism of acquiring polyploid nuclei, *vide infra*) and contain an intermediate DNA content. The PMkB respond to a variety of hematopoietic growth factors (IL-3, SCF, IL-6 and TPO) *in vitro*, maturing into single, large Mks [37,38]. Observations of the early phases of CFU-MK colony formation demonstrate that progenitor cells pass through a ProMKB stage during development thus confirming the parent:progeny relationship between ProMKBs and Mks [33]. Studies in animals document the responsiveness of these cells *in vivo*. ProMKBs are highly sensitive to thrombopoietic demand and are the first cells to increase in number following the induction of thrombocytopenia, or decrease following conditions of thrombocytosis [33,39]. Subsequently, expansion and reduction (respectively) in MK numbers are seen, again confirming the kinetic and developmental relationship between the ProMKBs and their more differentiated progeny. ProMKBs also are a heterogeneous group of cells, and during development increase in nuclear and cytoplasmic complexity.

Mature MKs

Morphologically recognizable MKs exist in three maturational stages as defined by their morphology. The megakaryoblast (Stage I) is characterized by high nuclear to cytoplasmic ratio and scanty basophilic cytoplasm, reflecting the large amounts of protein synthesis occurring in these cells. The Stage II is the cell in which both the cytoplasmic volume and number of platelet-specific granules increase. The granular or "platelet-shedding" MK (Stages III and IV) is the most mature of the MKs, and supposedly is the platelet-shedding cell [3,40]. It should be understood that these morphological classifications also represent a maturation progression and are, themselves, heterogeneous with respect to many other developmental characteristics such as antigenic expression, enzymatic content, and DNA content.

Platelets

The final event of MK development is the release of platelets into the circulation. Interestingly, the platelets were the first element of this lineage to be identified, and among the first of the blood cells observed. During maturation, a proliferation and invagination of the MK plasma membrane occurs, resulting in the development of a tubular network known as the demarcation membrane system (DMS). The DMS is thought to divide the MK cytoplasm into platelet fields, although its exact role in the formation of individual platelets remains obscure and, thus, controversial. Finally, MKs seem to extend pseudopods into the sinusoidal lumen from which platelets are shed into the circulation.

Regulation of MK Development

There are three areas in which physiological control over the MK lineage is relevant: the expansion of MK numbers (proliferation), the regulation of MK maturation, and the control of platelet-shedding [1,3]. The role of cytokines in the first two of these areas has been clearly defined.. Increasing evidence suggests the importance of the ECM components to MK and/or platelet production.

MK-Active Cytokines

Harker and Finch first demonstrated that, *in vivo*, thrombocytopoiesis was regulated by alterations in both MK number and MK volume (mass) [8]. In the late 1970s and early 1980s investigators, struggling with crude sources of MK growth factor, discovered the *in vitro* correlates of the Harker and Finch hypothesis: that distinct factors (bioactivities) seem to regulate the proliferative and maturation events occurring during *in vitro* MK development [38,41-43]. The purification of these activities proved difficult, but the rapid identification and cloning of numerous human recombinant hematopoietic growth factors in the mid to late 1980s and early 1990s markedly improved our understanding of the cytokine control of megakaryocytopoiesis [1,3].

A number of cytokines have been shown to affect MK proliferation *in vitro*, highlighting the importance of growth factor redundancy and combinatorial control. The concept of combinatorial control is illustrated by studies in which multiple cytokines provide a better (*in vitro*) stimulus than single growth factors. Studies in which purified progenitor cells are cultured in defined, serum free, media indicate that as many as 2-7 recombinant hematopoietic growth factors have additive proliferative effects on MKs progenitor cell proliferation [26,41,44].

The most physiologically relevant class of interactions are growth factor combinations which are synergistic (i.e., pharmacologically non-additive). This type of control is biologically important as synergistic responses strongly suggest that differing intracellular signal transduction pathways are co-activated, leading to dramatic and rapid increases in proliferation. This has been clearly demonstrated in other developmental systems and for murine as well as human megakaryocytopoiesis[41,45,46].

Of the hematopoietic growth factors which affect MK proliferation, IL-3 is the most potent. It stimulates each of the three classes of MK progenitor cells, the immature cells, as well as the mature MKs [18,19,47]. However, the physiological role of IL-3 remains unclear. Exogenous IL-3 stimulates *in vivo* expansion of MK progenitor cells, but by itself, IL-3 has little (significant) effect on *in vivo* platelet production[48]. Moreover, IL-3 is only produced by antigen-activated T lymphocytes suggesting that its role in maintaining basal platelet production is minimal. Another pleiotropic cytokine affecting MK development is GM-CSF. GM-CSF stimulates development of BFU- MK and CFU-MK. However, parallel cell culture experiments demonstrate that its MK-stimulatory activity is approximately 1/100th of that of IL-3 [47]. Nonetheless, this protein functions as a MK-CSF and its actions are additive to those of IL-3, suggesting a single, converging intracellular, mitotic signaling pathway.

A number of growth factors have MK maturational activities, e.g., TPO, IL-6, IL-3, SCF, IL-1, IL-11, G-CSF, and leukemia inhibitory factor (LIF) [18,22,49-52]. While none of these purified and/or recombinant molecules are MK lineage-specific, some are synergistic co-regulators. Such auxiliary growth factors were first defined *in vitro* as cytokines that lack the solitary ability to simulate MK proliferation, but do function as co-regulators to augment MK development [18,41,53]. Of hematopoietic growth factors identified, only a few fall into this category: SCF, IL-1α, IL-6, and IL-11. IL-11 has multiple effects on *in vivo* and *in vitro* megakaryocytopoiesis [18,51,54,55]. It not only affects IL-3 dependent MK colony formation, but also has a potent effect on MK maturation. Neben et al has shown that recombinant human IL-11 when administered *in vivo* to mice results in increased numbers of MK progenitors, increased MK DNA content (polyploidy), and increased peripheral platelet counts [56]. Recently, IL-11 was approved for use in humans for the treatment of chemotherapy-induced thrombocytopenia. Another MK maturational-promoter is IL-6 [44,50]. This cytokine stimulates MK maturation and its actions (are partially) additive to those of IL-3. Although *in vivo* IL-6 stimulates platelet production and speeds recovery from thrombocytopenia in animals, its actions may be via the secondary activation of accessory (stromal) cells [55,57].

Finally, a number of cytokines (e.g., TGF-β, platelet factor 4, certain interferons) can inhibit megakaryocytopoiesis. Platelets release specific and general inhibitors of megakaryocytopoiesis, such as TGF-β and platelet factor 4 [58-60]. However, the physiological role for platelet-derived inhibitors is unclear. Theoretically, one would hypothesize that increased platelet destruction should stimulate, rather than inhibit, platelet production raising the paradoxical situation of increasing inhibitors with increased platelet destruction. Other inhibitors such as the interferons also inhibit MK development [61].

Thrombopoietin (TPO)

TPO was classically defined as an activity in the plasma of thrombocytopenic animals or humans that, when transferred to a secondary recipient, stimulates platelet production (as monitored by radio-labeled amino acid incorporation) [62-64]. For three decades, multiple unsuccessful attempts were made to isolate TPO. The search for TPO began in earnest following studies which indicated that a rare, and poorly understood, member of an orphan-receptor family was involved in MK development. Vignon et al cloned the human and murine homologues of the v-mpl oncogene that is transduced by the myeloproliferative leukemia virus [65,66]. The c-mpl gene encodes a protein with strong homologies to the highly conserved hematopoietin receptor superfamily, and is expressed in low levels in cells of hematopoietic origin [67]. Methia et al used reverse-transcriptase-based PCR studies to demonstrate c-mpl expression in CD34[+] cells, MKs, and platelets[67]. This data clearly indicated a role for this receptor in megakaryocytopoiesis, and further suggested that the as yet unidentified mpl ligand may be the elusive TPO.

Guided by the Wendling observations, a number of groups cloned TPO (1994)[68-72]. The TPO gene encodes a protein with a predicted molecular weight of 31-35kDa, with the amino terminal domain having homology to EPO. The genomic structure of TPO spans 6-8 kilobases, and consists of approximately 8 axons and 6 introns, with the protein encoded by axons 3-7 [74,75]. Localization studies have mapped human TPO to chromosome 3, within the region of 3q26-28 [74]. Analysis of the promoter region of this gene shows binding sites for several important transcriptional activating factors including GATA-1 and Ets family members [75,76]. A splice variant of the TPO gene exists as a result of a 4 nucleotide deletion within the EPO homology domain [72,73,75]. These studies demonstrated a profound effect of TPO on the MK lineage. Administration of TPO results in an increase in the frequency of MKs in the bone marrow and spleen, an increase in MK size and DNA content, an increase in MK/platelet-specific antigenic markers, and an increase in circulating platelet concentration by a factor of 3- to 10-fold [69-71].

Numerous studies over the past 30 years demonstrated an inverse relationship between the levels of circulating TPO and platelet mass. The access to recombinant or purified TPO, and the availability of gene knockout animals, has allowed the further dissection of this relationship at the cellular and molecular level. Data from these studies best fit the model in which the predominant feed-back mechanism regulating TPO concentration is its binding to platelets and/or MKs. Thus, during periods of normal homeostasis, platelet counts (i.e., mass) remain constant and circulating TPO is at its basal concentration. By contrast, reduction of the platelet mass results in a fall in the binding and degradation of TPO by c-mpl-positive cells, and an increased concentration of "free" TPO. Conversely, during conditions such as rebound thrombocytosis or primary thrombocythemia, elevated platelet/MK mass serves as a "sink", reducing the levels of circulating TPO to achieve homeostasis. (Fig.1) Thus, TPO production in most circumstances remains constant, and its concentration is regulated by the total mass of platelets/MKs available to bind and degrade this protein. Gene inactivation studies demonstrate that TPO and its receptor (c-mpl) are the primary regulators of thrombocytopoiesis [77-82]. Thus, TPO-deficient and c-mpl-deficient mice show an approximate 85% reduction in the number of circulating platelets, as well as markedly reduced bone marrow MK numbers [77,78]. Studies of TPO concentration in c-mpl-deficient mice show increased levels, and gene-dose effects in TPO-deficient animals (i.e., TPO$^{+/-}$ vs. TPO$^{-/-}$) also demonstrates this relationship [82]. Confirming these *in vivo* observations, a number of studies demonstrate the interaction of TPO with platelets. Purified native TPO binds to platelets and, conversely, platelet infusions during times of thrombocytopenia leads to reductions in the elevated levels of TPO [81,82]. Studies of platelets from c-mpl-deficient mice indicate that they fail to bind (radiolabeled) TPO, whereas normal platelets bind, internalize, and degrade this protein [81-84]. Likewise, the administration of washed, normal platelets to c-mpl-deficient animals causes a transient reduction in their (high) TPO levels [82]. Consistent with these observations, platelets have been shown to express high-affinity TPO receptors with an affinity of 200-560 pM and between 20-200 receptors per platelet [82,85]. MK mass appears to be a major determinant of TPO levels. Individuals with thrombocytopenia due to peripheral destruction have normal TPO concentrations due to the presence of increased MK numbers, while levels are markedly elevated following chemotherapy or in aplastic anemia patients [86-88]. TPO is produced by the adult and fetal liver, and the adult kidney and its mRNA levels are not altered in these organs by changes in platelet concentration. However, a secondary, or alternative, mechanism of regulating TPO concentration seems to exist within the stroma of bone marrow and spleen, that is activated during periods of thrombocytopenia [89]. In these organs, TPO is transcriptionally activated during thrombocytopenia resulting in an increase in TPO mRNA, and, presumably, protein.

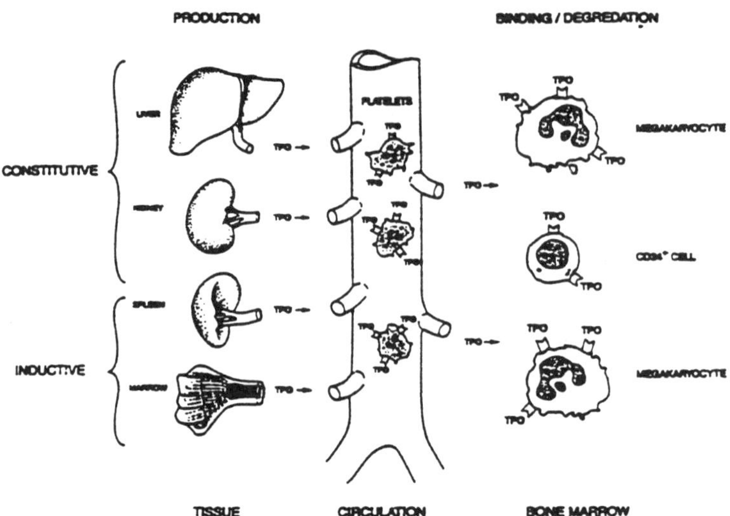

Figure 1. Regulation of Thrombopoietin Production. TPO is constitutively produced in the liver, kidney, and perhaps the spleen. During times of increased thrombocytopenic demand, the bone marrow and spleen seem to increase their expression of TPO, thus contributing to platelet production. TPO, in turn, is bound by circulating platelets, as well as megakaryocytes and other c-mpl positive cells in the bone marrow and other sites of hemato/thrombocytopoiesis (see text). From Long and Hoffman with permission [145].

The regulation of TPO concentration, therefore, can be thought of in terms of having both constitutive and inducible components (Figure 1). The liver, kidney, and perhaps the spleen, constitutively produce TPO, and its levels are regulated by the total mass of platelets and MKs. However, during times of thrombopoietic stress, increased TPO expression by the spleen and bone marrow presumably contribute to platelet production.

The cellular targets of TPO are diverse. C-mpl-receptors are expressed on both MKs and platelets, as well as hematopoietic stem/progenitor cells. In mice, TPO affects early stem/progenitor cells as shown by its stimulation of the expansion of a very immature precursor both *in vitro* and *in vivo* [91-93]. TPO thus stimulates both murine and human long-term repopulating cells, as well as phenotypically defined primitive hematopoietic stem cells [93]. In isolated populations of immunologically-defined primitive human hematopoietic cells, TPO generates CD41+ MKs (alone or in conjunction with other cytokines such as IL-3 or SCF) [92]. This capacity is observed at the single cell level thus demonstrating the direct effect of TPO on hematopoietic stem/progenitor cells.

TPO is required for full maturation of the MK lineage. TPO also synergizes with other members of the hematopoietin receptor superfamily to augment MK development. Under serum-free conditions, TPO stimulates CD34+ cells (either alone or in combination with other cytokines such as IL-3, EPO, or SCF) to produce MKs[94,95]. MK progenitor cells show variable response to TPO (alone or in combination with other cytokines) suggesting that these cells have a differential sensitivity to this growth factor [94,96]. More mature progenitor cells (as defined by co-expression of CD34 and CD41) or the transitional ProMKB (in single cell culture) respond with either maturational development or a limited degree of proliferation [97]. Interestingly, although the resulting single MKs are mature, and of high ploidy, 60% show ultrastructural defects in the formation of the DMS and/or alpha-granule synthesis, whereas the remainder are ultrastructurally indistinguishable from normal bone marrow MKs. It is interesting to note that, in serum-free culture, TPO fails to support full MK development, even when target cells are stimulated with high concentrations of TPO. Thus, few TPO-stimulated human MKs reach ploidy levels $\geq$16C [71]. Even the use of more mature CD34$^+$ CD41$^+$ cells as a starting population, generates CD41$^+$ cells predominantly with a low DNA content [98,99]. The limited ability of human CD34$^+$ stem/progenitor cells to generate high ploidy MKs is in sharp contrast to the experience in the murine system, where 35-55% of *ex vivo*-generated MKs are high ploidy cells [100]. Such observations suggest that other growth factors or microenvironmental signals are required for full polyploidization of human MKs and, hence, for MK maturation. The availability of recombinant TPO also allows the generation of intact, functional platelets *in vitro*, thus facilitating studies of this poorly understood aspect of MK development.[101] Interestingly, the administration of TPO to platelets *in vitro* does not stimulate platelet aggregation [102]. Rather, its pre-administration (*in vivo* or *in vitro*) "primes" platelet aggregation increasing platelet responsiveness to various agonists such as ADP, epinephrine, thrombin, and collagen[103,104].

Extracellular Influences and Cell Interactions

Blood cells develop within the marrow in the context of their interactions with neighboring cells and extracellular molecules. Within the last decade, a number of investigations demonstrated that stromal cells and ECM are dynamic and inductive (or permissive) components of all developing cellular systems. With respect to hematopoiesis, numerous studies have shown that hematopoietic progenitors cells interact with growth factors, accessory cells such as T cells, stromal cells, and ECM components [9]. This developmental network is further complicated by observations that stromal cells express membrane-associated growth factors [105,106], and that ECM both binds hematopoietic growth factors and presents these cytokines in a biologically functional manner [107,108].

Both cell:cell and cell:ECM communications among developing MKs are poorly understood. Structurally, mature (platelet-shedding) MKs are located on the abluminal surface of the bone marrow sinusoid. MKs are thought to extend pseudopods through or between sinusoidal endothelial cells, thus allowing sheer forces to fragment platelets into the circulation [109]. Both the location and putative mechanism of platelet-shedding imply that MK:ECM or MK:endothelial cell interactions are important to thrombocytopoiesis. Isolated MKs adhere to (bovine corneal endothelial) cell-derived ECM and proplatelet-like structures are induced under these conditions [110]. As well, MKs adhere to collagen and secrete both a collagenase and a gelatinase suggesting a possible mechanism for pseudopod infiltration of the surrounding EDM [11,110].

Studies of MK progenitor cells show that cell:ECM relationships are important to MK proliferation. Approximately 30% of CFU-MK cells in bone marrow adhere to the ECM proteins fibronectin or thrombospondin (TSP). Interestingly, 60-80% of primitive BFU-MK attach to TSP, whereas they fail to bind to fibronectin [10]. Therefore, primitive MK progenitor cells show both altered expression of cytoadhesion molecule attachment and altered responsiveness to complex matrix:cytokine regulatory signals.

MKs are known to transmigrate through bone marrow endothelial cells and release platelets within the sinusoidal space or lung capillaries [112]. Recently, the chemokine, stromal derived factor-1 has been shown to induce the transendothelial migration of mature Mks [113]. The receptor for stromal derived factor-1 is the G-protein coupled chemokine receptor CXCR4 which is expressed by mature MKs. The expression of CXCR4 by mature MKs may be the critical cellular signal needed for transmigration of MKs and platelet formation [112,113].

MK Cell Cycle Control and Endomitosis

Unlike other cells, MKs continue to synthesize DNA during differentiation. During this process, MKs become polypoid having a DNA content of 8C to 128C , where 2C is the DNA content of a somatic cell [114-116]. MKs are not multinucleate cells, but contain this increased DNA content within a single, albeit highly lobulated, nucleus[117,118]. Tritiated thymidine incorporation has been utilized to demonstrate that mature (Stage II and Stage III) MKs do not take up this label, thus showing they are not undergoing DNA synthesis [119,120]. Stage I MKs are the only recognizable cells capable of synthesizing DNA, but only 20-40% of these cells do so. Following a prolonged exposure to tritiated thymidine, 100% of the MKs are labelled indicating that the majority of DNA synthesis occurs in the immediate precursor of the megakaryoblast (the ProMKB). The cell cycle of MKs thus is different from other cells in that the normal cell cycle progression is abolished. However, this release from normal cell cycle control does not imply that MK DNA synthesis is dysregulated. The acquisition of a polyploid nucleus is tightly or globally controlled, as MKs show progressive doublings of their DNA content and no intermediate ploidy classes (e.g., 3C, 6C) are seen.

Two observations indicate that formation of a polyploid nucleus requires alterations in the MK cell cycle. As mentioned earlier, ProMKBs actively synthesize DNA, for a prolonged period [119,120]. Second, megakaryoblasts do not go through the usual processes of mitosis, as few, if any, cells reach metaphase and none progress into anaphase or telophase. As important as these observations are, they are based on either morphological evidence, or the analysis of a limited number of MKs. Indeed, the term that is usually applied to this process is endomitosis, a morphological classification [121]. The definition of endomitosis refers to the replication of nuclear elements within an intact nuclear envelope without subsequent chromosomal movement or cytokinesis. This term is best used to describe MK polyploidization [117]. Frequently, the term endoreduplication is erroneously applied to MKs. Endoreduplication is the mechanism which results in polytenic (diplo- and quatro-chromosome number) cells in insects, and is a chromosome duplication cycle not associated with endomitotic-like changes [121].

Given that the polyploid nature of MKs is unique among mammalian bone marrow cells, the question arises as to the biological significance of this altered DNA content. A related question is whether or not polyploidization occurs as a prerequisite to, or a consequence of, the increased MK in cell volume occurring within these cells. It is know that MK DNA content is related to MK cell size and thus to the eventual numbers of platelets produced [117,122]. A number of studies have documented the effect of thrombocytopenic demand on MKs. For example, acute thrombocytopenia results in an increased DNA content prior to increased platelet production [117]. Likewise, increments in cytoplasmic volume and cytoplasmic maturation occur predominantly, if not completely, in Stage II and Stage III MKs, which do not appear to synthesize DNA [117,122]. Therefore, whatever its functional significance, polyploidization precedes the increase in MK cell volume. This association of increased DNA content and increased cell volume implies that the large DNA content in MKs is somehow relevant to the process of platelet formation. For example, increased DNA content may be associated with increased mRNA expression which, in turn, might promote the degree of biosynthesis required for platelet formation. While this remains to be proven, it is clear that MKs synthesize increased amounts of DNA prior to increases in cytoplasmic maturation.

Two classes, or families of proteins control progression through the cell cycle in mammalian cells. These are the cell division kinases (also known as cyclin-dependent kinases, CDK), and the cyclins, so named for their cyclical synthesis and degradation. Together, these two classes of proteins form a protein-kinase complex in which the catalytic unit is a CDK, and the regulatory unit is a cyclin. Different CDK complexes regulate cell cycle progression [123,124]. The role of these kinase complexes in cell cycle control is complex. Currently, seven members of the cyclin gene family have been identified, as well as at least seven distinct CDK genes [125-127]. The role of the kinase known as cdc2, and its cognate cyclin (B) is best understood. Together, these proteins form a mitosis-initiating cdc2 kinase complex which is also known as Maturation (or Mitosis) Promoting Factor. The cdc2/cyclin B kinase complex regulates the initiation of mitosis at the G_2/M transition as well as subsequent events such as spindle fiber formation and cytokinesis. Among the CDK proteins, cdk2 plays an important role in regulating both G_1/S transit, and S-phase progression. A number of regulatory cyclins are complexed with cdk2; cyclin E plays a role in G_1 progression and in G_1/S transit; cyclin A is essential for both S phase and the initiation of DNA replication [-132] The cdk2/cyclin E complex is assembled in mid-G_1 and its associated kinase activity peaks in late G_1 and early S phase, whereas cdk2/cyclin A activity is maximal in S phase [128,133]. Another family of cyclins, the G_1 cyclins (D-type cyclins in mammals) together with cdk4 or cdk6, are important in timing G_1 progression, as well as in G_1/S transit [134]. The D-cyclins are partially cell-type specific, and most cells express cyclin D3 and either D1 or D2 [135]. Interestingly, the D-type cyclins also bind with cdk2 [136].

The precise role of CDK and cyclin proteins in MK endomitosis is unknown. Nonetheless, a general hypothesis can be put forward concerning the biochemical control of the endomitotic cell cycle. Mitosis must be altered in order to accommodate an increased DNA content within a single nucleus, and the S-phase must be modified to prevent (or weaken) its interdependency with the M-phase. Not too surprisingly, MKs have alterations at the two control (or restriction) points evident in all cycling cells. They have a prolonged S-phase period and synthesize increased amounts of DNA (i.e., they are altered in G_1 or S phase), and they undergo an abrogation of mitosis (M-phase). Interestingly, in most diploid cells, the cdc2/cyclin B complex kinase activity peaks in early metaphase [137]. This is just the point at which MKs fail to progress through mitosis. Moreover, recent observations demonstrate the stabilizing mutations of the cyclin B gene (e.g., the loss of its n-terminal domain) results in persistence of this protein, the sustained presence of which leads to mitotic arrest [138,139].

Human erythroleukemia (HEL) cells model endomitosis while becoming megakaryocytic during phorbol diester-induced MK differentiation [140]. Datta and co-workers have shown that the mitotic arrest occurring in these polyploid cells involves novel biochemical alterations in the cdc2/cyclin β1 complex: a marked reduction in cdc2 protein levels, and an elevated and sustained expression of cyclin β1 [141]. As a result, endomitotic cells lack cdc2/cyclin β1-associated H1-histone kinase activity. Constitutive over-expression of cdc2 in endomitotic cells failed to re-initiate normal mitotic events even though cdc2 was present in a 10-fold excess. This was due to an inability of cyclin-B1 to physically associate with cdc2. Thus during MK differentiation of HEL cells, mitosis is abrogated during endomitosis due to the absence of cdc2 and the failure to form active cdc2/cyclin β kinase complexes, resulting in a disassociation of mitosis from the completion of S-phase. Similar results were seen by Zhang and co-workers who demonstrated a decreased cdc2/cyclin β kinase activity in polyploid MKs [142].

Polyploid HEL cells also represent a useful model for examining endomitotic S-phase control, as their cell cycle machinery must be modulated in order to allow the acquisition of high levels of DNA content (ploidy) within a single nucleus, and to allow the re-replication of newly synthesized DNA without an intervening mitosis. In order to evaluate the mechanisms of S-phase control during the process of polyploidization, Datta et al also investigated the events occurring in CDK complexes during the induction of MK differentiation in human erythroleukemia (HEL) cells [141]. During polyploidization, megakaryocytic HEL cells undergo a dramatic shift in the subunit composition of G_1- and S-phase associated CDK complexes, and an increase in their specific activities. In particular, cyclin D3 protein levels are increased (due to both a change in D3 mRNA levels, and a stabilization of its half-life), and there is a marked increase in cdk2/cyclin D3 kinase activity throughout the period of endomitosis [143]. Moreover, these changes occur within the context of an up-regulated function of cdk2/cyclin E complexes that are associated with both G_1/S transit and S-phase progression [143]. The cyclin D observations are consistent with studies by Wang et al showing that anti-sense cyclin D3 oligonucleotides abrogated MK development[144].

Conclusion

A hierarchy of human megakaryocyte (MK) progenitor cells have been defined by means of studies of *in vitro* megakaryocytopoiesis. These MK progenitors can be distinguished by their cellular phenotype, physical characteristics, chemosensitivity, the cytokines required to induce progenitor cell derived colony formation, kinetics of colony formation, and the size of the colonies that each progenitor cell subclass is capable of producing. A sequential developmental relationship between these various cellular subpopulations has been defined. MKs and their precursors express a number of developmentally regulated antigenic determinants. These cell surface antigens allow for the isolation and purification of marrow cells enriched for MK progenitor cells. The hallmark of MK maturation is the development of a single large lobulated polyploid nucleus. MKs continue to synthesize DNA during differentiation. The formation of a polyploid MK nucleus requires specific alterations of cell cycle machinery. The molecular basis of this unique cellular process is currently being explored. The ligand for Mpl has recently been recognized to be thrombopoietin (TPO), the long sought after proliferation and differentiation factor for MK development. TPO is the primary physiological regulator of platelet production. The physiology of TPO production and degradation has been only recently clarified.

References

1. Hoffman R. Regulation of megakaryocytopoiesis. Blood 74:1196-1212, 1989
2. Long MW. Population heterogeneity among cells of the MK lineage. Stem Cells 11:33-40, 1993
3. Bruno E, Hoffman R. Human megakaryocyte progenitor cells. Sem Hematol 35:183-192, 1998
4. Gordon MS, Hoffman R. Growth factors affecting human thrombocytopoiesis: Potential agents for the treatment of thrombocytopenia. Blood 80:302-307, 1992
5. Long MW, Dixit V. Thrombospondin functions as a cytoadhesion molecule for human hematopoietic progenitor cells. Blood 75:311-2319, 1990
6. Long MW, Briddell RA, Walter AU, et al. Human hematopoietic stem cells adherence to cytokines and matrix molecules. J Clin Invest 90:251-255, 1992
7. Bruno E, Luikart SD, Long MW, et al. Marrow-derived heparan/sulfate proteoglycan mediates the adhesion of hematopoietic progenitor cells to cytokines. Exp Hemat 23:1212-1217, 1995
8. Harker LA, Finch CA. Thrombokinetics in man. J Clin Invest 48:963-974, 1969
9. Long MW: Blood cell cytoadhesion molecules. Exp Hematol 20:288-301, 1992
10. Leven RM, Yee T. Collagenase production by guinea pig megakaryocytes in vitro. Exp Hematol 18:743-747, 1990
11. Eldor A. Fuks Z, Levine RF, Vlodavsky I. Measurement of platelet and megakaryocyte interaction with the subendothelial extracellular matrix. Methods Enzymol 169:76-9, 1989
12. Hansen M, Pedersen NT. Circulating megakaryocytes in patients with pulmonary inflammation and in patients subjected to cholecystectomy. Scand J Haematol 23:211-216, 1979
13. Zauli G, Vitale L, Brunelli MA, Bagnara GP. Prevalence of the primitive megakaryocyte progenitors (BFU-meg) in adult human peripheral blood. Exp. Hematol 20:850-854, 1992
14. Grouls V, Helpap B. Megakaryocytopoiesis in the spleen of growing rats. Am J Anat 157:429-432, 1980
15. Kaufman KM, Ario R, Pollack S, et al. Origin of pulmonary megakaryocytes. Blood 25:767, 1965
16. Long MW, Gragowski LL, Heffner CH, et al. Phorbol esters stimulate the development of an early murine progenitor cell. The burst forming unit-megakaryocyte. J Clin Invest 1985;76:431-438
17. Briddell RA, Brandt JE, Straneva JE, et al. Characterization of the human burst forming unit-megakaryocyte. Blood 74:145-151, 1989
18. Jackson H, Williams N, Bertoncello I, et al. Classes of primitive murine megakaryocytic progenitor cells. Exp Hematol 22:954-958, 1994
19. Bruno E, Murray LJ, DiGusto R, et al. Detection of a primitive megakaryocyte progenitor cell in human fetal bone marrow. Exp Hematol 24:552-558, 1996
20. Murray LJ, Bruno E, Yeo EL, et al. CDw109 antibody 8A3 identifies a minor subset of CD34[+] fetal bone marrow cells that includes multilineage and megakaryocyte progenitor cells as well as hematopoietic stem cells. Blood 84:237a, 1994

21. Briddell RA, Hoffman R. Cytokine regulation of the human burst forming unit-megakaryocyte. Blood 76:516-522, 1990

22. Hunt P: A bipotential megakaryocyte/erythrocyte progenitor cell. The link between erythropoiesis and megakaryopoiesis becomes stronger. J Lab Med 125:303-304, 1995

23. Debili N, Coulombel L, Croisille L, et al. Characterization of a bipotent erythro-megakaryocytic progenitor in human bone marrow. Blood 88:1284-1296, 1996

24. Telamula M, Katahira J, Hoshino S, et al. Effect of recombinant growth factors on human megakaryocyte colony formation in serum-free cultures. Exp Hematol 17:1011-1016, 1989

25. Bruno E, Miller ME, Hoffman R. Interacting cytokines regulate *in vitro* human megakaryocytopoiesis. Blood 73:67-77, 1989

26. Debili N, Massè JM, Katz A, et al. Effects of the recombinant hematopoietic growth factors interleukin 3, interleukin 6, stem cell factor, and leukemia inhibitory factor on the megakaryocytic differentiation of CD34$^+$ cells. Blood 82:84-95, 1993

27. McNiece IK, Langley KE, Zsebo KM, et al. Recombinant stem cell factor synergizes with GM-CSF, G-CSF, IL-3 and EPO to stimulate human progenitor cells of the myeloid and erythroid lineages. Exp Hematol 19:226-231, 1991

27. Murray LJ, Mandich D, Bruno E, et al. Fetal bone marrow CD34+ CD41+ cells are enriched for multipotent hematopoietic progenitors, but not for pluripotent stem cells. Exp Hematol 24:236-245, 1996

28. Papayannopoulou T, Brice M, Farrer D, et al. Insights into the cellular mechanisms of erythropoietin-TPO synergy. Exp Hematol 24:660-699 , 1996

29. Debili N, Issaad C, Massè JM, et al. Expression of CD34 and platelet glycoproteins during human megakaryocytic differentiation. Blood 80:3022-3035, 1992

30. Louache F, Debili N, Marandin A, et al. Expression of CD4 by human hematopoietic progenitors. Blood 84:3344-3355, 1994

31. Dolzhansvy A, Basch RS, Karpatkin S. Development of human megakaryocytes: I. Hematopoietic progenitors (CD34+ bone marrow cells) are enriched with megakaryocytes expressing CD4. Blood 87:1353-1360, 1996

32. Zauli G, Furlini G, Vitale M, et al. A subset of human CD34+ hematopoietic progenitors express low levels of CD4, the high affinity receptor for human immunodeficiency Virus-Type 1. Blood 84:1896-1905, 1994

33. Long MW, Williams N, McDonald TP. Immature megakaryocytes in the mouse: in vitro relationship to megakaryocyte progenitor cells and mature megakaryocytes. J Cell Physiol 112:339-344, 1982

34. Jackson CW. Cholinesterase as a possible marker for early cells of the megakaryocytic series. Blood 42:413-421, 1973

35. Rabellino EM, Levene RB, Leung LLK, Nachman RL. Human megakaryocytes. II. Expression of platelet proteins in early marrow megakaryocytes. J Exp Med 154:88-100, 1981

36. Rabellino EM, Nachman RL, Williams N, et al: Human megakaryocytes. I. Characterization of the membrane and cytoplasmic components of isolated marrow megakaryocytes. J Exp Med 149:1273-1287, 1979

37. Vainchenker W, Guichard J, Deschamps J F, et al: Megakaryocyte cultures in the chronic phase and in the blast crisis of chronic myeloid leukaemia: Studies on the differentiation of the megakaryocyte progenitors and on the maturation of megakaryocytes in vitro. Br J Haematol 51:131146, 1982

38. Long MW, Williams N, Ebbe S. Immature megakaryocytes in the mouse: Physical characteristics, cell cycle status, and in vitro responsiveness to thrombopoietic stimulatory factor. Blood 59:569-575, 1982

39. Long MW, Henry RL: Thrombocytosis-induced suppression of small acetylcholinesterase positive cells in bone marrow of rats. Blood 54:1339, 1979

40. Long MW: Megakaryocyte differentiation events. Sem Hematol 35:192-199, 1998

41. Long MW, Hutchinson RJ, Gragowski LL, Heffner CH, Emerson SG. Synergistic regulation of human megakaryocyte development. J Clin Invest 82:1779-1786, 1998

42. Williams N, Jackson H. Regulation of the proliferation of murine megakaryocyte progenitor cells by cell cycle. Blood 52:163-170, 1978

43. Hoffman R, Yang HH, Bruno E, Straneva JE. Purification and partial characterization of a megakaryocyte colony-stimulating factor from human plasma. J Clin Invest 75:1174-1182, 1985

44. Quesenberry PJ, McGrath HE, Williams ME, et al. Multifactor stimulation of megkaryocytopoiesis: effects of interleukin 6. Exp Hematol 19:35-41, 1991

45. Long MW, Heffner CH, Gragowski LL. Cholera toxin and phorbol diesters synergistically modulate

murine hematopoietic progenitor cell proliferation. Exp Hematol 1988;16:195-200

46. Yoshimasa T, Sibley DR, Bouvier M, et al. Cross-talk between cellular signalling pathways suggested by phorbol-ester-induced adenylate cyclase phosphorylation. Nature 327:67-70, 1987

47. Emerson SG, Yang YC, Clark SC, Long MW. Human recombinant granulocyte-macrophage colony stimulating factor and interleukin 3 have overlapping but distinct activities. J Clin Invest 82:12821287, 1988

48. Lindemann A, Ganser A, Herrmann F, et al. Biologic effects of recombinant human interleukin-3 in vivo. J Clin Oncol 9:2120-2127, 1991

49. Ishibashi T, Burstein SA. Interleukin 3 promotes the differentiation of isolated single megakaryocytes. Blood 67:1512-1514, 1986

50. Kimura H, Ishibashi T, Uchida T, et al. Interleukin 6 is a differentiation factor for human megakaryocytes n vitro. Eur J Immunol 20:1927-1931, 1992

51. Bruno E, Briddell RA, Cooper RJ, Hoffman R. Effects of recombinant interleukin 11 on human megakaryocyte progenitor cells. Exp Hematol 19:378-381, 1991

52. McNiece IK, McGrath HE, Quesenberry PJ. Granulocyte colony-stimulating factor augments in vitro megakaryocyte colony formation by interleukin-3. Exp. Hematol 16:807-810, 1988

53. Debili N, Hegyi E, Navarro S, et al. In vitro effects of hematopoietic growth factors on the proliferation, endoreplication, and maturation of human megakaryocytes. Blood 77:2326-2338, 1997

54. Du XX, Williams PA: Interleukin 11. A multifunctional growth factor derived from the hematopoietic microenvironment. Blood 81:27-34, 1993

55. Bruno E, Hoffman R. Effect of interleukin 6 on in vitro human megakaryocytopoiesis: its interaction with other cytokines. Exp Hematol 17: 1038-1043, 1989

56. Neben TY, Loebelenz J, Hayes L, et al. Recombinant human interleukin-11 stimulates megakaryocytopoiesis and increases peripheral platelets in normal and splenectomized mice. Blood 81:901-908, 1993

57. Herodin F, Mestries JC, Janodet D, et al. Recombinant glycosylated human interleukin-6 accelerates peripheral blood platelet count recovery in radiation-induced bone marrow depression in baboons. Blood 80:688-695, 1992

58. Ishibashi T, Miller SL, Burstein SA. Type beta transforming growth factor s a potent inhibitor of murine megakaryocytopoiesis in vitro. Blood 69: 1737-1741, 1987

59. Kuter DJ, Gminski DM, Rosenberg RB. Transformig growth factor-B inhibits megakaryocyte growth and endomitosis. Blood 79:619-626, 1992

60. Gewirtz AM, Calabretta B, Rucinski B, et al. Inhibition of human megakaryocytopoiesis in vitro by platelet factor 4 (PF4) and a synthetic COOH-terminal PF4 peptide. J Clin Invest 83:1477-1486, 1989

61. Griffin CG, Grant BW: Effects of recombinant interferons on human megakaryocyte growth. Exp Hematol 18:1013-1018, 1990

62. Odell TT Jr, McDonald TP, Detwilder TC. Stimulation of platelet production by serum of platelet-depleted rats. Proc Soc Exp Biol Med 108:428, 1965

63. Spector B. In vivo transfer of a thrombopoietic factor. Proc Soc Exp Biol Med 1961;108:146

64. Schulman I, Abildgaard CF, Cornet JA, et al. Studies on thrombopoiesis. II. Assay of human plasma thrombopoietic activity. J Pediatr 66:604, 1965

65. Vigon I, Florindo C, Fichelson S, et al. Characterization of the murine Mpl proto-oncogene, a member of the hematopoietic cytokine receptor family: molecular cloning, chromosomal location and evidence for a function in cell growth. Oncog 8;2607-2615, 1993

66. Vigon I, Mornon JP, Cocault L, et al. Molecular cloning and characterization of MPL, the human homolog of the v-mpl oncogene: identification of a member of the hematopoietic growth factor receptor superfamily. Proc Natl Acad Sci USA 89:5640-5644, 1992

67. Methia N, Lauache F, Vainchenker W, Wendling F. Oligodeoxynucleotides antisense to the proto-oncogene C-mpl specifically inhibit in vitro megakaryocytopoiesis. Blood 82: 1395-1401, 1993

68. Lok S, Kaushansky K, Holly RD, et al: Cloning and expression of murine thrombopoietin cDNA and stimulation of platelet production in vivo. Nature 369:565-568, 1994

69. De Sauvage FJ, Hass PE, Spencer SD, et al: Stimulation of megakaryocytopoiesis and thrombopoiesis by the c-Mpl ligand, Nature 369:533-538, 1994

70. Kaushansky K, Lok S, Holly RD, et al: Promotion of megakaryocyte progenitor expansion and differentiation by the cMpl ligand thrombopoietin. Nature 369:568-571, 1994

71. Wendling F, Maraskovsky E, Debili N, et al: cMpl ligand is a humoral regulator of megakaryocytopoiesis. Nature 369:571-574, 1994

72. Bartley TD, Bogenberger J, Hunt P, et al: Identification and cloning of megakaryocyte growth and development factor that is a ligand fort he cytokine receptor mpl. Cell 77:1117-1124, 1994

73. Chang MS, NcNinch J, Basu R, et al: Cloning and characterization of the human megakaryocyte growth and development factor (MGDF) gene. J Biol Chem 275:511-514, 1995

74 Foster DC, Sprecher CA, Grant FJ, et al: Human thrombopoietin. Gene structure cDNA sequence, expression, and chromosomal localization. Proc Natl Acad Sci USA 91:13023-13027, 1997

75. Gurney AL, Kuang WJ, Xie MH, et al: Genomic structure, chromosomal localization, and conserved alternative splice forms of thrombopoietin. Blood 85:981-988, 1995

76. Deveaux S, Filipe A, Lemarchandel V, et al: Analysis of the thrombopoietin receptor (MPL) promoter implicates GATA and Ets proteins in the coregulation of megakaryocyte-specific genes. Blood 87:4678-4685, 1996

77. Gurney AL, Carver-Moore K, de Sauvage FJ, Moore MW. Thrombocytopenia in c-mpl-deficient mice. Science 265:1445-1447, 1994

78. Carver-Moore K, Broxmeyer HE, Luoh SM, et al: Low levels of erythroid and myeloid progenitors in thrombopoietin and c-mpl-deficient mice. Blood 88:803-808, 1996

79. Alxander WS, Roberts AW, Nicola NA, et al. Deficiencies in progenitor cells of multiple hematopoietic lineages and defective megakaryocytopoiesis in mice lacking the thrombopoietic receptor c-Mpl. Blood 87:2162-2170, 1996

80. de Sauvage FJ, Carver-Moore K, Luoh SM, et al: Physiological regulation of early and late stages of megakaryocytopoiesis by thrombopoietin. J Exp Med 183:651-656, 1996

81. Fielder PJ, Gurney AL, Stefanich E, et al: Regulation of thrombopoietin levels by c-mpl-mediated binding to platelets. Blood 87:2154-2161, 1996

83. Kuter DJ, Rosenberg RD. The reciprocal relationship of thrombopoietin (c-Mpl ligand) to changes in the platelet mass during busulfan-induced thrombocytopenia n the rabbit. Blood 85:2720-2730, 1995

84. Stoffel R, Wiestner A, Skoda RC. Thrombopoietin in thrombocytopenic mice; evidence against regulation at the mRNA level and for a direct regulatory role of platelets. Blood 1996;87:567-573

85. Boudy VC, Lin NL, Sabath DF, et al. Human Platelets display high-affinity receptors for thrombopoietin. Blood 89:1896-1904, 1997

86. Emmons RV, Reid DM, Cohen RL, et al: Human thrombopoietin levels are high when thrombocytopenia is due to megakaryocyte deficiency and low when due to increased platelet destruction. Blood 87:4068-4071, 1996

87. Tahara T, Usuki K, Sato H, et al: A sensitive sandwich ELISA for measuring thrombopoietin in human serum: serum thrombopoietin levels in healthy volunteers and in patients with hematopoietic disorders. Br J Haematol 93:783-788, 1996

88. Shivdasani RA, Fielder P, Keller GA, et al. Regulation of the serum concentration of thrombopoietin in thrombocytopenic NF-E2 knockout mice. Blood 90:1821-1827, 1997

89. McCarty JM, Sprugel KH, Fox NE, et al. Murine thrombopoietin mRNA levels are modulated by platelet count. Blood 86:3668-3675, 1997

90. Sangaran R, Markovic B, Chong BH. Localization and regulation of thrombopoietin mRNA expression in human kidney, liver, bone marrow, and spleen using in situ hybridization. Blood 89:101-107, 1997

91. Zeiger FC, de Sauvage F, Widner HR, et al: In vitro megakaryocytopoietic and thrombopoietic activity of c-mpl ligand (TPO) on purified murine hematopoietic stem cells. Blood 84:4045-4952, 1996

92. Young JC, Bruno E. Luens KM, et al. Thrombopoietin stimulates megakaryocytopoiesis, myelopoiesis, and expansion of CD34+ progenitor cells from single CD34+Thy- 1+Lin- primitive progenitor cells. Blood 88:1619-1631, 1996

93. Sitnicka E, Lin N, Priestley GV, et al. The effect of thrombopoietin on the proliferation and differentiation of murine hematopoietic stem cells. Blood 87:4998-5005, 1996

94. Angchaisuksiri P, Carlson PL, Dessypris EN. Effects of recombinant human thrombopoietin on megakaryocyte colony formation and megakaryocyte ploidy by human CD34+ cells in a serum-free system. Br J Haematol 93:13-17, 1996

95. Kaushansky K, Broudy VC, Grossmann A, et al: Thrombopoietin expands erythroid progenitors, increases red cell production, and enhances erythroid recovery after myelosuppressive therapy. J Clin Invest 96:1683-1687, 1995

96. Kaushansky K, Broudy VC, Lin N, et al: Thrombopoietin, the Mpl ligand, is essential for full megakaryocyte development. Proc Natl Acad Sci USA 92:3234-3238, 1992

97. Debili N, Wendling F, Katz A, et al: The Mpl-ligand or thrombopoietin or megakaryocyte growth and differentiative factor has both direct proliferative and differentiative activities on human megakaryocyte progenitors. Blood 86:2516-2525, 1995

98. Bertolini F, Battaglia M, Pedrazzoli P, et al: Megakaryocytic progenitors can be generated ex vivo and safely administered to autologous peripheral blood progenitor cell transplant recipients. Blood 89:2679-2688, 1997

99. Dolzhansky A, Basch RS, Karpatkin S. The development of human megakaryocytes: III. Development of mature megakaryocytes from highly purified committed progenitors in synthetic culture media and inhibition of thrombopoietin-induced polyploidization by interleukin-3. Blood 89:426-434, 1997

100. Wendling F, Maraskovsiy E, Delili N, et al: C-mpl ligand is a humoral regulator of megakaryocytopoiesis. Nature 369:571-574, 1994

101. Choi ES, Nichol JL, Hokom MM, Hornkohl AC, Hunt P. Platelets generated in vitro from proplatelet-displaying human megakaryocytes are functional. Blood 85:402-413, 1995

102. Peng J, Friese P, Wolf RF, et al: Relative reactivity of platelets from thrombopoietin- and interleukin-6-treated dogs. Blood 87:4158-4163, 1997

103. Oda A, Miyakawa Y, Druker BJ, et al: Thrombopoietin primes human platelet aggregation induced by shear stress and by multiple agonists. Blood 87:4664-4670, 1996

104. Chen J, Herceg-Harjacek L, Gropman JE, Grabarek J. Regulation of platelet activation in vitro by the c-Mpl ligand, thrombopoietin. Blood 86:4054-4062, 1995

105. Yamazaki K, Roberts RA, Sponcer E, et al. Cellular interactions between 3T3 cells and interleukin-3-dependent multipotent haemopoietic cells: a model system for stromal-cell-mediated haemopoiesis. J Cell Physiol 139:301-312, 1989

106. Anderson DM, Lyman SD, Baird A, et al: Molecular cloning of mast cell growth factor, a hematopoietin that is active in both membrane bound and soluble forms. Cell 63:235-243, 1990

107. Gordon MY, Riley GP, Watt SM, Greaves MF. Compartmentalization of a haematopoietic growth factor (GM-CSF) by glycosaminoglycans in the bone marrow microenvironment. Nature 326:403-405, 1987

108. Roberts R, Galagher J, Spooncer E, et al. Heparan sulphate bound growth factors: a mechanism for stromal cell mediated haemopoiesis. Nature 332:376-378, 1988

109. Zucker-Franklin D, Petursson SR. Thrombocytopoiesis: Analysis by membrane tracer and freeze-fracture studies on fresh human and cultured mouse megakaryocytes. J Cell Biochem 99:390-402, 1984

110. Tablin F, Castro M, Levin RM. Blood platelet formation in vitro. The role of the cytoskeleton in megakaryocyte fragmentation. J Cell Sci 97:59-70, 1990

111. Long MW, Dixit VM. Thrombospondin functions as a cytoadhesion molecule for human hematopoietic progenitor cells. Blood 75:2311-2318, 1990

112. Fielder PJ, Hass P, Nagel M, Stefanich E, Widner R, Bennett GL, Keller GA, de Sauvage FJ, Eaton D. Human platelets as a model for the binding and degradation of thrombopoietin. Blood 89:2782-2788, 1997

113. Cohen-Solal K, Villeval JL, Titeux M, et al. Constitutive expression of Mpl ligand transcripts during thrombocytopenia or thrombocytosis. Blood 88:2578-2584, 1996

112. Mohle RM, Moore MAS, Nachman RL, Rafii S. Transendothelial migration of CD34+ and mature hematopoietic cells an in vitro study using a human bone marrow endothelial cell line. Blood 89:72-80, 1997

113. Hamada T, Mohle R, Hesselgesser J, et al. Transendothelial migration of megakaryocytes n response to stromal derived factor-1 enhances platelet formation. Blood 90: 360a, 1997.

114. Odel TT, Jackson CD, Friday TJ. Megkaryocytopoiesis in rats with special reference to polyploidy. Blood 335:775-782, 1970

115. Odell TT Jr, Jackson CW. Polyploidy and maturation of rat megakaryocytes. Blood 32:102-110, 1968

116. Odell TT Jr, Jackson CW, Gosslee DG. Maturation of rat megakaryocytes studies by microspectrophotometric measurement of DNA. Proc Soc Exp Biol Med 119:1194-1199, 1965

117. Ebbe S. Biology of megakaryocytes. Prog Hemostasis and Thromb. 3:211-229, 1976

118. De Leval M, Paulus JM. "Megakaryocytes: uninucleate plurinucleate cells?" In *Platelet Kinetics*, Paulus JM, ed:. Amsterdam, North Holland, 1971

119. Ebbe S, Stohlman F Jr. Megakaryocytopoiesis in the rat. Blood 26:20-35, 1965

120. Feinendegen LE, Odartchenko N, Cottier H, Bond VP. Kinetics of megakaryocyte proliferation.

Proc Soc Exp Biol Med 111:177-182, 1962
121. Therman E, Sarto GE, Stubblefield PA. Endomitosis: A reappraisal. Hum Genet 63:13-18, 1983
122. Ebbe S, Stohlman F Jr, Overcash J, Donovan J, Howard DF. Megakaryocyte size in thrombocytopenic and normal rats. Blood 32:383-392, 1968
123. Riabowol K, Draetta G, Brixuela L, et al. The cdc2 kinase is a nuclear protein that is essential for mitosis in mammalian cells. Cell 57:393-401, 1989
124. Pines J, Hunter T. Isolation of a human cyclin cDNA: Evidence for cyclin mRNA and protein regulation in the cell cycle and for interaction with p34-CDC2. Cell 1989;58:833-846
125. Hunter T, Pines. Cyclins and cancer. Cell 66:1071-1074, 1991
126. Matsushime H, Roussel M, Ashmun R, Sherr C. Colony-stimulating factor 1 regulates novel cyclins during the G1 phase of the cell cycle. Cell 65:701-713, 1991
127. Meyerson M, Enders GH, Wu C-L, et al. A family of human cdc2-related protein kinases. EMBO J 11:2909-2917, 1992
128. Ohtsubo M, Theodoras AM, Schumacher J, et al. Human cyclin E, a nuclear protein essential for the G1-to-S phase transition. Mol Cell Biol 15:2612-2624, 1995
129. Pagano M, Pepperkok R, Verde F, Ansorge W, Draetta G. Cyclin A is required at two points n the human cell cycle. EMBO J 11:961-971, 1992
130. Dou QP, levin AH, Zhao S, Pardee AB. Cyclin E and cyclin A as candidates for the restriction point protein. Cancer Res 53:1493-1497, 1993
131. Dulic V, Lees E, Reed SI. Association of human cyclin E with a periodic G1-S phase protein kinase. Science 257:1958-1961, 1992
132. Girard F, Strausfeld U, Fernandez A, Lamb NJ. Cyclin A is required for the onset of DNA replication in mammalian fibroblasts. Cell 676:1169-1179, 1992
133. Koff A, Griordino A, Desai D, et al. Formulation and activation of a cyclin E-cdk2 complex during G1 phase of the human cell cycle. Science 257:1689-1694, 1992
134. Matshushime H, Ewen ME, Strom DK, et al. Identification and properties of an atypical catalytic subunit (p34 psk-j3/cdk4) for mammalian D type G1 cyclins. Cell 71:323-334, 1992
135. Hunter T, Pines J. Cyclins and cancer II: Cyclin D and CDK inhibitors come of age. Cell 79:573-582, 1994
136. Xiong Y, Zhang H, Beach D. D type cyclin associate with multiple protein kinases and the DNA replication and repair factor PCNA. Cell 71:505-514, 1992
137. Draetta G, Beach D. Activation of cdc2 protein kinase during mitosis in human cells: cell-cycle-dependent phosphorylation and subunit rearrangement. Cell 54:17-26, 1988
138. Luca FC, Shibuya ED, Dohrmann CE, Ruderman JV. Both Cyclin A delta 60 and B delta 97 are stable and arrest cells in M-phase, but only cyclin B delta 97 turns on cyclin destruction. EMBO J 10:4311-4320, 1991
138. Gallant P, Nigg EA. Cyclin B2 undergoes cell cycle-dependent nuclear translocation and, when expressed as a non-destructible mutant, causes mitotic arrest in HeLa cells. J Cell Biochem 117:213-224, 1992
140. Long MW, Heffner CH, williams JL, Peters C, Prochownik EV. Regulation of megakaryocyte potential in human erythroleukemia cells. J. Clin Invest 85:1072-1084, 1990
141. Datta N, Williams JL, Long MW. Alterations in cyclin-dependent kinase complex formation during the acquisition of polyploid DNA content. Mol Biol Cell 7:209-223, 1996
142. Zhang Y, Wang Z, Ravid K. The cell cycle in polyploid megakaryocytes is associated with reduced activity of cyclin B1-dependent cdc2 kinase. J Biol Chem 271:4266-4266, 1996
143. Datta NS, Long MW. The role of cyclin D3- and cyclin E- cell division kinase complexes in megakaryocyte endomitosis. Blood (abstr);82:209, 1993
144. Wang Z, Zhang Y, Kamen D, Lees E, Ravid K. Cyclin D3 is essential for megakaryocytopoiesis, Blood 865:3783-3788, 1995
145. Long MW, Hoffman R. "Megakaryocytopoiesis." In Hematology Basic Principles and Practice, R. Hoffman, EJ Benz Jr, HJ Cohen, P McGlave, L Silberstein, B Furie, S Shattil, eds. New York, NY: WB Saunders, (In press), 1999

13. The Effects of Multilineage Cytokines on Platelet Recovery

Ravi Vij, John DiPersio

Introduction

Current models of hematopoiesis stress the stochastic rather than the instructive nature of stem cells differentiation[1]. These models suggest that the differentiation of pluripotent stem cells is determined by intrinsic transcriptional factors and not by the presence of extrinsic growth factors or their receptors. Growth factors only provide proliferative and activation signals once lineage commitment has been established. Consistent with the stochastic model, it is known that early and aberrant expression of growth factor receptors on hematopoietic precursors does not alter the lineage commitment of these cells[2].

It is now known that thrombopoietin (TPO) is critical for the production of normal numbers of megakaryocytes (MK) and platelets in pre-clinical models[3-7]. The biology of TPO and the preclinical and clinical studies with TPO are reviewed elsewhere in this book. However, evidence that TPO is not absolutely essential for the production of platelets comes from TPO and/ or TPO receptor (c-mpl) gene knock-out mice (TPO -/- and c-mpl -/-) which have megakaryocyte and platelet levels 5-15% of littermate controls[8-10]. This suggests that other cytokines may promote megakaryocyte and platelet development. It is of interest to note that the bone-marrow cellularity of TPO -/- and c-mpl -/- mice is normal, though there is a decrease in early progenitors, suggesting that TPO and its receptor may have an essential role in the maintenance and expansion of early progenitors.

The thrombopoietic cytokines can be divided into two broad functional categories. The first group includes cytokines which induce the proliferation of early committed megakaryocytic progenitor cells such as megakaryocyte burst-forming cells (MK-BFC) and megakaryocyte colony forming cells (MK-CFC)[11-14]. The MK-BFC have a high proliferative capacity giving rise to large colonies of megakaryocytes (40- 500 cells/ colony) comprised of single or multiple foci. The MK-CFC represent a heterogeneous population of cells that vary in their proliferation potential, giving rise to smaller colonies of megakaryocytes (16-32 cells). The second group of cytokines comprise those which stimulate the maturation of megakaryocytes resulting in terminal differentiation and platelet production.

Over the last decade we have greatly expanded our knowledge of cytokines involved in the regulation of thrombopoiesis (Figure 1). However, it must be noted that most of the studies using these cytokines have been done in a variety of different culture systems and in different species. Only recently have cultures been initiated with purified progenitors in serum free media. Inspite of our increased understanding, it remains difficult to identify those cytokines which have a predominant effect on early versus later stages of megakaryocyte differentiation.

In this chapter, we will review the effects of selected multi-lineage cytokines which have a role in megakaryocyte and platelet development. We will briefly discuss the preclinical data and focus primarily on the effects of these cytokines in clinical trials.

Finally, we will discuss the potential uses and limitations of these growth factors as thrombopoietins in clinical medicine.

Interleukin-11 (IL-11)

<u>Molecular Biology</u>. Interleukin 11 was originally isolated from primate bone-marrow fibroblasts[15]. The human IL-11 gene was isolated from a human lung fibroblast cell line and encodes a 19 kilodalton (kD) protein comprised of 178 amino acids[16,17]. This gene is located on chromosome 19. IL-11 is structurally related to Interleukin-6 (IL-6), Leukemia Inhibitory Factor (LIF), Oncostatin M (OSM) and Ciliary Neurotropic Factor (CNTF). These cytokines exhibit a similar alpha helical structure, and similar exon/intron structure at the DNA level, suggesting their evolution from a single primitive gene. Consistent with this notion is the homology between the receptors for each of these cytokines. The receptors consist of a cytokine binding subunit, and at least one associated common subunit gp130[18-26]. This subunit appears to be essential for signal transduction.

IL-11 binds specifically to a heterodimeric receptor complex consisting of a low affinity IL-11 binding subunit (α) and gp130 which induces downstream signaling events. Presently it is known that there are two α subunits (IL-11Rα-1 and IL-11Rα-2), both of which have been mapped to a 200 kilobase pair region on chromosome 9 p13[27]. The genes for IL-11Rα-1 and IL-11Rα-2 have 99% homology. Although IL-11Rα-1 is expressed ubiquitiously, the expression of IL-11Rα-2 is limited to the testes, thymus and lymph nodes. The role of the IL-11Rα-2 isoform is currently unclear, but in vitro studies suggest that it functions in a similar fashion to IL-11Rα-1 on stable expression in Ba/F3 cells[28].

Preclinical Studies

<u>In Vitro Data.</u> Interleukin-11 has a wide spectrum of in vitro biological activities in hematopoietic, lymphopoietic, hepatic, adipose, neuronal and osteoclast tissues, either alone or in synergy with other hematopoietic growth factors[29]. The primary activity of IL-11 in hematopoiesis is based upon its maturational effect on MK precursors. Specifically, IL-11 increases the ploidy of MK, resulting in increased platelet production[30-32].

Interleukin-11 alone does not stimulate MK progenitors to form colonies in serum free cultures [33]. However, in the presence of other cytokines, IL-11 has been shown to support MK, lymphohematopoietic and erythroid progenitor colonies[34-40]. It now appears that the MK colony formation activity of IL-11 alone or when used in combination with Interleukin-3 and Stem Cell Factor (SCF) is dependent upon TPO[41-43]. Anti-TPO antiserum has been shown to reduce IL-11 stimulated megakaryocyte colony formation by 90% (anti-IL-3 antiserum effects a 28% reduction in colony formation). The megakaryocyte colony forming activity of IL-11 in combination with

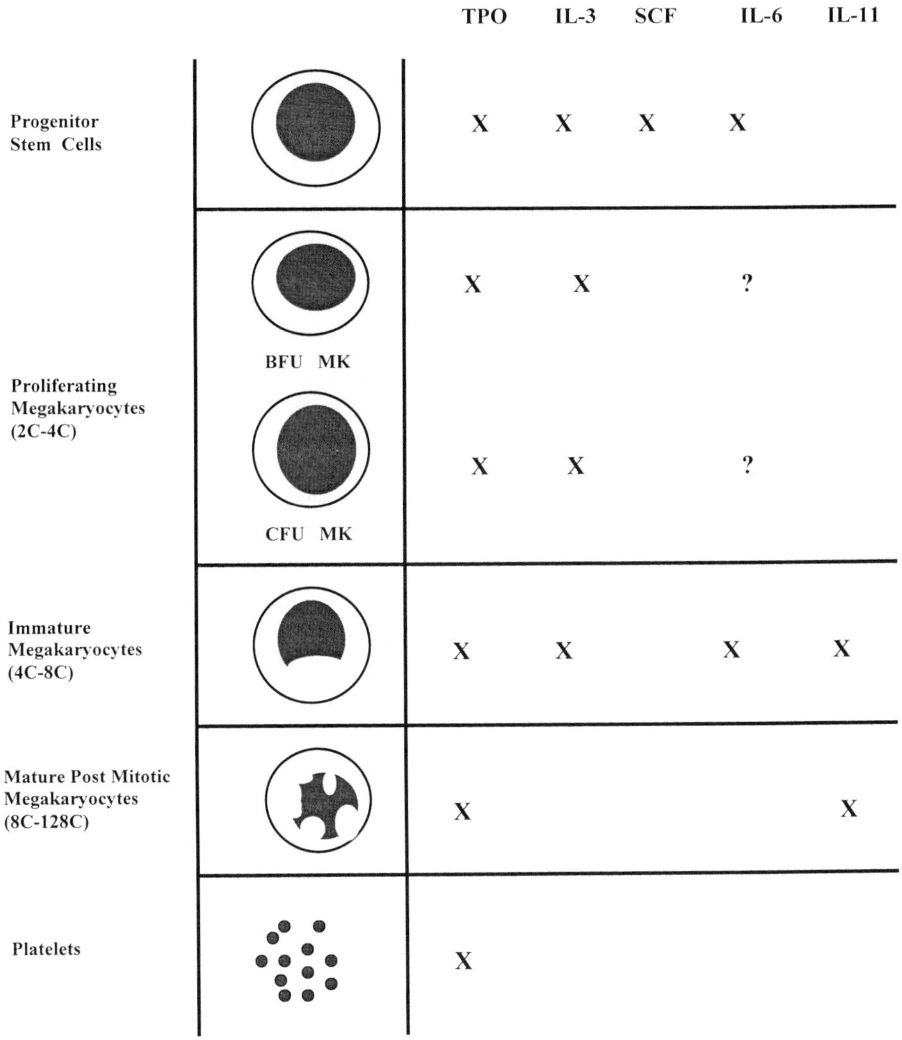

		TPO	IL-3	SCF	IL-6	IL-11
Progenitor Stem Cells		X	X	X	X	
Proliferating Megakaryocytes (2C-4C)	BFU MK	X	X		?	
	CFU MK	X	X		?	
Immature Megakaryocytes (4C-8C)		X	X		X	X
Mature Post Mitotic Megakaryocytes (8C-128C)		X				X
Platelets		X				

Figure1. Postulated sites of action of selected multilineage cytokines involved in thrombopoiesis.

IL-3 or SCF is also reduced by the absence of TPO. Recently however, there have been reports that IL-11 promotes megakaryocyte development independent of endogenous or exogenously added TPO[44].

<u>In Vivo Data</u>. It is known that adult mice with targeted mutation of the interleukin-11 receptor (IL-11r α) display normal hematopoiesis[45]. However, in mice and non-human primate models, IL-11 has been shown to stimulate platelet production in a dose related manner[11, 46-52]. Platelet counts peaked at 14-21 days after initiation of IL-11. The combination of IL-11 and Granulocyte Colony Stimulating Factor (G-CSF) or IL-11 and SCF was shown to have synergistic effects on expanding MK progenitors in vivo using a murine pre-clinical model[53]. The combination of IL-11 and either IL-3 or Granulocyte-Macrophage Colony Stimulating Factor (GM-CSF), when evaluated in normal non human primates increased circulating platelets when compared to the administration of primates with individual cytokines alone[54].

IL-11 has been shown to ameliorate thrombocytopenia in myelosuppressed animals[55-62]. IL-11 and TPO demonstrated synergy, improving platelet recovery in mice treated with a combination of chemotherapy and radiation[63,64]. The combination of IL-11 and IL-3 was shown to have a radioprotective effect and enhance recovery of platelets in irradiated mice[65].

A novel activity of IL-11 noted in a chemotherapy/radiotherapy murine model was the enhanced recovery of small intestinal mucosal epithelial cells[66]. This translated into an increase in survival in mice treated with rhIL-11 at a dose of 250mcg/kg/d subcutaneously (s.c): 64% vs 27% in the control group. The increase in survival was associated with decreased bacterial foci in the liver, spleen and mesentery. The mechanism by which IL-11 decreases gastrointestinal toxicity is unclear. In the above study it was shown that there was an increased mitotic index of gut crypt cells[66]. Other in vitro studies have shown that IL-11 can directly interact with gastrointestinal epithelial cells and reversibly inhibit the proliferation of intestinal stem cell lines[67-69].

Clinical studies

In an initial phase I trial in patients with breast cancer, cohorts of three to five women were treated with five different doses of rhIL-11 (10, 25, 50, 75, 100 mcg/kg/d s.c)[70]. Recombinant human IL-11 was administered for 14 days during "cycle 0" prior to chemotherapy. Patients subsequently received up to four cycles of chemotherapy followed by rhIL-11 at their assigned dose. The maximum tolerated dose was found to be 75 mcg/kg. The dose limiting toxicites were myalgias, arthralgias and fatigue. A therapy related anemia was seen at all doses. The anemia was thought to be secondary to plasma volume expansion. Recombinant human IL-11 was associated with a mean 76%, 93%, 108% and 185% increase in platelet counts at doses of 10, 25, 50 and 75mcg/kg s.c, respectively. Bone marrow effects included increases in MK ploidy at all doses and a mild increase in both the number of MK progenitors as well as the number of bone marrow MK at the 75mcg/kg dose. Following chemotherapy, a decrease in the degree of thrombocytopenia (platelet counts $\leq$ 50,000/ mm^3 was noted at doses$\geq$ 25mcg/kg, when compared to historical controls and patients treated at the 10mcg/kg dose level.

A multicenter phase I/II trial testing the combination of rhIL-11 and rhG-CSF following ICE chemotherapy in pediatric patients with solid tumors demonstrated that this combination accelerated platelet recovery and decreased the number of platelet transfusions[71]. In this study rhIL-11 was tolerated without evidence of grade III/IV toxicity at 100mcg/kg/d.

Two phase III trials using rhIL-11 have been reported. In a multicenter randomized placebo controlled trial, 93 patients were treated as part of a secondary prophylaxis study[72]. Patients were eligible for this trial if they developed chemotherapy-induced severe thrombocytopenia (defined as a platelet count $< 20,000/ \text{ mm}^3$) and had received at least one platelet transfusion during the preceding cycle of therapy. Following the subsequent cycle of chemotherapy, patients received either rhIL-11 at a dose of 25 or 50mcg/kg/d s.c or placebo for 14 to 21 days starting day 1 after chemotherapy. Approximately 30% of the patients treated with rhIL-11 at a dose of 50mcg/kg/d did not require platelet transfusions, compared to only 4% of the placebo patients (p<0.05). Patients receiving 25mcg/kg/d demonstrated a trend towards requiring fewer platelet transfusions, though this was not statistically significant. The difference in the median number of transfusions required among the patients receiving rhIL-11 at a dose of 50mcg/kg compared with those receiving placebo did not achieve statistical significance. The mean number of platelet transfusions required per patient was 2.2 for each of the rhIL-11 groups and 3.4 for the placebo group; this difference was not statistically significant. Among patients receiving either dose of rhIL-11, the median duration of platelet counts less than 20,000, 50,000, and $100,000/ \text{ mm}^3$ were not statistically significant. Though grade III toxicity was rare, side effects at the 50mcg/kg dose occurred in a significant proportion of patients and included edema (55%), dizziness (48%), dyspnea (48%), fever (38%), headaches (31%), tachycardia (28%), rash (24%), palpitations (21%). Six patients each experienced syncope/near-syncope and atrial arrhythmias.

A second phase III placebo controlled study evaluated the effectiveness of rhIL-11 and rhG-CSF in reducing platelet transfusions after the first and second cycles of dose intensive cyclophosphamide and doxorubicin chemotherapy in patients with breast cancer[73]. The patients were stratified by whether or not they had received prior chemotherapy. Patients were randomized to treatment with placebo or rhIL-11 at a dose of 50mcg/kg/d s.c for 10 or 17 days after the first two cycles of chemotherapy. Seventy-seven patients were randomized. Approximately 68% of the patients who received rhIL-11 did not require transfusions, compared with 41% of controls (p=0.04). No statistically significant difference in the number of platelets transfused and duration of thrombocytopenia could be demonstrated after the first cycle. Treatment with rhIL-11 after the second cycle of chemotherapy significantly reduced the mean number of platelet transfusions administered in the assessable group (0.8 vs 2.2; p=0.04). The mean time to platelet recovery $\geq 20,000/\text{mm}^3$ (2.5 days vs 6.4 days; p= 0.03) and $\geq 50,000/\text{mm}^3$ (9.3 days vs 13.0 days; p=0.01) was also significantly reduced. The time to platelet recovery $\geq 100,000/\text{mm}^3$ was however not statistically significant. In the rhIL-11 group 71% of the transfusions were single donor platelets, compared with only 51% in the placebo group. Significant toxicities included peripheral edema (63%), dyspnea (48%), pleural effusions (18%), and conjunctival injection (25%).

IL-11 was studied in patients who received autologous bone marrow transplantation (ABMT) following myeloablative therapy. A randomized double blind placebo controlled phase II study, showed that the platelet transfusion requirement and duration of thrombocytopenia were similar for the rhIL-11 and placebo arms[74].This study published only in abstract form included patients who received either peripheral blood stem cells (PBSC) or bone marrow stem cells. It is not clear if the groups were identical regarding the number of bone marrow and peripheral blood stem cell infusions or balanced regarding the number of CD34+ cells infused.

The combined administration of escalating doses of rhIL-11 with rhG-CSF at 5mcg/kg/d was studied in breast cancer patients receiving high dose cyclophosphamide, BCNU and thiotepa followed by ABMT[75]. The dose limiting toxicity was atrial arrhythmias and fluid retention at an IL-11 dose of 75mcg/kg/d. There were no significant trends identified suggesting a decrease in platelet utilization or a shorter duration of thrombocytopenia.

Interleukin-3 (IL-3)

<u>Molecular Biology</u>. Interleukin-3 or multi-CSF is a glycoprotein produced primarily by T lymphocytes. It has a molecular weight ranging from 14 to 28 kD[76-77]. The gene for IL-3 is located on the long arm of chromosome 5, proximal to the genes encoding GM-CSF and IL-5[78]. All three cytokines share similar structural features at the protein, DNA and genomic levels suggesting evolution from a common ancestral gene. These three cytokines all have an impact on eosinophil production and survival. This is consistent with the observation that clinical trials using these cytokines show objective eosinophilia and similar toxicities. The receptor complex for IL-3 is a heterodimer consisting of a low affinity IL-3 binding subunit (IL-3Rα) and a signaling subunit (β) which is common to the GM-CSF, IL-3, and IL-5 receptor complexes.

Preclinical Studies

<u>In Vitro</u>. IL-3 stimulates the proliferation and differentiation of both multipotent hematopoietic stem cells, as well as committed progenitor cells of the erythroid, granulocytic, macrophage, MK, eosinophilic, basophilic and mast cell lineages[79-91]. Furthermore, it prevents apoptosis of progenitor cells and promotes the specialized function of differentiated cells such as eosinophils, macrophages, mast cells and tissue basophils[92].

In MK colony forming assays, the combination of IL-3 and TPO has been shown to maximize Colony Forming Units (CFU-MK) in culture[41-43]. IL-3 alone induces approximately 40% of the maximal CFU-MK, seen when progenitors are stimulated in vitro with both IL-3 and TPO. Optimum concentrations of TPO alone can support 75% of the maximal CFU-MK in vitro. Colonies supported by TPO alone are invariably small to medium in size, with 3-20 large MK per colony. In contrast, colonies that develop in the presence of IL-3 often contain up to 200 MK. It was therefore hypothesized that IL-3 acts on developmentally more immature CFU-MK than does TPO. IL-6 and IL-11 also augment the number of MK colonies in IL-3 containing cultures, but not to the level seen with TPO. In addition TPO leads to the development of platelet-specific granules, demarcation membranes and platelet fields.

However, IL-3-induced MK fail to display any ultrastructural features of MK differentiation. The addition of IL-11 leads to modest demarcation, but only poorly formed platelet-specific granules, and few if any platelet fields.

<u>In Vivo Data</u>.   IL-3 in murine and non-human primate in vivo models demonstrated a modest stimulatory effect on megakaryopoiesis[93-99]. However, in non-human primates administration of human IL-3 following chemotherapy, failed to demonstrate any effect on megakaryocytopoiesis[100]. These negative results may have, in part, been due to the fact that human and not primate IL-3 was tested. [101,102]. It is well known that significantly higher concentrations of human cytokines are needed to produce therapeutic effects in primates. In addition non-human primates have been shown to generate neutralizing antibodies to human cytokines. These may have blunted the therapeutic effect seen in these studies.

Clinical Trials

Initial phase I trials with rhIL-3 were conducted in patients with bone-marrow failure syndromes[103-107]. It was the first multi-potential hematopoietic growth factor to demonstrate reproducible multilineage clinical hematologic activity with acceptable toxicity. The benefit however was minimal and transient.

In cancer patients, several phase I /II studies showed that the thrombopoietic activity of rhIL-3 is modest at best[108-114]. These studies established that the dose limiting toxicity of rhIL-3 was headaches which occurred at a dose of 15mcg/kg/d[6]. Other side-effects noted were fever, flu-like symptoms, nausea, skin rash, flushing, facial erythema and urticaria.

Recombinant human IL-3 was compared to placebo in a multicenter phase III trial 179 patients with non-Hodgkin's Lymphoma and Hodgkins Disease were treated with Ifosfamide, Epirubicin and Etoposide (IEV) [115]. This was followed by either rhIL-3 at a dose of 10mcg/kg/d s.c or placebo on days 4-15. Analysis of the data revealed that the requirement for transfusions was not significantly different in the two groups.

IL-3+GM-CSF/ IL-3+IL-6 Combination Therapy

Preclinical Studies

The effects of treatment with IL-3 in combination with GM-CSF were evaluated in vitro and in animal models[116-125]. The rationale for this combination was based on early in vitro analyses and pre-clinical studies which demonstrated that IL-3 stimulates early progenitor cells which can then be stimulated to proliferate in response to a second factor acting on differentiated precursors. In non-human primates, the co-administration of IL-3 and GM-CSF was more effective in enhancing recovery of both platelets and neutrophils after chemotherapy than the sequential administration of IL-3 followed by GM-CSF.

IL-3 and IL-6 act synergistically to support the proliferation of murine multipotent progenitor cells in culture[126]. Sequential administration of IL-3 and IL-6 to non-human primates given sublethal doses of radiation resulted in a significantly enhanced platelet recovery compared with primates co-administered IL-3 and IL-6 or with primates given placebo control. However, the sequential administration of IL-3 and IL-6 did not significantly enhance platelet recovery over either IL-6 or IL-3 as monotherapy, though the duration of thrombocytopenia was shortened [127]. One must interpret these results with caution as these may be due to a small number of animals treated. In addition the co-administration of IL-3 and IL-6 was no better than administration of IL-6 alone in a non-human primate model of hepsulpham-induced thrombocytopenia[128].

Clinical Trials

In a phase I study in patients with advanced solid tumors, the sequential administration of rhIL-3 (at doses of 125 and 250mcg/m^2 s.c days 1-5) and rhGM-CSF (at 250mcg/m^2 sc days 1-10) following rhIL-3, was compared to treatment with rhIL-3 alone (at the same doses for 15 days). Sequential treatment with rhIL-3 and rhGM-CSF was found to be as effective as treatment with rhIL-3 alone in stimulating platelet counts[129].

In a phase I/II trial, 36 patients with advanced malignancies were treated with VP-16, ifosfamide and cisplatin (VIP) chemotherapy[130]. This was followed by the sequential administration of rhIL-3 at a dose of 250mcg/ m^2 s.c (days 1-5) and rhGM-CSF at 250mcg/m^2 s.c (days 6-15). Control patients received either rhGM-CSF alone (days 1-15) or were treated with placebo control. This clinical trial demonstrated that platelet recovery did not differ significantly between the three treatment groups.

In a separate study, the sequential administration of rhIL-3 followed by rhGM-CSF was compared to the co-administration of rhIL-3 and rhGM-CSF in women with breast cancer receiving chemotherapy. Recombinant human IL-3 and rhGM-CSF alone were also investigated[131]. The sequential use of rhIL-3 and rhGM-CSF was associated with higher platelet nadirs, shorter duration of platelet counts < 50,000/ mm^3 and need for fewer platelet transfusions. Since IL-3 and GM-CSF share the same receptor β subunit, it possible that simultaneous administration may decrease the efficacy, due to competition among these cytokines for the same β subunit[132].

A phase III multicenter trial compared the sequential administration of rhIL-3 and rhGM-CSF to rhGM-CSF alone in patients undergoing ABMT[133]. After transplant patients were randomized to receive either rhIL-3 at a dose of 2.5mcg/kg/d s.c for 10 days and rhGM-CSF at 250mcg/m^2/d IV after IL3 (day 11 to ANC $\geq$ 1500/ mm3), or rhGM-CSF alone until the ANC was $\geq$ 1500/ mm^3 for 3 days. No statistically significant difference was seen in the median time to platelet recovery $\geq$20,000/ mm^3 or ANC $\geq$ 500/ mm^3.

PIXY321

<u>Molecular Biology</u>. PIXY321 is a fusion protein consisting of the active domains of rhGM-CSF and rhIL-3 coupled by a flexible amino acid linker sequence allowing the binding domains to fold into their native conformation[134,135]. The rationale for creating such a molecule was based on the different but complementary patterns of response generated by GM-CSF and IL-3.

Preclinical Studies

Receptor binding studies show that PIXY321 binds to cell lines that express specific receptors for GM-CSF or IL-3 with affinities similar to the native growth factors[134,136]. PIXY321 is a potent stimulator of multipotential and lineage-restricted progenitors, including colony-forming unit-granulocyte-erythroid-monocyte-megakaryocyte (CFU-GEMM) and colony-forming unit-granulocyte-macrophage (CFU-GM)[137, 138]. In addition PIXY321 was shown to enhance the rate of platelet recovery in sublethally irradiated non-human primates by five days post irradiation, when compared with human serum albumin or GM-CSF [139,140]. Its major advantage is that two growth factors can be administered as a single agent.

Clinical studies

In a phase I/II trial patients with sarcoma were administered PIXY321 over 14 days during " cycle 0" prior to chemotherapy[141]. The patients again received PIXY321 after cycle no 2 of cyclophosphamide, doxorubicin and dacarbazine chemotherapy. Even at the highest dose of 1000mcg/kg/d dose limiting toxicity was not encountered. Though the majority of side effects were mild (grade I toxicity) , local skin reactions at the injection site were seen in 100% of patients. Other side effects included headache (54%), myalgia (42%), malaise (50%), bone pain (25%), fever (17%), and nausea (21%). When given prior to chemotherapy, modest increases in platelet counts were observed. The increase in platelets was gradual and platelet counts peaked at a median of day 20. PIXY321 at doses of 500 to 1000 mcg/m^2/d s.c after the second cycle of chemotherapy significantly reduced the mean nadir platelet count and mean time to recovery of platelets to $\geq$ 100,000/ mm^3. However, severe thrombocytopenia (nadir platelet count < 20,000/ mm^3) was still observed following cycle no 2. The need for platelet transfusion was also not altered in the two cycles.

Randomized trials have failed to demonstrate a benefit with PIXY321. In one trial, fifty-three patients with advanced breast cancer were randomized to receive either PIXY321 375mcg/m^2 s.c twice daily, or rhGM-CSF 250 mcg/m s.c daily after chemotherapy[142]. No differences in the platelet nadir, duration of thrombocytopenia, or need for platelet transfusions were observed. PIXY321 was less well tolerated than GM-CSF; more patients developed chills and local skin reactions and more patients stopped PIXY321 due to intolerance. Similarly, no convincing benefit could be shown in a randomized phase II study of PIXY321 vs rhG-CSF when administered following DHAP as salvage therapy for lymphoma[143]. Results of a randomized double-blind trial of PIXY321 vs GM-CSF in patients with non Hodgkins Lymphoma (NHL) undergoing ABMT were also disappointing[144].

Stem Cell Factor (SCF)

<u>Molecular Biology</u>. Stem Cell Factor (also known as the Steel Factor, Mast Cell Growth Factor or kit ligand) is a ligand for the receptor encoded by the c-kit proto-oncogene[145-150]. It is constitutively produced by endothelial cells and by fibroblasts. Keratinocytes in normal skin and epithelial cells in the gut also produce SCF, and the

SCF protein can be detected in the thymus. It is normally found in two forms (1) a soluble glycoprotein which circulates as a non covalently bonded dimer with a molecular weight of 18.5 kD and (2) a membrane bound molecule that is expressed on stromal cells in the bone marrow microenvironment[151-156]. Membrane bound SCF may facilitate homing of hematopoietic progenitor cells to the marrow[157-159]. SCF has structural homology with Macrophage Colony Stimulating Factor (M-CSF) and the recently identified flk-2/ flt-3 ligand[160-162].

The c-kit receptor is a 145 kD glycoprotein and has been given the designation CD117[163-167]. It is a member of the type III receptor tyrosine kinase family. These receptors are characterized by five immunoglobulin like repeats in the extracellular domain, a single short membrane spanning domain, and a cytoplasmic domain with tyrosine kinase activity. Other members of this family include the flk-2/ flt-3, M-CSF and PDGF receptors. Binding of SCF to its receptor triggers receptor homodimerization and intermolecular tyrosine phosphorylation of the receptor. This creates docking sites for a number of SH2- (SRC homology domain 2) and PID- (phosphotyrosine interaction domain) containing signal transduction molecules. The c-kit receptor is broadly distributed within the hierarchy of hematopoietic cells and is especially common on early progenitor cells[168, 169].

Preclinical Studies

<u>In Vitro Data</u>. SCF has been shown to enhance colony formation by primitive cell populations. It displays synergistic activity with other cytokines on myeloid, erythroid and megakaryocytic progenitors. Purified SCF alone is a poor stimulus of MK colony formation. However in the presence of TPO, IL-3, IL-6, GM-CSF and IL-11, MK colony formation is increased[91, 170-179]. When a soluble form of the mpl receptor was used to neutralize the biological activity of TPO produced by stromal elements in whole marrow culture systems, the MK formation ability of SCF was virtually eliminated.

<u>In Vivo Data</u>. In mice, a variety of naturally occurring mutations at the Sl locus or the W locus which encode SCF and the c-kit receptor, respectively, have been identified[149-151, 180-182]. Absence of the SCF protein (the Sl mutation) or absence of the c-kit receptor (the W mutation) results in death in utero or in the perinatal period with severe macrocytic anemia. The Sld mutation results in the production of soluble SCF with absence of the transmembrane form. Sl/Sld mice are viable but have severe macrocytic anemia and an abnormal megakaryopoiesis. This is characterized by a decrease in megakaryocyte numbers but an increase in megakaryocyte size, leading to a normal platelet count. The mutant mice also have markedly reduced tissue mast cells.

Animal studies have shown that SCF displays multilineage activity in vivo that includes expansion of the stem cell compartment[183-189]. Although the administration of SCF to non-human primates increased the number of megakaryocytes in the bone marrow, the platelet count did not increase. SCF did increase the marrow cellularity and absolute numbers of CFU-GM and BFU-E. Increases in erythrocytes and white blood cell subsets in peripheral blood were also observed.

Clinical studies

In a phase I/II multicenter trial, patients with NHL undergoing autologous PBSC transplant, were randomized to receive either rhG-CSF at a dose of 10 mcg/kg/d s.c or a combination of rhSCF at 5, 10, 15 mcg/kg/d with rhG-CSF at 10mcg/kg/d s.c to mobilize PBSC[190]. Following stem cell infusion, the median time to recovery of platelets $\geq$ 20,000/ mm3 was similar in both arms. However, when heavily pretreated patients were compared to non-heavily pretreated patients, there was a trend towards more rapid platelet recovery for those receiving the combination of rhSCF and rhG-CSF. Therapy with rhSCF was associated with local cutaneous effects at the injection sites, including erythema, swelling and hyperpigmentation. The latter is thought to be due to an effect on melanocytes. In phase I trials with rhSCF doses of 25 and 50mcg/kg/d, systemic toxicities including respiratory and cutaneous symptoms were observed. These were attributed to the effects of rhSCF on tissue mast cells[191, 192]. Therefore, in subsequent studies, all patients received anti-allergy prophylaxis with H1/ H2 blockade, bronchodilators and pseudoephedrine.

In a large phase II trial, 215 patients with high risk breast cancer undergoing ABMT were randomized to receive either rhG-CSF alone at a dose of 10mcg/kg/d s.c for 7 days or the combination of rhG-CSF at 10mcg/kg/d s.c and rhSCF at 5 to 30mcg/kg/d s.c for 7, 10 or 13 days. The median number of CD34+ cells collected was greater for patients receiving the combination of rhSCF and rhG-CSF. However, the median time to platelet and granulocyte recovery following transplantation was the same in all cohorts[193].

A phase II study compared the combination of rhSCF 20mcg/kg/d and rhG-CSF 10mcg/kg/d to rhG-CSF alone at 10mcg/kg/d in heavily pre-treated patients with NHL or Hodgkin's Disease (HD). Growth factors were started on day 1 and continued until $\geq$ 5.0x10^6/kg CD34+ cells were collected or 5 days of apheresis were completed[194]. Although the administration of rhSCF was reported to significantly improve the number of CD34+ cells collected, data on platelet recovery was not provided.

Recently, a phase III study of PBSC mobilization using either rhSCF 20mcg/kg/d s.c in combination with rhG-CSF at 10mcg/kg/d s.c or G-CSF alone 10mcg/kg/d s.c in patients with high risk breast cancer has been reported. By day 5 of leukapheresis 67% of the patients who received rhSCF in combination with rhGCSF (n= 85) compared to 48% of those receiving rhG-CSF alone reached a target collection of 5x 10^6 CD34+ progenitor cells. However, the time to platelet recovery was equivalent in the two groups[195]. Data on the effects on platelet counts during the pre-pheresis phase was not published. Mild injection site reactions, primarily erythema and pruritis were seen in 88% of the patients who received combination therapy.

Interleukin-6 (IL-6)

<u>Molecular Biology</u>. Interleukin-6 was originally identified as a B-cell differentiation factor[196]. A series of subsequent studies have shown that it also acts on T-cells, hepatocytes, hematopoietic progenitor cells and even neuronal cells[197, 198]. Biochemically, it is a 21- to 30- kD glycoprotein of 212 amino acids. The gene which encodes IL-6 is located on chromosome 7[199]. The Interleukin-6 receptor (IL-6R) has

a low affinity ligand binding subunit (IL6-Rα)[200, 201]. This subunit has an extracellular region which consists of an Ig-like domain. The intracytoplasmic region of the α subunit lacks any known signal transduction motif. Binding of IL-6 to IL-6Rα triggers the hetrodimerization of a non-ligand binding 130 kD signal-transduction molecule, gp130. As mentioned in the discussion of IL-11, gp130 is a common cytokine signal transducer for the IL-6 family of cytokines including IL-11, LIF, OSM, CNTF and IL-6.

Preclinical Studies

<u>In Vitro Data</u>. IL-6 has both proliferative and maturational effects on hematopoietic precursors. IL-6 increases the mean MK ploidy, without increasing the number of CFU-MK [91, 202-214]. Since both IL-6 and its receptor are expressed by megakaryocytes and megakaryocyte cell lines, it is postulated that IL-6 participates in an autocrine regulatory loop controlling post mitotic megakaryocyte development[210, 215].

<u>In Vivo Data</u>. IL-6 deficient knock-out mice do not develop thrombocytopenia[216]. However, when IL-6 was administered to mice and non-human primates increases in platelet counts, MK size and ploidy were observed[96, 217-225]. Aberrant megakaryocytic ultrastructural features were seen after IL-6 administration[221]. There was excessive membrane formation, without clear-cut demarcation of platelet territories, a marked decrease in granules, and aberrant distribution of heterochromatin in the nucleus. In animal models of either chemotherapy or radiation induced marrow aplasia, IL-6 was shown to reduce both the depth and the duration of thrombocytopenia.[226-230].The co-administration of IL-6 and IL-3, IL-6 and G-CSF or IL-6 and GM-CSF in myelosuppressed animal models has produced variable results compared to the individual cytokines alone[98, 231-234]. Co-incident with its stimulation of thrombopoiesis, IL-6 also stimulated physiologic changes characteristic of an acute inflammatory response[222].

Clinical Studies

In humans, serum IL-6 levels are increased in reactive thrombocytosis associated with rheumatoid arthritis or secondary thrombocytosis due to iron deficiency anemia[235, 236]. This suggests that this cytokine may be responsible for pathological megakaryopoiesis. However, no correlation between IL-6 and platelet levels has been found. This is in contrast to published data demonstrating that IL-11 and TPO have an inverse relationship with platelet counts [237].

When evaluated in phaseI/II studies in patients with a wide variety of cancers it was established that rhIL-6 can be safely administered at a dose of 10mcg/kg/d [238-245]. The side-effect profile of rhIL-6 was dose related. At doses < 2.5mcg/kg/d side-effects consisted of fever, headache, myalgia and local erythema. Starting at 2.5mcg/kg/d, these side-effects were compounded by nausea, reversible increase in liver enzymes and anemia[239]. Flu-like symptoms were controlled up to a dose of 10mcg/kg/d with acetaminophen. Hepatotoxicity and cardiac arrhythmias were found to occur at an IL-6 dose of 30mcg/kg/d[247]. The anemia associated with rhIL-6 is rapid in onset, dose dependent and quickly reversible after cessation of rhIL-6 therapy. The anemia is thought to be caused by an increase in plasma volume[248].

Phase I/II studies in patients with malignancies administered rhIL-6 before any chemotherapy have demonstrated variable results. One study showed that increases in platelet counts occurred only at rhIL-6 doses above the maximum tolerated dose of $\geq$ 10mcg/kg/d[238]. The thrombopoietic effect was delayed with platelet counts actually decreasing during therapy . Bone marrow samples obtained after rhIL-6 treatment failed to show an increase in the number of MK. Megakaryocyte ploidy was however increased. Other studies have shown a dose related elevation in platelet counts in patients receiving rhIL-6 at doses of 2.5-10mcg/kg/d with peak platelet counts achieved between days 8 to 15 [240, 245]. Following the administration of chemotherapy, phase I/II studies showed that the absolute nadirs of platelet counts were not significantly different between patients receiving placebo and IL-6 doses of up to10mcg/kg/d[240, 241].

In a phase I trial in patients with myelodysplastic syndromes and thrombocytopenia the maximum tolerated dose for rhIL-6 was found to be 3.75mcg/kg/d. In this study, it was observed that rhIL-6 had limited thrombopoietic activity and significant toxicity[246]. In another phase I multicenter trial, when rhIL-6 was administered after ABMT for advanced breast cancer, the maximum tolerated dose of rhIL-6 was 1mcg/kg/d. In this trial, dose limiting (grade IV) hyperbilirubinemia occurred at a dose of 3mcg/kg/d or greater[247].

The combination of rhIL-6 and rhG-CSF was studied in two phaseI/II studies[249, 250]. Preliminary results showed that rhIL-6 can be tolerated at a dose of 10mcg/kg/d with rhG-CSF administered at a dose of 5mcg/kg/d. In the first study, there was no statistically significant difference in platelet nadirs between patients treated with the combination of rhIL-6 and rhG-CSF vs rhG-CSF alone[249]. However, a trend towards a shorter duration of thrombocytopenia was noted (1.75d vs 2.6d). In the second study in patients receiving rhG-CSF alone, 21% of cycles were associated with platelet counts $\leq$ 20,000/mm^3 and required platelet transfusions. vs 15% of cycles in patients receiving the combination of rhIL-6 and rhG-CSF[250]. These differences are not statistically significant.

Other Cytokines:

Granulocyte-Macrophage Colony Stimulating Factor (GM-CSF)

The administration of GM-CSF to non-human primates resulted in increased MK ploidy and size, but did not increase the number of MK or platelets[251]. In human trials the effect of rhGM-CSF administration on thrombopoiesis, either in bone marrow failure states or chemotherapy-treated patients, has been largely negative[253-256]. In fact, thrombocytopenia has been reported as an adverse event in some clinical studies[257-259]. In a canine model, rhGM-CSF induced thrombocytopenia has been shown to be associated with shortened platelet survival[260].This is postulated to be due to a non-immune mechanism resulting from GM-CSF induced activation of the monocyte-macrophage system in the spleen and liver.

Interleukin-1 (IL-1)

Invitro, IL-1 has been shown to stimulate the production of M-CSF, G-CSF, GM-CSF, Tumor Necrosis Factor (TNF), and IL-6. IL-1 increases the number of early myeloid precursors. In mice IL-1 enhances the generation of myeloid, MK and early erythroid precursors. IL-1 has also been shown to protect mice from lethal irradiation and enhance myeloid recovery in mice and non-human primate models. Clinical trials with IL-1 have demonstrated its ability to promote platelet production[261-263]. However the toxicity of IL-1 has been a major impediment to its potentially broad applicability.

Leukemia-Inhibitory Factor (LIF) And Oncostatin-M (OSM)

As mentioned earlier LIF and OSM are pleiotropic cytokines that belong to the IL-6 family of structurally related cytokines. In vitro studies reveal that LIF when used alone, promotes MK maturation. When combined with IL-3, LIF stimulates increased MK colony formation as well[31, 91, 264, 265]. When administered to normal mice and non-human primates, it increased the number of bone marrow progenitor cells as well as the circulating platelet count[266, 267]. In a non-human primate model of radiation-induced myelosuppression, LIF decreased the duration of thrombocytopenia significantly[268].

In vitro OSM potentiates colony formation induced by IL-3[269]. In addition OSM may promote maturation of megakaryocytes as has been noted for IL-6 and IL-11. In myelosuppressed mice administration of OSM was found to accelerate platelet recovery. However, it was shown to be ineffective when administered to non-human primates after myelosuppressive irradiation.

Daniplestim (SC-55494)

Daniplestim is an IL-3 analog which has a high affinity for the human IL-3 receptor. It retains the multilineage hematopoietic activity of IL-3, with less intrinsic inflammatory activity[270] . In a non-human primate model of radiation-induced myelosuppression, Daniplestim was found to reduce significantly the duration of thrombocytopenia when compared to placebo treated control animals[271, 272]. Phase II /III human studies in combination with G-CSF are currently underway to mobilize PBSC and to minimize post chemotherapy pancytopenia.

Myelopoietins (SC-68420 And SC-70935)

The myelopoietins are a class of chimeric cytokines which consist of a genetically engineered truncated IL-3 analog, an IgG2b linker, and a genetic variant of G-CSF[273-275]. They bind to human IL-3 and G-CSF receptors with high affinity. In addition, they stimulate less leukotriene and TNF-α production than native rhIL-3 suggesting that these agents may have less pro-inflammatory activity. In a non-human primate model of myelosuppression, myelopoietin decreased the duration of thrombocytopenia and platelet nadir[276]. These myelopoietins are currently being evaluated in phaseI/II trials in patients undergoing stem cell mobilization and to minimize pancytopenia after myelosuppressive chemotherapy.

Promegapoietin (SC-71858)

Promegapoietin is a genetically engineered chimeric protein which combines IL-3 ligand and recombinant human c-mpl agonist activities[277,278]. When tested in non-human primates it was reported to be effective in reducing the platelet nadir and hasten the time to platelet recovery after myelosuppressive radiation therapy[279]. Phase I/II clinical trials are currently underway to test promegapoietin, both as a PBSC mobilization agent and in the post-chemotherapy and ABMT setting to minimize treatment associated thrombocytopenia.

Fms-like tyrosine kinase 3 ligand (Flt3L)

Flt3 is a class III tyrosine receptor kinase that is preferentially expressed on primitive hematopoietic progenitor cells[161,162]. Several studies have shown that Flt-3L synergizes with a number of other growth factors to induce the proliferation CD34+ cells from human bone marrow and to enhance the formation of committed progenitor colonies (CFU-GEMM and CFU-GM)[280]. Although Flt3L alone and in combination with G-CSF can promote the mobilization of PBSC in mice and primates, no obvious changes in platelet counts were noted in initial published abstracts[280, 281].

Flt3L and TPO appear to act synergistically on murine and human stem cells to stimulate multilineage growth in vitro[282].In spite of this, Flt3L has very little direct effect on megakaryopoiesis since Flt3L -/- knockout mice do not have any abnormalities in megakaryocyte or platelet production[283]. Flt3L alone, or in combination with IL-3, SCF, or TPO has no effect on in vitro growth of murine megakaryocyte progenitor cells[284]. In addition, Flt3L alone has no effect on megakaryocyte ploidy nor does it enhance the effect of TPO on megakaryocyte ploidy[284]. Human trials with Flt3L, both as an enhancer of PBSC mobilization and as a dendritic cell activator and anti-tumor agent are currently underway.

Negative Regulators of Megakaryopoiesis

Data concerning the substances capable of inhibiting platelet progenitor proliferation have recently become available. Most inhibitors are produced by megakaryocytes and platelets themselves. These negative regulators include Transforming Growth Factor β-1 (TGF β-1), Platelet Factor 4 (PF4) and other CXC chemokine family members, as well as interferon-α and thrombin. Whether chemokines elaborated by ancillary cells in the marrow microenvironment play a role in the autocrine or paracrine regulation of megakaryopoiesis has yet to be determined.

TGF β-1 is probably the most potent inhibitor of megakaryopoiesis[285-287]. It is a pleiotropic cytokine and a constituent of platelet alpha-granules. In human and murine in-vitro systems, its effect on MK progenitors is direct and irreversible[288]. In vivo experiments have also shown that it lowers platelet counts.

Chemokines are a family of proteins comprising 70-100 amino-acid peptides that contain four highly conserved cysteine residues[289, 290]. This family of chemokines is divided into two sub-groups: (1) CXC or alpha chemokines (PF-4, β-Thromboglobulin, Interleukin-8, Neutrophil Activating Peptide-2) and (2) CC or beta chemokines (C 10, Macrophage-Inhibiting Proteins: MIP-1 α, MIP-1 β). PF-4 is a platelet specific CXC chemokine that is released from α-granules when platelets are activated. PF-4 and other chemokines have inhibitory effects on in vitro megakaryocyte colony formation[291-296]. An in vivo inhibitory effect of PF4 on murine megakaryopoiesis and granulopoiesis has been demonstrated in mice.

Thrombin has been shown to inhibit selectively megakaryocyte progenitor cell growth[297]. This is probably due to the release of some inhibitors, particularly those derived from platelets.

Interferon-α has been reported to inhibit megakaryocyte colony formation in vitro[298, 299]. Clinical studies in Essential Thrombocythemia have confirmed the inhibitory effect of Interferon-α on the proliferation of MK progenitors and thrombopoiesis[300].

Potential Clinical Applications of Thrombopoietic Growth Factors

Cytokines may be used (1) to reduce the need for platelet transfusions (2) to increase the yield of platelets obtained by apheresis from normal volunteer or family donors and (3) to enhance the mobilization of PBSCs. We shall briefly address the potential for the use of thrombopoietic growth factors in the first two of these areas.

Reduction Of Platelet Transfusions

It is estimated that 8.3 million units of platelets were transfused in the United States in 1992. There has been an increase in such transfusions of 5 to 7 percent annually since 1987 [301]. It is hoped that the use of thrombopoietins will reduce the need for platelet transfusions and consequently, the incidence of infections, allo-immunization and other potential adverse reactions related to the transfusion of platelets[302-304].

Currently there are wide variations in clinical practice concerning criteria for administering platelet transfusions. Though results of the bleeding-time test become abnormal when the platelet count falls below 100,000/ mm3, spontaneous small-vessel bleeding does not increase until the platelet count is less than 5000/ mm3[305]. In the past a platelet count of 20,000/ mm^3 was the most quoted figure for the use of prophylactic platelet transfusions[306]. This recommendation was based predominantly on a study that established no threshold value that prevented all bleeding; furthermore many patients on the study were treated with aspirin[306]. Recent studies have however established that the threshold to prevent bleeding can safely be set at a platelet count of 10,000/ mm^3 [308-312].

To evaluate the potential benefit of any thrombopoietin randomized trials will be necessary. Therefore, it is critical to identify groups of patients who require platelet transfusions as part of their treatment. There are four such groups of patients: i) those receiving myeloablative therapy with stem cell support, ii) those receiving induction or post-remission consolidation therapy for acute leukemia, iii) those undergoing intensive chemotherapy for solid tumors or lymphomas and iv) those with marrow failure states like aplastic anemia, myelodysplastic syndromes and myelofibrosis.

Stem Cell Transplantation. There has been a dramatic increase in the use of stem cell transplants with intensive chemotherapy for patients with hematologic malignancies and solid tumors. However, in most patients there is only transient thrombocytopenia with a predictable return of platelet counts by day 10 to 14 post stem cell infusion, provided the product has an adequate number of CD34+ progenitor cells. This is especially true with peripheral blood increasingly replacing bone marrow as a source of stem cells in the autologous setting. In our own institution an average of only 4.5 and 5.5 units of single donor platelets are transfused to patients undergoing autologous and allogeneic PBSC transplants respectively. This suggests that even with severely myeloablative regimens the need for platelet transfusions is modest at best. It may therefore be difficult to improve on these results even with an effective thrombopoietic factor.

Acute Leukemia. All patients with acute myeloid leukemia (AML) receiving initial induction therapy and most adults receiving induction therapy for acute lymphoblastic leukemia (ALL) require large numbers of platelet transfusions. Because adult AML is a relatively common disorder with subgroups of patients being cured after therapy, this is an important subgroup of patients in which to evaluate the benefit of thrombopoietic agents. Unfortunately, most thrombopoietic cytokines require approximately two weeks to exert their effect, making it necessary to administer cytokines concurrent with or even perhaps preceding chemotherapy. However, there has been concern regarding co-administration of hematopoietic stimulatory factors and chemotherapy because of the possibility that normal precursors may be recruited into cycle with enhanced cytotoxicity from the chemotherapy. In addition, it is still unclear if these cytokines can enhance leukemia cell growth. Besides, the presence of several confounding factors like thrombocytopenia secondary to residual leukemia, sepsis and alloimmunization can complicate the analysis of clinical trials. In patients receiving post-remission consolidation chemotherapy, it may be difficult to demonstrate a statistically significant reduction in the number of platelet transfusions given because of the small number of transfusions required and the fewer number of patients enrolled on these studies.

Solid Tumors. In the case of solid tumors, the role of dose intensive chemotherapy regimens capable of causing significant thrombocytopenia is still limited at best. Patients receiving standard chemotherapy regimens for solid tumors infrequently require platelet transfusions.

Marrow Failure States. In many patients with myelodysplasia and aplastic anemia, severe thrombocytopenia is a major cause of morbidity. However, available data shows that both groups of patients have markedly impaired marrow function and decreased ability to respond to growth factors.

Platelet Donation

The concept of administering thrombopoietic cytokines to volunteer or family platelet donors is based on the knowledge that both the yield of platelets obtained from apheresis and the expected increments are directly related to the donor's pre-collection platelet count. Donor safety issues related to pre-medication and the potential for thrombotic episodes are however paramount. Another potential use of thrombopoietins is to obtain autologous platelets for alloimmunized patients who are in remission after chemotherapy but who require further courses of intensive therapy.

Current Status of Multilineage Cytokines in Clinical Medicine

Recombinant human IL-11 (opreleukin, Neumega) was recently approved by the FDA for the prevention of severe thrombocytopenia and reduction of the need for platelet transfusions following myelosuppressive chemotherapy in patients with non-myeloid malignancies who are at high risk of developing severe thrombocytopenia. In addition, based on the potent effects of IL-11 observed in animal models demonstrating a decrease in gastrointestinal epithelial damage, it is possible that a major advantage of IL-11 may be its simultaneous beneficial effects on both bone marrow and gastrointestinal toxicities of chemotherapy and radiation .

Before endorsing the use of opreleukin it is however essential to perform a cost-benefit analysis to assess its true worth. According to the randomized trial of rhIL-11 vs placebo, 21% of rhIL-11 treated patients who completed the second cycle of chemotherapy required platelet transfusions, compared with 48% of placebo-treated patients[5]. In the evaluable subgroup, the mean number of platelet transfusions required by patients who received rhIL-11 was 0.8 and that for placebo treated patients was 2.2. Assuming that a unit of single donor platelets costs $500, this translates into savings of $40,000 per 100 patients treated. The cost of a dose of opreleukin for a 70kg individual is approximately $225. This translates into an expenditure of approximately $380,000 per 100 patients treated (assuming 17 days of s.c injections). The cost benefit analysis would be even less favorable if one were to administer opreleukin prophylactically starting with the first cycle of chemotherapy, as was done in the randomized trial. Opreleukin therefore, currently does not appear to be a financially viable alternative to platelet transfusions especially since the rates of serious bleeding complications in patients given prophylactic platelet transfusions for platelet counts < 10-20,000/ mm^3 is very low.

Unfortunately the other multilineage cytokines appear even less promising. As a result of the lack of convincing benefit, interest in the use of rhIL-3 and rhSCF as post chemotherapy cytokines has waned. Trials with IL-3 analogues and IL-3/G-CSF chimeric molecules are however ongoing.

Recombinant human IL-6 was the first "maturational" cytokine to enter clinical trials. In addition, because of its immunomodulating functions, IL-6 has also been evaluated as a potential anti-tumor agent. Unfortunately the dilemma of greater toxicity at higher more effective doses has made the clinical development of IL-6 difficult. It is hoped that the use of shorter durations of higher dose therapy might allow for improved tolerance.

In summary there appears to be limited clinical indication for thrombopoietins in clinical medicine. Also, because of the above detailed problems, it will be difficult to show benefit for the use of thrombopoietins in clinical medicine. The growth factor that appears most promising is TPO. It is currently being evaluated in clinical trials and if approved for clinical use, enthusiasm for the development of multilineage cytokines as thrombopoietins is likely to diminish further.

References

1. Ogawa M. Differentiation and proliferation of hematopoietic stem cells. Blood 81: 2844, 1993.
2. Stoffel R, Ledermann B, de Sauvage FJ.: Evidence for a selective-permissive role of cytokine receptors in hematopoietic cell fate decisions. Blood 90: 123a (abstr), 1997.
3. deSauvage FJ, Hass PE, Spencer SD, et al.: Stimulation of megakaryocytopoiesis and thrombopoiesis by the c-mpl ligand. Nature 369: 533, 1994.
4. Lok S, Kaushansky K, Holly RD, et al.: Cloning and expression of murine thrombopoietin cDNA and stimulation of platelet production in vivo. Nature 369: 565, 1994.
5. Wendling F, Maraskovsky E, Debill N, et al.: c-mpl ligand is a humoral regulator of megakaryocytopoiesis. Nature 369: 571, 1994.
6. Bartley TD, Bogenberger J, Hunt P, et al.: Identification and cloning of a megakaryocyte growth and development factor that is a ligand for the cytokine receptor mpl. Cell 77: 1117, 1994.
7. Kuter DJ, Beeler DL, Rosenberg RD.: The purification of megapoietin: a physiologic regulator of megakaryocyte growth and platelet production. Proc Natl Acad Sci USA 91:11104, 1994.
8. Gurney Al, Carver Moore K, de Sauvage FJ, et al.: Thrombocytopenia in c-mpl-deficient mice. Science 265: 1445, 1994.
9. de Sauvage FJ, Caever-Moore K, Luoh SM, et al.: Physiological regulation of early and late stages of megakaryocytopoiesis by thrombopoietin. J Exp Med 183: 651, 1996.
10. Kimura S, Roberts AW, Metcalf D, et al.: Hematopoietic stem cell deficiencies in mice lacking c-mpl, the receptor for thrombopoietin. Proc Natl Acad Sci USA 95: 1195, 1998.
11. Levin J, Levin FC, Penington DG, et al.: Measurement of ploidy distribution in megakaryocyte colonies obtained from culture with studies of the effects of thrombocytopenia. Blood 57: 287. 1981.
12. Long MW, Gragowski LL, Heffner CH, et al.: Phorbol diesters stimulate the development of an early murine progenitor cell. The burst forming unit-megakaryocyte. J Clin Invest 76: 431, 1985.
13. Long MW, Heffner CH, Gragowski LL. In vitro differences in responsiveness of early (BFU-Mk) and late (CFU-Mk) murine megakaryocyte progenitor cells. Prog Clin Biol Res 215: 179, 1986.
14. Kuriya S, Ogata K, Yamada T, et al.: Three stages of differentiation in mouse megakaryocyte progenitor cells(CFU-Meg). Exp Hematol 18: 416, 1990.
15. Paul SR, Bennet F, Calvetti JA, et al.: Molecular cloning of a cDNA encoding interleukin 11, a stromal derived lymphopoietic and hematopoietic cytokine. Proc Natl Acad Sci USA 87: 7512, 1990.
16. Ohsumi J, Miyadai I, Ishikawa-Ohsumi H, et al.: Adipogenesis inhibitory factor. A novel inhibitory regulator of adipose conversion in bone marrow. FEBS Letter 288: 13, 1991.
17. McKinley D, Wu Q, Yang-Feng T, et al.: Genomic sequence and chromosomal location of human interleukin (IL)-11 gene. Genomics 13: 814, 1992.
18. Hibi M, Murakami M, Saito M, et al.: Molecular cloning and expression of an IL-6 signal transducer, gp130. Cell 63: 1149, 1990.
19. Bazan JF.: Structural design and molecular evolution of a cytokine receptor superfamily. Proc Natl Acad Sci USA 87: 6934, 1990.
20. Gearing DP, Comeau MR, Friend DJ, et al.: The IL-6 signal transducer, gp130: an oncostatin M receptor and affinity converter for the LIF receptor. Science 255 1434, 1992.
21. Ip NY, Nye SH, Boulton TG, et al.: CNTF and LIF act on neuronal cells via shared signaling pathways that involve the IL-6 signaling pathways that involve the IL-6 signal transducing receptor component gp130. Cell 69:1121, 1992.
22. Liu J, Modrell A, Aruffo A, et al.: Interleukin-6 signal transducer gp130 mediates oncostatin M signaling. J Biol Chem 267: 16763, 1992.
23. Yin T, Taga T, Tsang M LS, et al.:Involvement of interleukin-6 signal transducer gp130 in interleukin-11 mediated signal transduction. J Immunol 151: 2555, 1993.
24. Davis S, Aldrich TH, Stahl N, et al.: LIFR beta and gp130 as heterodimerizing signal transducers of the tripartite CNTF receptor. Science 260: 1805, 1993.
25. Fourcin M, Chevalier S, Leburn J-J, et al.: Involvement of gp130/interleukin-6 receptor transducing component in interleukin-11 receptor. Eur J Immunol 24: 277, 1994.
26. Nandurkar HH, Hilton D, Nathan P, et al.: The human IL-11 receptor requires gp130 for signaling: demonstration by molecular cloning of the receptor. Oncogene 12: 585, 1996.
27. Robb L, Hilton DJ, Brook-Carter PT et al.: Identification of a second murine interleukin-11 receptor alpha-chain gene (IL11R α) with a restricted pattern of expression. Genomics 40: 387,

1997.

28. Lebeau B, Montero Julian FA, Wijdenes J, et al.: Reconstitution of two isoforms of the human interleukin-11 receptor and comparison of their functional properties. FEBS Letter 407: 141, 1997.

29. Du XX, Williams DA.: Interleukin-11: a multifunctional growth factor derived from the hematopoietic environment. Blood 83: 2023, 1994.

30. Teramura M, Kobyashi S, Hoshino S, et al.: Interleukin-11 enhances human megakaryocytopoiesis in vitro. Blood 79 327, 1992.

31. Burstein SA, Mei RL, Henthorn J, et al.: Leukemia inhibitory factor and interleukin-11 promote maturation of murine and human megakaryocytes in vitro. J Cell Physio 153: 305, 1992.

32. Goldman SJ.: Preclinical biology of interleukin 11: a multifunctional hematopoietic cytokine with potent thrombopoietic activity. Stem Cells 13: 462, 1995.

33. Yonermura Y, Kawakita M, Masuda T, et al.: Effect of recombinant human interleukin 11 on rat megakaryopoiesis in vivo: comparative study with interleukin 6. Brit J Haematol 84: 16, 1993.

34. Briddell RA, Hoffman R.: Cytokine regulation of the human burst-forming unit- megakaryocyte. Blood 76: 516, 1990.

35. Musashi M, Yang Y-C, Paul SR, et al.: Direct and synergistic effects of interleukin 11 on murine hemopoiesis in culture. Proc Natl Acad Sci USA 1991 88: 765.

36. Bruno E, Bridell RA, Cooper RJ, et al.: Effects of recombinant interleukin 11 on human megakaryocyte progenitor cells. Exp Hematol 19: 378, 1991.

37. Musashi M, Clark SC, Sudo T, et al.: Synergistic interactions between interleukin-11 and interleukin-4 in support of proliferation of primitive hematopoietic progenitors of mice. Blood 78: 1448, 1991.

38. Hirayama F, Shih J-P, Awgulewitsch A, et al.: Clonal proliferation of murine lymphohematopoietic progenitors in culture. Proc Natl Acad Sci USA 89: 5907, 1992.

39. Neben S, Donaldson D, Sieff C, et al.: Synergistic effects of interleukin-11 with other growth factors on the expansion of murine hematopoietic progenitors and maintenance of stem cells in liquid culture. Exp Hematol 22: 353, 1994.

40. Broudy VC, Lin NL, Kaushansky K.: Thrombopoietin (c-mpl ligand) acts synergistically with erythropoietin, stem cell factor and interleukin-11 to enhance murine megakaryocytic colony growth and increase megakaryocyte ploidy in vitro. Blood 85: 1719, 1995.

41. Kaushansky K, Broudy VC, Lin N, et al.: Thrombopoietin, the mpl ligand, is essential for full megakaryocyte development. Proc Natl Acad Sci USA 92: 3234, 1995.

42. Kaushansky K, Nimer SD, Gordon MS, et al.: Megakaryocyte growth factors: role in pathophysiology and results of clinical trials. Hematology- 1996 Education Program of the American Society of Hematology 147, 1996.

43. Murray LJ, Bruno E, Zucker-Franklin D, et al.: Thrombopoietin induction of megakaryocytopoiesis from purified subpopulations of human CD34+ cells including primitive CD34+Thy-1+Lin- cells. Exp Hematol (In press.), 1998.

44. Weich NS, Wang A, Fitzgerald M, et al.: Recombinant human interleukin-11 directly promotes megakaryocytopoiesis in vitro. Blood 90: 3893, 1997.

45. Nandurkar HH, Rob L, Tarlinton D, et al.: Adult mice with targeted mutation of the interleukin-11 receptor (IL-11R α) display normal hematopoiesis. Blood 90: 2148, 1997.

46. Neben TY, Loebelenz J, Hayes L, et al.: Recombinant human interleukin-11 stimulates megakaryocytopoiesis and increases peripheral platelets in normal and splenectomized mice. Blood 81: 901, 1993.

47. Hangoc G, Yin T, Cooper S, et al.: In vivo effects of recombinant interleukin-11 on myelopoiesis in mice. Blood 81: 965, 1993.

48. Bree A, Schlerman F, Timony G, et al.: Pharmacokinetics and thrombopoietic effects of recombinant human interleukin-11 (rhIL-11) in nonhuman primates and rodents. Blood 78: 132a (abstr), 1991.

49. Goldman S, Loebelanz J, McCarthy K, et al.: Recombinant human interleukin-11 (rhIL-11) stimulates megakaryocyte maturation and increase in peripheral platelet numbers in vivo. Blood 78: 518a (abstr), 1991.

50. Goldman SJ, Neben TY, Ouinto C, et al.: Constant subcutaneous infusion of recombinant human interleukin-11 induces stem cell mobilization and causes prolonged elevation of peripheral platelets. Blood 80: 91a (abstr), 1992.

51. Ault KA, Knowles C, G oldman S.: Recombinant human IL-11 induces increases in reticulated platelets and platelet count in mice. Blood 80: 91a (abstr), 1992.

52.   Kaviani MD, Mason LE, Bree AG, et al.: Effects of recombinant human interleukin 11 on the activation and morphology of peripheral blood platelets and megakaryocytes in nonhuman primates. Blood   88: 26a (abstr), 1996.

53.   Cairo MS, Plunkett JM, Nguyen A, et al.: Effects of interleukin-11 and G-CSF on in vivo neonatal rat hematopoiesis: induction of thrombocytosis by IL-11 and enhancement of neutrophilia by IL-11+ G-CSF. Blood   80: 411a (abstr), 1992.

54.   Schlermnan F, Bree A, Schaub R ,et al.: Effects of subcutaneous administration of recombinant human granulocyte macrophage colony stimulating factor (rhGM-CSF) alone , or rhIL-11 in combination with recombinant human interleukin-3 (rhIL-3) or rhGM-CSF in nonhuman primates. Blood   80: 64a. (abstr), 1992

55.   Du XX, Neben T, Goldman S, et al.: Effects of recombinant human interleukin-11 on hematopoietic reconstitution in transplant mice   acceleration of recovery of peripheral blood neutrophils and platelets. Blood   81: 27, 1993.

56.   Du XX, Keller D, Maze R, et al.: Comparative effects of in vivo treatment using interleukin-11 and stem cell factor on reconstitution in mice after bone marrow transplantation. Blood   82: 1016, 1993.

57.   Witsell A, Mauch P, Neben TY, et al.: Constant subcutaneous infusion of recombinant human interleukin-11 induces stem cell mobilization and causes prolonged elevation of platelets. J Cell Biochem Suppl 17B: 71, 1993.

58.   Leonard JP, Quinto CM, Kozitza MK, et al.: Recombinant human interleukin-11 stimulates multilineage hematopoietic recovery in mice after a myelosuppressive regimen of sublethal irradiation and carboplatin. Blood   83: 1499, 1994.

59.   Maze R, Moritz T, Williams DA.: Increased survival and multilineage hematopoietic production from delayed and severe myelosuppressive effects of a nitrosourea with recombinant interleukin-11 (IL-11). Cancer Res 54: 4947, 1994.

60.   Nash RA, Siedel K, Storb R, et al.: Effects of rhIL-11 on normal dogs and after sublethal radiation. Exp Hematol 23: 389, 1995.

61.   Leonard JP, Neben TY, Ouinto C, et al.: Recombinant human interleukin-11 (rhIL-11) accelerates peripheral platelet and RBC recovery following combined sublethal irradiation and carboplatin treatment in mice. Blood   80: 91a (abstr), 1992.

62.   Du XX, Keller D, Goldman S, et al.: Functional effects of interleukin-11 treatment in vivo following bone marrow transplantation(BMT) and combined modality therapy in mice. Exp Hematol 20: 768a (abstr), 1992.

63.   Du XX, Keller D, Maze R, et al.: Comparative effects of in vivo treatment using interleukin-11 and stem cell factor on reconstitution in mice after bone marrow transplantation. Blood   82: 1016, 1993.

64.   Yonemura Y, Kawakita M, Miyake H, et al.: Effects of interleukin-11 on carboplatin-induced thrombocytopenia in rats and in combination with stem cell factor. Int J Hemat 65: 397, 1997.

65.   Galmiche MC, Vogel CA, Delaloye AB, et al.: Combined effects of interleukin-3 and interleukin-11 on hematopoiesis in irradiated mice. Exp Hemat. 24: 1298, 1996.

66.   Du XX, Doerschuk A, Orazi A, et al.: A bone marrow stromal derived growth factor, interleukin-11, stimulates recovery of small intestinal mucosal cells after cytoablative therapy. Blood   83: 33, 1994.

67.   Booth C, Potten CS.: Effects of IL-11 on the growth of intestinal epithelial cells in vitro. Cell Prolif 28: 581, 1995.

68.   Peterson RL, Bozza MM, Dorner AJ.: Interleukin-11 induces intestinal epithelial growth arrest through effects on retinoblastoma phosphorylation. Am J Path 149: 895, 1996.

69.   Peterson RL, Trepicchio WL, Bozza MM, et al.: G1 growth arrest and reduced proliferation of intestinal epithelial cells induced by rhIL-11 may mediate protection against mucositis. Blood   86: 311a 1(suppl 1, abstr), 1995.

70.   Gordon M, McCaskill-Stevens W, Battiato L, et al.: A phase I trial of recombinant human interleukin-11 (Neumega rhIL-11 growth factor) in women with breast cancer receiving chemotherapy. Blood 87: 3615, 1996.

71.   Kirov I, Goldman S, Blazer B, et al.: Recombinant human interleukin 11 (Neumega) is tolerated at double the adult dose and enhances hematopoietic recovery following ifosfamide, carboplatin and etoposide (ICE) chemotherapy in children: Correlation with rapid clearence, lack of induction of inflammatory cytokines and mobilization of early progenitor cells. Blood 90: 581a (abstr), 1997.

72.   Tepler I, Elias L, Smith III JW, et al.: A randomized placebo-controlled trial of recombinant human

interleukin-11 in cancer patients with severe thrombocytopenia due to chemotherapy. Blood 87: 3607, 1996.

73. Isaacs C, Robert NJ, Bailey FA, et al.: Randomized placebo controlled study of recombinant human interleukin-11 to prevent chemotherapy induced thrombocytopenia in patients with breast cancer receiving dose intensive cyclophosphamide and doxorubicin. J Clin Oncol 15(11): 3368, 1997.

74. Hussein A, Fisher D, Vrendenburgh J, et al.: Phase 2 trial of Neumega rhIL-11 in patients with breast cancer after high-dose chemotherapy with bone marrow and peripheral blood stem cell support. Blood 300a (abstract), 1996.

75. Champlin RE, Mehra R, Kaye JA, et al.: Recombinant human interleukin eleven (rhIL-11) following autologous BMT for breast cancer. Blood 84: 395a (abstract), 1994

76. Yang YC, Ciarletta AB, Temple PA, et al.: Human IL-3 (multi-CSF): identification by expression cloning of a novel hematopoietic growth factor related to murine IL-3. Cell 47: 3, 1986.

77. Otsuka T, Miyajima A, Brown N, et al.: Isolation and characterization of an expressible cDNA encoding human IL-3. J Immunol 140: 2288, 1988.

78. Yang Y-C, Kovacic S, Kriz R, et al.: The human genes for GM-CSF and IL-3 are closely linked in tandem on chromosome 5. Blood 71: 958, 1988.

79. Ishibashi T, Burstein SA.: Interleukin-3 promotes the differentiation of isolated single megakaryocytes. Blood 67: 1512, 1986.

80. Burstein SA.: Interleukin 3 promotes maturation of murine megakaryocytes in vitro. Blood Cells11: 469, 1986.

81. Lopez AF, To LB, Yang YC, et al.: Stimulation of proliferation, differentiation, and function of human cells by interleukin-3. Proc Natl Acad Sci USA 84: 2761, 1987.

82. Leary AG, Yang Y-C, Clark SC, et al.: Recombinant gibbon interleukin 3 supports formation of human multilineage colonies and blast cell colonies in culture: comparison with recombinant human granulocyte-macrophage colony-stimulating factor. Blood 70: 1343, 1987.

83. Sealand S, Caux C, Favre C, et al.: Effects of recombinant human interleukin 3 on CD34-enriched normal hematopoietic progenitors and on myeloblastic leukemia cells. Blood 72: 1580, 1988.

84. Sonoda Y, Yang Y-C, Wong GG, et al.: Analysis in serum-free culture of the targets of recombinant human hematopoietic growth factors :interleukin 3 and granulocyte/macrophage-colony-stimulating factor are specific for early developmental stages. Proc Natl Acad Sci USA 85: 4360, 1988.

85. Bruno E, Briddell R, Hoffman R.: Effect of recombinant and purified hematopoietic growth factors on human megakaryocyte colony formation. Exp Hematol 70: 371, 1988.

86. Lu L, Briddell RA, Graham CD, et al.: Effect of recombinant and purified human hematopoietic growth factors on in vitro colony formation by enriched populations of megakaryocyte progenitor cells. Br J Haematol 70: 149, 1988.

87. Teramura M, Katahira J, Hoshino S, et al.: Clonal growth of human megakaryocyte progenitors in serum-free cultures: effect of recombinant human interleukin 3. Exp Hematol 16:843-848, 1988.

88. Segal GM, Stueve T, Adamson JW.: Analysis of murine megakaryocyte colony size and ploidy: effects of interleukin-3. J Cell Physiol 137: 537, 1988.

89. Mazur EM, Cohen JL, Bogart L, et al.: Recombinant gibbon interleukin-3 stimulates megakaryocyte colony growth in vitro from human peripheral blood progenitor cells. J Cell Physiol 136: 439, 1988.

90. Sieff CA, Ekern SC, Nathan DG, et al.: Combinations of recombinant colony stimulating factors are required for optimal hematopoietic differentiation in serum deprived culture. Blood 73:688., 1989

91. Debili N, Masse JM, Katz A, et al.: Effects of the recombinant hematopoietic growth factors interleukin-3, interleukin-6, stem cell factor, leukemia inhibitory factor, on megakaryocytic differentiation of CD34+ cells. Blood 82: 84, 1993.

92. Williams GT, Smith CA, Spooncer E, et al.: Haematopoietic colony stimulating factors promote cell survival by suppressing apoptosis. Nature 343: 76, 1990.

93. Kindler V, Thorens B, de Kossodo S, et al.: Stimulation of hematopoiesis in vivo by recombinant bacterial murine interleukin-3. Proc Natl Acad Sci USA 83: 1001, 1986.

94. Metcalf D, Begley CG, Johnson GR, et al.: Effects of purified bacterially synthesized murine multi-CSF (IL-3) on hematopolesis in normal adult mice. Blood 68: 46, 1986.

95. Krumwieh D, Seiler FR.: In vivo effects of recombinant colony stimulating factors on hematopoiesis in cynomolgus monkeys. Transplant Proc 21: 2964, 1989.

96. Carrington PA, Hill RJ, Stenberg PE, et al.: Multiple in vivo effects of interleukin-3 and interleukin 6 on murine megakaryocytopoiesis. Blood 77: 34, 1991.

97.   Monroy RL, Davis TA, Donahue RE, et al.: In vivo stimulation of platelet production in a primate model using IL-1 and IL-3. Exp Hematol 19: 629, 1991.

98.   Geissler K, Valent P, Bettelheim P, et al.: In vivo synergism of recombinant human interleukin 3 and recombinant human interleukin 6 on thrombopoiesis in primates. Blood 79: 1155, 1992.

99.   Carrington PA, Hill RJ, Levin J, et al.: Effects of interleukin 3 and interleukin 6 on platelet recovery in mice treated with 5-flourouracil. Exp Hematol 20: 462, 1992.

100. Gillio AP, Gasparetto C, Laver J, et al.: Effects of interleukin 3 on hematopoietic recovery after 5-fluorouracil or cyclophosphamide treatment of cynomolgus primates. J Clin Invest 85: 1560, 1990.

101. Burger H, van Leen RW, Dorssers LCJ, et al.: Species specificity of human interleukin 3 demonstrated by cloning and expression of the homologous rhesus monkey (Macaca mulatta) gene. Blood 76: 2229, 1990.

102. Wagemaker G, van Gils FCJM, Burger H, et al.: Highly increased production of bone marrow - derived blood cells by administration of homologous interleukin 3 to rhesus monkeys. Blood 76: 2235, 1990.

103. Ganser A, Siepelt G, Lindemann A, et al.: Effects of recombinant human interleukin 3 in patients with myelodysplastic syndromes. Blood 76: 455, 1990.

104. Ganser A, Lindemann A, Siepelt G, et al.: Effects of recombinant human interleukin 3 in patients with normal hematopoiesis and in patients with bone marrow failure. Blood 76: 666., 1990

105. Ganser A, Lindemann A, Siepelt G, et al.: Effects of recombinant human interleukin 3 in aplastic anemia. Blood 76: 1287, 1990.

106. Kurzrock R, Talpaz M, Estrov Z, et al.: Phase I study of recombinant human Interleukin 3 in patients with bone marrow failure. J Clin Oncol 9: 1241, 1991.

107. Lindemann A, Ganser A, Hermann F, et al.: Biologic effects of recombinant human interleukin-3 in vivo. J Clin Oncol 9: 2120, 1991.

108. Biesma B, Willemse PHB, Mulder NH, et al.: Effects of interleukin 3 after chemotherapy for advanced ovarian cancer. Blood 80 1141, 1992.

109. Postmus PE, Gietema JA, Damsma O, et al.: Effects of recombinant human interleukin 3 in patients with relapsed small cell lung cancer treated with chemotherapy: a dose finding study. J Clin Oncol 10: 1131, 1992.

110. Raemaekers J, van Imhoff G, Fibbe W, et al.: A randomized, double blind, placebo-controlled, phaseI/II study on human recombinant interleukin 3 after DHAP chemotherapy in patients with relapsed malignant lymphoma. Blood 78: 162 (abstr), 1991.

111. Demetri GD,Young DC, Merica E, et al.: Clinical effects of interleukin 3 in patients with advanced sarcomas:a phase I/II trial. Blood 78: 5 (abstr), 1991.

112. D'Hondt V, Canon JL, Humblet Y, et al.: Dose dependent IL-3 stimulation of thrombopoiesis and neutropoiesis in patients with small cell lung carcinoma (SCLC) before and after chemotherapy (CT): a placebo controlled randomized phase Ib study. Proc Am Soc Clin Oncol 11: 381a (abstr), 1992.

113. Tepler I, Elias A, Young D, et al.: Use of recombinant human interleukin 3 (IL-3) after "ICE" chemotherapy for non-small cell lung cancer (NSCLC): effects on hematological recovery. Proc Am Assoc Cancer Res 11: 296a (abstr), 1992.

114. Ceribelli A, Fossata C, Gamucci T, et al.: Interleukin 3 (IL-3) by 120-hour continuous infusion (c.i) after myelosuppressive chemotherapy (CT): a phase I study. Proc Am Assoc Cancer Res 33: 231a (abstr), 1992.

115. Gerhartz H, Mandelli F, Philip T, et al.: Randomized phase III study of interleukin-3 in IEV-chemotherapy of relapsing lymphomas. Blood 86: 202a (abstr), 1995.

116. Robinson BE, McGrath HE, Quesenberry PJ.: Recombinant murine granulocyte macrophage colony-stimulating factor has megakaryocyte colony-stimulating activity and augments megakaryocyte colony stimulation by interleukin 3. J Clin Invest 79: 1648, 1987.

117. Paquette RL, Zhou JY, Yang YC, et al.: Recombinant gibbon interleukin-3 acts synergistically with recombinant human G-CSF and GM-CSF in vitro. Blood 71: 1596, 1988.

118. Emerson SG, Yang YC, Clark SC, et al.: Human recombinant granulocyte-macrophage colony stimulating factor and interleukin-3 have overlapping but distinct hematopoietic activities. J Clin Invest 82: 1282, 1988.

119. Quesenberry PJ, Ihle JN, McGrath E.: The effect of interleukin-3 and GM-CSA-2 on megakaryocyte and myeloid clonal colony formation. Blood 1995 65: 214.

120. Broxmeyer HE, Williams DE, Hangoc G, et al.: Synergistic myelopoietic actions in vivo after

administration to mice of combinations of purified natural murine colony-stimulating factor 1, recombinant murine interleukin 3, and recombinant murine granulocyte/macrophage colony stimulating factor. Proc Natl Acad Sci USA 84: 3871, 1987.

121. Donahue RE, Seehra J, Metzger M, et al.: Human IL-3 and GM-CSF act synergistically in stimulating hematopoiesis in primates. Science 241: 1820, 1988.

122. Mayer P, Valent P, Schmidt G, et al.: The in vivo effects of recombinant human interleukin 3 demonstration of basophil differentiation factor, histamine-producing activity, and priming of GM-CSF-responsive progenitors in non-human primates. Blood 74: 613, 1989.

123. Giessler K, Valent P, Mayer P, et al.: Recombinant human interleukin-3 expands the pool of circulating hemopoietic progenitor cells in primates: synergism with recombinant human granulocyte/macrophage colony-stimulating factor. Blood 75: 2305, 1990.

124. Stahl CP, Winton EF, Monroe MC, et al.: Differential effects of sequential, simultaneous and single agent interleukin-3 and granulocyte-macrophage colony-stimulating factor on megakaryocyte maturation and platelet response in primates. Blood 80: 2479, 1991.

125. Farese AM, Williams DE, Seiler FR, et al.: Combination protocols of cytokine therapy with interleukin-3 and granulocyte-macrophage colony-stimulating factor in a primate model of radiation-induced marrow aplasia. Blood 82: 3012, 1993.

126. Ikebuchi K, Wong GG, Clark SC, et al.: Interleukin 6 enhancement of interleukin 3-dependant proliferation of multipotential hemopoietic progenitors. Proc Natl Acad Sci USA. 84: 9035, 1987.

127. MacVittie TJ, Farese AM, Patchen ML, et al.: Therapeutic efficacy of recombinant interleukin-6 (IL-6) alone and combined with recombinant human IL-3 in a nonhuman primate model of high-dose, sublethal radiation-induced marrow aplasia. Blood 84: 2515, 1994.

128. Winton EF, Srinivasiah J, et al.: Effect of recombinant human interleukin-6 (rhIL-6) and rhIL-3 on hematopoietic regeneration as demonstrated in a nonhuman primate chemotherapy model. Blood 84: 65, 1994.

129. Ganser A, Lindemann A, Ottman OG, et al.: Sequential in vivo treatment with two recombinant human hematopoietic growth factors (interleukin 3 and granulocyte-macrophage colony-stimulating factor) as a new therapeutic modality to stimulate hematopoiesis: results of a phase I study. Blood 79: 2583, 1992.

130. Brugger W, Frisch J, Schulz G, et al.: Sequential administration of interleukin-3 and granulocyte-macrophage colony-stimulating factor following standard-dose combination chemotherapy with etoposide, ifosfamide, and cisplatin. J Clin Oncol 10: 1452, 1992.

131. O'Shaughnessy J, Venzon D, Gossard M, et al.: A phase I study of sequential versus concurrent interleukin-3 and granulocyte-macrophage colony stimulating factor in advanced breast cancer patients treated with FLAC (5-fluorouracil, leucovorin, doxorubicin, cyclophosphamide) chemotherapy. Blood 86: 2913, 1995.

132. Taketazu F, Chiba S, Shibuya K, et al.: IL-3 specifically inhibits GM-CSF binding to the higher affinity receptor. J Cell Physiol 146:251-257, 1991.

133. Fay JW, Felser JM, Abboud C, et al.: Sequential administration of recombinant human interleukin-3 (IL-3) and granulocyte-macrophage colony stimulating factor (GM-CSF) after autologous bone marrow transplantation (ABMT) therapy for lymphoma: results of a phase III multicenter study. Blood 86: 222a (abstr), 1995.

134. Williams DE, Park LS, Broxmeyer HE, et al.: Hybrid cytokines as hematopoietic growth factors. Intl J Cell Clon 9: 542, 1991.

135. Williams DE, Park LS.: Hematopoietic effects of a granulocyte-macrophage colony-stimulating factor/interleukin-3 fusion protein. Cancer 10: 2705, 1991.

136. Curtis BM, Williams DE, Broxmeyer HE, et al.: Enhanced hematopoietic activity of a human granulocyte/macrophage colony-stimulating factor-interleukin 3 fusion protein. Proc Natl Acad Sci USA 88: 5809, 1991.

137. Bruno E, Briddell RA, Copper RJ, et al.: Recombinant GM-CSF/IL-3 fusion protein: its effect on in vitro human megakaryocytopoiesis. Exp Hematol 20: 494, 1992.

138. Broxmeyer HE, Benninger L, Cooper S, et al.: Effects of in vivo treatment with PIXY (GM-CSF/IL-3 fusion protein) on proliferation kinetics of bone marrow and blood myeloid progenitor cells in patients with sarcoma. Exp Hematol 23: 335, 1995.

139. Williams DE, Dunn JT, Park LS et al.: A GM-CSF/IL-3 fusion protein promotes neutrophil and platelet recovery in sublethally irradiated rhesus monkeys. Biotechnology Therapeutics 4: 17, 1993.

140. Williams DE, Farese A, MacVittie TJ.: PIXY321, but not GM-CSF plus IL-3, promotes

hematopoietic reconstitution following lethal irradiation. Blood 82: 366a (abstr), 1993.

141.	Vadhan-Raj S, Papadopoulos NE, Burgess MA, et al.: Effects of PIXY321, a granulocyte-macrophage colony stimulating factor interleukin-3 fusion protein, on chemotherapy-induced multilineage myelosuppression in patients with sarcoma. J Clin Onc 12: 715, 1994.

142.	O'Shaughnessy J, Tolcher A, Risenberg D, et al.: Prospective randomized trial of 5-fluorouracil, leucovorin, doxorubicin, and cyclophosphamide chemotherapy in combination with interleukin-3/granulocyte-macrophage colony-stimulating factor fusion protein (PIXY321) versus GM-CSF in patients with advanced breast cancer. Blood 87: 2205, 1996.

143.	Schuster M, Beveridge M, Sosman J, et al.: Randomized phase II study of PIXY321 or Neupogen in combination with DHAP as salvage therapy for lymphoma. Blood 86:204a (abstr), 1995.

144.	Vose J, Pandite L, Beveridge R, et al.: Phase III study comparing PIXY321 and GM-CSF following autologous bone marrow transplantation in patients with non-hodgkin's lymphoma. Blood 86: 972a (abstr), 1995.

145.	Williams DE, Eisenman J, Baird A, et al.: Identification of a ligand for the c-kit proto-oncogene. Cell 63: 167, 1990.

146.	Flanagan JG, Leder P.: The kit ligand a cell surface molecule altered in steel mutant fibroblasts. Cell 63: 185, 1990.

147.	Zsebo KM, Wypych J, McNiece IK, et al.: Identification, purification and biological characterization of hematopoietic stem cell factor from buffalo rat liver-conditioned medium. Cell 63:195, 1990.

148.	Martin FH, Suggs SV, Langley KE, et al.: Primary structure and functional expression of rat and human stem cell factor DNAs. Cell 63: 203, 1990.

149.	Zsebo KM, Williams DA, Geissler EN, et al.: Stem cell factor is encoded at the Sl locus of the mouse and is the ligand for the c-kit tyrosine kinase receptor. Cell 63: 213, 1990.

150.	Huang E, Nocka K, Beier DR, et al.: The hematopoietic growth factor KL is encoded by the Sl locus and is the ligand of the c-kit receptor gene product of the W locus. Cell 63:225, 1990.

151.	Tan JC, Nocka K, Ray P.: The dominant W42 spotting phenotype results from a missense mutation in the c-kit receptor kinase. Science 247: 209, 1990.

152.	Anderson DM, Lyman SD, Baird A, et al.: Molecular cloning of mast cell growth factor, a hematopoietin that is active in both membrane bound and soluble forms. Cell 63: 235, 1990.

153.	Flanagan JG, Chan DC, Leder P.: Transmembrane form of the kit ligand growth factor is determined by alternative splicing and is missing in the sld mutant. Cell 64: 1025, 1991.

154.	Toksoz D, Zsebo KM, Smith KA, et al.: Support of human hematopoiesis in long-term bone marrow cultures by murine stromal cells selectively expressing the membrane-bound and secreted forms of the human homolog of the steel gene product, stem cell factor. Proc Natl Acad Sci USA 89:7350, 1992.

155.	Miyazawa K, Williams DA, Gotoh A, et al.: Membrane-bound steel factor induces more persistent tyrosine kinase activation and longer life span of c-kit gene-encoded protein than its soluble form. Blood 85: 641, 1995.

156.	Huss R, Hong DS, Beckham C, et al.: Ultrastructural localization of stem cell factor in canine marrow-derived stromal cells. Exp Hematol. 23: 33, 1995.

157.	Rameshwar P, Gascon P.: Substance P (SP) mediates production of stem cell factor and interleukin-1 in bone marrow stroma: potential autoregulatory role for these cytokines in SP receptor expression and induction. Blood 86: 482, 1995.

158.	Funk PE, Stephan RP, Witte PL, et al.: Vascular cell adhesion molecule 1-positive reticular cells express interleukin-7 and stem cell factor in the bone marrow. Blood 86: 2661, 1995.

159.	Fleischman RA, Simpson F, Gallardo T, et al.: Isolation of endothelial-like stromal cells that express kit ligand and support in vitro hematopoiesis. Exp Hematol. 23: 1407, 1995.

160.	Bazan JF.: Genetic and structural homology of stem cell factor and macrophage colony-stimulating factor. Cell 65: 9, 1991.

161.	Lyman SD, James L, Vanden Bos T, et al.: Molecular cloning of a ligand for the flt3/flk-2 tyrosine kinase receptor: a proliferative factor for primitive hematopoietic cells. Cell 75: 1157, 1993.

162.	Hannum C, Culpepper J, Campbell D, et al. Ligand for flt3/flk2 receptor tyrosine kinase regulates growth of haematopoietic stem cells and is encoded by variant RNAs. Nature 368: 643, 1994.

163.	Yarden Y, Kuang W-J, Yang-Feng T, et al.: Human proto-oncogene c-kit: a new cell surface receptor tyrosine kinase for an unidentified ligand. EMBO J. 6: 3341, 1987.

164.	Qiu F, Ray P, Brown K, et al.: Relationship with the CSF-1/PDGF receptor kinase family-oncogenic activation of v-kit involves deletion of extracellular domain and C terminus. EMBO J.

7: 1003, 1988.
165. Ullrich A, Schlessinger J, et al.: Signal transduction by receptors with tyrosine kinase activity. Cell 61: 203, 1990.
166. Heldin C-H.: Dimerization of cell surface receptors in signal transduction. Cell 80: 213, 1995.
167. Besmer P, Murphy JE, George PC, et al.: A new acute transforming feline retrovirus and relationship of its oncogene v-kit with the protein kinase gene family. Nature 320: 415, 1996.
168. Okada S, Nakauchi H, Nagayoshi K, et al.: Enrichment and characterization of murine hematopoietic stem cells that express c-kit molecule. Blood 78 1706, 1991.
169. Ogawa M, Matsuzaki Y, Nishikawa S, et al.: Expression and function of c-kit in hemopoietic progenitor cells. J Exp Med. 174: 63, 1991.
170. Metcalf D, Nicola NA.: Direct proliferation actions of stem cell factor on murine bone marrow cells in vitro: effects of combination with colony-stimulating factors. Proc Natl Acad Sci USA 88: 6239, 1991.
171. Bernstein ID, Andrews RG, Zsebo KM, et al.: Recombinant human stem cell factor enhances the formation of colonies by CD34+ and CD34+ Lin- cells and the generation of colony-forming cell progeny from CD34+ lin- cells cultured with IL-3, G-CSF, or GM-CSF. Blood 77: 2316, 1991.
172. Briddell RA, Bruno E, Cooper RJ, et al.: Effects of c-kit ligand on in vitro human megakaryocytopoiesis. Blood 78: 2854, 1991.
173. McNiece IK, Langley KE, Zsebo KM, et al.: Recombinant human stem cell factor synergises with GM-CSF, G-CSF, IL-3 and epo to stimulate human progenitor cells of the myeloid and erythroid lineages. Exp Hematol. 19: 226, 1991.
174. Avraham H, Vannier E, Cowley S, et al.: Effects of the stem cell factor, c-kit ligand on human megakaryocytic cells. Blood 79: 365, 1992.
175. Debili N, Masse J-M, Katz A, et al.: Effects of the recombinant hematopoietic growth factors interleukin-3, interleukin-6, stem cell factor, and leukemia inhibitory factor on the megakaryocytic differentiation of CD34+ cells. Blood 82: 84, 1993.
176. Ulich TR, Yi ES, Yin SM , et al.: Hematologic effects of stem cell factor alone and in combination with G-CSF and GM-CSF in vivo and in vitro in rodents. Int Rev Exp Pathol.: 34:215, 1993.
177. Brandt JE, Bhalla K, Hoffman R.: Effects of interleukin-3 and c-kit ligand on the survival of various classes of human hematopoietic progenitor cells. Blood 83: 1507, 1994.
178. Grabarek J, Groopman JE, Lyles YR, et al.: Human kit ligand (stem cell factor) modulates platelet activation in vitro. J Biol Chem. 269: 21718, 1994.
179. Broudy VC, Lin NL, Kaushansky K.: Thrombopoietin (c-mpl ligand) acts synergistically with erythropoietin, stem cell factor, and interleukin-11 to enhance murine megakaryocyte colony growth and increases megakaryocyte ploidy in vitro. Blood 85: 1719, 1995.
180. Russell ES.: Hereditary anemias of the mouse: A review for geneticists. Adv Genet. 1981 20: 357.
181. Copeland NG, Gilbert DJ, Cho BC, et al.: Mast cell growth factor maps near the steel locus on mouse chromosome 10 and is deleted in a number of steel alleles. Cell 63:175, 1990.
182. Brannan CI, Lyman SD, Williams DE, et al.: Steel-dickie mutation encodes a c-kit ligand lacking transmembrane and cytoplasmic domains. Proc Natl Acad Sci USA 88 : 4771, 1991.
183. Molineux G, Migdalska A, Szmitkowski M, et al.: The effects on hematopoiesis of recombinant stem cell factor (ligand for c-kit) administered in vivo to mice either alone or in combination with granulocyte colony-stimulating factor. Blood 78: 961, 1991.
184. Andrews RG, Knitter GH, Bartelmez SH, et al.: Recombinant human stem cell factor, a c-kit ligand, stimulates hematopoiesis in primates. Blood 78:1975, 1991.
185. Andrews RG, Bartelmez SH, Knitter GH, et al.: A c-kit ligand, recombinant human stem cell factor, mediates reversible expansion of multiple CD34+ colony-forming cell types in blood and marrow of baboons. Blood 80: 920, 1992.
186. Pietsch T, Kyas U, Steffens U, et al.: Effects of human stem cell factor (c-kit ligand) on proliferation of myeloid leukemia cells: heterogeneity in response and synergy with other hematopoietic growth factors. Blood 80: 1199, 1992.
187. Andrews RG, Bensinger WI, Knitter GH, et al.: The ligand for c-kit, stem cell factor, stimulates the circulation of cells that engraft lethally irradiated baboons. Blood 80: 2715, 1992.
188. Bodine DM, Seidel NE, Zsebo KM, et al.: In vivo administration of stem cell factor to mice increases the absolute number of pluripotent hematopoietic stem cells. Blood 82: 445, 1993.
189. Briddell RA, Hartley CA, Smith KA, et al.: Recombinant rat stem cell factor synergizes with recombinant human granulocyte-stimulating factor in vivo in mice to mobilize peripheral blood progenitor cells that have enhanced repopulating potential. Blood 82: 1720, 1993.

190. Moskowitz C, Stiff P, Gordon M, et al.: The influence of extensive prior chemotherapy on the mobilization of peripheral blood progenitor cells (PBSC) using stem cell factor (rhSCF) and filgrastim (rmetHuG-CSF) on hematologic recovery post cyclophosphamide, BCNU, and VP-16 (CBV) in patients with relapsed non-hodgkins lymphoma (NHL):An interim analysis. Blood 96: 107a (abstr).

191. Crawford J, Lau D, Erwin R, et al.: A phase I trial of recombinant methionyl human stem cell factor (SCF) in patients (pts) with advanced non-small cell lung carcinoma (NSCLC). Proc Am Soc Clin Oncol. 12: 135 (abstr), 1993.

192. Demetri GD, Costa JJ, Hayes DF, et al.: A phase I trial of recombinant methionyl human stem cell factor (SCF) in patients with advanced breast carcinoma pre- and post- chemotherapy (chemo) with cyclophosphamide (C) and doxorubicin (A). Proc Am Soc Clin Oncol. 12: 142 (abstr), 1993.

193. Glaspy JA, Shpall EJ, LeMaistre C.F, et al.: Peripheral blood progenitor cell mobilization using stem cell factor in combination with filgrastim in breast cancer patients. Blood 90: 2939, 1997.

194. Stiff P, Gingrich R, Luger S, et al.: Improved PBSC collection using STEMGEN (stem cell factor, SCF) and Filgrastim (G-CSF) compared to G-CSF alone in heavily pretreated lymphoma (NHL) and Hodgkin's Disease (HD) patients (pts). Blood 90: 591a (abstr), 1997.

195. Shpall EJ, Wheeler CA, Turner SA, et al.: A randomized phase 3 study of PBSC mobilization by stem cell factor (SCF, Stemgen) and Filgrastim in patients with high risk breast cancer. Blood 2627 (abstr), 1997.

196. Hirano T, Yasukawa K, Harada H, et al. Complementary DNA for a novel human interleukin (BSF-2) that induces B lymphocytes to produce immunoglobulin. Nature 324: 73, 1986.

197. Kishimoto T.: The biology of interleukin-6.Blood 74: 1, 1989.

198. Hirano T, Akira S, Taga T, et al.: Biological and clinical aspects of interleukin-6. Immunol Today. 11: 443, 1990.

199. Sehgal PB, Zilberstein A, Ruggieri R-M, et al.: Human chromosome 7 carries the beta2 interferon gene. Proc Natl Acad Sci USA 83: 5219, 1986.

200. Yamasaki K, Taga T, Hirata Y, et al.: Cloning and expression of the human interleukin-6 (BSF-2/ IFN b 2) receptor. Science 241: 825, 1988.

201. Taga T, Hibi M, Hirata Y, et al.: Interleukin-6 triggers the association of its receptor with a possible signal transducer, gp130. Cell : 58: 573, 1989.

202. Bruno E, Briddell R, Hoffman R, et al.: Effect of recombinant and purified hematopoietic growth factors on human megakaryocyte colony formation. Exp Hematol. 16: 371, 1988.

203. Bruno E, Hoffman R.: Effects of interleukin-6 on in vitro human megakaryocytopoiesis: its interactions with other cytokines. Exp Hematol. 17: 1038, 1989.

204. Warren MK, Conroy LB, Rose JS.: The role of interleukin 6 and interleukin 1 in megakaryocytic development. Exp Hematol. 17: 1095, 1989.

205. Lotem J, Shabo Y, Sachs L.: Regulation of megakaryocyte development by interleukin-6. Blood 74: 1545, 1989.

206. Ishibashi T, Kimura H, Uchida T, et al.: Human IL-6 is a direct promoter of maturation of megakaryocytes in vitro. Proc Natl Acad Sci. 86: 5953-5957, 1989.

207. Koike K, Nakahata T, Kubo T, et al.: Interleukin-6 enhances murine megakaryocytopoiesis in serum-free culture. Blood 75: 2286, 1990.

208. Williams N, De Giorgio T, Banu N, et al.: Recombinant interleukin-6 stimulates immature murine megakaryocytes. Exp Hematol. 18: 69, 1990.

209. Kimura H, Ishibashi T, Uchida T, et al.: Interleukin 6 is a differentiation factor for human megakaryocytes in vitro. Eur J Immunol. 20: 1927, 1990 .

210. Navarro S, Debili N, Le Couedic, et al.: Interleukin-6 and its receptor are expressed by human megakaryocytes. In vitro effects on proliferation and endoreplication. Blood 77: 461, 1991.

211. Imai T, Koike K, Kubo T et al.: Interleukin-6 supports human megakaryocytic proliferation and differentiation in vitro. Blood 78: 1969, 1991.

212. Navarro S, Mitjavila MT, Katz , et al: Expression of Interleukin 6 and its specific receptor by untreated and PMA-stimulated human erythroid and megakaryocytic cell lines. Exp Hematol. 19: 11, 1991.

213. Bruno E, Cooper R, Briddell R, et al.: Further examination of the effects of recombinant cytokines on the proliferation of human megakaryocyte progenitor cells. Blood 77: 2339, 1991.

214. Quesenberry PJ, McGrath HE, Williams ME, et al.: Multifactor stimulation of megakaryocytopoiesis effects of interleukin 6. Exp Hematol. 19: 35, 1991.

215. Wickenhauser C, Lorenzen J, Thiele J, et al. Secretion of cytokines (interleukins-1 α, -3, and -6

and granulocyte-macrophage colony-stimulating factor) by normal human bone marrow megakaryocytes. Blood 85: 685, 1995.

216.	Kopf M, Lamers M, Bluethman H, et al. IL-6 deficient mice show immunologic abnormalities. Nature 376: 339, 1994.

217.	Ishibashi T, Kimura H, Shikama Y, et al.: Interleukin-6 is a potent thrombopoietic factor in vivo in mice. Blood 74: 1241, 1989.

218.	Asano S, Okano A, Ozawa K, et al.: In vivo effects of recombinant human interleukin-6 in primates: Stimulated production of human platelets. Blood 75:1602, 1990.

219.	Pojda Z, Tsuboi A.: In vivo effects of human recombinant interleukin-6 on hemopoietic stem and progenitor cells and circulating blood cells in normal mice. Exp Hematol. 18: 1034.

220.	Hill RJ, Warren MK, Stenberg P, et al.: Stimulation of megakaryocytopoiesis in mice by human recombinant interleukin-6. Blood 77: 42, 1991.

221.	Stahl C, Zucker-Franklin D, Evatt B, et al.: Effects of human interleukin-6 on megakaryocyte development and thrombocytopoiesis in primates. Blood 78:1467, 1991.

222.	Mayer P, Geissler K, Valent P, et al.: Recombinant human interleukin-6 is a potent inducer of the acute phase response and elevates the blood platelets in non-human primates. Exp Hematol. 19: 688, 1991.

223.	Ishibashi T, Shikama Y, Kimura H.: Thrombopoietic effects of interleukin-6 in long-term administration in mice. Exp Hematol. 21 640, 1993.

224.	Selig C, Kreja L, Muller H, et al.: Hematologic effects of recombinant human interleukin-6 in dogs exposed to a total-body radiation dose of 2.4 Gy. Exp Hematol. 22: 551, 1994.

225.	Inoue H, Kadoya T, Kabaya K, et al.: A highly enhanced thrombopoietic activity by monmethoxypolyethylene glycol modified recombinant human interleukin-6. J Lab Clin Med. 124: 529, 1994.

226.	Takatsuki F, Okano A, Suzuki C, et al.: Interleukin 6 perfusion stimulates reconstitution of the immune and hematopoietic systems ater 5-fluorouracil treatment. Cancer Res. 18: 2885, 1990.

227.	Patchen ML, MacVittie TJ, Williams JL, et al.: Administration of interleukin 6 stimulates multilineage hematopoiesis and accelerates recovery from radiation-induced hematopoietic depression. Blood 77: 472, 1991.

228.	Burstein SA, Downs T, Friese P, et al.: Thrombocytopoiesis in normal and sublethally irradiated dogs: response to human interleukin-6. Blood 80: 420, 1992.

229.	Herodin F, Mestries JC, Janodet D, et al.: Recombinant glycosylated human interleukin-6 accelerates peripheral blood platelet count recovery in radiation-induced bone marrow depression in baboons. Blood 80: 688, 1992.

230.	Zeidler C, Kanz L, Hurkuck F, et al.: In vivo effects of interleukin-6 on thrombopoiesis in healthy and irradiated primates. Blood 80: 2740, 1992 .

231.	Leven RM, Rodriguez A.: Immunomagnetic bead isolation of megakaryocytes from guinea-pig bone-marrow: effect of recombinant interleukin-6 on size, ploidy and cytoplasmic fragmentation. Br J Haematol. 77: 267, 1991.

232.	MacVittie TJ, Monroy RL, Patchen ML, et al.: Therapeutic use of recombinant human G-CSF in a canine model of sublethal and lethal whole body irradiation. Int J Radiat Biol. 57: 723, 1990.

233.	Farese AM, Myers LA, MacVittie TJ.: Therapeutic efficacy of the combined administration of either recombinant human interleukin-6 and rh-granulocyte colony stimulating factor or rh-granulocyte-macrophage colony stimulating factor in a primate model of radiation-induced marrow aplasia. Exp Hematol. 22: 684 (abstr), 1994.

234.	Gontor PW, Hillyer CD, Strobert EA, et al.: Enhanced post-chemotherapy platelet and neutrophil recovery using combination rhIL-6 and rhGM-CSF in a nonhuman primate model. Blood 82: 365a (abstr), 1993.

235.	de Benedetti F, Massa M, Robbioni P, et al.: Correlation of serum interleukin-6 levels with joint involvement and thrombocytosis in systemic juvenile rheumatoid arthritis. Arthritis Rheumatology. 34: 1158, 1991.

236.	Hollen CW, Henthorn J, Koziol J, et al.: Elevated serum interleukin-6 levels in patients with reactive thrombocytosis. Br J of Haematol. 76: 286, 1991.

237.	Chang M, Suen Y, Meng G, et al.: Differential mechanisms in the regulation of endogenous levels of thrombopoietin and interleukin-11 during thrombocytopenia: insight into the regulation of platelet production. Blood 88: 3354, 1996.

238.	Weber J, Yang J, Topalian S, et al.: Phase I trial of subcutaneous interleukin-6 in patients with advanced malignancies. J Clin Oncol. 11: 499, 1993.

239. van Gameren M, Willemse P, Mulder N, et al.: Effects of recombinant human interleukin-6 in cancer patients: a phase I-II study. Blood 84: 1434.

240. D'Hondt V, Humblet T, Baatout S, et al.: Thrombopoietic effects and toxicity of interleukin-6 in patients with ovarian cancer before and after chemotherapy: a multicenter placebo-controlled, randomized phase Ib study. Blood 1995 85: 2347, 1994.

241. Veldhuis G, Willemse P, Sleijfer D, et al.: Toxicity and efficacy of escalating dosages of recombinant human interleukin-6 after chemotherapy in patients with breast cancer or non-small-cell lung cancer. J Clin Oncol. 13: 2585, 1995.

242. Chang A, Boros L, Asbury R, et al.: Effects of interleukin-6 in cancer patients treated with ifosfamide, carboplatin, and etoposide. Proc Am Soc Clin Onc. 12:936a (abstr), 1993.

243. Samuels B, Bukowski R, Gordon M, et al.: Phase I study of rhIL-6 with chemotherapy in advanced sarcoma. Proc Am Soc Clin Onc. 12:298a (abstr), 1993.

244. Chang A, Boros L, Ashbury R, et al.: Effects of interleukin-6 in cancer patients treated with ifosfamide, carboplatin and etoposide. Proc Am Soc Clin Onc. 12:936a (abstr), 1993.

245. Atkins MB, Kappler K, Mier JW, et al.: Interleukin-6 associated anemia: determination of the underlying mechanism. Blood 86: 1288, 1995.

246. van Gameren MM, Willemse PHB, Mudler NH, et al.: Effects of recombinant human interleukin-6 in cancer patients: a phase I-II study. Blood 84: 1434.

247. Gordon MS, Neumanitis J, Hoffman R, et al.: A phase I trial of recombinant human interleukin-6 in patients with myelodysplastic syndromes and thrombocytopenia. Blood 85: 3066, 1995.

248. Lazarus HM, Winton EF, Williams SF, et al.: Phase I multicenter trial of interleukin 6 therapy after autologous bone marrow transplantation in advanced breast cancer. Bone Marrow Transplantation. 15: 935, 1995.

249. Hamm J, Crawford J, Figlin R, et al.: A phase I/II study of the simultaneous administration of recombinant human interleukin-6 (rhIL-6 E.coli) and Neupogen (rhG-CSF E.coli) following ICE chemotherapy in patients with advanced non-small cell lung cancer. Proc Am Soc Clin Onc. 13:1100a (abstr), 1994.

250. Budd G, Pelley R, Samuels B, et al.: Phase II randomized trial of simultaneous rhIL-6 and G-CSF following MAID chemotherapy in patients with sarcomas: Preliminary results. Proc Am Soc Clin Onc. 14: 694a (abstr), 1995.

251. Stahl CP, Winton EF, Monroe MC, et al.: Recombinant human granulocyte-macrophage colony-stimulating factor promotes megakaryocyte maturation in non-human primates. Exp Hematol. 19: 810, 1991

252. Mazur EM, Cohen JL, Wong GG et al. Modest stimulatory effect of recombinant human GM-CSF on colony growth from peripheral blood human megakaryocyte progenitor cells. Exp Hematol. 15: 1128, 1987.

253. Vadhan-Raj S, Keating M, Hittelman WN, et al.: Effects of recombinant human granulocyte-macrophage colony-stimulating factor in patients with myelodysplastic syndromes. N Engl J Med. 3178: 1545, 1987.

254. Lieschke GJ, Maher D, Cebon J, et al.: Effects of bacterially synthesized recombinant human granulocyte-macrophage colony-stimulating factor in patients with advanced malignancy. Ann Intern Med. 110: 357, 1989.

255. Ganser A, Volkers B, Greher J, et al.: Recombinant human granulocyte-macrophage colony-stimulating factor in patients with myelodysplastic syndromes: A phase I/II trial. Blood 73: 31, 1989.

256. Neumanitis J, Rabinowe S, Singer J, et al.: Recombinant granulocyte-macrophage colony-stimulating factor after autologous bone marrow transplantation for lymphoid cancer. N Engl J Med. 324: 1773, 1991.

257. Levine JD, Allan JD, Tessitore JH, et al.: Recombinant human granulocyte-macrophage colony-stimulating factor ameliorates zidovudine-induced neutropenia in patients with acquired immune deficiency syndrome (AIDS/AIDS related complex). Blood 78: 3148, 1991.

258. Bunn PA Jr, Browley J, Hazaka M, et al.: The role of GM-CSF in limited stage SCLC: a randomized phase III study of the Southwest Oncology Group (SWOG). Proc Am Soc Clin Oncol. 11: 292 (abstr), 1992.

259. Anasetti C, Anderson G, Applebaum FR, et al.: Phase III study of rhGM-CSF in allogeneic marrow transplantation from unrelated donors. Blood 82: 454a (abstr), 1993.

260. Nash RA, Burstein SA, Storb R, et al.: Thrombocytopenia in dogs induced by granulocyte-macrophage colony-stimulating factor: increased destruction of circulating platelets. Blood 86:

1765, 1995.
261.	Tewari A, Buhles W Jr, Starnes HF Jr.: Preliminary report: effects of interleukin-1 on platelet counts. Lancet. 336: 712, 1990.
262.	Crown J, Jakubowski A, Kemeny N, et al.: Phase I trial of recombinant human interleukin-1 beta alone and in combination with myelosuppressive doses of 5-fluorouracil in patients with gastrointestinal cancer. Blood 78: 1420, 1991.
263.	Smith II JW, Longo DL, Alvord WG, et al.: The effects of treatment with interleukin-1 α on platelet recovery after high dose carboplatin. N Eng J Med. 328: 756, 1993
264.	Leary AG, Wong GG, Clark SC, et al.: Leukemia inhibitory factor differentiation-inhibiting activity/human interleukin for DA cells augments proliferation of human hematopoietic stem cells. Blood 75: 1960, 1990.
265.	Metcalf D, Hilton D, Nicola NA.: Leukemia inhibitory factor can potentiate murine megakaryocyte production in vitro. Blood 77: 2150, 1991.
266.	Metcalf D, Nicola NA, Gearing DP.: Effects of injected leukemia inhibitory factor(LIF) on hemopoietic and other tissues in mice. Blood 76: 50, 1990.
267.	Mayer P, Geissler K, Ward M, et al.: Recombinant human leukemia inhibitory factor induces acute phase proteins and raises the platelet counts in non human primates. Blood 81: 3226, 1993.
268.	Farese AM, Myers LA, MacVittie TJ.: Therapeutic efficacy of recombinant human leukemia inhibitory factor in a primate model of radiation-induced marrow aplasia. Blood 84: 3675, 1994.
269.	Wallace PM, MacMaster JF, Rillena JR, et al.: Thrombocytopoietic properties of oncostatin M. Blood 86: 1310, 1995.
270.	Thomas JW, Baum CM, Hood WF, et al.: Potent interleukin-3 receptor agonist with selectively enhanced hematopoietic activity relative to recombinant human interleukin-3. Proc Natl Acad Sci USA 92: 3779, 1995.
271.	Farese AM, Herodin F, Baum C, et al.: Acceleration of hematopoietic reconstitution with a synthokine (SC-55494) after radiation-induced bone marrow aplasia. Blood 87: 581, 1996.
272.	MacVittie TJ, Farese AM, Heodin F, et al.: Combination therapy for radiation-induced bone marrow aplasia in nonhuman primates using Synthokine SC55494 and recombinant human granulocyte colony stimulating factor. Blood 87: 4129, 1996.
273.	Monahan JB, Hood WF, Joy WD, et al.: Functional characterization of SC 68420- a multifunctional agonist which activates both IL-3 and G-CSF receptors. Blood 86: 154a (abstr), 1995.
274.	McKearn JP, Hood WF, Monahan JB, et al.: Myelopoietin-A multifunctional agonist of human IL-3 and G-CSF receptors. Blood 86: 259a (abstr), 1995
275.	Beckmann MP, Heimfeld S, Fei R, et al.: Novel hematopoietic factors enhance ex vivo expansion of human CD34+ hematopoietic progenitor cells. Blood 86: 492a (abstr), 1995.
276.	MacVittie TJ, Farese AM, Grab LB, et al.: Stimulation of multilineage hematopoietic recovery in a nonhuman primate, bone marrow aplasia model by a multifunctional agonist of human IL-3 and G-CSF receptors. Blood 86: 499a (abstr), 1995.
277.	 Giri JG, Smith WG, Kahn LE, et al.: Promegapoietin, a chimeric growth factor for megakaryocyte and platelet restoration. Blood 90: 580a (abstr), 1997.
278.	Lin J, Nachtrieb E, Bensinger W, et al. Ex vivo expansion of myeloid and megakaryocytic progenitors using HS-5 stromal cell conditioned media plus promegapoietin. Blood 538a (abstr), 1997.
279.	Burnette BL, Wood DC, Duffin K, et al.: Biochemical characterization of promegapoietin, a chimeric growth factor for platelet producing cells. Blood 177b (abstr), 1997.
280.	Brasel K, McKenna HJ, Morrissey PJ, et al.: Hematologic effects of flt3 ligand in vivo in mice. Blood 88: 2004, 1996.
281.	Winton E, Bocur SZ, Bray RA, et al.: The hematopoietic effects of recombinant human (rhu) Flt3 ligand administered to nonhuman primates. Blood 86: 424a (abstr), 1995.
282.	Ramsfjell V, Borge OJ, Veiby OP, et al.: Thrombopoietin, but not erythropoietin, directly stimulates multilineage growth of primitive murine bone marrow progenitor cells in synergy with early acting cytokines: distinct interactions with the ligands for c-kit and FLT3. Blood 88: 4481, 1996.
283.	Mackarehtschian K, Hardin JD, Moore KA, et al.: Targeted disruption of the flk2/flt3 gene leads to deficiencies in primitive hematopoietic progenitors. Immunity 3 147, 1995.
284.	Turner AM, Lin NL, Issarachai S, et al.: FLT3 receptor expression on the surface of normal and malignant human hematopoietic cells. Blood 88: 3383, 1996.
285.	Mitjavila MT, Vinci G, Villeval JL, et al.: Human platelet alpha granules contain a non-specific

inhibitor of megakaryocyte colony formation: its relationship to type beta transforming growth factor (TGF beta). Journal of Cell Physio 1988 134: 93.

286. Moses HL, Yang EY, Pietenpol JA.: TGF-beta stimulation and inhibition of cell proliferation: new mechanistic insights. Cell   63: 245, 1990.

287. Kuter DJ, Gminski DM, Rosenberg RD.: Transforming growth factor beta inhibits megakaryocyte growth and endomitosis. Blood   79 :619, 1992.

288. Han ZC, Bellucci S, Wan HY, et al.: New insights into the regulation of megakaryocytopoiesis by hematopoietic and fibroblast growth factors and transforming growth factor beta 1. Br J of Haem 81: 1, 1992.

289. Ishibashi T, Miller S, Burnstein SA.: Type B transforming growth factor is a potent inhibitor of murine megakaryocytopoiesis in vitro. Blood 69:1737-1741, 1987

290. Mantovani A, Sozzani S.: Chemokines. Lancet. 343: 923, 1994.

291. Baggiolini M, Deward B, Moser B. Interleukin-8 and related chemotactic cytokines- CXC and CC chemokines. Adv in Immun 55: 97, 1994.

292. Gewirtz AM, Calabretta B, Rucinski et al.: Inhibition of human megakaryocytopoiesis in vitro by platelet factor 4 (PF4) and a synthetic COOH-terminal PF4 peptide. J of Clin Inv 83: 1477, 1989.

293. Han ZC, Bellucci S, Tenza D, et al.: Negative regulation of human megakaryocytopoiesis by human platelet factor 4 and beta-thromboglobulin: comparative analysis in bone marrow cultures from normal individuals and patients with essential thrombocythaemia and immune thrombocytopenic purpura. Br J of Haem 74: 395, 1990.

294. Han ZC, Sensebe L, Abgrall JF, et al.: Platelet factor 4 inhibits human megakaryocytopoiesis in vitro. Blood   75: 1234, 1990

295. Gewirtz AM, Zhang J, Ratajczak J, et al.: Chemokine regulation of megakaryocytopoiesis. Blood 86:2559, 1995.

296. Xi XD, Caen JP, Fournier, et al.: Direct and reversible inhibition of platelet factor 4 on megakaryocyte development from CD34+ cord blood cells: comparative studies with transforming growth factor beta1. Br J of Haem 93: 265, 1996.

297. Plantier JL, Berthier R, Rival Y, et al.: Evidence for a selective inhibitory effect of thrombin on megakaryocyte progenitor growth mediated by the thrombin receptor. Br J of Haem 87: 755, 1994.

298. Ganser A, Carlo-Stella C, Greher, et al.: Effect of recombinant interferon alpha and gamma on human bone-marrow derived megakaryocytic progenitor cells. Blood 70:1173, 1987.

299. Griffin CG, Grant BW.: Effects of recombinant interferons on human megakaryocyte growth. Exp Hematol 18: 1013, 1990.

300. Wadenvik H, Kutti J, Ridell B, et al.: The effect of alpha interferon on bone marrow megakaryocytes and platelet production rate in essential thrombocythemia. Blood   77: 2103, 1991.

301. Wallace EL, Surgenor DM, Hao HS, et al.: Collection and transfusion of blood and blood components in the United States, 1989. Transfusion 33: 139, 1993.

302. Anderson KC, Weinstein HJ. Transfusion-associated graft-versus-host disease. N Engl J Med 323: 315, 1990.

303. Dodd RY. The risk of transfusion-transmitted infection. N Eng J Med 327: 419, 1992.

304. Novotny VM, van Doorn R, Witvliet MD, et al. Occurrence of allogenic HLA and non-HLA antibodies after transfusion of prestorage filtered platelets and red blood cells: a prospective study. Blood   85: 1736, 1995.

305. Slichter SJ. Principles of platelet transfusion therapy. Hematology: basic principles and practice. 2nd ed. New York: Churchill Livingstone: 1987, 1995.

306. National Institutes of Health Consensus Conference. Platelet transfusion therapy. Transfus Med Rev 1: 195, 1987.

307. Gaydos LA, Freireich EJ, Mantel N. The quantitative relation between platelet count and hemorrhage in patients with acute leukemia. N Eng J Med 266:905, 1962.

308. Gmur J, Burger J, Schanz U, et al. Safety of stringent prophylactic platelet transfusion policy for patients with acute leukemia. Lancet 338: 1223-6, 1991.

309. Gil-Fernandez JJ, Alegre A, Fernandez-Villalta MJ, et al. Clinical results of a stringent policy on prophylactic platelet transfusion non-randomized comparative analysis in 190 bone marrow transplant patients from a single institution. Bone Marrow Transplant 18:931, 1996.

310. Wandt H, Frank M, Schneider C, et al.: The 10,000/microL trigger compared to 20,000/microL for prophylactic platelet transfusion in AML: a prospective comparative multicenter study. Blood   88: 443a (abstr) , 1996.

311.   Rebulla P, Finazzi G, Marangoni F, et al. The threshold for prophylactic platelet transfusions in

adults with acute myeloid leukemia. N Eng J Med 337: 1870, 1997.
312. Heckman KD, Weiner GJ, Davis CS, et al.: Randomized study of prophylactic platelet transfusion threshold during induction therapy for adult acute leukemia: 10,000/ microL versus 20,000/microL. J Clin Oncol 15: 1143, 1997.

14. Clinical Studies of Thrombopoietin

Russell L. Basser

Introduction

It was recognized soon after the discovery of the ligand to *c-mpl* that this was the long sought after central regulator of megakaryocytopoiesis and thrombopoiesis [1]. The native or biological form of Mpl ligand is referred to as thrombopoietin (TPO). Two formulations of Mpl ligand are in clinical development. Recombinant human *megakaryocyte growth and development factor* (rHu-MGDF) is a truncated form of Mpl ligand with identical biological activity. Pegylation of MGDF, in which it is coupled to poly-ethylene glycol to form PEG-rHuMGDF, results in a molecule that is approximately ten times more potent *in vivo* than non-pegylated MGDF [2]. PEG-rHuMGDF has been chosen as the agent for clinical use. A full length gycosylated form of thrombopoietin, *recombinant human TPO (rTPO)*, is also being developed.

Hematological Effects of Mpl Ligand Alone

The safety and biological activities of PEG-rHuMGDF were assessed in phase one studies in Australia [3-5] and the USA [6]. These initial trials were randomized, double-blinded and placebo controlled. In the Australian study, 17 patients with advanced cancer received either PEG-rHuMGDF (13 patients) or placebo (4 patients) alone prior to chemotherapy. PEG-rHuMGDF was administered by daily subcutaneous injection in sequential cohorts of 0.03 (n=3), 0.1 (n=3), 0.3 (n=4) and 1.0 (n=3) μg/kg/day. The placebo and lower 3 dose schedules were given for 10 days, whereas the highest dose was given for six, seven, and nine days because of early thrombocytosis. The functional characteristics of PEG-rHuMGDF produced platelets, and the mobilisation of peripheral blood progenitor cells were assessed.

A dose dependent increase in platelet counts was observed following the administration of PEG-rHuMGDF (Figure 1), although considerable individual variation in response was seen [3]. Patients receiving 0.3 and 1 μg/kg PEG-rHuMGDF had increases in platelet counts ranging from 51% to 584%. The maximum platelet count observed was less than 450 x 10^9/L in the 0.03 and 0.10 μg/kg/day groups, and 970 x 10^9/L and 1876 x 10^9/L, in the 0.3 and 1.0 μg/kg/day groups respectively. The platelet numbers began to increase from day 6 and continued to rise despite cessation of PEG-rHuMGDF. The peak count was reached between days 12 and 18, and platelets returned to normal between days 22 and 30. The rise in platelet counts in the lower dose cohorts was considerably less pronounced. However, an increase in bone-marrow megakaryocytes by up to 1.8-fold was observed in all PEG-rHuMGDF cohorts, suggesting that the molecule is biologically active even at the lowest dose level.

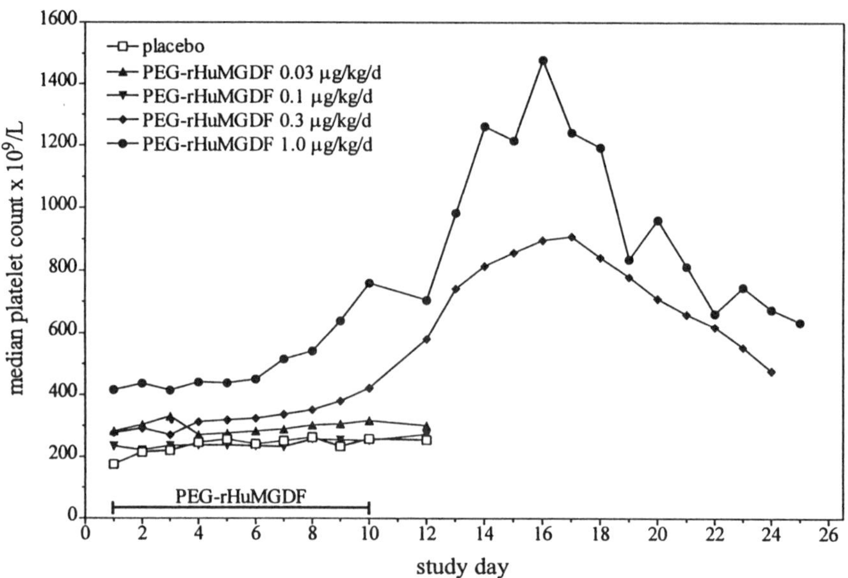

Figure 1. The effects of PEG-rHuMGDF (daily administration indicated by the bar) on platelet counts in patients receiving placebo, and 0.03, 0.1, 0.3, and 1.0 μg/kg/d of PEG-rHuMGDF. (From Basser et al. Thrombopoietic effects of pegylated recombinant human megakaryocyte growth and development factor (PEG-rHuMGDF) in patients with advanced cancer. Lancet 348:1279-1281, 1996.

The potency of PEG-rHuMGDF was also seen in the US study of identical design. In this study, seven patients with non-small cell lung cancer were treated with placebo or PEG-rHuMGDF 0.03 or 0.1 μg/kg/d for up to ten days. A significant rise in platelet count occurred even at these low doses [6].

In another study, a single dose of glycosylated rTPO was given alone to 12 patients with sarcoma at doses ranging from 0.3 to 2.4μg/kg [7]. There was a dose dependent increase in platelets, usually beginning on day 4 and peaking at a median of 12 days after the injection. Platelet counts peaked between 61% to 213% above baseline. Bone marrow megakaryocytes increased up to four-fold.

In the studies of PEG-rHuMGDF and rTPO, there was no increase in peripheral leukocyte counts or hematocrit.

Normal Platelet Donors

In view of the potency and low toxicity of PEG-rHuMGDF and rTPO, a potential use of these agents is to improve the efficiency of platelet collection from healthy volunteers. Early results of an investigation of the effects of PEG-rHuMGDF in this population were recently published in abstract form [8]. Kuter and colleagues showed that a single dose of PEG-rHuMGDF 1 μg/kg or 3 μg/kg enhanced apheresis platelet yield compared to placebo controls in a dose-dependent manner by approximately three-fold (in those donors given PEG-rHuMGDF 3 μg/kg). Furthermore, infusion of the platelets collected in PEG-rHuMGDF-treated donors into thrombocytopenia recipients resulted in a larger platelet increment than infusion of platelets from donors given placebo.

Mpl Ligand after Chemotherapy

<u>Single-Cycle Chemotherapy</u>: In a trial of 53 patients with non-small cell lung cancer, PEG-rHuMGDF 0.03 to 5.0 µg/kg/d or placebo (3:1 ratio) was given alone for up to 16 days after carboplatin (AUC=9) and paclitaxel (175mg/m^2) [6]. The platelet nadir was higher in patients given PEG-rHuMGDF than in the placebo group (188 x 10^9/L versus 111 x 10^9/L, p=0.013), and the time to recovery of baseline platelet count was shorter (14 days vs >21 days, p<0.001). No dose-response to PEG-rHuMGDF was observed (Figure 2). This study demonstrated that PEG-rHuMGDF was effective at

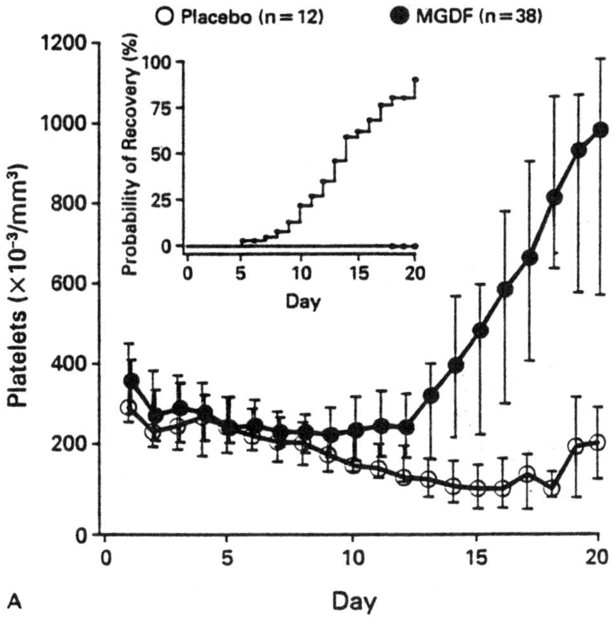

Figure 2. Platelet recovery (medians) after carboplatin and paclitaxel in patients with lung cancer receiving PEG-rHuMGDF (n=38) versus those given placebo (n=12). Error bars indicate interquartile ranges. (From Fanucchi et al. Effects of polyethylene glycol-conjugated recombinant human megakaryocyte growth and development factor on platelet counts after chemotherapy for lung cancer. N Engl J Med 1997, 336: 404-409 - Panel A of Figure 1, p406)

abrogating thrombocytopenia due to mildly myelosuppressive chemotherapy.

In another trial, PEG-rHuMGDF was given with filgrastim (granulocyte colony-stimulating factor) after moderately intensive chemotherapy. In this study [10], PEG-rHuMGDF or placebo (3:1 ratio) was given with filgrastim 5 µg/kg/d after carboplatin 600 mg/m^2 and cyclophosphamide 1200 mg/m^2 to 41 patients. Fifteen patients who had participated in the pre-chemotherapy trial received the same study drug and dose after chemotherapy. Study drug was given daily for up to 21 days at doses of 0.03, 0.1, 0.3 and 1.0 µg/kg/day commencing on the day after chemotherapy. In cohorts receiving 1, 3 or 5 µg/kg/day, the duration of PEG-rHuMGDF administration was shortened to seven days because of asymptomatic thrombocytosis in the previous dose levels. Filgrastim 5µg/kg/day was given until neutrophil recovery. In the absence of intolerable toxicity or disease progression, patients were able to receive the same chemotherapy at 28 day intervals. After the second and subsequent cycles of

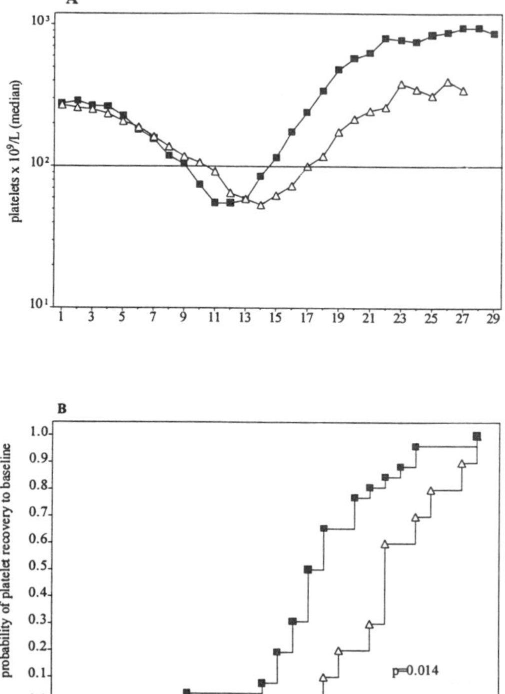

Figure 3. Platelet recovery after dose-intensive carboplatin and cyclophosphamide in patients receiving PEG-rHuMGDF 0.3 to 5.0 µg/kg (n=25) plus filgrastim versus those given filgrastim alone (n=10). Panel A shows platelet counts, while Panel B demonstrates the time of recovery to baseline (prechemotherapy) platelet levels. (From Basser et al. Randomised, blinded, placebo-controlled phase I trial of pegylated recombinant human megakaryocyte growth and development factor (PEG-rHuMGDF) with filgrastim after dose-intensive chemotherapy in patients with advanced cancer. Blood 1997; 89: 3118-3128).

chemotherapy, PEG-rHuMGDF was not given. Administration of PEG-rHuMGDF significantly enhanced platelet recovery when given in "effective" doses (0.3 to 5 μg/kg/d). In these patients (n=25), the platelet nadir occurred significantly earlier than in the placebo group (Figure 3A), analogous to the effect of G-CSF on neutrophil recovery following chemotherapy [11]. PEG-rHuMGDF did not influence the depth of the platelet nadir, but rather shortened the time to recovery of pre-treatment platelet count (median 17 days versus 22 days for the placebo group) (Figure 3B). PEG-rHuMGDF did not influence neutrophil recovery or red cell toxicity. Antibodies to PEG-MGDF were not detected in any patients.

A hint to the importance of scheduling of PEG-rHuMGDF was given by the observation that faster platelet recovery occurred in five patients who received PEG-rHuMGDF 0.3 or 1.0 μg/kg/d both before and after chemotherapy, compared with that of nine patients given 1.0 μg/kg/day only after chemotherapy. In addition, recovery of platelet count to normal following the second cycle of chemotherapy was significantly reduced in those patients who had received PEG-rHuMGDF after the first cycle compared to the placebo group (21 versus 24 days; p=0.013). This difference was greater in patients who experienced a shorter interval between cessation of PEG-rHuMGDF and commencement of the second cycle of chemotherapy [10].

These observations have led to further studies investigating the potential benefit in administering PEG-rHuMGDF prior to chemotherapy. However while early results from these studies have demonstrated an effect on platelet recovery from this approach, the clinical benefits have so far been modest [12].

<u>Multicycle Chemotherapy / High-Dose Chemotherapy</u>. Meeting reports of the use of PEG-rHuMGDF following treatment of relapsed non-Hodgkin's lymphoma [13] and lung cancer [14] showed PEG-rHuMGDF was effective in preventing cumulative thrombocytopenia during dose-intensive multicycle chemotherapy. In another report, rTPO was given only after the second cycle of high-dose carboplatin to patients with gynecological cancer. The incidence of severe thrombocytopenia was significantly reduced following the second cycle compared with the first cycle [15].

Initial results of the use of PEG-rHuMGDF in autologous bone marrow transplantation showed a promising reduction in the number of days to platelet recovery compared with placebo treated patients [16]. However, no beneficial effect has so far been demonstrable for the use of PEG-rHuMGDF in progenitor cell transplantation [17].

It is important to note that the reports cited in this section are phase I/II studies, and as such include small numbers of patients and present only preliminary data. Strong conclusions regarding the benefit of PEG-rHuMGDF / rTPO in these scenarios require more formal presentation of the results and studies directly addressing efficacy (rather than dose and scheduling).

Platelet Function

Preclinical observations that recombinant forms of Mpl ligand increase sensitivity of platelets to aggregating agents were not borne out by the clinical studies of PEG-rHuMGDF [4] or TPO [7]. Platelets produced following administration of multiple doses of PEG-rHuMGDF [4] or a single dose of rTPO[7] showed no altered tendency to aggregate and no changes in adenosine triphosphate-release responses *in vitro*. In addition, there was no change in the expression of P-selectin (a platelet-surface activation marker), or induction of the fibrinogen binding site on glycoprotein IIb/IIIa [4]. Importantly, the platelets were structurally and functionally normal [4]. In the PEG-rHuMGDF study, after aspirin was given to a patient because of asymptomatic thrombocytosis (platelet peaking at 1876 x 10^9/L) platelets responded with the expected inhibition of aggregation response and ATP release [4]. Furthermore, there were no changes in coagulation parameters. Similarly, no alteration of platelet function was obtained when PEG-rHuMGDF was given with filgrastim after chemotherapy [10].

Thus, administration of PEG-rHuMGDF or rTPO was associated with production of platelets which had a normal state of activation without an increased tendency to aggregate. The thrombocytosis induced by these cytokines therefore appears more akin to a reactive process than to that associated with a myeloproliferative disorder. In vitro abnormalities of platelet aggregation and clinical hemorrhagic and thrombotic events seldom occur in reactive thrombocytosis, but are quite common in patients with essential thrombocythemia [18, 19].

Progenitor Cell Mobilisation

<u>PEG-rHuMGDF / Thrombopoietin Alone</u>. Given the expression of *c-mpl* on a number CD34[+] cells, the observations of progenitor cell mobilization in preclinical models [20], and the unexpected observations during phase 1 studies of G-CSF [21], it might be expected that PEG-rHuMGDF and rTPO would display similar biological behaviour.

In contrast to the lineage-dominant effect of PEG-rHuMGDF on mature cell populations, a dose-dependant mobilization of progenitor cells of multiple lineages into the blood was observed following administration of $\geq 0.1\mu$g/kg PEG-rHuMGDF alone [5]. The most pronounced effect was seen on megakaryocyte colony-forming cells (Meg-CFC), where there was a maximum 30-fold increase. Although lesser in magnitude, mobilization of granulocyte-macrophage colony-forming cells (GM-CFC) and erythroid progenitor cells (BFU-E) was also seen at the two higher dose levels [5]. Multi-lineage mobilization was also observed after a single dose of rTPO [7, 22].

An interesting observation was that the kinetics of progenitor cell release from the marrow after PEG-rHuMGDF were unlike that of other lineage-dominant cytokines, such as G-CSF. Following administration of the latter, PBHPC levels rise almost immediately, peak at day 5 or 6, and fall when G-CSF is ceased. However, PEG-rHuMGDF resulted in a *late* and *sustained* rise in progenitor cells, so that increased levels were first detected only on day 8, and were generally greater on day 12, despite discontinuation of the cytokine several days earlier [5].

<u>PEG-rHuMGDF plus Filgrastim after Chemotherapy</u>. Administration of PEG-rHuMGDF in doses of 0.3 to 5.0μg/kg combined with filgrastim after chemotherapy significantly enhanced mobilization of PBHPC compared to placebo plus filgrastim [10]. Furthermore, higher peak levels of PBHPC were observed with increasing dose of PEG-rHuMGDF. In the 5μg/kg cohort, levels of GM-CFC were a up to 1000-fold greater than in the placebo group (Figure 4). PEG-rHuMGDF [3,6,10] and rTPO [7] were associated with minimal toxicity, whether given prior to or after chemotherapy. No

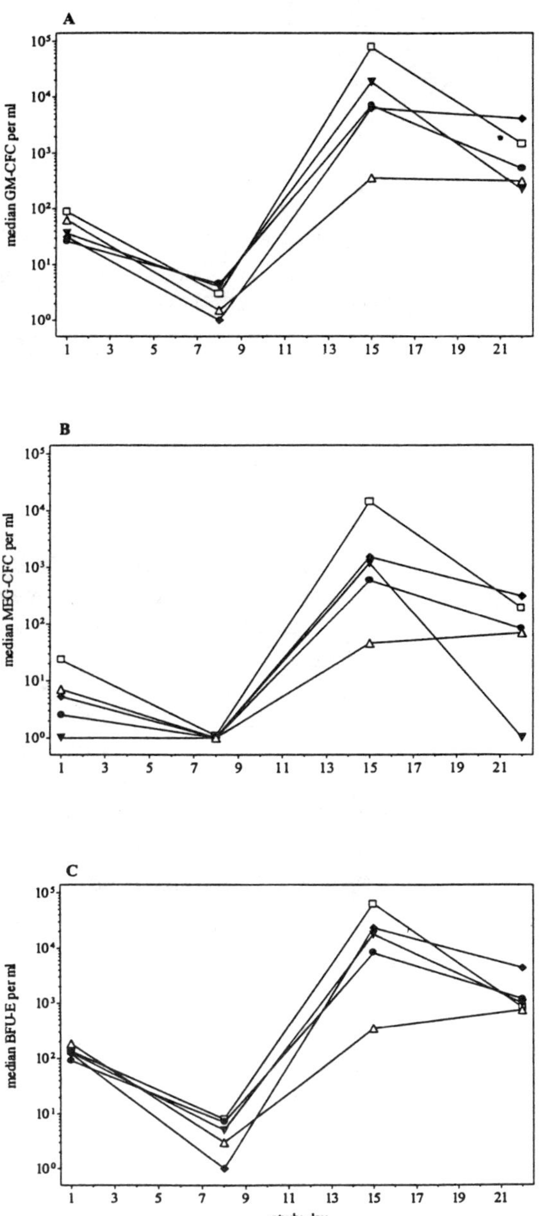

Figure 4. Peripheral blood progenitor cell mobilization (median) in p[...]nts receiving PEG-rHuMGDF 0.3 (▼, n=3), 1.0 μg/kg (◆, n=11), 3.0 μg/kg (●, n=7[...] 5.0 μg/kg (□, n=4), and placebo (Δ, n=10). GM-CFC are shown in Panel A, Meg-CFC in Panel B and BFU-E in Panel C. (From Basser et al. Randomised, blinded, placebo-controlled phase I trial of pegylated recombinant human megakaryocyte growth and development factor (PEG-rHuMGDF) with filgrastim after dose-intensive chemotherapy in patients with advanced cancer. Blood 1997; 89: 3118-3128).

275

changes in performance status, vital signs or body-weight were observed, and there were no changes in biochemical, renal or liver function tests. Unlike other, less potent thrombopoietic cytokines, there was no evidence of induction of an acute phase response.

Safety

A low incidence of thrombosis has been reported in studies of PEG-rHuMGDF and rTPO, but this is consistent with the expected rates of venous thromboembolism reported in patients with advanced cancer [23] and suggests that the risk of a thromboembolic event related to administration of these cytokines, if any, is low.

Conclusions

Early clinical studies with PEG-rHuMGDF and rTPO have demonstrated these agents enhance platelet recovery in patients receiving both single and multiple cycles of dose-intensive chemotherapy. Importantly, they are both associated with very few side effects, and concern regarding activation of platelets has not been borne out in these trials. However, important questions remain on the most effective dose and schedule with which to deliver these agents. Furthermore, there are not many clinical situations in which severe thrombocytopenia occurs. Apart from those mentioned in this chapter, the other major oncological cause of thrombocytopenia is acute leukemia and its treatment. It is unlikely that the future use of PEG-rHuMGDF or rTPO in treatment of cancer patients will be as broad as myeloid growth factors, such as G-CSF. Observations such as the efficacy of PEG-rHuMGDF in platelet donors and the mobilization of progenitor cells by both PEG-rHuMGDF and rTPO suggest these may be important clinical uses. In addition, clinical investigation is also warranted into non-oncologic causes of severe thrombocytopenia, including bone marrow failure states (such as aplastic anemia or myelodysplasia), cardiac surgery, chronic liver disease, immune thrombocytopenia and HIV infection. Results of such studies are eagerly anticipated.

References

1. Kaushansky K Thrombopoietin: The primary regulator of platelet production. Blood 86: 419-31, 1995.
2. Vilmer E, Guglielmi P, David V, et al. Predominant expression of circulating CD3+ lymphocytes bearing gamma T cell receptor in a prolonged immunodeficiency after allogeneic bone marrow transplantation. J.Clin.Invest. 82: 755-61, 1988.
3. Basser RL, Rasko JEJ, Clarke K, et al. Thrombopoietic effects of pegylated recombinant human megakaryocyte growth and development factor (PEG-rHuMGDF) in patients with advanced cancer. Lancet 348: 1279-81, 1996.
4. O'Malley CJ, Rasko JEJ, Basser RL, et al. Administration of pegylated recombinant human megakaryocyte growth and development factor to humans stimulates the production of functional platelets that show no evidence of *in vivo* activation. Blood 88: 3288-98, 1996.
5. Rasko JEJ, Basser RL, Boyd J, et al. Multilineage mobilization of peripheral blood progenitor cells in humans following administration of PEG-rHuMGDF. Br J Haematol 97: 871-80, 1997.
6. Fanucchi M, Glaspy J, Crawford J, et al. Effects of polyethylene glycol-conjugated recombinant human megakaryocyte growth and development factor on platelet counts after chemotherapy for lung

cancer. N.Engl.J.Med. 336: 404-9, 1997.

7. Vadhan-Raj S, Murray LJ, Bueso-Ramos C, et al. Stimulation of megakaryocyte and platelet production by a single dose of recombinant human thrombopoietin in patients with cancer. Ann Intern Med 126: 673-81, 1997.

8. Kuter D, McCullough J, Romo J, et al. Treatment of platelet (PLT) donors with pegylated recombinant human megakaryocyte growth and development factor (PEG-rHuMGDF) increases circulating PLT counts (CTS) and PLT apheresis yields and increases platelet incremements in recipients of PLT tranfusions. Blood 90 (suppl 1): 579a (Abstract), 1997.

9. Basser RL, Rasko JEJ, Clarke K, et al. Randomised, blinded, placebo-controlled phase I trial of pegylated recombinant human megakaryocyte growth and development factor (PEG-rHuMGDF) with filgrastim after dose-intensive chemotherapy in patients with advanced cancer. Blood 89: 3118-28, 1997.

10. Crawford J, Ozer H, Stoller R, et al. Reduction by granulocyte colony-stimulating factor of fever and neutropenia induced by chemotherapy in patients with small-cell lung cancer . N.Engl.J.Med. 325: 164-70, 1997.

11. Szer J, Basser R, Underhill C, et al. Reduction of thrombocytopenia (TCP) after multicycle, intensive chemotherapy by megakaryocyte growth and development factor (PEG-rHuMGDF). Pro Am Soc Clin Oncol 17: 76a (Abstract), 1998.

12. Moskowitz C, Nimer S, Gabrilove J, et al. A randomized, double-blind, placebo-controlled, dose-finding, efficacy and safety study of PEG-rHuMGDF (M) in non-Hodgkin's lymphoma (NHL) patients (pts) treated with ICE (ifosfamide, carboplatin and etoposide). Pro Am Soc Clin Oncol 17: 76a (Abstract), 1998.

13. Crawford J, Glaspy J, Belani C, et al. A randomized, placebo-controlled , blinded, dose scheduling trial of pegylated recombinant human megakaryocyte growth and development factor (PEG-rHMGDF) with filgrastim support in non-small cell lung cancer (NSCLC) patients treated with paclitaxel and carboplatin during multiple cycles of chemotherapy. Pro Am Soc Clin Oncol 17: 73a (Abstract), 1998.

14. Vadhan-Raj S, Verschraegen C, McGarry L, et al. Recombinant human thrombopoietin (rhTPO) attenuates high-dose carboplatin (C)-induced thrombocytopenia in patients with gynecologic malignancy. Blood 90 (suppl 1): 580a (Abstract), 1997.

15. Beveridge R, Schuster M, Waller E, et al. Randomized, double-blind, placebo-controlled trial of pegylated recombinant human growth and development factor (PEG-rHUMGDF) in breast cancer patients (Pts) following autologous bone marrow transplantation (ABMT). Blood 90 (suppl 1): 580a (Abstract), 1997.

16. Glaspy J, Vredenburgh J, Demetri GD, et al. Effects of PEGylated recombinant human megakaryocyte growth and development factor (PEG-rHuMGDF) before high-dose chemotherapy (HDC) with peripheral blood progenitor cell (PBPC) support. Blood 90 (Suppl 1): 580a (Abstract), 1997.

17. Ginsburg AD. Platelet function in patients with high platelet counts. Ann.Intern.Med. 82: 506-11, 1975.

18. Buss DH, Cashell AW, O'Connor ML, et al. Occurrence, etiology, and clinical significance of extreme thrombocytosis. Am.J.Med. 96: 247-53, 1994.

19. Kaushansky K, Lin N, Grossmann A, Humes J, et al. Thrombopoietin expands erythroid, granulocyte-macrophage, and megakaryocytic progenitor cells in normal and myelosuppressed mice. Exp.Hematol. 24: 265-69, 1996.

20. Duhrsen U, Villeval JL, Boyd J, et al. Effects of recombinant granulocyte colony-stimulating factor on hematopoietic progenitor cells in cancer patients. Blood 72: 2074-81, 1988.

21. Murray LJ, Luens KM, Estrada ME, et al. Thrombopoietin mobilizes CD34[+] cell subsets into peripheral blood and expands multilineage progenitors in bone marrow of cancer patients with normal hematopoiesis. Exp.Hematol. 26: 207-16, 1998.

22. Bunn PA, Jr., Ridgway EC . Paraneoplastic syndromes, *in* Cancer: Principles and Practice of Oncology (DeVita V.T., Jr., Hellman S. & Rosenberg S.A., eds.), J.B.Lippincott Co., Philadelphia, pp. 2026-71, 1993.

V

The Role of Cytokines to Enhance Cancer Chemotherapy

15. Dose Intensification in Solid Tumor Chemotherapy

Henrik van Deventer, Thomas Shea

Introduction

Since their introduction in the 1980's, colony-stimulating factors (CSFs) have been widely used to prevent episodes of febrile neutropenia in patients who have either had febrile neutropenia following chemotherapy (secondary prophylaxis) or who are at high risk for this complication (primary prophylaxis). Data from randomized controlled trials has confirmed that granulocyte colony-stimulating factor (G-CSF) can reduce the incidence and duration of febrile neutropenia in both settings [1,2,3]. This` reduction has been associated with a decrease in hospital duration and antibiotic use. However, none of these trials in solid tumor patients have demonstrated a reduction in mortality. This fact reflects the low pre-existing mortality associated with most chemotherapy-induced febrile neutropenia in the modern antibiotic era.

More recently, investigators have attempted to use CSFs to increase the dose intensity (DI) of cytotoxic therapy. Whereas chemotherapy designed without growth factors was predominantly limited by hematologic toxicity, G-CSF could ameliorate these side effects in more aggressive regimens. The survival benefit would result from improved chemotherapeutics rather than prevention of febrile neutropenia and its sequelae. Though this is an appealing strategy, the American Society of Clinical Oncology guidelines still do not recommend regular application of CSFs for this purpose outside of clinical trials [4].

This chapter summarizes the theoretical constructs and the clinical data pertaining to dose intensity and the use of growth factors. Most of the information presented applies to G-CSF since it is the most thoroughly investigated of the growth factors. The end of the chapter will focus on other growth factors including granulocyte macrophage colony-stimulating factor (GM-CSF) and megakaryocyte stimulating factors.

Principles of Dose Intensity

Dose and dose intensity as applied to chemotherapy regimens are defined below [5]. In general, these terms refer to single agents unless otherwise specified.

Dose (D): The amount of an agent (usually a drug) given during any one cycle.
Total Dose (TD): The sum of the doses from each cycle.
Actual Dose Intensity (ADI): Total Dose divided by the number of weeks of a regimen.
Intended Dose Intensity (IDI): The planned Total Dose divided by the scheduled number of weeks
Relative Dose Intensity (RDI): Actual Dose Intensity divided by the Intended Dose Intensity

Dose Intensity

The relative dose intensity for a combination regimen can be calculated by averaging the RDI of each agent.

For example, consider cyclophosphamide (750 mg/m^2 d1), doxorubicin (50 mg/m^2 d1), vincristine (1.4 mg/m^2 d1), and prednisone (100 mg d 1-5) (CHOP) given once every three weeks for six cycles. If a patient had received all six cycles on time without any dose reductions, then the above definitions as applied to cyclophosphamide would yield:

Dose (D) = 750 mg/m^2
Total Dose (TD) = 4,500 mg/m^2
Actual Dose Intensity (ADI) = 250 mg/m^2 per week
Relative Dose Intensity (RDI) = 1.0

If that same patient had been delayed by one week at cycle 3 and again at cycle 5, then the calculations would change as follows:

Dose (D) = 750 mg/m^2
Total Dose (TD) = 4,500 mg/m^2
Actual Dose Intensity (ADI) = 225 mg/m^2 per week
Relative Dose Intensity (RDI) = 0.9

If instead of delaying cycles 3 and 5, the practitioner decided to reduce the dose of each agent by 30%, the calculation would proceed as below:

Dose (D) = 750 mg/m^2 for weeks 1,2, 4, and 6
Dose (D) = 525 mg/m^2 for weeks 3 and 5
Total Dose (TD) = 4,050 mg/m^2
Actual Dose Intensity (ADI) = 225 mg/m^2 per week
Relative Dose Intensity (RDI) = 0.9

As a point of reference for future discussions about DI, consider the following perturbations on this common regimen:

CHOP given every four weeks for six cycles
RDI = 0.75
CHOP given with a cyclophosphamide dose of 1000 mg/m^2 every four weeks
RDI = 1.08

The terminology of dose intensity originated from studies of chemotherapeutics in animals and cell lines. These models were characterized by stable cellular kinetics where the fraction of dividing cells, length of cell cycle, and effects of chemotherapy remained constant. Skipper summarized these observations in his cell kill hypothesis that states a fixed number of tumor cells is killed for each dose of chemotherapy [6]. The effects of multiple agents are additive and the simple relationships depicted in the above examples are accurate.

In these models, larger doses of chemotherapy led to larger cell-kill fractions[5]. In fact, this dose-response relationship was often non-linear so that a doubling of the dose could lead to a ten-fold increase in the effect of some drugs [9]. High dose therapy tries to maximize cell killing by exploiting this phenomenon. To do so, doses are increased to a maximally tolerated level.

The Skipper model also predicts certain relationships between dose, dose intensity, and total dose. In order to eradicate tumor, the cell kill fraction must be larger than the fraction that recovers between doses. For small doses, frequent administration of chemotherapy will be required. High doses of chemotherapy could be administered less frequently with an equal or better chance for cure. These relationships suggest that patients undergoing palliative treatment would do best with smaller more frequent therapy that maximizes the total dose. Such a strategy avoids the side effects of high dose therapy while maintaining efficacy. On the other hand, patients who are candidates for cure may benefit from maximizing the DI.

Human tumors follow these models to a variable degree. Dose and dose intensity do correlate with response but not always to cure in most tumors. The relationship between total dose and the duration of response is not easy to demonstrate though some trials support this model. However, most tumors are far more difficult to eradicate than these dose intensity models would predict. Resistance to chemotherapy is the reason for this apparent dichotomy.

Kinetic resistance is the failure of chemotherapy to eliminate a tumor based on its size and growth characteristics [10]. Most tumors demonstrate Gompertzian growth where tumor doubling decreases with size. Hence when tumors are clinically apparent, they grow slowly; but, as treatment reduces their size, the growth rate increases. Such changes would necessitate more frequent dosing, which is not predicted by the above models. These growth characteristics are due to the smaller fraction of actively cycling cells in larger tumors. This leads to increased resistance to chemotherapeutic agents that target such cells.

Chemotherapy also fails because of cellular resistance. Such resistance can be seen in vitro among the different lines of the same cell type [5] as well as among different cell types using the same drug [6]. Resistance on a cellular level may occur as a result of decreased drug uptake, rapid efflux, deactivation, or evasion of a drug's cytotoxic effects. As a result, the cell kill fraction is not consistent with each dose, as the Skipper model would presume. Resistance is more evident in larger tumors because of the greater genetic variability and opportunity to acquire such mechanisms. In vivo, additional factors such as poor drug delivery to the tumor may compound the problem. Both cellular and kinetic resistance help explain the difficulties in treating a large tumor burden.

Dose intensive chemotherapy may still benefit patients despite the difficulties presented by resistance. In some cases, multiple agents given in non-cross resistant combinations can overcome cellular resistance as outlined in the Goldie-Coldman hypothesis. Such treatment has been well-established in Hodgkin's disease and in early stage breast cancer though it is not as well established for other tumor types. High dose therapy may also benefit patients by reducing the tumor burden quickly and lowering the opportunities for further genetic mutations. Larger cell kill fractions associated with higher dose therapy may also overcome kinetic resistance. For these reasons, investigators continue to pursue clinical benefit from higher dose therapy.

Clinical Rationale for Dose Intensity

There are essentially four types of clinical studies that support the practice of maximizing dose intensity. The first is a retrospective analysis that compare patients who received less than the intended dose of a given regimen to those that received the full dose within the same study. Such studies help establish the importance of maintaining the DI of a standard regimen. However, failure to complete all scheduled doses of a regimen may be a poor prognostic factor in itself and the conclusions are likely to be tautological. The second type of study is also retrospective and compares a current trial to historical controls. The control arm is usually an earlier trial where the intended dose was less than the dose in the study arm. These trials help to establish the advantage of DI greater than standard therapy. Though there may be less selection bias in this trial, differences in supportive care may introduce another form of bias.

There are two types of prospective trials: those that compare a standard regimen to a more intense regimen and those that compare a standard regimen to less intense therapy. There are only a few trials where patients have been randomized to either standard therapy or lower dose therapy. As will be discussed later, many of these do support the concept of maintaining a minimum or threshold level of dose intensity. The most common prospective trial remains standard therapy versus a more dose intense experimental arm.

The most prominent studies in dose intensity have been the result of autologous bone marrow transplantation (ABMT) and Stem Cell Transplantation (SCT) where the RDI may be five to ten times greater than standard treatment. If ABMT/SCT does not benefit patients, it seems unlikely that the increases of DI less than five will be significant. This statement should remain true provided the assumptions of the dose response relationship are accurate and the toxicity of ABMT/SCT does not neutralize any survival advantage.

The efficacy of ABMT/SCT has been established for a variety of malignancies. For patients with relapsed intermediate or high grade non Hodgkin's lymphoma, eight year event-free survival was 36% for those who underwent transplant versus 11% for those who did not [11]. Similar data is available for Hodgkin's disease [12]. For patients with relapsed or refractory germ cell tumors, SCT can result in a greater than 50% event free survival at three years when given as initial salvage therapy [13]. Such data helps establish these tumors as dose responsive.

The role of transplantation in other solid tumors is more controversial. ABMT/SCT does lead to a higher complete response rate versus standard therapy in metastatic breast cancer [8]. The survival benefit has not been well established and remains the subject of a series of on-going trials. Likewise, data on adjuvant treatment remains inconclusive[7, 15,16]. Transplantation is also associated with a higher complete response for small cell lung cancer [17], but the survival data remains disappointing. Reasons given for this ineffectiveness include reinfusion of tumor cells, inability to control local disease, and the contribution of pre-existing medical conditions. Other solid tumors are considered too chemoresistant for consideration of transplantation.

Most clinical trials with conventional therapy have enhanced the dose intensity by increasing the dose of chemotherapy. This leads to increases in the total dose, the dose intensity, and toxicity as well. Before examining the role of G-CSF in dose intensity, it is instructive to examine the trials that study each aspect of dosing separately.

Several adjuvant breast cancer trials have attempted to sort out the contribution of each of these dosing parameters. NASBP B-22 considered adjuvant chemotherapy in over 2,000 lymph node positive patients using the following dosing [18]:

	ARM 1	ARM 2	ARM 3
Doxorubicin (mg/m^2) q 3 wks	60 x 4	60 x 4	60 x 4
Cyclophosphamide (mg/m^2) q 3 wks	600 x 4	1200 x 2	1200 x 4

In this trial, the dose intensity of cyclophosphamide in ARM 1 is being compared to the increased dose intensity of ARMS 2 and 3. At the same time, the total dose of ARMS 1 and 2 can be compared to the increased total dose of ARM 3. Interestingly, there were no differences in disease free survival or overall survival in any of these groups. The CALGB ran a similar trial in over 1500 lymph node positive patients [19]. Their dosing schedule was as follows:

	ARM 1	ARM 2	ARM 3
Doxorubicin (mg/m^2) d1 q 4 wks	60 x 4	40 x 6	30 x 4
Cyclophosphamide (mg/m^2) d1 q 4 wks	600 x 4	400 x 6	300 x 4
Fluorouracil (mg/m^2) d 1, 15 q 4 wks	600 x 4	400 x 6	300 x 4

This is a study of three different dose intensities, which decrease in magnitude from ARM 1 to ARM 3. In addition, ARM 1 and ARM2 have equal total dose, which is twice that of ARM 3. The only significant differences in both disease free and overall survival came between ARM 1 and 3 and ARM 2 and 3. ARM 1 and 2 were not statistically different despite this large sample size. One might conclude that total dose is more important than dose intensity since differences in DI seem to make very little difference in ARM 1 and 2. Unfortunately, this trial is more of an indictment against "under dosing" with chemotherapy than it is a champion for dose intensification. Though these are both elegant trials, the contribution of total dose and dose intensity to the efficacy of chemotherapy remains an under-explored area.

Using G-CSF to Increase Dose Intensity

G-CSF can be used to maximize chemotherapy in one of three ways. First, G-CSF can be used to increase dose intensity by diminishing the myelotoxicity associated with increased doses or increased frequency. In this case, G-CSF would be used to enhance the curative potential of the regimen. Second, G-CSF can be used to maintain dosing of a standard regimen. The division between the first and second use is a bit arbitrary and depends on the definition of the "standard regimen". A standard regimen as defined here is one that can be administered to most patients without significant myelotoxicity. G-CSF can be used in those patients who were otherwise unable to complete standard chemotherapy without severe bone marrow suppression. Again the intent would be to give these patients the full benefit of the regimen for possible cure rather than compromising the dose. Finally, G-CSF can be used to increase the total dose of a cytotoxic agent by extending the duration of effective therapy. Unlike the previous uses, the main endpoint would be palliation with the possible extension of overall survival.

There have been over 40 phase I and II trials in the past five years that have looked at the feasibility of using G-CSF to increase dose intensity in solid tumors. Trials in which the contribution of G-CSF to dose intensity can be directly evaluated are listed in Table 1. The design for most of these studies is dose escalation without G-CSF until a maximum tolerated dose (MTD) is reached. G-CSF is then begun in the subsequent cohort and additional dose escalation is undertaken. Augmentation of dose intensity ranges from 1.0 to 2.0 with the majority being less than 1.5. Occasionally trials will generate much higher doses of chemotherapy with G-CSF. Usually this occurs in trials where only a few cycles are given or where greater toxicity is accepted.

To compare the dose intensity of a G-CSF based regimen to one that does not use G-CSF, the number and frequency of the cycles actually administered must be given in the trial data. Often times this information is not available making the analysis difficult. Many of these trials are also paclitaxel based, which reflects the enthusiasm for this drug over the past five years. Nevertheless, other reviewers have noted similar increases in DI with G-CSF over the past ten years [20,21].

Studies that attempt to increase dose intensity by decreasing the interval between treatment are less common. Phase II studies have demonstrated that the interval of many three and four week regimens can be reduced by one week. Dose intensity is increased up to a factor of 1.33 and 1.5 respectively. In actual practice these levels are not reached because many patients cannot tolerate them[22-28]. A few phase I studies have attempted to decrease the dosing interval to less than two weeks.

Smith et. al. looked at cohorts of 21 days, 15 days, and 10 days for the administration of CHOP with G-CSF [29]. Several dose-limiting toxicities (DLTs) were reached in the Q 15 day group including mucositis and infections. Sawada undertook an even more aggressive approach by administering CHOP as soon as the WBC count was > 10,000 [30]. With G-CSF support, CHOP could be given every 14.7 days. Cumulative hematologic toxicity is a significant concern for these regimens as will be discussed later in this chapter.

G-CSF and other growth factors have also encouraged the development of novel combinations of chemotherapeutics as well as the revival of older regimens that were abandoned because of their myelosuppression. The data from these trials does demonstrate an improvement in compliance as measured by the ability to deliver chemotherapy as initially scheduled. Expressed in the terms of dose intensity, the RDI with G-CSF is closer to 1.0. However, the improvement in dose intensity is usually no greater than 20%.

The above data generally supports the feasibility of using G-CSF to increase dose intensity though the increase is relatively modest. However, such increases are generally not associated with improvement in survival (see Table 2).

There are several possible reasons for this lack of efficacy. First, multiple drug regimens may be inferior to multiple single agents given in series. Administration of single agents sequentially may expose the cancer to the full extent of the dose response curve for each agent. Such a position is currently untested though trials with breast cancer patients are underway. Second, G-CSF may not permit a sufficient increase in DI. G-CSF is effective in decreasing neutropenia but many patients will

Table I. Phase I Trials using G-CSF

Ref.	Disease	n	Treatment	MTD w/o G-CSF (mg/m²)	MTD w/G-CSF (mg/m²)	Increase (expressed as a factor)	Dose Limiting Toxicity
Du Bois [68]	Advanced Ovarian	33	Paclitaxel (3 hr)	185	185	1.0	Neutropenia
			Carboplatin (q 3wk x4-6)	AUC = 6	AUC = 6	1.0 Avg = 1.0	
Fanning [49]	Advanced Ovarian	30	Cisplatin Etoposide Ifosfamide (q 4wk x 6)	105 300 3,000	105 360 3,600	1.0 1.2 1.2 Avg = 1.13	Thrombocytopenia
O'Reilly [70]	Refractory Recurrent Ovarian	22	Topotecan Paclitaxel (q 3wk x 5)	0.6 (d1-5)* 135	1.25(d1-5) 135	2.0 1.0 Avg = 1.5	Neutropenia Thrombocytopenia
Belani [71]	Stage IV Lung Cancer	26	Paclitaxel (24hr) Carboplatin (q3 x 6)	135 AUC = 5	135 AUC = 9	1.0 1.8 Avg = 1.4	Thrombocytopenia
Georgiadis [72]	Advanced Lung Cancer	50	Paclitaxel (96h) Cisplatin (q3 x 8)	120 80	160 80	1.33 1.0 Avg = 1.17	Neutropenia
Lilenbaum [73]	Metastatic	45	Paclitaxel (3hr) Topotecan (q 3 x 3-4)	80 1.0 (d1-5)	230 1.0	2.875 1.0 Avg = 1.93	Neutropenia Neuromuscular
Murren [74]	Refractory	26	Cytoxan Topotecan (q3 x 2)	600 0.75 (d1-5)	600 1.0	1.0 1.33 Avg = 1.17	Hematologic
Huber [75]	Solid Tumor	41	Paclitaxel (24h) Methotrexate (q3 x ?)	85 23	135 40	1.59 1.74 Avg = 1.66	Neutropenia
Schiller [76]	Advanced Untreated	35	Paclitaxel (3hr) (q 3 x 3)	210	250	1.19 Avg = 1.19	Neuropathy

Extrapolated Data

continue to have problems with other hematologic toxicities such as thrombocytopenia as well as with non-hematologic complications. Finally, the dose response hypothesis may not apply to certain malignancies for reasons outlined in the first section.

As reviewed by Antoine and Khayat, there have been no breast cancer trials to date that have shown an improvement in overall survival with an increase of dose intensity up to 2.5 in either the adjuvant or metastatic setting [14]. More recent attempts have been made to increase both the cyclophosphamide and the adriamycin doses in standard adjuvant therapy without benefit [31,32]. Though the addition of paclitaxel to these regimens is beneficial, increasing the dose of this drug has not been effective as demonstrated in a recent metastatic breast cancer trial [33]. These results may have been predicted given the difficulties in establishing a survival advantage with transplantation and its higher degree of dose intensity.

There have been no recent randomized trials that have increased the doses of standard chemotherapy for lymphoma. G-CSF does permit increases in DI up to 1.68 in more aggressive chemotherapeutic regimens [34]. None of these increases have been associated with an improvement in survival in randomized trials. Whereas the increases in DI appear to be correlated with survival in transplantation, this relationship cannot be established with the use of G-CSF.

The relationship between DI and small cell lung cancer has been intriguing ever since Ariagada showed a modest increase in survival of limited stage patients by increasing the doses of cisplatinum by 20% and cyclophosphamide by 25% in the first cycle only [35].

Most subsequent studies, however, have not been able to show an improvement[17]. For example, Ihde compared a regimen of standard cisplatin and etoposide to one with an ncreased DI of 46%. The survival was the same in both groups though the toxicity was more profound in the high dose arm [36].

The CODE (cisplatin, vincristine, doxorubicin, and etoposide) and VICE (vincristine, ifosfamide, carboplatin, and etoposide) trials are two small cell cancer regimens that are often cited as counter examples to this trend. In the CODE trial, patients received a complex alternating week chemotherapy schedule and were randomized to either G-CSF or placebo [37]. The median survival for those in the G-CSF arm was 59 weeks compared to 32 weeks for those without G-CSF. Two large trials in the U.S. and Japan subsequently compared this regimen with G-CSF to standard CAV/EP (cyclophosphamide, doxorubicin, and vincristine/ etoposide and cisplatin). No significant difference in mortality could be found[5]. The VICE regimen was administered when the patients' counts recovered from the previous cycle. This occurs around day 22 to 23 without G-CSF and on day 20 to 21 with G-CSF. The RDI of the overall regimen improved with G-CSF from 1.18 to 1.25 (p=0.03) with the largest differences occurring in earlier cycles. Though there were more deaths due to complications of therapy in the G-CSF arm (17.6% vs. 3.2%), the overall two-year survival was improved (32% vs 15%). This study has been criticized because VICE is considered by many to be a q three-week regimen and the control arm may have been underdosed. Had the criteria for administering chemotherapy been lowered slightly the differences in RDI and survival may have been non-significant.

In light of these criticisms, this trial may not support the use of G-CSF as a means of dose intensification; however, it does support the concept of dose intensity. This

Table 2. Randomized Trials Using G-CSF

Reference	Disease	n	Regimen	Dose Intensity	Overall Response	Survival	G-CSF Advantage ?
Zinzani [77]	High Grade Lymphoma (> 60 yo)		VNCOP-B VNCOP-B+G-CSF	85% 95% (NS)	80% 83%	30 mth: 64% 30 mth: 62%	No
Pettengell [78]	High Grade Lymphoma	39 40	VAPEC-B VAPEC-B+G-CSF	83% 96% (p<0.02)	92% 90% (NS)	1 yr: 80% (both groups)	No
Gisselbrecht [79]	Poor Prognosis Lymphoma	87 82	LNH-84 LNH-84 + G-CSF	80.1% 93.3% p<0.0001	67% 71% (NS)	3 yr: 71% 3 yr: 67% (NS)	No
Miles [80]	Small Cell Good Prognosis	17 23	CE/IA CE/IA + G-CSF	82% 84% (NS)	71% 74%	NR	No
Woll [81]	Small Cell Good Prognosis	59 63	VICE VICE+G-CSF	1.13 1.34 p=0.001	93.5% 94.1% (NS)	2 yr: 15% 2 yr: 32%	Yes
Thatcher[50]	Small Cell	202 201	ACE q3 wks x 6 ACE+G-CSF q2 wks x 6	NR 1.33	86% 89%	1 yr: 39% 1 yr: 47%	Yes
Negoro [82]	Small Cell Extensive Stage	31 32	CODE CODE+G-CSF	72% 83%	84% 96% (NS)	2 yr: 6.5 % 2 yr: 31.3%	Yes
Henderson [83]	Adjuvant Tx of Breast Ca	3170*	A=60/C=600 A=75/C=600 A=90/C=600+G-CSF	NR	NS	NS	No
Bonomi [84]	Advanced Non Small Cell Lung Cancer	194 187 190	CE Cisplatin/Paclitaxel CP + G-CSF	NR	12% 26% 31% (2,3 to 1: p<0.001)	NR	No
Fossa [85]	Poor Prognosis Germ Cell	130 129	BEP/EP or BOP/VIP BEP/EP or BOP/VIP+G-CSF	92% v 98% Etoposide 90% v 97% Ifosfamide (p<0.01)		1 yr: 70.8% 1 yr:76.0%	No
Omura [86]	Advanced Ovarian	163 171	Paclitaxel: 175 Paclitaxel 250 + G-CSF	NR NR	27.5% 36.0%	MS: 12.5 m MS: 11.9 m (NS)	No

* Total number of patients in trial, number in each group not specified.

NR=Not reported; NS = Not significant

finding is a bit surprising given the experience with small cell cancer in transplantation. The inadequacy of transplantation may be due to greater toxicity rather than the inefficacy of increased dose intensity. Toxicity is likely to have a greater impact on these patients given their older age and usual co-morbid conditions. When applying this principle to patients, one must keep in mind that both the VICE trial and the Ariagada trial included predominantly limited stage patients. In addition, the differences in dose intensity were predominantly found in the early cycles.

Two germ cell trials that randomized patients with respect to G-CSF did not show any statistically significant improvement in survival [38,39]. This is consistent with data from other phase II and III trials that have failed to show a meaningful improvement in survival with an increase in DI of 1.5 or less [40]. Given the effectiveness of current chemotherapy and the safety of SCT in the event of relapse, there seems to be little justification for increasing DI using growth factors.

Using G-CSF to Maintain Dose Intensity

Though the above data indicates that there is little benefit to increasing the DI from 1.0 to 1.5 in most solid tumors, there may be a substantial advantage in increasing the DI from 0.6 to 1.0 in an individual patient. Such clinical reasoning assumes the existence of a threshold dose. Doses above the threshold result in response whereas lower doses lead to progressive disease. In the terms of the cell kill hypothesis, the cellular fraction that dies is smaller than the fraction which proliferates during a cycle of chemotherapy. This dynamic results in progressive tumor growth despite chemotherapy.

Determining whether G-CSF can have an impact by maintaining dose intensity is difficult given the relatively small number of patients who are unable to tolerate standard regimens. This occurs because most chemotherapy regimens can be administered without G-CSF and with an acceptable toxicity profile. Investigation into the benefits of G-CSF for such patients depends predominantly on subgroup and/or retrospective analysis.

Though this data is not extensive, G-CSF does seem to be effective in maintaining dose intensity. de Graaf followed 123 patients with lymph node positive breast cancer receiving CMF chemotherapy. The patients received G-CSF if their white blood count recovery was not adequate at the time of their next treatment. 23 patients qualified for growth factor but did not receive it. Of these, only 45% achieved a DI >0.85 compared to 74% who qualified and did receive G-CSF [41]. In breast cancer patients who had had two or more dose delays, G-CSF allowed them to complete their regimen with a DI of 0.94 [42]. Likewise, lymphoma patients could increase dose intensity with CHOP and CHOP hybrid regimens from 87.8% to 99.5% [43].

At what dose intensity should a clinician consider using growth factors? The answer in part depends on the goal of therapy. For curative regimens, maintaining DI with CSFs is probably worth the cost and potential side effects. On the other hand, CSFs should only be used in palliative therapy if the DI attained results in symptomatic relief and there is reason to believe that lower doses of chemotherapy would provide less effective palliation. The actual levels of DI are difficult to cull from the literature since there are few studies that compare lower doses of chemotherapy with standard doses. Table 3 lists some of the studies that do make such comparisons.

Bonadonna and Valgussa showed as early as 1981 that improved relapse-free survival was associated with maintenance of a DI of at least 0.85 in a retrospective study [44]. As previously discussed, the CALGB trial that randomized stage II breast cancer patients to varying intensities of CAF showed that a DI of 0.5 led to a decline in overall and disease free survival when compared to a DI of 1.3 [19]. Similar trials have not been undertaken with AC chemotherapy.

Retrospective analysis of patients with germ cell cancer treated with PVB showed a survival benefit for those with an RDI > 0.9 [45]. There were large differences in administered dose in this trial with the average RDI of non responders equal to 0.32 and the responders equal to 0.9. In small cell lung cancer, a decrease in DI to 0.75 was associated with decreased survival [46]. In a randomized trial of CAE with or without G-CSF, DI of 0.88 had no less survival than a DI of 0.96[2]. For most regimens, maintaining DI > 0.85 appears to be justified.

Using G-CSF to Increase the Total Dose for Palliation

For patients who are not candidates for cure, the role of G-CSF is less clear. Increasing dose intensity is unlikely to be helpful once a response is attained. Maintaining this response with regular cycles of chemotherapy has been accomplished for some cancers but not all. For patients who appear to be responding to such a maintenance program, G-CSF and other growth factors may allow for further cycles and an increase in total dose. Since most studies concentrate on cure, there are very few studies that examine the efficacy of such an approach.

Metastatic breast cancer appears to be the most amenable to maintenance chemotherapy. There are several phase I and II trials looking at the feasibility of weekly chemotherapy with low dose growth factor support. Many of these regimens are administered with few side effects except for myelotoxicity. In a randomized trial by Muhonen et. al., patients were randomized to MMM (mitoxantrone, methotrexate, and mitomycin) given on a Q42 day regimen either with or without G-CSF. Patients on G-CSF received more cycles of chemotherapy and had a survival of 10.4 months versus 6.5 months [47].

Maintenance therapy for small cell lung cancer has been disappointing. There has been one trial comparing six cycles of VAC with 14 cycles that showed improved survival in patients with extensive disease. However the majority of the randomized studies have not found such a relationship [48].

More studies are needed in this area before regular recommendations can be made.

Adverse Effects of Regular G-CSF Use

G-CSF can lead to profound hematologic toxicity in two ways. First, clinicians are able to administer higher and potentially more toxic doses of chemotherapy because of the reduced level of neutropenia associated with G-CSF. Second, administration of G-CSF shortly before or at the time of chemotherapy can lead to increased pancytopenia by heightening the effects of chemotherapy on actively cycling progenitors. The result may be anemia and thrombocytopenia that requires transfusional support. This side effect in particular should be considered when administering G-CSF for palliative purposes.

Several of the phase I trials that used G-CSF to increase the DI were limited by anemia and thrombocytopenia. For example, using a three-drug regimen that included cisplatin, Fanning increased the dose of etoposide and ifosfamide by 20% with G-CSF in stage III and IV ovarian cancer patients. The result of this increase was a rate of thrombocytopenia of 50% [49]. In a randomized trial of non-small cell lung cancer patients receiving ACE (doxorubicin, cyclophosphamide, and etoposide) every two weeks with G-CSF compared to those receiving it every three weeks, rates of thrombocytopenia were 43% vs. 7% [50].

The myelosuppressive effect also appears to be cumulative. Both Colucci [51] and Bissett [52] using levofolinic, 5 FU, and cyclophosphamide paired with mitoxantrone or epirubicin respectively showed a correlation between the number of cycles administered and the drop in hemoglobin, platelets, and absolute neutrophil count. The cumulative nature of this toxicity in all three cell lines suggests G-CSF is not protecting stem cells from the effects of chemotherapy. Stem cell damage is also reflected in a trial of patients randomized to either intensified CHOP with G-CSF versus standard therapy. In this trial, patients received CHOP when their peripheral counts recovered. The intensive therapy was associated with a significant delay in engraftment when these patients came to transplant [53].

Whether increased hematologic toxicity is simply the result of increased chemotherapy dosing or is aggravated by G-CSF in some other way is not clear. Administering G-CSF during or just prior to chemotherapy appears to exacerbate the toxicity associated with cytotoxic therapy. In a randomized trial of 37 women with either advanced or metastatic breast cancer, G-CSF given five days prior and seven days after chemotherapy led to grade IV neutropenia in 74% of the cycles and grade IV thrombocytopenia in 54%. This compares to 66% and 6% in patients who received G-CSF only after chemotherapy. Both groups were treated with equal amounts of cyclophosphamide and adriamycin [54]. Primitive progenitor cells are stimulated to undergo cell division during the administration of G-CSF and may be more sensitive to the effects of chemotherapy [55,56]. This and other data suggest that chemotherapy should not be administered for at least 48 hours after the G-CSF is stopped. For cycles that are every three weeks or more, such a stipulation is not a problem. The use of G-CSF in weekly and biweekly regimens is more problematic. Possible long term hematologic toxicity should considered when starting such a regimen.

Interestingly, most of the DLT for newer regimens have been hematologic despite the introduction of G-CSF. This may reflect better understanding of current agents as well as better supportive care. Of course, some regimens are limited by non hematological DLT. For example, the dose of MVAC (methotrexate, vinblastine, doxorubicin, and cisplatin) cannot be increased as a result of significant non-hematologic toxicity [89]. 72-hour paclitaxel infusion with cyclophsophamide for both previously treated [57] and untreated [58] patients with metastatic breast cancer was limited by diarrhea, typhlitis, and mucositis.

Table 3. Trials that Establish a Threshold Dose

Reference	Disease	n	Type of Study	Regimen (mg/m^2)	Dose Intensity	Outcome
Miyanaga[45]	Advanced Germ Cell	33	Retrospective	PVB	1.09 0.97 0.69	CR PR PD/NC
Cohen[46]	Advanced Small Cell Lung	9 23	Prospective	CCNU 50, Cytoxan 500, Mtx 10 CCNU 100, Cytoxan 1000, Mtx 15	NR	1 yr: 11.1% 1 yr: 30.4%
Trillet-Lenoir[2]	Untreated Small Cell Lung	64 65	Randomized	ADE ADE+G-CSF	0.88 0.96	OR 79% MS10.4 m OR 87% MS 12.4 m (NS)
Bonadonna[44]	Breast Cancer	901	Retrospective	CMF	* >85% 65-84% <65%	5 yr: 80% 5 yr: 72% 5 yr 67%
Wood[19]	Stage II Breast Ca	513 507 509	Randomized	C 600 x 4; A 60 x 4; F 600 x 4 C 400 x 6; A 40 x 6; F 400 x 6 C 300 x 4; A 30 x 4; F 300 x 4	** 1.5 1.0 0.75	3 yr: 92% 3 yr: 90% 3 yr: 84% p≤0.05: 3 vs 1 or 2
Tannock[88]	Metastatic Breast Cancer		Randomized	C 600 q3; M 40 q3; F 600 C 300 q3; M 20 q 3; F 600	** 1.0 0.66	MS: 15.6 m MS 12.8 m p = 0.026

* Percentage of the total dose received
** Expressed as intended DI

Granulocyte Macrophage Colony-Stimulating Factor

Historically GM-CSF has not been as effective as G-CSF in ameliorating neutropenia associated with chemotherapy. The initial ASCO guidelines considered five randomized trials when assessing the efficacy of GM-CSF for primary prophylaxis. Two studies in small cell lung cancer [94,95] and one in germ cell tumors [90] showed no difference in febrile neutropenia, antibiotic use, or hospitalization. Though DI and overall survival were secondary endpoints, there was also no significant difference in dose intensity or survival between the placebo and GM-CSF arms. The two trials that showed an advantage for prophylactic administration were in selected lymphoma patients including one study that was limited to HIV patients. The data for use in secondary prevention is limited to a non-randomized trial that showed a decrease in grade IV neutropenia from six days to three days [62].

Early comparisons of GM-CSF and G-CSF were biased in part by the side effect profile of GM-CSF. Though GM-CSF is still more likely to cause a viral-like syndrome, this side effect was substantially more frequent and severe when the E Coli derived recombinant product was used as opposed to the currently approved yeast derived compound. Since most trials reported intention-to-treat data only, it was difficult to know how much poor compliance affected the results. The difference in DI between GM arms and controls in most trials is less than 50%. This appears to be slightly less than G-CSF but direct comparisons of the two are few. Mamounas et. al. did show G-CSF was associated with less neutropenia than GM-CSF in a non-randomized trial. More recently, Beveridge randomized 181 afebrile patients to G-CSF or GM-CSF when their neutrophil count was < 500/μl. There were no significant differences in hospitalization, antibiotic use, or time to neutrophil recovery (i.e. absolute neutrophil count > 1,000) seen in the two groups [63]. No trial using GM-CSF in solid tumor patients has demonstrated an improvement in survival though one trial of older patients with acute myelogenous leukemia has [64]. A summary of trials using GM-CSF is given on Table 4.

Other Growth Factors

There are ten randomized studies evaluating the value of recombinant human erythropoietin in chemotherapy patients. Many of these studies establish the effectiveness of erythropoietin in increasing hemoglobin by 1 to 2 g/dl, decreasing the transfusion requirement on a cohort level, and improving the quality of life of a patient. Since the effects of chemotherapy on red cells tends to be less acute, less severe, and rarely life threatening, anemia is never listed as a DLT. Therefore, rHu EPO is not used as an adjunct in dose intensity. The most cost-effective use for erythropoietin is likely to be treatment for symptomatic, transfusion dependent

Table 4.Randomized trials using GM-CSF.

Ref.	Disease	n	Regimen	DI	OR	Survival	GM-CSF advantage
Logothetis [89]	Metastatic or unresectable urothelial	23 25	Escalated MVAC Escalated MVAC + GM-CSF	61% 66% (NS)	85% (Combined) (NS)	5 yr NED:20% 5 yr NED: 28% (NS)	No
Bajorin [90]	Poor prognosis germ cell	49 55	VIP or VeIP VIP or VeIP + GM-CSF	86.4% 89.2% (NS)	NR	NR	No
Yau [91]	Advanced BrCa/NHL	28 28	DICEP DICEP + GM-CSF	36%* 43%* (NS)	60% 75% (NS)	NR	No
Kaplan [92]	HIV + NHL	98 94	Low dose m-BACOD Std dose m-BACOD + GM-CSF	0.9-1.0 1.3-1.4	69% 78% (NS)	MS:35 wks MS:31 wks	No
Gerhartz [93]	High Grade NHL	90 92	COP-BLAM COP-BLAM + GM-CSF	81% 85%	81% 85% (NS)	(NS)	No
Hamm [94]	Untreated small cell lung	74 74	CAE CAE+GM-CSF	78.3% 78.1% (NS)	NR	NR	No
Bunn [95]	Limited stage small cell	60 61	VP-16/CDDP/RT VP-16/CDDP/RT+GM-CSF	85.5% 75.4% (p<0.01)	86% 73% (p=0.29)	MS:17 mths MS:14 mths (p=0.15)	No
Steward [96]	Small cell (≤3adverse factors)	149 151	V-ICE V-ICE+GM-CSF	Improved (NS)	84% 83% (NS)	MS:53.6 wks MS:55.4 wks (NS)	No
Bajetta [97]	Advanced Gastric	30 32	FEP FEP+GM-CSF	92% 125% (p=0.0001)	34% (NS)	MS:9 mths	No

* Completion of 3 cycles
DI= dose intensity; OR = overall response; NR = not reported; NS = not significant

patients following chemotherapy. This approach has been validated in non-Hodgkin's lymphoma and myeloma patients [65].

Several of the trials that use G-CSF or GM-CSF to increase dose intensity have been complicated by thrombocytopenia. Currently Interleukin 11 (IL-11) and recombinant megakaryocyte growth and development factor (MGDF) are undergoing clinical testing as megakaryocyte-stimulating factors. IL-11 does decrease platelet transfusion requirement in a dose dependent manner. Its contribution to dose intensity in part depends on the definition of dose limiting toxicity. In the Isaacs [66] trial, DI of cyclophosphamide and doxorubicin was 3.29 versus standard AC. In this dose intensive trial, however, 32% of these patients still required platelets despite IL-11. In this case, IL-11 adds to DI only if a 50% platelet transfusion requirement is unacceptable. Though thrombocytopenia can be complicated by life threatening bleeding episodes, these are less common than the life threatening complications of neutropenia. Finding a survival advantage with this medication may be difficult.

MGDF is a newer agent and has been studied in only one small randomized trial to date [67]. This trial also showed a dose dependent reduction in platelet transfusion requirements. When given in combination with G-CSF, there was an increase in RDI though long-term follow up and survival data is not available. This trial may be more clinically applicable when assessing MGDFs contribution to DI since the use of this agent prevented the need for platelet transfusion. More trials will be needed before any reasonable conclusions can be drawn.

Summary

Dose intense chemotherapy attempts to exploit relationships seen between the dose of an agent and the response to that agent. Higher doses are associated with higher responses as measured by cell death in vitro. In patients, a dose response curve is observed at higher doses of chemotherapy when measuring complete and partial response rates. Unfortunately, this has not translated into higher cure rates for most cancers.

G-CSF can increase the dose intensity of most regimens from 1.5 to 2.0. Thus far, this increase in DI has not been associated with improvements in overall survival or disease free survival. G-CSF can increase the DI to > 0.85 in the small number of patients who may not otherwise tolerate therapy. This level is an appropriate target DI based on the above literature and likely offers a survival advantage for those patients. Proving this is difficult given the small number of patients who fall into this category.

G-CSF could conceivably be used to increase the total dose of chemotherapy. This may be advantageous in the palliative setting where total dose but not dose intensity has been correlated with survival. Unfortunately, there are very few trials that allow the clinician to decide if this approach is worthwhile.

These advantages must be weighed against potential adverse effects of G-CSF. Patients on G-CSF have a greater problem with cumulative bone marrow toxicity and thrombocytopenia. This is due to both the higher dose of chemotherapy as well as increased sensitization of progenitor cells that occurs with G-CSF administration. Care must be taken particularly if G-CSF is given within 48 hours of the next chemotherapeutic dose. Non hematologic toxicity may be more common in patients on G-CSF though this very much depends on the chosen regimen.

Differences in efficacy between G-CSF and GM-CSF are small. Currently, G-CSF is in greater use as reflected by the trial information. Megakaryocyte growth factors are in the early stages of development and testing. The degree to which these agents can improve DI depends in part on the level of thrombocytopenia one is willing to accept. Their contribution to the survival of cancer patients will be the focus of many trials to come.

References

1. Crawford J, Ozer H, Stollr R, et al. Reduction by granulocyte colony stimulating factor of fever and neutropenia induced by chemotherapy in patients with small-cell lung. N Eng J Med 325:164, 1991.
2. Trilet-Lenoir V, Green J, Manegold C, et al. Recombinant granulocyte colony stimulating factor reduces the infectious complications of cytotoxic chemotherapy. Eur J Cancer 29A:319, 1993.
3. Pettengill R, Gurney H, Radford JA, et al. Granulocyte colony-stimulating factor to prevent dose-limiting neutropenia in non-Hodgkin's lymphoma: A randomized controlled trial. Blood 80:1430, 1992.
4. Update of recommendations for the use of hematopoietic colony-stimulating factors: Evidence-based clinical practice guidelines. American Society of Clinical Oncology. J Clin Oncol 14:1957, 1996.
5. Murray N. Importance of dose and dose intensity in the treatment of small-cell lung cancer. Cancer Chemother Pharmacol 40:S58, 1997.
6. Skipper HE, Schabel FM Jr, Wilcox WS. On the criteria and kinetics associated with "curability" of experimental leukemia. Cancer Chemother Rep 35:3-9, 1964.
7. Peters WP, Dansey R. New concepts in the treatment of breast cancer using high-dose chemotherapy. Cancer Chemother Pharmacol 40:S88, 1997.
8. Bezwoda WR. High-dose chemotherapy with hematopoietic rescue in breast cancer: From theory to practice. Cancer Chemother Pharmacol 40:S79, 1997.
9. Murray N, The importance of dose and dose intensity in lung cancer chemotherapy. Semin Oncol 14:S4, 1987.
10. Saijo N, Nishio K, Kubota N, et al. 7-Ethyl-10-4(1-piperdino)-1- piperdinocarbonyloxy camp-thothecin: Mechanism of resistance and clinical trials. Cancer Chemother Pharmacol 342:S112, 1995.
11. Philip T, Guglielmi C, Hagenbeek A, et al. Autologous bone marrow transplantation as compared with salvage chemotherapy in relapses of chemotherapy-sensitive non-hodgkin's lymphoma. N Eng J Med 333:1540, 1995.
12. Linch DC, Winfield D, Goldstone AH, et al. Dose intensification with autologous bone-marrow transplantation in relapsed and resistant Hodgkin's disease: Results of a BNLI randomized trial. Lancet 341:1051, 1993.
13. Bhatia S, Cornetta K, Broun R, et al. High dose chemotherapy with peripheral stem cell or autologous bone marrow transplant as initial salvage chemotherapy for testicular cancer. Proc ASCO 17:1239, 1998.
14. Antoine EC, Khayat D. European School of Oncology European consensus on the use of granulocyte colony-stimulating factor: The example of breast cancer. Cancer Chemother Pharmacol 38:S103, 1996.
15. Rhodenhuis S, Richel DJ, van der Wall E, et al. A randomized trial of high-dose chemotherapy and hematopoietic progenitor cell support in operable breast cancer with extensive axillary lymph node involvement. Proc ASCO 17:470, 1998.
16. Hortobagyi GN, Buzdar AU, Champlin R, et al. Lack of efficacy of adjuvant high-dose tandem combination chemotherapy for high risk primary breast cancer - a randomized trial. Proc ASCO 17:471, 1998.
17. Elias A. Dose-intensive therapy in lung cancer. Cancer Chemother Pharmacol 40:64, 1997.
18. Fisher B, Anderson S, Wickerham DL, et al. Increased intensification and total dose of cyclophosphamide in a doxorubicin-cyclophosphamide regimen of the treatment of primary breast cancer: Findings from National Surgical Adjuvant Breast and Bowel Project B-22. J Clin Oncol 15:1858, 1997.

19. Wood WC, Budman DR, Korzun AH, et al. Dose and dose intensity of adjuvant chemotherapy for stage II, node-positive breast carcinoma. N Eng J Med 331:139, 1994.

20. Ganser A, Karthaus M. Clinical use of hematopietic growth fctors. Curr Opinion Oncol 8:254, 1996.

21. Elias AD, Dose-intensive therapy for small cell lung cancer. Chest 107:261S, 1995.

22. Thatcher N, Sambrook RJ, Stephens J, et al. Dose intensification with G-CSF improves survival in small cell lung cancer patients: Results of a randomized trial. Proc ASCO 17:1754, 1998.

23. Woll PJ, Hodgetts J, Lomax L, et al. Can cytotoxic dose-intensity be increased by using granulocyte colony-stimulating factor? A randomized controlled trial of lenograstim in small-cell lung cancer. J Clin Oncol 13:652, 1995.

24. Planting AS, de Wit R, van der Burg ME, et al. Phase II study of a closely spaced ifosfamide-cisplatin schedule with the addition of G-CSF in advanced non-small-cell lung cancer and malignant melanoma. Ann Oncol 7:1080, 1996.

25. Scinto AF, Ferraresi V, Campioni N, et al. Accelerated chemotherapy with high-dose epirubicin and cyclophosphamide plus r-met-HuG-CSF in locally advanced and metastatic breast cancer. Ann Oncol 6:665, 1995.

26. Ferguson JE, Dodwell DJ, Seymour AM, et al. High dose, dose-intensive chemotherapy with doxorubicin and cyclophosphamide for the treatment of advanced breast cancer. Br J Cancer 67:825, 1993.

27. Piccart MJ, Bruning P, Wildiers J, et al. An EORTC pilot study of filgrastim (recombinant human granulocyte colony-stimulating factor) as support to a high dose-intensive epirubicin-cyclophosphamide regimen in chemotherapy-naive patients with locally advanced or metastatic breast cancer. Ann Oncol 6:673, 1995.

28. Thatcher N, Anderson H, Bleehen NM, et al. The feasibility of using glycosylated recombinant human granulocyte colony-stimulating factor (G-CSF) to increase the planned dose intensity of doxorubicin, cyclophosphamide and etoposide (ACE) in the treatment of small cell lung cancer. Medical Research Council Lung Cancer Working Party. Eur J Cancer 31A:152, 1995.

29. Smith GM, Child JA, Cullen MH, et al. A phase I trial to assess the value of recombinant human granulocyte colony stimulating factor (R-MeTHuG, filgrastim) in accelerating the dose rate of chemotherapy for intermediate and high-grade non-Hodgkin's lymphoma (NHL). The Central Lymphoma Group. Hematol Oncol 14:193,1996.

30. Sawada KI, Sata N, Kohno M, et al. Efficacy of delayed granulocyte colony-stimulating factor after full dose CHOP therapy in non-Hodgkin's lymphoma: A pilot study for a leukocyte count oriented regimen. Leuk Lymphoma 20:103, 1995.

31. Dimitrov N, Anderson S, Fisher B, et al. Dose intensification and increased total dose of adjuvant chemotherapy for breast cancer. Findings fromnNSAP B-22. Proc ASCO 13:58, 1994.

32. Henderson IC, Berry D, Demetri G, et al. Improved disease-free and overall survival from the addition of sequential paclitaxel but not from escalation of doxorubicin dose level in the adjuvant chemotherapy of patients with node positive primary breast cancer. Proc ASCO 17:390A, 1998.

33. Winder E, Berry D, Duggin D, et al. Failure of higher dose paclitaxel to improve outcome in patients with metastatic breast cancer - results from CALGB 9342. Proc ASCO 17:388, 1998.

34. Shipp MA, Neuberg D. High-dose CHOP as initial therapy for patients with poor prognosis aggressive non-hodgkin's lymphoma: A dose-finding pilot study. J Clin Oncol 13:2916, 1995.

35. Arriagada R, Le Chevalier T, Pignon JP, et al. Initial chemotherapeutic doses and survival in patients with limited small-cell lung cancer. N Eng J Med 329:1848, 1993.

36. Ihde DC, Mulshine Jl, Kramer BS, et al. Prospective randomized comparison of high-dose and standard-dose etoposide and cisplatin chemotherapy in patients with extensive-stage small-cell lung cancer. J Clin Oncol 12:2022, 1994.

37. Negoro S, Masuda N, Furuse K, et al. Dose-intensive chemotherapy in extensive-stage small-cell lung cancer. Cancer Chemother Pharmacol 40:70, 1997.

38. Fossa SD, Kaye SB, Meed GM, et al. Filgrastim during combination chemotherapy of patients with poor-prognosis metastatic germ cell malignancy. European Organization for Research and Treatment of Cancer, Genito-Urinary Group, and the Medical Research Council Testicular Cancer Working Party, Cambridge, United Kingdom. J Clin Oncol 16:716, 1998.

39. Fossa S, Kaye SB, Meed GM, et al. An MRC/EORTC randomized trial in poor prognosis metastatic teratoma, comparing treatment with/without filgrastrim (G-CSF). Proc ASCO 14:656, 1995.

40. Boekmeyer C, Kuczyk MA, Kohne H, et al. Hematopoietic growth factors and treatment of testicular cancer: Biological interactions, routine use and dose-intensive chemotherapy. Ann Hematol 72:1, 1996.

41. De Graaf H, Willemse PH, Bong SB, et al. Dose intensity of standard adjuvant CMF with granulocyte colony-stimulating factor for premenopausal patients with node-positive breast cancer.

42. Ribas A, Albanell J, Bellmunt J, et al. Frequent dose delays and growth factor requirements with the sequential doxorubicin-CMF schedule. Acta Oncol 36:701, 1997.

43. Silvestri F, Velisig M, Fanim R, et al. Granulocyte colony-stimulating factor (G-CSF) allows the delivery of effective doses of CHOP and CVP regimens in non-Hodgkin lymphomas. Leuk Lymphoma 16:465, 1995.

44. Bonadonna G, Valagussa P. Dose-response effect of adjuvant chemotherapy in breast cancer. N Eng J Med 304:10, 1981.

45. Miyanaga N, Akaza H, Hattori K, et al. The importance of dose intensity in chemotherapy of advanced testicular cancer. Urol Int 54:220, 1995.

46. Cohen MH, Creaven PJ, Fossieck BE Jr, et al. Intensive chemotherapy of small cell bronchogenic carcinoma. Cancer Treat Rep 61:349, 1977.

47. Muhonen T, Jantunen I, Pertovaara H, et al. Prophylactic filgrastim (G-CSF) during mitomycin-C, mitoxantrone, and methotrexate (MMM) treatment for metastatic breast cancer: A randomized study. Am J Clin Oncol 19:232, 1996.

48. Saka H, Shimokata K. Chemotherapy for small-cell lung cancer: More is not better. Cancer Chemother Pharmacol 40:S107, 1997.

49. Fanning J, Hilgers RD. Prophylactic granulocyte colony-stimulating factor allows escalation of chemotherapeutic dose intensity in advanced epithelial ovarian cancer. Gynecol Oncol 63:323, 1996.

50. Thatcher N, Sambrook RJ, Stephens RJ, et al. Dose intensification (DI) with G-CSF improves survival in small cell lung cancer (SCLC): Results of a randomized trial. Proc ASCO 17:456a, abstract #1754, 1998.

51. Colucci G, Giotta F, Gebbia V, et al. Dose intensification of mitoxantrone in combination with levofolinic acid, fluorouracil, cyclophosphamide and granulocyte colony stimulating factor support in advanced untreated breast cancer patients. A multicentric phase II study of the Souther Italy Oncology Group. Anticancer Drugs 8:257, 1997.

52. Bissett D, Jodrell D, Harnett AN, et al. Phase I study of accelerated FEC with granulocyte colony-stimulating factor (Lenograstim) support. Br J Cancer 71:1279, 1995.

53. Freedman A, Neuberg D, Mauch P, et al. Cyclophosphamide, doxorubicin, vincristine, prednisone dose intensification with granulocyte colony-stimulating factor markedly depletes stem cell reserve for autologous bone marrow transplantation. Blood 90:4996, 1997.

54. de Wit R, Verweij J, Bontenbal M, et al. Adverse effect on bone marrow protection of prechemotherapy granulocyte colony-stimulating factor support . J Natl Cancer Inst 88:1393, 1996.

55. Hansen PB, Johnsen HE, Ralfkiaer E, et al. Short-term rhG-CSF priming before chemotherapy does mobilize blood progenitors but does not prevent chemotherapy induced myelotoxicity: A randomized study of patients with non-Hodgkin's lymphomas. Leuk Lymphoma 19:453, 1995.

56. Lieschke GJ, Burgess AW. Granulocyte colony-stimulating factor and granulocyte-macrophage colony-stimulating factor (2). N Eng J Med 327:99, 1992.

57. Kennedy MJ, Zahurak ML, Donehower RC, et al. Phase I and pharmacologic study of sequences of paclitaxel and cyclophosphamide supported by granulocyte colony-stimulating factor in women with previously treated metastatic breast cancer. J Clin Oncol 14:783, 1996.

58. BR73 Fisherman JS, Cowan KH, Noone M, et al. Phase I/II study of 72-hour infusional paclitaxel and doxorubicin with granulocyte colony-stimulating factor in patients with metastatic breast cancer. J Clin Oncol 14:774, 1996.

59. Hamm JT, Schiller J, Oken MM, et al. Dose ranging study of recombinant human granulocyte-macrophage colony stimulating factor in small cell lung cancer. Proc ASCO 12:1118, 1993.

60. Bunn PA, Crowley J, Hazuka M, et al. The role of GM-CSF in limited stage small cell lung cancer. A randomized Phase III study of the Southwest Oncology Group (SWOG). Proc ASCO 11:974, 1992.

61. Nichol C, Bajorin D, Schmoll HJ, et al. VIP chemotherapy with/without GM-CSF for poor risk, relapsed, or refractory germ cell tumors. Proc ASCO 10:532, 1991.

62. Vadhan-Raj S, Broxmeyer HE, Hittelmannn WN, et al. Abrogating chemotherapy induced myelosuppression by GM-CSF: Optimizing the schedule. Proc ASCO 10:1241, 1991.

63. Beveridge RA, Miller JA, Kales AN, et al. A comparison of efficacy of Sargramostim and Filgrastim in the therapeutic setting of chemotherpay induced myelosuppression. Ca Invest 16:366, 1998.

64. Rowe JM, Anderson J, Mazza JJ, et al. Phase III randomized placebo-controlled study of yeast derived GM-CSF in adult patients (55-70 years) with AML. Blood 82:329a, 1993.

65. Osterborg A, Boogarts MA, Cimino R, et al. Recombinant human erythropoietin in transfusion-

dependent anemic patients with multiple myeloma and non-Hodgkin's lymphoma - a multicenter study. Blood 87:2675, 1996.

66. Isaacs C, Robert NJ, Bailey FA, et al. Randomized placebo-controlled study of recombinant human interleukin-11 to prevent chemotherapy-induced thrombocytopenia in patients with breast cancer receiving dose-intensive cyclophosphamide and doxorubicin. J Clin Oncol 15:3368, 1997.

67. Moskowitz C, Nimer J, Gabrilove A, et al. A randomized double blinded, placebo controlled, dose finding, efficacy and safety study of PEG-rHuMGDF in non-Hodgkin's lymphoma patients treated with ICE. Proc ASCO 17:295, 1998.

68. du Bois A, Luck HJ, Bauknecht T, et al. Phase I/II study of the combination of carboplatin and paclitaxed as first-line chemotherapy in patients with advanced epithelial ovarian cancer. Ann Oncol 8:355, 1997.

69. Fanning J, Hilgers RD. Prophylactic granulocyte colony-stimulating factor allows escalation of chemotherapeutic dose intensity in advanced epithelial ovarian cancer. Gynecol Oncol 63:323, 1996.

70. O'Reilly S, Fleming GF, Barker SD, et al. Phase I trial and pharmacologic trial of sequences of paclitaxel and topotecan in previously treated ovarian epithelial malignancies: A Gynecologic Oncology Group study. J Clin Oncol 15:177, 1997.

71. Belani CP, Aisner J, Hiponia D, et al. Paclitaxel and Carboplatin with and without Filgrastrim support in patients with metastatic non-small cell lung cancer. Semin Oncol 22:7, 1995.

72. Georgiadia MS, Schuller BS, Brown JE, et al. Paclitaxel by 96-hour continuous infusion in combination with cisplatin: A phase I trial in patients with advanced lung cancer. J Clin Oncol 15:735, 1997.

73. Lilenbaum RC, Ratain MJ, Miller AA, et al. Phase I study of paclitaxel and topotecan in patients with advanced tumors: A cancer and leukemia group B study. J Clin Oncol 13:2230, 1995.

74. Murren JR, Anderson S, Fedele J, et al. Dose-escalation and pharmacodynamic study of topotecan in combination with cyclophosphamide in patients with refractory cancer. J Clin Oncol 15:148, 1997.

75. Huber MH, Lee JS, Newman RA, et al. A phase I investigation of the sequential use of methotrexate and paclitaxel with and without G-CSF for the treatment of solid tumors. Ann Oncol 7:59, 1996.

76. Schiller JH, Storer B, Tutsch K, et al. A phase I trial of 3-hour infusions of paclitaxel with or without granulocyte colony-stimulating factor. Semin Inc 21:9, 1994.

77. Zinzani PL, Pavone E, Storti S, et al. Randomized trial with or without granulocyte colony-stimulating factor as adjunct to induction VNCOPB treatment of elderly high-grade non-Hodgkin's lymphoma. Blood 89:3974, 1997.

78. Pettengell R, Gurney H, Radford JA, et al. Granulocyte colony-stimulating factor to prevent dose-limiting neutropenia in non-Hodgkin's lymphoma: A randomized controlled trial. Blood 80:1430, 1992.

79. Gisselbrecht C, Haioun C, Lepage E, et al. Placebo-controlled phase III study of lenograstim (glycosylated recombinant human granulocyte colony-stimulating factor) in aggressive non-Hodgkin's lymphoma: Factors influencing chemotherapy administration. Groupe d'Etude des Lymphomes de l'adulte leuk lymphoma 25:289, 1997.

80. Miles DW, Forarty O, Ash CM, et al. Received dose intensity: A randomized trial of weekly chemotherapy with and without granulocyte colony-stimulating factor in small cell lung cancer. J Clin Oncol 12:77, 1994.

81. Woll PJ, Hodgetts J, Lomax L, et al. Can cytotoxic dose-intensity be increased by using granulocyte colony-stimulating factor? A randomized controlled trial of lenograstim in small-cell lung cancer.

82. Negoro S, Masuda N, Furuse K, et al. Dose-intensive chemotherapy in extensive-stage small-cell lung cancer. Cancer Chemother Pharmacol 40:S70, 1997.

83. Henderson IC, Berry D, Demetri G, et al. Improved disease free survival from the addition of sequential paclitaxel but not from the escalation of doxorubicin dose level in the adjuvant chemotherapy of patients with node positive breast cancer. Proc ASCO 17:101a, 1998.

84. Bonomi P, Kim K, Kusler J, et al. Cisplatin/Etoposide vs paclitaxel/cisplatin/G-CSF vs paclitaxel/cisplatin in non-small-cell lung cancer. Oncol 11:9, 1997.

85. Fossa SD, Kaye SB, Meed GM, et al. Filgrastim during combination chemotherapy of patients with poor-prognosis metastatic germ cell malignancy. European Organization for Research and Treatment of cancer, Genito-Urinary Group, and the Medical Research Council Testicular Cancer Working Party, Cambridge, United Kingdon. J Clin Oncol 16:716, 1998.

86. Omura GA, Brady MF, Delmore JE, et al. A randomized trial of paclitaxel at 2 dose levels and filgrastrim at 2 dose levels. Proc ASCO 15:280, 1996.

87. Cohen MH, Creaven PJ, Fossieck BE, et al. Intensive chemotherapy of small cell bronchogenic

carcinoma. Canc Treat Rep 61:349, 1977.

88. Tannock IF, Boyd NF, DeBoer G, et al. A randomized trial of two dose levels of cyclophosphamide, methotrexate, and fluorouracil chemotherapy for patients with metastatic breast cancer [see comments]. J Clin Oncol 6:1377, 1988.

89. Logothetis CJ, Finn LD, Smith T, et al. Escalated MVAC with and without reacombinant granulocyte-macrophage colony-stimulating factor for the initial treatment of advanced malignant urothelial tumors: Results of a randomized trial. J Clin Oncol 13:2272, 1995.

90. Bajorin DF, Nichols CR, Schmoll HJ, et al. Recombinant human granulocyte-macrophage colony-stimulating factor as an adjunct to conventional-dose ifosfamide-based chemotherapy for patients with advanced or relapsed germ cell tumors: A randomized trial. J Clin Oncol 13:79, 1995.

91. Yau J, Neidhart J, Triozzi P, et al. Randomized placebo-controlled trial of granulocyte-macrophage colony-stimulating factor support for dose-intensive cyclophosphamide, etoposide, and cisplatin. Am J Hematol 51:289, 1996.

92. Kaplan L, Straus D, testa M, et al. Low-dose compared with standard-dose m-BACOD chemotherapy for non-Hodgkin's lymphoma associated with human immunodeficiency virus infection. N Eng J Med 336:1641, 1997.

93. Gerhartz H, Engelhard M, Meusers P, et al. Randomized, double-blind, placebo-controlled, phase III study of recombinant human granulocyte-macrophage colony-stimulating factor as adjunct to induction treatmetn of high-grade malignant non-Hodgkin's lymphoma. Blood 82:2329, 1993.

94. Hamm J, Schiller J, Oen M, et al. Granulocyte-macrophage colony-stimulating factor in small cell carcinoma of the lung: Preliminary analysis of a randomized controlled trial. Proc ASCO 10:255, 1991.

95. Bunn P, Crowley J, Kelly K, et al. Chemoradiotherapy with or without granulocyte-macrophage colony-stimulating factor in the treatment of limited-stage small cell lung cancer: A prospective phase II randomized study of the Southwest Oncology Group. J Clin Oncol 13:1632, 1995.

96. Steward W, von Pawel J, Gatzemeier U, et al. Effects of granulocyte-macrophage colony-stimulating factor and dose intensification of V-ICE chemotherapy in small cell lung cancer: A prospective randomized study of 300 patients. J Clin Oncol 16:642, 1998.

97. Bajetta E, DiBartolomeo M, Carnaghi C, et al. FEP regimen in advanced gastric cancer, with and without low-dose GM-CSF: An Italian trial in Medical Oncology study. Br J Cancer 77:1149, 1998/

16. Conventional and High Dose Chemotherapy for Lymphomas

Koen W. van Besien

Introduction

One of the more promising developments in the treatment of non-Hodgkin's lymphoma (NHL) is the use of intensive chemotherapy regimens with marrow or blood stem cell support. Such regimens are based on the concept that dose-escalation can overcome intrinsic tumor cell resistance[1]. Initially, high dose chemotherapy regimens were tested in patients with recurrent and refractory disease. Although impressive response rates were observed in NHL and a fraction of durable remissions, the toxicity of high dose therapy was substantial, preventing its widespread use and generating uncertainty about the value of this treatment in general [2]. More recently, the use of recombinant cytokines and of peripheral blood stem cells has led to faster and more reliable hematologic recovery, thereby reducing the toxicity associated with high-dose chemotherapy. Treatment-related mortality of less than 5% is now routinely achieved.We will discuss the more recent evolutions in the use of high-dose chemotherapy for the treatment of NHL. We will structure our discussion according to disease histology and take into account the different natural histories of various lymphoid disorders and their outcome with conventional treatment modalities.

Intermediate grade NHL

<u>Conventional chemotherapy and salvage treatment in intermediate grade NHL</u>: Anhracycline containing regimens and specifically the CHOP regimen have been the mainstay of treatment for aggressive NHL since the 1970's [3,4]. Overall, approximately 70% to 80% of patients with aggressive NHL respond to CHOP, but many will relapse and only approximately 40% of patients can be cured. The 1970's and early '80's saw the testing of numerous so called third-generation regimens built on the CHOP backbone but with the addition of other drugs. Despite encouraging early results, four large randomized multi-center studies failed to show in a more representative population a significant advantage for any of these regimens [5-8]. Two other reports indicate a statistically significant benefit for the second generation regimens [9,10]. However, any benefit of such regimens is likely to be influenced by the selection of patients participating in the study and is unlikely to be very large.

A large number of trials of conventional dose salvage chemotherapy which are mainly based on the use of non-cross resistant chemotherapeutic agents have been reported as well. Platinum- and/or ifosfamide containing regimens result in response rates in approximately 60% of the patients [11,12]. However, only approximately 10% of the remissions obtained with salvage chemotherapy are durable. The large majority of patients will progress either during or shortly after completion of chemotherapy.

High dose chemotherapy and autologous transplantation for patients with recurrent NHL The frustration with lack of durable responses to conventional salvage chemotherapy led to the investigation of high-dose chemotherapy in aggressive NHL. Early results indicated that patients with chemosensitive recurrences were more likely to benefit from these approaches than patients with chemotherapy-refractory disease[13,14]. A randomized study (Parma study) confirmed that durable remissions could be obtained in approximately 50% of patients with chemosensitive recurrences, which was significantly better than what was obtained with conventional doses of DHAP chemotherapy [15]. These data have been recently updated and continue to show a benefit for patients undergoing high-dose chemotherapy [16].

A number of different conditioning regimens have been used for high-dose chemotherapy in NHL. The majority are based on combinations of chemotherapeutic agents. The most commonly used regimens are BEAC (BCNU, etoposide, ara-C and cyclophosphamide) [17], CBV (cyclophosphamide, BCNU and etoposide)[18] or BEAM (BCNU, etoposide, ara-C and high-dose melphalan)[19,20]. Others have used combinations of alkylating agents with total body irradiation [21-23]. Sometimes busulfan containing regimens are used [24,25]. Conditioning regimens for autologous transplantation have not been evaluated in a randomized fashion, and it is unclear whether any particular regimen is superior in terms of anti-tumor activity. For practical purposes, many centers have abandoned the use of TBI in conditioning regimens for patients with aggressive lymphoma. It requires sophisticated and time consuming radiation technology and is often not applicable for patients who have previously received involved field radiation. Among chemotherapy regimens, it appears that high dose melphalan containing regimens which lack the cardiac and urinary tract toxicity of cyclophosphamide are somewhat better tolerated and at least equally effective [26].

High dose chemotherapy is superior to standard chemotherapy for the treatment of recurrent lymphoma. Nonetheless, recurrence rates are high after high-dose chemotherapy and more effective approaches are needed. Some of these include the treatment of minimal residual disease by the administration of post-transplant interleukin-2 or interferon, or the induction of autologous graft versus host disease. Others have evaluated the use of allogeneic transplantation. It is beyond the scope of this chapter to describe these approaches in detail.

One particular approach that has been facilitated by the use of recombinant cytokines is the administration of multiple cycles of dose-intense chemotherapy with growth factor and/or stem cell support. With such an approach, one hopes to optimally exploit dose-intensity [27]. This treatment strategy has become possible thanks to the availability of blood stem cell progenitors, which can be collected in much larger numbers than was possible with a bone marrow harvest. The administration of recombinant cytokines after dose-intense chemotherapy allows rapid hematologic recovery and consequently a rapid succession of treatment cycles.

Long et al [28], treated 19 patients with metastatic breast cancer and 6 patients with refractory NHL with etoposide 2 gm/m^2 and G-CSF. Stem cells were collected upon recovery of counts. Patients were then treated with four cycles of mitoxantrone 18 mg/m^2, thiotepa 150-200 mg/m^2 and cyclophosphamide 4500-5000 mg/m^2 as a 48 hour continuous infusion, followed by infusion of one quarter of their progenitor cells 48 hours later. All patients also received G-CSF 5 mcg per kg after every chemotherapy cycle. The treatment was in general well tolerated, with only one treatment-related death among these 26 heavily pre-treated patients. Two of the six patients with NHL remain progression-free.

Rodriguez et al. administered ifosfamide 10 gm/m^2 with etoposide 900 mg/m^2 followed three weeks later by ifosfamide 10 gm/m^2 with mitoxantrone 20 mg/m^2 [29]. Stem cells were collected upon recovery from the first cycle of chemotherapy. Patients also received G-CSF 5 mcg/kg with each cycle of chemotherapy. Prior to mobilization, the dose was increased to 10 mcg/kg. Patients who achieved a complete remission after the two cycles of induction chemotherapy underwent consolidation with high dose BEAM and stem cell support. Those who had achieved only a partial remission underwent two sequential high- dose chemotherapy consolidations. The first one consisted of cyclophosphamide 4.5 gm/m^2, etoposide 1200 mg/m^2 and cisplatinum 135 mg/m^2 with stem cell rescue. The second one consisted of BEAM with stem cell rescue. Most of the agents used for salvage in this regimen are not used for standard front line chemotherapy and therefore patients may be less likely to have developed resistance to these regimens. Experience has been accrued with 44 patients. The response rate is approximately 80%. Approximately 50% of all the patients have achieved durable remissions. Only one treatment related death occurred. These data indicate that repetitive cycles of high-dose chemotherapy can be safely administered to patients with recurrent lymphoma. Response rates are higher and the proportion of durable responses may be increased when compared with less intensive reinduction regimens.

<u>High dose chemotherapy as initial treatment in aggressive NHL</u>. Prognostic models allow a prediction of the efficacy of conventional chemotherapy in individual patients with large cell lymphoma. The most commonly used model is the International Prognostic Index, in which a score of 1 to 5 is assigned to each patient based on <u>a</u>ge, <u>p</u>erformance status, serum <u>L</u>DH, involvement of <u>e</u>xtranodal sites and <u>s</u>tage (mnemonic APLES) [30].

CHOP is highly effective in subsets of patients with good prognostic features, which includes those under the age of sixty with an age-adjusted international index of 0 or 1. For such patients the expected CR rate with a conventional anthracycline containing regimen, or with combinations of chemotherapy and radiation is at least 80% and two thirds of the remissions are durable [30]. By contrast, among patients with several adverse prognostic features, neither CHOP nor any of its derivatives are likely to result in high durable remission rates.

Several large randomized studies have evaluated the use of intensive chemotherapy with stem cell support in patients with such poor risk features [31-36]. In a large French study [37], patients with poor prognostic features who achieved complete remission after 4 induction cycles of conventional chemotherapy were randomized to intensification with autologous transplantation or to continued chemotherapy. The conditioning regimen for transplantation was CBV and patients received bone marrow. Only 30% of the autologous transplant patients received growth factor after transplantation. The three year disease free survival rate was 52% (45%-59%) in the sequential chemotherapy arm and 59% (52%-66%) in the autologous BMT arm, which was not significantly different (P=0.46). Upon re-analysis of the data, approximately 50% of the patients were found to be in a high intermediate or high risk category as defined by the international prognostic index. For these patients, five year disease free survival was 39% after conventional chemotherapy versus 59% after autologous BMT, suggesting a benefit from autologous transplant among those with more advanced disease (*P*=0.01). In a Dutch study [38], patients with stage II-IV lymphoma who had a partial remission after 3 induction cycles of CHOP chemotherapy, but no bone marrow involvement, were randomized to either 3 additional cycles of CHOP or to autologous BMT after conditioning with cyclophosphamide and TBI. Sixty-nine patients were randomized, 34 to autologous BMT, 35 to CHOP chemotherapy. In this study no benefit in either survival or disease-free survival could be shown for autologous transplantation [39]. By contrast, Martelli et al, randomized forty-nine patients whose response to front line treatment was only a partial remission to receive either DHAP chemotherapy or high-dose chemotherapy and autologous stem cell transplantation [40]. The complete response rate was significantly higher for patients undergoing high dose chemotherapy (96% vs 59% P<.001). Disease-free survival at three years was 73% in the ABMT group vs 52% in the DHAP group (P=NS). The difference was not statistically significant due to the small numbers of patients randomized.

Gianni et al. reported a comparison between MACOP-B versus an innovative high dose sequential chemotherapy program, supported by growth factors and autografting for patients with bulky or advanced stage diffuse large B-cell lymphoma, but without bone marrow involvement [41]. In this study, patients randomized to the investigational arm were treated with rapidly alternating cycles of non-cross resistant chemotherapy. They initially received one cycle of standard doses of doxorubicin, vincristine and prednisone. This was followed by one cycle of cyclophosphamide 7 gm/m^2 with growth factor (G-CSF or GM-CSF) rescue. This course of chemotherapy was used for stem cell mobilization. Subsequently patients received vincristine 1.4 gm/m2 and high dose methotrexate 8 gm/m^2 with leucovorin rescue. The fourth course consisted of etoposide 2 gm/m^2 with growth factor rescue. The last treatment cycle consisted of high-dose melphalan 120-140 mg/m^2 with TBI with stem cell rescue and growth factor support. Because of toxicity associated with melphalan-TBI, the regimen was subsequently changed to mitoxantrone 60 mg/m^2 with melphalan 180 mg/m^2 and stem cell rescue. In a group of patients with bulky disease, they found an improved survival and disease-free survival for patients undergoing high dose chemotherapy. Event-free survival at six years was 76% for those assigned to high-dose chemotherapy vs 49% for those treated with MACOP-B.

These data suggest that high-dose chemotherapy improves the outcome of younger patients with NHL and some adverse prognostic features, such as bulky disease, by approximately 10% to 20%. The most impressive data were reported by Gianni et al. They demonstrated the feasibility and potential for long-term disease-free survival using an intensive chemotherapy protocol. The Dutch and French studies were designed earlier and used bone marrow rather than stem cell rescue. This resulted in a higher percentage of patients that could not complete the treatment, because of considerations of toxicity, patient refusal or inability to collect bone marrow.

The results from Gianni et al were confirmed in a pilot study by Schenkein et al.[42], in a group of 32 poor prognostic patients (28 with intermediate grade and 4 with high grade non-Hodgkin's lymphoma.) . Overall and disease-free survival in this study were 78% and 69% respectively. Stoppa et al. [35] used a slightly different strategy. They treated 20 patients with poor prognostic features (age adjusted IPI 2 or 3) with six consecutive cycles of an innovative chemotherapy regimen. The first three cycles consisted of cyclophosphamide 3 gm/m^2, doxorubicin 75 mg/m^2 and vincristine 2 mg plus steroids. All patients also received G-CSF 300 mcg/day. Stem cells were collected after each of these chemotherapy cycles. Cycle four through six consisted of the same drugs with the addition of etoposide 300 mg/m^2 on day 2 and cisplatin 100 mg/m^2. Stem cells were reinfused after cycle four through six and G-CSF 300 mcg daily administered. The cycles of chemotherapy were planned 21 days apart. Only one treatment-related death occurred in this study. The two year failure free survival was 56%.

The rapid administration of dose-intensive chemotherapy therefore appears to benefit at least some patients with poor prognostic features. Most studies are however limited to younger patients, with good performance status. Few, if any patients with bone marrow involvement are enrolled. Whether intensification will also benefit the elderly and those with even more advanced disease, remains to be seen. Haioun et al recently reported the preliminary results of a pilot trial of double autologous transplant in younger patients with very poor prognostic features. 36% had bone marrow involvement and 48% had an age-adjusted IPI of 3. Thirty one patients were evaluable. Only 24 had a response to the induction regimen and underwent the first autologous transplant. Nineteen underwent a second autologous transplant. With a follow-up of 9 to 19 months, only 11 patients remain free of disease. These data suggest that in patients with very poor prognostic features, the administration of truly dose-intensive therapy may be more difficult and less efficacious.

Mantle cell lymphoma

<u>Natural history and conventional management of mantle cell NHL</u>. Mantle cell lymphoma is a B-cell lymphoma originating from a normal counterpart in the mantle of the lymphoid follicle [43]. The disease is associated with t(11;14)(q13;q32) and rearrangement of bcl-1 in a large percentage of cases. In the past, the disease was often confused with either CLL or diffuse large cell lymphoma. In the past five years, the disease has been recognized more reliably and the clinical features better described. Patients often present with widespread disease; bone marrow involvement and peripheral blood involvement are common as is involvement of the gastro-intestinal tract [43-49]. Despite morphologic and phenotypic similarities to CLL, the prognosis of mantle cell lymphoma is worse than that of CLL or of follicular lymphoma. In general the responses to chemotherapy are also less durable than those achieved in other types of diffuse lymphoma [44-48]. Estimated 10 year survival in a recent series was only 8%[46].

<u>Intensive chemotherapy for mantle cell lymphoma</u>. Because of the the poor long-term survival in mantle cell lymphoma, many centers, have recommended autologous or allogeneic transplantation as consolidation of remission [43,50,51]. Encouraging early results have been reported after autologous transplantation [52].

Blay et al [53], reported on 18 patients with diffuse centrocytic lymphoma, including nine who had a confirmed diagnosis of mantle cell lymphoma, who underwent autologous transplantation in partial or complete remission. The conditioning regimen contained TBI in 11 cases and was BCNU-based in six. One patient received a combination of etoposide, carboplatin and ara-C. Seven patients received bone marrow and 12 received G-CSF stimulated peripheral blood progenitor cells. With a median follow-up of 30 months, progression-free survival was 75%.Dreger et al. reported on 12 patients with stage III/IV mantle cell lymphoma who received two cycles of induction with Dexa-BEAM, followed by consolidation with autologous transplantation [54]. Six patients received TBI containing regimens and two received high dose chemotherapy regimens. With a median follow-up of 12 months post -transplant, all patients were alive and in remission.Khouri et al, reported on 25 patients with aggressive mantle cell lymphoma who underwent transplant in first remission [50]. Nine received autologous transplants and four underwent allogeneic transplantation. Conditioning for transplantation consisted of cyclophosphamide and TBI. One patient died from interstitial pneumonitis. With a median follow-up of six months, 11 patients remained free of disease.Finally, Stewart et al. reported nine patients with mantle cell lymphoma in relapse who underwent autologous transplantation and achieved a two year disease free survival of 34% [51]. Haas et al reported on 13 patients. With a median follow-up of 18 months, disease-free survival was 74%.

Follow-up in all of these studies is rather limited. In contrast, the Dana-Farber group, in a retrospective analysis of 26 patients with recurrent or refractory mantle cell lymphoma, found a very high recurrence rate after autologous transplantation [55]. By two years after transplantation, more than half of the patients had relapsed. The high recurrence rate may be due to the high percentage of occult bone marrow involvement in these patients and the inability to achieve adequate purging of the marrow. In four mantle cell lymphoma patients in whom no resdual lymphoma was infused (including 2 allogeneic and one syngeneic recipient), only one patient relapsed. This series casts serious doubts on the long-term curative potential of autologous transplantation in mantle cell lymphoma, at least with currently available purging methodology.

Follicular lymphomas

<u>Conventional treatment for follicular lymphoma</u>. The median survival of patients affected by follicular lymphoma is 7 to 9 years. This disorder is therefore considerably more indolent than the intermediate and high grade lymphomas. Follicular lymphoma usually responds well to initial chemotherapy, but patients almost invariably relapse. At the time of first recurrence, the median life expectancy decreases to approximately 4 years and it decreases with subsequent recurrences [56,57]. Newer treatments include nucleoside analogs (fludarabine or 2CDA) or the monoclonal rituximab. None of these treatments are however expected to be curative in this disorder. Treatment with interferon either as maintenance or during induction induces a prolongation of disease free survival and probably also of survival but is not curative [58,59].

Small lymphocytic lymphoma is very similar in morphology and phenotype to CLL, but clinically it behaves more like follicular lymphoma and has often been treated as such. Most of the results of conventional chemotherapy and autologous transplantation in follicular lymphoma can probably be applied to small lymphocytic lymphoma as well, although specific data on this disorder are not available.

<u>Myeloablative therapy for follicular lymphoma</u>. Several groups have used autologous BMT in recurrent low grade lymphoma [60-63]. The patients usually had chemosensitive recurrences and underwent autologous BMT after achieving a second

complete remission or a good partial remission. Because of the frequent involvement of the bone marrow with lymphoma, purging procedures were used in some of the studies. Conditioning contained TBI in most of the patients.

Freedman et al. [60] reported 69 patients with low grade B-cell non Hodgkin lymphoma with chemosensitive relapse or partial remission who underwent autologous BMT. Fifty-one had low grade lymphoma at the time of transplantation, and 18 had transformed histology. The bone marrow was treated with a cocktail of monoclonal antibodies combined with complement. Conditioning consisted of high dose cyclophosphamide and TBI. Actuarial disease free survival was estimated at 53% for those with low grade histologies. Those in complete remission at the time of bone marrow transplant had a significantly better outcome than those in partial remission. With prolonged follow-up however, the difference in outcome between those transplanted in CR vs those transplanted in PR is not significant any longer [64]. In subsequent studies the Dana-Farber group demonstrated the association between persistence of lymphoma cells in the marrow infusate and disease recurrence [65]. Rohatiner et al.[61] reported 64 patients with recurrent follicular lymphoma who underwent autologous BMT as consolidation of second or subsequent remission. The marrow mononuclear cell component was treated in vitro with three cycles of the monoclonal anti-CD20 and complement. Conditioning consisted of high dose cyclophosphamide and TBI. With a median follow-up of three years, the disease free survival was 50%. This does not take into account treatment-related deaths. As there were three early deaths and four cases of secondary leukemia/MDS, this may be a somewhat optimistic estimate. Duration of remission was improved compared with historical controls, but survival was not significantly different.

Bastion et al. [62], reported a series of 60 patients with poor prognosis follicular lymphoma who underwent autologous stem cell transplantation. Twelve patients were in first partial remission, 34 were in second partial or complete remission and 14 had more advanced disease (i.e, multiple recurrences). Sixteen patients had histologic transformation. Different conditioning regimens were used, but included TBI in 46 of the 60 patients. Chemotherapy mobilized peripheral blood progenitor cells were used as stem cell source. Purging was not used. There were five treatment-related deaths, all occurring in patients with advanced disease. At a median follow-up of 21 months, the estimated two year failure-free survival was 53%. Patients with multiple recurrences and those with transformed disease had a worse outcome.

Bierman et al [63], reported one hundred patients who underwent unpurged autologous bone marrow (N=13) or cytokine mobilized stem cell transplantation (N=87) for recurrent or refractory follicle center lymphomas. Fifty seven patients had a chemotherapy sensitive recurrence, twelve had refractory disease and in thirty one cases chemosensitivity was either untested or unknown. Different conditioning regimens were used, but included TBI in 77 of the 100 patients. There were eight deaths in the first 100 days after transplantation, and six non-relapse deaths between 102 and 912 days after transplantation. With a median follow-up of 2.6 years, failure-free survival at 4 years was estimated at 44%. The only factor associated with overall survival and failure free survival was the number of chemotherapy regimens received prior to transplantation.

These studies and a number of other smaller studies as well as registry analysis,[66] indicate the feasibility of high dose chemotherapy and autologous transplantation in patients with follicular lymphoma. Treatment-related mortality appears to be a function of patient selection. In patients with minimal prior treatment, the early treatment related mortality is usually less than 5%. In patients who are more heavily pretreated, the treatment-related mortality is higher, there are commonly problems with delayed engraftment and overall outcome is worse. It is therefore generally accepted that, as in other disorders, high dose chemotherapy should be pursued sooner rather than later in the course of the disease. But even in relatively selected patients, there has been a continued pattern of relapse after autologous BMT for recurrent NHL. It is therefore not entirely certain whether the survival is improved after autologous transplantation in indolent NHL [57,67]. Another potential long-term problem has been the high rate of secondary myelodysplasia in long term survivors after autotransplants in this disease.

Despite these concerns, the results of autologous transplantation in recurrent disease have been sufficiently encouraging to explore its use as consolidation treatment in patients with poor prognosis disease in first remission. Freedman et al, reported a phase II study of 83 patients with poor prognosis follicular lymphoma who underwent consolidation with autologous transplantation after six to eight cycles of induction chemotherapy with CHOP. With a median follow-up of 45 months, disease-free survival at three years was expected to be 63%. Unfortunately, there was no indication of a plateau in the disease-free survival curve and there was a high rate of secondary MDS/leukemia. In a similar patient group, Horning et al., recently reported a 67% event-free survival at five years after autologous transplantation.[68] Longer follow-up will be necessary to establish whether or not this treatment is curative in a subset of patients.

Burkitt's disease and lymphoblastic lymphoma

<u>Conventional treatment for high-grade lymphoma</u>. Diffuse small non-cleaved cell lymphoma and lymphoblastic lymphoma are very aggressive malignancies that often affect children and young adults. Diffuse small non-cleaved cell lymphoma is associated with chromosomal translocations involving the myc oncogene and immunoglobulin genes [69]. Clinically the disease is extremely aggressive: patients present with rapidly proliferating tumors, and frequent bone marrow and peripheral blood involvement. A number of intensive treatment regimens designed for pediatric B-cell ALL have recently been used in adult Burkitt's lymphoma. The prognosis has steadily improved even for patients who present with CNS involvement [70], and it is now generally agreed upon that Burkitt's disease particularly those with bone marrow involvement or with Ann Arbor stage IV disease should be treated similarly to B cell ALL [71-76]. As in B-cell ALL, maintenance therapy is probably unnecessary and the major components of treatment appear to be high doses of alkylating agents and high dose methotrexate [77].

Most cases of lymphoblastic lymphoma are T-cell malignancies of thymic origin and are TdT-positive [78]. Young adults and children are the most commonly affected and present with large mediastinal masses, commonly associated with bone marrow and peripheral blood involvement. The disease is closely related to T-cell ALL and should be treated as such, even in the occasional case presenting with isolated mediastinal involvement [79-82]. Cure rates with such treatment are in the order of 40%.

<u>High dose chemotherapy for Burkitt's disease and lymphoblastic lymphoma</u>. High dose chemotherapy and autologous transplantation have been used both for consolidation of first remission and for treatment of recurrent disease in patients with high grade lymphoma. Numerous studies have shown the curative potential of high-dose chemotherapy for patients with recurrent high grade lymphoma [83-88]. In a case-control study from the European Bone Marrow Transplant registry, patients with lymphoblastic lymphoma derived an additional benefit from allogeneic transplantation [89].

A high incidence of durable complete remissions has also been observed among patients with high grade lymphoma who were consolidated with autologous transplantation in first remission [86,90-93]. Until recently, no formal comparisons between modern conventional chemotherapy and high dose intensification had been carried out and it was impossible to rule out that the excellent outcomes after autotransplant were due to patient selection vs true benefit of chemotherapy. This continues to be the case for diffuse small non-cleaved lymphoma. A recent prospective randomized study has however evaluated conventional chemotherapy vs autologous transplantation in lymphoblastic lymphoma [94]. 65 patients were randomized, 31 to autologous stem cell transplantation and 35 to conventional chemotherapy. With a median follow-up of 12 months there was a 45% reduction in risk for recurrence among those undergoing autologous transplantation (P=0.082).

Conclusions

High-dose chemotherapy plays an important and increasing role in the treatment of malignant lymphoma. Many issues of toxicity have been resolved and high-dose chemotherapy is becoming an increasingly attractive option. Further progress is needed to better define and expand its indications.

References

1. Frei E, III, Canellos GP: Dose: a critical factor in cancer chemotherapy. Am J Med 69:585, 1980
2. Coiffier B, Philip T, Burnett AK, Symann ML: Consensus conference on intensive chemotherapy plus hematopoietic stem cell transplantation in malignancies, Lyon, June 4-6, 1993. Ann Oncol 5:19, 1994
3. Gottlieb JA, Gutterman JU, McCredie KB, et al. Chemotherapy of malignant lymphoma with adriamycin. Cancer Res 33:3024, 1973
4. McKelvey EM, Gottlieb JA, Wilson HE, et al. Hydroxyldaunomycin (adriamycin) combination chemotherapy in malignant lymphoma. Cancer 38:1484, 1976
5. Fisher RI, Gaynor ER, Dahlberg S, et al. Comparison of a standard regimen (CHOP) with three intensive chemotherapy regimens for advanced non-Hodgkin's lymphoma. N Engl J Med 328:1002, 1993
6. Gordon LI, Harrington D, Andersen J, et al. Comparison of a second-generation combination chemotherapeutic regimen (m-BACOD) with a standard regimen (CHOP) for advanced diffuse non-Hodgkin's lymphoma. N Engl J Med 327:1342, 1992
7. Sertoli MR, Santini G, Chisesi T, et al. MACOP-B versus ProMACE-MOPP in the treatment of advanced diffuse non-Hodgkin's lymphoma: results of a prospective randomized trial by the non-Hodgkin's Lymphoma Cooperative Study Group. J Clin Oncol 12:1366, 1994
8. Cooper IA, Wolf MM, Robertson TI, et al. Randomized comparison of MACOP-B with CHOP in patients with intermediate-grade non-Hodgkin's lymphoma. The Australian and New Zealand Lymphoma Group. J Clin Oncol 12:769, 1994
9. Wolf M, Matthews JP, Stone J, et al. Long-term survival advantage of MACOP-B over CHOP in intermediate-grade non-Hodgkin's lymphoma. The Australian and New Zealand Lymphoma Group. Ann

Oncol 8 Suppl 1:71, 1997

10. Meerwaldt JH, Carde P, Somers R, et al. Persistent improved results after adding vincristine and bleomycin to a cyclophosphamide/hydroxorubicin/Vm-26/prednisone combination (CHVmP) in stage III-IV intermediate- and high-grade non-Hodgkin's lymphoma. The EORTC Lymphoma Cooperative Group. Ann Oncol 8 Suppl 1:67, 1997

11. Velasquez WS, McLaughlin P, Tucker S, et al. ESHAP-an effective chemotherapy regimen in refractory and relapsing lymphoma: a 4 year follow-up study. J Clin Oncol 12:1169, 1994

12. Rodriguez MA, Cabanillas FC, Velasquez W, et al. Results of a salvage treatment program for relapsing lymphoma: MINE consolidated with ESHAP. J Clin Oncol 13:1734, 1995

13. Philip T, Armitage JO, Spitzer G, et al. High-dose therapy and autologous bone marrow transplantation after failure of conventional chemotherapy in adults with intermediate grade or high-grade-non-Hodgkin's lymphoma. N Engl J Med 316:1493, 1987

14. Takvorian T, Canellos CP, Ritz J, et al. Prolonged disease-free survival after autologous bone marrow transplantation in patients with non-Hodgkin's lymphoma with a poor prognosis. N Engl J Med 316:1499, 1987

15. Philip T, Guglielmi C, Hagenbeek A, et al. Autologous bone marrow transplantation as compared with salvage chemotherapy in relapses of chemotherapy-sensitive non-Hodgkin's lymphoma. N Engl J Med 333:1540, 1995

16. Philip T, Gomez F, Guglielmi C, et al. Long term outcome of relapsed non-Hodgkin's lymphoma patients included in the PARMA trial: incidence of late relapses, long-term toxicity and impact of the international prognostic index (IPI) at relapse. ASCO Proceedings 17:62, 1998 (abstr.)

17. Rapoport AP, Rowe JM, Kouides PA, et al. One hundred autotransplants for relapsed or refractory Hodgkin's disease and lymphoma: Value of pretransplant disease status for predicting outcome. J Clin Oncol 11:2351, 1993

18. Wheeler C, Strawderman M, Ayash L, et al. Prognostic factors for treatment outcome in autotransplantation of intermediate-grade and high-grade non-Hodgkin's lymphoma with cyclophosphamide, carmustine, and etoposide. J Clin Oncol 11:1085, 1993

19. Gribben JG, Goldstone AH, Linch DC, et al. Effectiveness of high-dose combination chemotherapy and autologous bone marrow transplantation for patients with non-Hodgkin's lymphomas who are still responsive to conventional-dose therapy. J Clin Oncol 7:1621, 1989

20. Colombat P, Gorin N-C, Lemonnier M-P, et al. The role of autologous bone marrow transplantation in 46 adult patients with non-Hodgkin's lymphomas. J Clin Oncol 8:630, 1990

21. Gulati SC, Shank B, Black P, et al. Autologous bone marrow transplantation for patients with poor-prognosis lymphoma. J Clin Oncol 6:1303, 1988

22. Weisdorf DJ, Haake R, Miller WJ, et al. Autologous bone marrow transplantation for progressive non-Hodgkin's lymphoma: Clinical impact of immunophenotype and *in vitro* purging. Bone Marrow Transplant 8:135, 1991

23. Vose JM, Anderson JR, Kessinger A, et al. High-dose chemotherapy and autologous hematopoietic stem-cell transplantation for aggressive non-Hodgkin's lymphoma. J Clin Oncol 11:1846, 1993

24. Przepiorka D, Nath R, Ippoliti C, et al. A phase I-II study of high-dose thiotepa, busulfan and cyclophosphamide as a preparative regimen for autologous transplantation for malignant lymphoma. Leuk Lymphoma 17:427, 1995

25. Kroger N, Hoffknecht M, Hanel M, et al. Busulfan, cyclophosphamide and etoposide as high-dose conditioning therapy in patients with malignant lymphoma and prior dose-limiting radiation therapy. Bone Marrow Transplant 21:1171, 1998

26. Van Besien KW, Tabocoff J, Rodriguez MA, et al. Intensive chemotherapy with the BEAC regimen and autologous bone marrow transplantation in patients with refractory or recurrent intermediate grade and immunoblastic lymphoma; toxicity, long-term follow-up and identification of prognostic factors. Bone Marrow Transplant 15:549, 1995

27. Hryniuk WM, Goodyear M: The calculation of received dose intensity. J Clin Oncol 8:1935, 1990

28. Long GD, Negrin RS, Hoyle CF, et al. Multiple cycles of high dose chemotherapy supported by hematopoietic progenitor cells as treatment for patients with advanced malignancies. Cancer 76:860, 1995

29. van Besien K, Rodriguez M, Amin K, et al. Intensive reinduction with high-dose ifosfamide/VP16 and ifosfamide/novantrone followed by BEAM and stem cell transplant for patients with recurrent lymphoma. ASCO Proceedings 16:21a, 1997 (abstr.)

30. The International Non-Hodgkin's Lymphoma Prognostic Factors Project: A predictive model for aggressive non-Hodgkin's lymphoma. N Engl J Med 329:987, 1993

31. Dreyfus F, Leblond V, Belanger C, et al. Peripheral blood stem cell collection and autografting in high

risk lymphomas. Bone Marrow Transplant 10:409, 1992

32. Nademanee A, Schmidt GM, O'Donnell MR, et al. High-dose chemoradiotherapy followed by autologous bone marrow transplantation as consolidation therapy during first complete remission in adult patients with poor-risk aggressive lymphoma: A pilot study. Blood 80:1130, 1992

33. Freedman AS, Takvorian T, Neuberg D, et al. Autologous bone marrow transplantation in poor-prognosis intermediate-grade and high-grade B-cell non-Hodgkin's lymphoma in first remission: A pilot study. J Clin Oncol 11:931, 1993

34. Vitolo U, Cortellazzo S, Liberati AM, et al. Intensified and high-dose chemotherapy with granulocyte colony-stimulating factor and autologous stem cell transplantation support as first line therapy in high-risk diffuse large-cell lymphomas. J Clin Oncol 15:491, 1997

35. Stoppa AM, Bouabdallah R, Chabannon C, et al. Intensive sequential chemotherapy with repeated blood stem-cell support for untreated poor-prognosis non-Hodgkin's lymphoma [see comments]. J Clin Oncol 15:1722, 1997

36. Nademanee A, Molina A, O'Donnell M, et al. Results of high-dose therapy and autologous bone marrow/stem cell transplantation during remission in poor-risk intermediate and high-grade lymphoma: international index high and high-intermediate risk group. Blood 90:3844, 1997

37. Haioun C, Lepage E, Gisselbrecht C, et al. Comparison of autologous bone marrow transplantation with sequential chemotherapy for intermediate-grade and high-grade non-Hodgkin's lymphoma in first complete remission: a study of 464 Patients. J Clin Oncol 12:2543, 1994

38. Verdonck LF, Van Putten WLJ, Hagenbeek A, et al. Comparison of CHOP chemotherapy with autologous bone marrow transplantation for slowly responding patients with aggressive non-Hodgkin's lymphoma. N Engl J Med 332:1045, 1995

39. Haioun C, Lepage E, Gisselbrecht C, et al. Benefit of autologous bone marrow transplantation over sequential chemotherapy in poor-risk aggressive non-Hodgkin's lymphoma: updated results of the prospective study LNH87-2. Groupe d'Etude des Lymphomes de l'Adulte. J Clin Oncol 15:1131, 1997

40. Martelli M, Vignetti M, Zinzani PL, et al. High-dose chemotherapy followed by autologous bone marrow transplantation versus dexamethasone, cisplatin, and cytarabine in aggressive non-Hodgkin's lymphoma with partial response to front-line chemotherapy: a prospective randomized italian multicenter study. J Clin Oncol 14:534, 1996

41. Gianni AM, Bregni M, Siena S, et al. High dose chemotherapy and autologous bone marrow transplantation compared with MACOP-B in aggressive B-cell lymphoma. N Engl J Med 336:1290, 1997

42. Schenkein DP, Roitman D, Miller KB, et al. A phase II multicenter trial of high-dose sequential chemotherapy and peripheral blood stem cell transplantation as initial therapy for patients with high-risk non-Hodgkin's lymphoma. Biol Blood Marrow Transplant 3:210, 1997

43. Weisenburger DD, Armitage JO: Mantle cell lymphoma: an entity comes of age. Blood 87:4483, 1996

44. Majlis A, Pugh WC, Rodriguez MA, et al. Mantle cell lymphoma:correlation of clinical outcome and biologic features with three histologic variants. J Clin Oncol 15:1664, 1997

45. Shivdasani RA, Hess JL, Skarin AT, Pinkus GT: Intermediate lymphocytic lymphoma: clinical and pathologic features of a recently characterized subtype of non-Hodgkin's lymphoma. J Clin Oncol 11:802, 1993

46. Fisher RI, Dahlberg S, Nathwani BN, et al. A clinical analysis of two indolent lymphoma entities: mantle cell lymphoma and marginal zone lymphoma (including the mucosa-associated lymphoid tissue and monocytoid B-cell subcategories): a Southwest Oncology Group study. Blood 85:1075, 1995

47. Velders GA, Kluin-Nelemans JC, De Boer CJ, et al. Mantle-cell lymphoma: a population-based clinical study. J Clin Oncol 14:1269, 1996

48. Teodorovic I, Pittaluga S, Kluin-Nelemans JC, et al. Efficacy of four different regimens in 64 mantle-cell lymphoma cases: clinicopathologic comparison with 498 other non-Hodgkin's lymphoma subtypes. European Organization for the Research and Treatment of Cancer Lymphoma Cooperative Group. J Clin Oncol 13:2819, 1995

49. Duggan MJ, Weisenburger DD, Ye YL, et al. Mantle zone lymphoma. A clinicopathologic study of 22 cases. Cancer 66:522, 1990

50. Khouri I, Romaguera J, Kantarjian H, et al. Hyper-cvad and high dose methotrexate/ara-c (hd mtx-ara-c) followed by stem cell transplantation for aggressive mantle cell lymphoma (mcl). Blood 88 Suppl 1:122a, 1996 (abstr.)

51. Stewart DA, Vose JM, Weisenburger DD, et al. The role of high-dose therapy and autologous hematopoietic stem cell transplantation for mantle cell lymphoma. Ann Oncol 6:263, 1995

52. Coiffier B: Which treatment for mantle cell lymphoma in 1998? J Clin Oncol 16:3, 1998

53. Blay J-Y, Sebban C, Surbiguet C, et al. High-dose chemotherapy with hematopoietic stem cell

transplantation in patients with mantle cell or diffuse centrocytic non-Hodgkin's lymphoma. A single center experience on 18 patients. Bone Marrow Transplant 21:51, 1998

54. Dreger P, von Neuhoff N, Kuse R, et al. Sequential high-dose therapy and autologous stem cell transplantation for treatment of mantle cell lymphoma. Ann Oncol 8:401, 1997

55. Andersen N, Donovan JW, Borus JS, et al. Failure of immunologic purging in mantle cell lymphoma assessed by polymerase chain reaction detection of minimal residual disease. Blood 90:4212, 1997

56. Spinolo JA, Cabanillas F, Dixon DO, et al. Therapy of relapsed or refractory low-grade follicular lymphomas: factors associated with complete remission, survival and time to treatment failure. Ann Oncol 3:227, 1992

57. Weisdorf DJ, Andersen JW, Glick JH, Oken MM: Survival after relapse of low-grade non-Hodgkin's lymphoma: implications for marrow transplantation. J Clin Oncol 10:942, 1992

58. Solal-Celigny P, Lepage E, Brousse N, et al: Doxorubicin-Containing Regimen With or Without Interferon Alfa-2b for Advanced Follicular Lymphomas: Final Analysis of Survival and Toxicity in the Groupe d'Etude des lymphomes Folliculaires 86 Trial. J Clin Oncol 16:2232, 1998

59. Rohatiner A, Gregory W, Peterson B, et al. A meta-analysis of randomised trials evaluating the role of interferon as treatment for follicular lymphoma. Proc Am Soc Clin Oncol 17:abst 11, 1998

60. Freedman AS, Ritz J, Neuberg D, et al. Autologous bone marrow transplantation in 69 patients with a history of low-grade B-cell non-Hodgkin's lymphoma. Blood 77:2524, 1991

61. Rohatiner AZS, Johnson PWM, Price CGA, et al. Myeloablative therapy with autologous bone marrow transplantation as consolidation therapy for recurrent follicular lymphoma. J Clin Oncol 12:1177, 1994

62. Bastion Y, Brice P, Haioun C, et al. Intensive therapy with peripheral blood progenitor cell transplantation in 60 patients with poor-prognosis follicular lymphoma. Blood 86:3257, 1995

63. Bierman PJ, Vose JM, Anderson JR, et al. High-dose therapy with autologous hematopoietic rescue for follicular low-grade non-Hodgkin's lymphoma. J Clin Oncol 15:445, 1997

64. Freedman AS, Nadler LM: Which patients with relapsed non-Hodgkin's lymphoma benefit from high-dose therapy and hematopoietic stem-cell transplantation. J Clin Oncol 11:1841, 1993

65. Gribben JG, Freedman AS, Neuberg D, et al. Immunologic purging of marrow assessed by PCR before autologous bone marrow transplantation for B-cell lymphoma. N Engl J Med 325:1525, 1991

66. Williams CD, Goldstone AH, Pearce RM, et all. Purging of bone marrow in autologous bone marrow transplantation for non-Hodgkin's lymphoma: a case-matched comparison with unpurged cases by the European Blood and Marrow Transplant Lymphoma Registry. J Clin Oncol 14:2454, 1996

67. Johnson PWM, Rohatiner AZS, Whelan JS, et al. Patterns of survival in patients with recurrent follicular lymphoma: a 20-year study from a single center. J Clin Oncol 13:140, 1995

68. Hoppe RT: The role of radiation therapy in the management of non-hodgkin's lymphoma. Cancer 55:2176, 1985

69. Magrath IT, Shiramizu B: Biology and treatment of small non-cleaved cell lymphoma. Oncology 3:41, 1989

70. Haddy TB, Adde MA, Magrath IT: CNS involvement in small noncleaved-cell lymphoma: is CNS disease per se a poor prognostic sign? J Clin Oncol 9:1973, 1991

71. Magrath IT, Adde M, Shad A, et al. Adults and children with small non-cleaved cell lymphoma have a similar excellent outcome when treated with the same chemotherapy regimen. J Clin Oncol 14:925, 1996

72. Todeschini G, Tecchio C, Degani D, et al. Eighty-one percent event-free survival in advanced Burkitt's lymphom/leukemia: no differences in outcome between pediatric and adult patients treated with the same intensive pediatric protocol. Ann Oncol 8 (suppl10:S77, 1997

73. Ostronoff M, Soussain C, Zambon E, et al. Burkitt's lymphoma in adults: a retrospective study of 46 cases. Nouv Rev Fr Hematol 34:389, 1992

74. Soussain C, Patte C, Ostronoff M, et al. Small noncleaved cell lymphoma and leukemia in adults. A retrospective study of 65 adults treated with the LMB pediatric protocols. Blood 85:664, 1995

75. Straus DJ, Wong GY, Liu J, et al. Small non-cleaved-cell lymphoma (undifferentiated lymphoma, Burkitt's type) in American adults: Results with treatment designed for acute lymphoblastic leukemia. Am J Med 90:328, 1991

76. McMaster ML, Greer JP, Greco FA, et al. Effective treatment of small-noncleaved-cell lymphoma with high-intensity, brief-duration chemotherapy. J Clin Oncol 9:941, 1991

77. Hoelzer D, Ludwig WD, Thiel E, et al. Improved outcome in adult b-cell acute lymphoblastic leukemia. Blood 87:495, 1996

78. Picozzi VJ, Coleman N: Lymphoblastic lymphoma. Sem Onc 17:96, 1990

79. Slater DE, Mertelsmann R, Koriner B: Lymphoblastic lymphoma in adults. J Clin Oncol 4:57, 1986

80. Eden OB, Hann I, Imeson J, et al. Treatment of advanced stage T cell lymphoblastic lymphoma: Results

of the United Kingdom Children's Cancer Study Group (UKCCSG) protocol 8503. Brit J Haematol 82:310, 1992

81. Bernasconi C, Brusamolino E, Lazzarino M, et al. Lymphoblastic lymphoma in adult patients: clinicopathological features and response to intensive multiagent chemotherapy analogous to that used in acute lymphoblastic leukemia. Ann Oncol 1:141, 1990

82. Morel P, Lepage E, Brice P, et al. Prognosis and treatment of lymphoblastic lymphoma in adults: A report on 80 patients. J Clin Oncol 10:1078, 1992

83. Hartmann O, Pein F, Beaujean F, et al. High-dose polychemotherapy with autologous bone marrow transplantation in children with relapsed lymphomas. J Clin Oncol 2:979, 1984

84. Philip T, Biron P, Herve P, et al. Massive BACT chemotherapy with autologous bone marrow transplantation in 17 cases of non-Hodgkin's malignant lymphoma with a very bad prognosis. Eur J Cancer Clin Oncol 19:1371, 1983

85. Philip T, Biron P, Philip I, et al. Massive therapie and autologous bone marrow transplantation in pediatric and young adults with Burkitt's lymphoma (30 courses on 28 patients: a 5 year experience). Eur J Cancer Clin Oncol 22:1015, 1986

86. Sweetenham JW, Liberti G, Pearce R, et al. High-dose therapy and autologous bone marrow transplantation for adult patients with lymphoblastic lymphoma: results of the European group for bone marrow transplantation. J Clin Oncol 12:1358, 1994

87. Appelbaum FR, Deisseroth AB, Graw RG, et al. Prolonged complete remission following high dose chemotherapy of Burkitt's lymphoma in relapse. Cancer 41:10559, 1978

88. Abdel-Reheim FA, Edwards E, Arber DA: Utility of a rapid polymerase chain reaction panel for the detection of molecular changes in B-cell lymphoma. Arch Pathol Lab Med 120:357, 1996

89. Chopra R, Goldstone AH, Pearce R, et al. Autologous versus allogeneic bone marrow transplantation for non-Hodgkin's lymphoma: a case-controlled analysis of the European Bone Marrow Transplant Group registry data. J Clin Oncol 10:1690, 1992

90. Sweetenham JW, Pearce R, Taghipour G, et al. Adult Burkitt's and Burkitt-like non-Hodgkin's lymphoma--outcome for patients treated with high-dose therapy and autologous stem-cell transplantation in first remission or at relapse: results from the European Group for Blood and Marrow Transplantation. J Clin Oncol 14:2465, 1996

91. Baro J, Richard C, Sierra J, et al. Autologous bone marrow transplantation in 22 adult patients with lymphoblastic lymphoma responsive to conventional dose chemotherapy. Bone Marrow Transplant 10:33, 1992

92. Santini G, Congiu AM, Coser P, et al. Autologous bone marrow transplantation for adult advanced stage lymphoblastic lymphoma in first CR. A study of the NHLCSG. Leukemia 5 Suppl. 1:42, 1991

93. Verdonck LF, Dekker AW, de Gast GC, et al. Autologous bone marrow transplantation for adult poor-risk lymphoblastic lymphoma in first remission. J Clin Oncol 10:644, 1992

94. Sweetenham JW, Santini G, Simnett S, et al. Autologous stem cell transplantation in first remission improves relapse free survival in adult patients with lymphoblastic lymphoma: results from a randomized trial of the European group for blood and marrow and transplantation and the UK lymphoma group. ASCO Proceedings 17:abst 63, 1998 (abstr.)

17. Hematopoietic Growth Factors in Acute Leukemia

Richard M. Stone

Introduction

The clinical use of hematopoietic growth factors (HGFs) in the acute leukemias has been associated both with great promise and significant pitfalls. The myeloid growth factors offered the potential to decrease complications of the highly myelosuppressive chemotherapy required to successfully treat acute leukemias. However, because the HGFs were shown to stimulate proliferation of myeloblasts [1], these agents came relatively late to be tested in clinical trials of supportive care in acute myeloid leukemias. Once both GM-CSF and G-CSF were shown not to possess clinically apparent leukemogenic activity, large randomized trials were conducted with generally positive, but not dramatically beneficial results. The very ability of the HGFs to interact with leukemia cells could, by inducing DNA synthesis, sensitize the cells to the cytotoxic effects of cell-cycle active chemotherapy [2]. This so-called priming strategy has been explored in a preliminary fashion, but with generally disappointing results. The challenge ahead is to develop better ways to use existing HGFs and to integrate newer agents in this category into effective clinical strategies.

Use of HGFs as Post-chemotherapy Support

Significant effort has been directed to determine whether HGFs are useful supportive agents during the induction or initial treatment of patients with acute leukemia. In addition to potential nonhematopoietic side effects, the evaluation of growth-factor safety requires assurance that leukemic proliferation is not promoted. Most trials that attempted to determine the efficacy of HGFs in AML induction have focused on elderly patients because of a CR rate (40% to 50%) poorer than that observed in younger patients (70%) [3]. Older patients have a greater likelihood of failure from death during the period of chemotherapy-induced bone marrow aplasia [4], possibly due to a relatively low endogenous stem-cell reserve or poor end-organ tolerance of myelosuppressive complications. When the results of prospective randomized trials are compared, it is important to recognize that they differ in several ways including the type of growth factor used (either G-CSF or GM-CSF derived from *Escherichia coli* or from yeast [glycosylated]); the growth-factor stopping rules; the specific drugs and doses used for induction therapy; whether bone marrow hypoplasia was required prior to the initiation of growth factor therapy; whether newly diagnosed (either primary or secondary) or relapsed/refractory cases were included; and whether the factors were administered before or during chemotherapy, or both.

<u>Supportive Care: GM-CSF in AML</u> Preliminary studies in which GM-CSF was administered after chemotherapy to patients with AML at high risk of relapse suggested that the drug was reasonably well-tolerated and did not lead to an appreciable increase in disease resistance. Two preliminary studies compared the outcome to historical controls: the study performed in Germany[5] (n=30; yeast-derived GM-CSF) concluded that the rate of complete remission was superior while the trial conducted at MD Anderson [6] (n=12; <u>E. coli</u>-derived GM-CSF) showed little, if any benefit. Large prospective randomized studies were required to more precisely determine the role of GM-CSF in induction therapy.

Two major American cooperative group studies (Table 1) which attempted to determine the role of GM-CSF as a supportive agent in AML had superficially similar

Table 1.   **Supportive Care in AML: Randomized studies with GM-CSF used after induction chemotherapy.**

Author (Group)	Age	HGF	N	Chemo	Results
Rowe [7] (ECOG)	55-70	(if hypoplastic marrow) d10 (yeast, Sargramostim) to recov [ANC > 1500 x 3d]	124	Dnr 60 dl-3 ARA-C 100 dl-7	CR D OS NPdur G 60 6% 10.6 24d P 44 15% 4.8 28d
Stone [8] (CALGB)	≥ 60	d8 (E.coli) to recov. [ANC >500/mlx1d	388	Dnr 45 dl-3 ARA-C 200 dl-7	CR D OS NPdur G 51 27% 8.4 23d P 54 23% 10.8 25d

ANC=absolute neutrophil count; Npdur=neutropenia duration; recov=recovery; Dnr=daunorubicin; CR=complete remission; (chemo doses are mg/m^2); D=hypoplastic deaths; OS=overall survival in months; G=G-CSF; P=placebo

designs, but reached opposite conclusions. In the study conducted by the Eastern Cooperative Oncology Group (ECOG)[7], 124 patients 55-70 years old with de novo AML received induction therapy consisting of daunorubicin 60mg/m^2/d for three days and cytosine arabinoside 100mg/m^2/d for seven days. On day 10, if the marrow aspirate was aplastic without leukemia, patients were randomized to receive GM-CSF (Sargramostim; yeast-derived [glycosylated] GM-CSF) or placebo at 250µg/m^2 intravenously daily until the ANC exceeded 1500/µl for 3 days. The CR rate was marginally higher in the GM-CSF arm (60% vs. 44%; p=.08) and was associated with a 4 day reduction in the time that the neutrophil count was below 500/µl. While the disease-free survival in both cohorts was similar, the overall survival was better for those who received GM-CSF which was also administered after the single protocol-dictated post-remission therapy cycle (10.6 vs. 4.8 months). The improvement in outcome in the GM-CSF arm could have been due to a slight reduction in the likelihood of treatment-related mortality. Patients who received GM-CSF had fewer severe infections, fewer fatal infections, and fewer deaths associated with fungal pneumonia (2% vs. 19%). This benefit could have been due merely to the reduction in the duration of neutropenia, to an effect of GM-CSF on monocyte function, or to chance. This ECOG study provided the basis for the FDA to approve GM-CSF as a supportive agent in older patients with AML.

A large study conducted by the CALGB[8] failed to detect significant clinical benefit for GM-CSF as a supportive agent. 388 patients 60 years of age or older with de novo AML were randomly assigned to receive placebo or GM-CSF ($5\mu g/kg$ of E. coli-derived recombinant drug over 6hr intravenously daily) until the neutrophil count exceeded $1000/\mu l$ beginning on the day after an induction regimen consisting of daunorubicin $45mg/m^2/d$ for 3 days plus ara-c $200mg/m^2/d$ for 7 days. While there was a 2 day reduction in the duration of neutropenia, there was no other clinical benefit: the CR rate (52%), infectious death rate (25%) and the overall survival (approximately 9 months) were not different in the two arms. Approximately one-third of patients receiving GM-CSF had the study drug discontinued prematurely due to perceived toxicity from the agent. However, a similar number of patients on the placebo arm also had the experimental infusion discontinued because the investigator perceived that the patient was experiencing GM-CSF associated toxicity. This finding stresses the difficulty in ascribing side effects to a given drug in a sick leukemia patient. Even if the results only in those patients who completed the study drug infusion due to count recovery were analyzed, there was still no important benefit associated with GM-CSF.

The reasons for the apparent different outcomes between the two studies could be the degree of myelosuppression (a higher dose of daunorubicin in the ECOG study), that documentation of hypoplasia was required in ECOG study before the growth factor could be given, or the use of glycosylated GM-CSF in the ECOG study. It is also possible that the beneficial results were due to chance in the smaller sized ECOG trial.

<u>Supportive Care: G-CSF in AML</u>. A preliminary trial conducted by Ohno[9] suggested that G-CSF could be used safely and effectively to reduce the duration of neutropenia in patients with relapsed or refractory acute leukemia. This encouraging data prompted three large studies (Table 2) in which adults with newly diagnosed AML were randomized to receive either G-CSF or placebo at the conclusion of induction therapy. Although the induction regimens differed slightly among the studies, G-CSF or placebo was initiated after the conclusion of chemotherapy and continued until counts recovered. The results suggested that G-CSF is associated with reproducible benefits in shortening the duration of neutropenia and perhaps antibiotic usage and days in the hospital, but there was no effect on the more important parameters of reduction in infectious deaths or improvement in disease-free or overall survival.

The French Cooperative AML Group [10] enrolled 173 patients 65 years of age or older with de novo AML who received 4 days of daunorubicin in combination with 7 days of ara-C and either G-CSF or placebo beginning on day 9 until neutrophil recovery. Those receiving G-CSF experienced a significantly higher CR rate (70%) compared to those receiving placebo (47%) and had a reduction in the duration of neutropenia from 27 to 21 days. However, the likelihood of severe infection, toxic death, or disease-free or overall survival was unchanged. Although a primary antileukemic effect associated with G-CSF might be inferred from these results, since disease-free survival was not influenced, it is quite possible that the growth factor caused the assessment of remission bone marrow examinations to be altered. In a trial conducted by the Southwest Oncology Group [11] 234 patients aged 50 years and older with de novo or secondary AML received 3 days daunorubicin and 7 days of ara-C, followed by G-CSF or placebo on day 10. Although the duration of neutropenia was reduced by 4 days, no improvement in CR rate, decrease in the number of fatal infections, significant shortening of the hospital duration, or effect on overall survival was noted. An Amgen-Roche-sponsored trial conducted by a European cooperative group revealed similar results [12]. A 5-day regimen of VP 16 was administered in addition to a standard anthracycline/ara-C combination, with G-CSF being started at the conclusion of the chemotherapy. Although the CR rate and overall survival were identical in the two treatment arms, a 5-day reduction in the duration of neutropenia and hospital stay as well as lower antibiotic use represented real benefits. An economic analysis would be required to determine if the savings in hospitalization reduction justifies the routine use of this expensive growth factor in all patients.

Table 2.   **Supportive Care in AML: Randomized studies with G-CSF.**

Author (Group)	Age	HGF	N	Chemo	Results
Godwin [11] (SWOG)	≥ 55 median 60	d11 (E.coli: Filgrastim) to recov [ANC > 1000 x 1d, then taper]	124	Dnr 60 dl-3 Ara-C 100 dl-7	CR D OS NPdur G 41 20 6 24d P 50 19 9 27d
Heil [12] (Amgen-Roche)	> 16 median 54	d8 (E.coli: Filgrastim) to recov. [28d max.; ANC >1,000x3d]	388	Dnr 45 d1-3 Ara-C 200 d1-7	CR D OS NPdur G 69 8 10 20d P 68 10 9 25d
Dombret [10] (AML CSG)	> 65	d8 (glycosylated, lenograstim) to recov [28d max.; ANC >1,00 x 3d]	173	Dnr 45 d1-4 Ara-C 200 d1-7	CR D OS NPdur G 70 23 9 21d P 40 27 9 27d

recov=recovery; max=maximun; Dnr=daunorubicin; CR=complete remission; D=hypoplastic deaths; OS=overall survival in months; Npdur=neutropenic duration; G=G-CSF; P=placebo; ANC=absolute neutrophil count, AML CSG= AML cooperative study group

Surprisingly little attention has been paid to the use of HGFs as support after post-remission consolidation chemotherapy. However, a CALGB trial described a significant decrease in the number of neutropenic days when G-CSF was added after a mitozantrone/diazoquone regimen [13].

<u>Supportive Care: G-CSF in Acute Lymphoblastic Leukemia (ALL)</u>. With regard to the treatment of ALL, concerns about HGFs stimulating leukemic proliferation are markedly diminished. Given the lack of expression of growth factor receptors for either G- or GM-CSF on lymphoid cells (either benign or malignant) the use of

myeloid growth factors to reduce the myelosuppresive complications of induction or post-remission therapy for patients with ALL should yield issues much more similar to those encountered in the treatment of patients with lymphomas or solid tumors. Despite these considerations, there have been few clinical trials performed with HGFs in patients with ALL. However, the available trials do suggest that G-CSF does have a potentially important, albeit limited, role in preventing certain specific complications associated with chemotherapy, particularly the number of days of neutropenia.

Modern combination chemotherapy in association with central nervous prophylaxis has led to the cure of at least 70% of children who develop ALL. Infectious complications still remain a barrier to successful treatment in a finite number of sick children. The St. Jude Children's Research Hospital Group [14] performed a prospective randomized trial in which a 164 children with ALL were randomized to receive placebo or G-CSF (10µ/kg daily subcutaneously) beginning one day after the completion of remission induction therapy and continuing until the neutrophil count was greater than or equal to 1,000/µ for two days. G-CSF treatment did not significantly lower the rate of patients developing or being hospitalized for febrile neutropenia nor was it associated with an improvement in key clinical parameters such as event free or overall survival. Importantly, just as has been seen in most of the trials with this agent in AML, G-CSF was not associated with reduction in the incidence of severe or life-threatening infections. However, patients treated with G-CSF did experience a shorter median hospital stay (6 versus 10 days, p=0.11) and fewer documented infections (12 versus 27, p=0.009). Despite these reductions, an economic analysis suggested that G-CSF did not lower the total cost of supportive care. As such, while the routine use of G-CSF in children with ALL is probably safe, its benefit is limited. Interestingly, patients randomized to the G-CSF arm were able to start their consolidation chemotherapy at a significantly earlier time. Again, despite this apparent increase in dose intensity, no benefits in anti-leukemic efficacy were noted. The reasons why G-CSF failed to effect a significant reduction in the treatment of severe infections may again be, as was noted in patients with AML, an inability of the growth factor to ablate the period of severe and profound neutropenia which occurs at a time when mucosal barriers are also disrupted. An important finding also derived from the St. Jude's trial was the fact that G-CSF was not associated with an increase in secondary epipodophyllotoxin associated AML.

The Cancer and Leukemia Group B [15] performed a trial in which G-CSF or a placebo was begun on day four after cyclophosphamide/daunorubicin/vincristine/ prednisone/L-asparaginase induction therapy was given to 194 adults with ALL. Just as in the trial in childhood ALL, there was a significant reduction in the duration of neutropenia after induction therapy. This effect was particularly pronounced in older patients. The complete remission rate, infectious death rate, and event free survival rate were unaffected. Perhaps because the myelosuppression after post-remission (intensification) chemotherapy was less pronounced, the effect of G-CSF in the early post-remission setting was less marked than after induction therapy. Based on these results, subsequent CALGB protocols which have asked different questions, have included the routine administration of G-CSF beginning on day four during induction but have not mandated the use of G-CSF during post remission therapy. Other trials using G-CSF in adults with ALL have reached similar conclusions [16]. Consequently, it is probably reasonable to use this growth factor as an adjunctive treatment for the intense myelosuppressive chemotherapies for ALL in adults and children. HGFs in this setting probably provide the same magnitude of benefit associated with their use after other intensive chemotherapeutic regimens, such as high dose cyclophosphamide/doxorubicin for treatment of breast cancer. However, it seems doubtful that the use of growth factors in ALL will lead to an improvement in cure rates.

Use of HGFs to Enhance Chemotherapeutic Efficacy

<u>GM-CSF as a priming agent in AML</u>. Preliminary studies offered conflicting results as to the potential benefit of concurrent use of growth factors and induction therapy in AML [17, 18]. The American cooperative group trials with GM-CSF during induction therapy evaluated the drug in a purely supportive role after chemotherapy. At least 4 European groups have sought to test whether or not this growth factor might also have a role in sensitizing leukemic cells to chemotherapy. The mechanism of sensitization was postulated to be: 1) increase in the percentage of blasts in S-phase rendering them more sensitive to S-phase anti-leukemic drugs such as cytarabine and/or 2) increase in the incorporation of ara-C into DNA by increased formation of ara-CTP. Especially since older individuals have intrinsically resistant disease, a strategy aimed at enhancing the effectiveness of existing chemotherapy agents is attractive. However, the four European trials [19-22] (Table 3) in which GM-CSF was given before or during

Table 3.   **Supportive Care in AML GM-CSF: Placebo controlled trials.**

Author (Group)	Age	HGF	N	Chemo	Results
Heil [21] (German)	≥ 18 median 50	d-2 (E.coli) to recov [ANC>500/µl x 3d]	80	Ara-C 100 d1-8 Dnr 60 d3-5 VP-16 100 d4-8	<u>CR D OS NPdur</u> G 81 16 19 20.5d P 79 17 31 19.5d
Zittoun [19] (EORTC)	15-60	d-1 to 7 or 7 (E.coli) to recov or d-1 to recov [ANC >1,000/µl]	102	Dnr 45 d1-3 Ara-C 200 d1-7	<u>CR D OS NPdur</u> n 77 8 NA 25 d 60 4 NA 22 a 44 4 NA 22 d/a 42 8 NA 19.5
Lowenberg [20] (EORTC)	> 61	d-1 (E.coli) to recov. [ANC >500/µl]	318	Dnr 30 d1-34 Ara-C 200 d1-7	<u>CR D OS NPdur</u> G 56 14 22 23d P 55 13 22 25d
Lowenberg [22] (HOVON-SAKK)	15-60	d-1 to 7 (E.coli) or d-1 to recov or D8 to recov or none [recov to ANC>500/µl x 3 d]	274	Dnr 45 d1-3 Ara-C 200 d1-7	<u>CR D OS NPdur</u> n 75 10 41 27d d 80 10 30 27d a 77 10 46 24d d/a 77 10 37 24d

recov=recovery; maximum; Dnr=daunorubicin; CR=complete remission; D=hypoplastic deaths; OS=overall survival in months in percentage; Npdur=neutropenic duration in days; G=G-CSF; P=placebo; ANC=absolute neutrophil count, AML CSG= AML cooperative study group; d= during; a=after; d/a=during/after; n = neither during or after.

induction therapy each failed to show a complete remission rate, disease free-survival, or overall survival benefit associated with the use of the HGF. Moreover, a trial in which patients with relapsed AML were randomized to receive high dose ara-C re-induction therapy also failed to show any demonstrable benefit [23].

    <u>G-CSF as a priming agent in AML</u>. In a similar fashion to that observed with GM-CSF, G-CSF administration to patients with AML can increase the number of cells in S-phase [24]. Whether such a biological effect can be exploited clinically is less clear. A randomized prospective double-blind controlled study in which G-CSF or placebo was administered starting 2 days before induction therapy in 58 patients with relapsed/refractory AML until neutrophil recovery demonstrated a trend toward a better CR rate (50 vs 37, p=0.306) in the G-CSF group [25] but the disease-free and overall survival rates were not affected. It does not seem likely that this strategy will be pursued further by most investigators.

HGFs in the Treatment of Patients with Myelodysplasia (MDS)

The myelodysplastic syndromes are a heterogeneous group of bone marrow stem-cell disorders characterized by hypercellular bone marrow and peripheral blood cytopenias. Although, until recently [26], most clinicians were reluctant to use AML-type intensive chemotherapy in patients with MDS outside the context of the clinical trial, supportive care remains the norm for therapy of MDS. Although not the focus of this chapter, there have been numerous trials (Table 4) in which GM-CSF [27,28], G-CSF [29,30], and

Table 4. Selected trials of HGFs in MDS

Author (Ref)	Patients	HGF	Results
Greenberg[36]	70 RAEB 32 RAEBT	G-CSF vs Obs	100% vs. 0% increased ANC No survival benefit Survival decreased with G-CSF [10 vs 21] in RAEB group
Negrin[42]	38 RA/RARS 17 RAEB/T	G-CSF 1 µg/kg/d or greater 14d later EPO added at 300 µg/kg/d	48% RBC responders
Negrin[30]	2 RA 17 RAEB/T	G-CSF 0.1-3.0 µg/kg/d	16/18 with at least 5x increased ANC
Gaenser[27]	5 RA 6 RAEB/T	GM-CSF 15-150 µg/m² IV	8/11 increased ANC 4/11 transient increased blasts
Stein[32]	20 RA/RAEB	EPO 1200-1600 µg/kg 2 x wk IV	4/20 RBC responses

ANC=absolute neutrophil count, RAEB=refractory anemia with excess blasts; RAEBT=refractory anemia with excess blasts in transformation; obs=observation, EPO=erythropoietin; RA=refractory anemia; RARS=refractory anemia with ringed sideroblasts erythropoietin [31,32] have been administered to patients with MDS without concommitant use of chemotherapy. Obviously, given the potential for stimulation of leukemic proliferation, those patients with MDS whose bone marrows or peripheral blood displayed excess myeloblasts were carefully scrutinized to exclude the possibility of conversion to AML; indeed, in some of the earlier trials in which GM-CSF [27] was given to promote a higher white count in patients with MDS, there was a transient conversion to AML. However, it seemed not to be clinically important, since the percentage of myeloblasts decreased upon discontinuation of the agent [33,34]. In fact, trials performed in the 1980's clearly documented a neutrophil response rate in the 70% range for patients with MDS treated with either G- or GM-CSF. In some cases, it was suggested that the use of the myeloid growth factors could repair the intrinsically poor bactericidal function of neutrophils [35]. Nonetheless, myeloid growth factors are not routinely used in the supportive management of patients with MDS because their long term benefits have never been documented. The only randomized trial (G-CSF vs. observation in patients with advanced MDS) documented a high response rate associated with the growth factor, but there was no impact on survival and a possible deleterious effect on conversion to AML in certain patient subsets [36]. Moreover, most patients with MDS do not suffer from repeated bouts of infection (and in these there could be a clinical case made for the use of G-CSF) but rather from the ravages of anemia and thromobocytopenia.

There are currently no growth factor-based approaches to deal with the thrombocytopenia that plagues many patients with MDS. Clinical trials with interleukin-3 and interleukin-6 [37-39], growth factors which stimulate relatively primitive bone marrow progenitor cells are capable of increasing the platelet counts in a minority of patients so treated. However, these agents are associated with a significant incidence of secondary cytokine-mediated systemic effects that have limited, if not precluded, further clinical development. The thrombopoietic agent currently approved for use in ameliorating the thrombocytopenia associated with chemotherapy-induced aplasia, interleukin-11 [40], has not been tested in patients with MDS or acute leukemia. Recombinant thrombopoietin, (in both native and pegylated forms), the cytokine centrally important in maintaining platelet homeostasis, is undergoing clinical development at this time in patients with AML undergoing induction chemotnerapy. A preliminary report concerning the administration of the pegylated version of thrombopoietin after induction chemotherapy to adults with AML was disappointing: the use of this agent was not associated with a reduction in the duration of thrombocytopenia nor in the number of platelet transfusions administered [41]. Given the limited available data, the prospects for ameliorating the severe thrombocytopenia in MDS or the thrombocytopenia induced by induction chemotherapy in acute leukemia are not promising.

Compared with efforts to reduce thrombocytopenia in patients with MDS, by utilization of a HGF, much more data is available regarding the use of erythropoietin to improve the hematocrit and decrease the red cell transfusion requirement. Problems associated with severe anemia that characterizes about 90% of patients with MDS include decreased quality of life, congestive heart failure and secondary hemochromatosis. Erythropoietin alone may improve the anemia in MDS in approximately 20% of patients [31,32]. The response rate may be even lower in patients with refractory anemia with ringed sideroblasts and may be somewhat higher in those who have a relatively low endogenous erythropoietin level or have not yet required a red cell transfusion [32]. Based on *in vitro* studies which demonstrate that erythropoietin in combination with other early acting or myeloid cytokines may have a synergistic effect on erythropoiesis [42], several clinical trials have purported to show a benefit in terms of improvement of anemia when erythropoietin and G-CSF are used in combination. Response rates for improvement of anemia have been as high as 40% in several preliminary reports and, withdrawal of G-CSF has been associated with a loss in the erythropoietic response that was observed when both agents were used together [43, 44]. A recently published randomized phase II trial[5] evaluated two alternative treatment strategies: G-CSF for 4 weeks followed by the combination of EPO plus G-CSF for 12 weeks or EPO for 8 weeks followed by the combination of G-CSF plus EPO for 10 weeks. The overall response rate to G-CSF plus EPO was 38% which seemed to confirm previous studies. The response rate for improvement of anemia did not differ in the two alternative treatment schedules.

Since no therapeutic approach, other than bone marrow transplantation in the relatively young patient with MDS, has been shown to conclusively alter the natural history of this condition, it is recommended that patients with this condition be enrolled on a clinical trial whenever possible. However, patients with MDS treated supportively should have a serum erythropoietin level measured. If the serum EPO level is below 500 m IV/ml a four to eight week trial of erythropoietin (doses of 10,000 to 20,000 subcutaneously daily have been used); if no response has been observed it is reasonable to add G-CSF for a period of four weeks. The use of myeloid growth factors alone should not be considered routine; however they might be considered for those patients with MDS who have repeated bouts of infection.

Summary

While the concerns regarding the potential leukemic simulatory effect of G- and GM-CSF have been dissipated by many clinical trials, their promise as agents which could either enhance chemotherapeutic efficacy or reduce mortality from infection have not been realized. Nonetheless, much like in the case of their use after intensive chemotherapy in myeloablative therapy or inpatients with solid tumors, or lymphomas the myeloid growth factors will routinely reduce the duration of neutropenia. Several recent reviews [46-48] emphasize these points. The emphasis in the treatment of patients with acute leukemia must now shift to other therapeutic strategies including new chemotherapy drug development, reversal of drug resistance, and immunotherapeutic approaches.

References

1.   Lowenberg B, Touw I: Hematopoietic Growth Factors and their receptors in acute leukemia. Blood 81: 281-292, 1993
2.   Tafuri A, Andreef M: Kinetic rationale for cytokine-induced treatment of myeloblastic leukemia followed by cycle-specific chemotherapy in vitro. Leukemia 4:826-834, 1990
3.   Mayer RJ, Davis RB, Schiffer CA, et al: Intesive postremission chemotherapy in adults with acute

myeloid leukemia. N Engl J Med 331:896-903, 1994

4. Stone RM, Mayer RJ: The approach to the elderly patient with acute myeloid leukemia. Hematol Oncol Clin North Am 7: 65-79, 1993

5. Buchner T, Hiddeman W, Koenigsman M, et al: Human granulocyte-macrophage colony-stimulating factor after chemotherapy in patients with acute myeloid leukemia at higher age or after relapse. Blood 78: 1190-1197, 1991

6. Estey E, Dixon D, Kantarjian H: Treatment of poor-prognosis newly diagnosed acute myeloid leukemia with ara-C and recombinant human granulocyte-macrophage colony-stimulating factor. Blood 75: 1766-1769, 1990

7. Rowe J, Andersen J, Mazza, et al: A randomized placebo-controlled phase II study of (> 55 to 70 years of age) with acute myelogenous leukemia: a study of the eastern cooperative oncology group (E1490). Blood 86: 457-462, 1995

8. Stone R, Berg D, George S, et al: Granulocyte-macrophage colony-stimulating factor after initial chemotherapy for elderly patients with primary acute myelogeneous leukemia. N Engl J Med 332: 1671-1677, 1995

9. Ohno R, Tomonaga M, Kobayashi T et al: Effect of granulocyte colony-stimulating factor after intensive induction therapy in relapsed or refractory acute leukemia. N Engl J Med 323: 871-876, 1990

10. Dombret H, Chastang C, Fenaux P, et al: A controlled study of recombinant human granulocyte-stimulating factor in elderly patients after treatment for acute myelogeneous leukemia. N Engl J of Med 332 1678-1683, 1995

11. Godwin J, Kopecky K, Head D, et al: A double-blind placebo-controlled trial of granulocyte colony-stimulating factor in elderly patients with previously untreated acute myeloid leukemia: a southwest oncology group (9031). Blood 91: 3607-3615, 1998

12. Heil G, Hoelzer D, Sanz et al: A randomized, double-blind, placebo-controlled, phase II study of filgrastim in remission induction and consolidation therapy for adults with de novo acute myeloid leukemia. Blood 90: 4710-4718, 1997

13. Moore J, Dodge R, Amrein P, et al: Granulocyte-colony stimulating factor (fligrastim) accelerates granulocyte recovery after intensive postremission chemotherapy for acute myeloid leukemia with aziridinyl benzoquinone and mitoxantrone: cancer and leukemia group B study 9022. Blood 89: 780-788, 1997

14. Pui C, Boyett J, Hughes W, et al: Human granulocyte colony stimulating factor after induction chemotherapy in children with acute lymphoblastic leukemia. N Engl J Med 336: 1781, 1997

15. Larson R, Dodge R, Linker et al: A randomized controlled trial of filgrastim during remission induction and consolidation chemotherapy for adults with acute lymphoblastic leukemia: CALGB study 9111. Blood 92 1556-1564, 1998

16. Ottmann OG, Hoelzer D, Gracien E, et al: Concomitant granulocyte colony-stimulating factor and induction chemoradiotherapy in adult acute lymphoblastic leukemia: A randomized phase II trial. Blood 86: 444, 1995

17. Bettleheim P, Valent P, Andreef M: Recombinant human granulocyte-macrophage colony-stimulating factor in combination with standard induction chemotherapy in de novo acute myeloid leukemia. Blood 77: 700-711, 1991

18. Estey E, Thall P, Kantarjian H, et al: Treatment of newly diagnosed acute myelogenous leukemia with granulocyte-macrophage colony-stimulating factor (GM-CSF) before and during continuous-infusion high-dose ara-C + daunorubicin: comparison to patients treated without GM-CSF. Blood 79: 2246-2255, 1992

19. Zittoun R, Suciu S, Mandelli F, et al: Granulocyte-Macrophage colony-stimulating factor associated with induction treatment of acute myelogenous leukemia: a randomized trial by the european organization for research and treatment of cancer leukemia cooperative group. J Clin Oncol 41: 2150-2159, 1996

20. Lowenberg B., Suciu S, Archimbaud et al: Using of recombinant granulocyte-macrophage colony-stimulating factor during and after remission induction chemotherapy in patients aged 61 years and older with acute myeloid leukemia (AML): final report of AML-11, a phase III randomized study of the leukemia cooperative group of european organization for the research and treatment of cancer (EORTC-LCG) and the Dutch elgian Hemato-oncology cooperative group (HOVON). Blood 90: 2952-2961, 1997

21. Heil G, Chadid L, Hoelzer D: GM-CSF in a double-blind randomized, placebo controlled trial in therapy of sdult patients with de novo acute myeloid leukemia (AML): Leukemia 9: 3-9, 1995

22. Lowenberg B, Boogaerts M, Daenen S, et al: Value of different modalities of granulocyte-macrophage colony-stimulating factor applied during or after induction therapy of acute myeloid leukemia. J Clin Oncol   15: 3496-3506, 1997

23. Peterson BA, Gerge SL, Bhalla, et al: A phase II trial with or without GM-CSF administered before and during high dose cytarabine in patients with relapsed refractory acute myelogenous leukemia. Proc ASCO   15: 504, 1996

24. Baer M, Bernstein S, Brunetto V: Biological effects of recombinant human granulocyte colony-stimulating factor in patients with untreated acute myeloid leukemia: Blood   87: 1484-1494, 1996

25. Ohno R, Naoe T, Kanamaru A, et al: A double-blind controlled study of granulocyte colony-stimulating factor started two days before induction chemotherapy in refractory acute myeloid leukemia. Blood   83: 2086-2092, 1994

26. Estey e, Thall P, Beran M, et al: Effect of diagnosis (refractory anemia with excess blasts, refractory anemia with excess blasts in transformation, or acute myeloid leukemia [AML] on outcome of AML-type chemotherapy. Blood   90: 2969-2977, 1997

27. Ganser A, Volkers B, Greher J, et al: Recombinant human granulocyte-macrophage colony-stimulating factor in patients with myelodysplastic syndromes - a phase I/II trial. Blood   73: 31-37, 1989

28. Vadhan-Raj S, Keating M, LeMaistre, et al: Effects of recombinant human granulocyte-macrophage colony-stimulatingfactor in patients with myelodysplastic syndromes. N Engl J Med 317: 1545, 1987

29. Kobayashi Y, Okabe T, Ozawa K, et al: Treatment of myelodysplastic syndromes with recombinant human granulocyte colony-stimulating factor: a primary report. Am J Med   86: 178-182, 1989

30. Negrin R, Haeuber D, Nagler A, et al: Maintenance treatment of patients with myelodysplastic syndromes using recombinant human granulocyte colony-stimulating factor. Blood   76: 36-43, 1990

31. GoyA, Belanger C, Casadevall N: High dose of intravenous recombinant erythropoietin for the treatment of anemia in myelodysplastic syndrome. Brit J Hem atol 84: 232-237, 1993

32. Stein R, Abels R, Krantz S: Pharmacologic doses of recombinant human erythropoietin in the treatment of myelodysplastic syndromes. Blood   78: 1658-1663, 1991

33. Greenberg P: Treatment of myelodysplastic syndromes with hempoietic growth factors. Sem Oncol 19: 106-114, 1992

34. Ganser A, Hoelzer: Clinical use of hematopoietic growth factors in the myelodysplastic syndromes. Sem Hem   33: 186-195, 1996

35. You A, Kitagawa S, Okabe T: Recombinant human granulocyte colony-stimulating factor repairs the abnormalities of neutrophils in patients with myelodysplastic syndromes and chronic myelogenous leukemia. Blood 70: 404-411, 1987

36. Greenberg P, Taylor K, Larson R: Phase II randomized multicenter trial of G-CSF vs, observation for myelodysplastic syndromes (MDS). Blood 82:196a, 1993

37. Kurzrock R, Talpaz M, Estrov, et al: Phase I study of recombinant human interleukin-3 in patients with bone marrow failure. J Clin Oncol 9: 1241-1250, 1991

38. Ganser A, Lindemann A, Seipelt G, et al: Effect of recombinant human interleukin-3 in patients withnormal hematopoiesis and in patients with bone marrow failure. Blood   76: 666, 1990

39. Gordon M, Nemunaitis J, Hoffman R, et al: A phase I trial of recombinant human interleukin-6 in patients with myelodysplastic syndromes and thrombocytopenia. Blood 85: 3066-3076, 1995

40. Tepler I, Elias L, Smith J, et al: A randomized placebo-controlled trial of recombinant human interleukin-11 in cancer patients with severe thrombocytopenia due to chemotherapy. Blood 87: 3607-3614, 1996

41. Geissler E, Kabrna S, Stengg I, et al: Recombinant human magakaryocyte growth and development factor augments moblization of hematopoietic progenitor cells post chemotherapy in patients with acute myeloid leukemia. Blood   1997 90: 98a

42. Negrin R, Stein R, Doherty K, et al: Maintenance treatment of the anemia of myelodysplastic syndromes with recombinant human granulocyte colony-stimulating factor and erythropoietin: evidence of in vitro synergy. Blood 87: 4076-4081, 1996

43. Negrin RS, Stein R, Vardiman J, et al: Treatment of the anemaia of myelodysplastic syndromes using recombinant human granulocyte colony-stimulating factor in combination with erythropoietin. Blood 82: 737-743, 1993

44. Hellstrom-Lindberg E. Birgegard G, Carlsson M, et al: A combination of granulocyte colony-stimulating factor and erythropoietin may syngergistically improve the anemia in patients with myelodysplastic syndromes. Leuk Lymph   11: 221-228, 1993

45. Hellstrom-Lindberg E, Ahlgren T, Beguin,Y, et al: Treatment of anemia in myelodysplastic syndromes

with granulocyte colony-stimulating factor plus erythropoietin: results from a randomized phase II study and long-term follow-up of 71 patients. Blood 92: 68-75, 1998
46. Estey E: Use of colony-stimulating factors in the treatment of acute myeloid leukemia. Blood 83: 2015-2019, 1994
47. Geller R: Use of cytokines in the treatment of acute myelocytic leukemia: a critical review. J Clin Oncol 14: 1371-1382, 1996
48. Schiffer C: Hematopoietic growth factors as adjuncts to the treatment of acute myeloid leukemia. Blood 88: 3675-3685, 1996

VI

Management of Marrow Failure States

18. Cytokines for the Treatment of Myelodysplastic Syndromes and Other Bone Marrow Failure States

Robert S. Negrin M.D.

Introduction

In this chapter the biological rationale and potential clinical utility of cytokines and colony stimulating factors (CSFs) for the treatment of myelodysplastic syndromes (MDS) and other bone marrow failure states such as aplastic anemia (AA), Fanconi's Anemia, Diamond-Blackfan Syndrome and bone marrow suppression from drug therapy will be discussed. Since the application of CSFs has been more extensively studied in MDS and AA patients these disorders will be stressed. The rationale for the use of CSFs in these disorders is clear since they all represent difficult disease situations where bone marrow dysfunction or failure results in cytopenias. The goal of CSF therapy has been to correct those cytopenias without causing toxicity or progression of disease. In all of these clinical situations there are limitations to the efficacy of this form of therapy and these will be discussed.

Myelodysplastic Syndromes (MDS)

MDS provides a clinical model for the study of the evolution of a relatively benign disorder to one which is frankly leukemic, i.e. acute myelogenous leukemia (AML). Because this disease affects predominantly elderly individuals its management has posed certain therapeutic challenges; namely, to support the complications of the patient's dominant cytopenia without excessive toxicity. The CSFs, mainly granulocyte-colony stimulating factor (G-CSF), granulocyte-macrophage colony stimulating factor (GM-CSF) and erythropoietin (EPO) have been evaluated clinically in an effort to improve the management of MDS patients.

In MDS, defective proliferation of hematopoietic precursors has been suggested to be due to decreased production or responsiveness to hematopoietic growth factors. In addition, MDS precursors have an increased rate of apoptosis [1]. The identification of recurring chromosomal abnormalities, primarily involving chromosomes 5,7 and 8 have suggested potential genetic lesions which provide unique insights into this disease. Because some leukemic cells will proliferate by the addition of CSFs in vitro[2-4] there has been concern about the possibility of progression of disease in MDS patients. In vitro studies have been performed on bone marrow cells extracted from MDS patients where it has been demonstrated that CSF therapy in vitro improved the otherwise abnormal growth patterns. These in-vitro findings have suggested the possible efficacy of CSFs in this clinical setting and have led to therapeutic trials [5].

Clinical Characteristics of Patients with MDS

Patients with MDS have characteristic clinical features which include chronic cytopenias and cellular dysfunction with dysplastic morphologic features. Patients with these disorders are at increased risk for infection, bleeding, symptomatic anemia, as well as transformation to AML [6-8]. This disorder has been subclassified by marrow morphologic criteria (mainly the proportion of marrow blasts) into five sub-types by the French-American-British (FAB) group which are useful for prognostic purposes[9]. These subtypes include refractory anemia (RA), refractory anemia with ringed sideroblasts (RARS), refractory anemia with excess blasts (RAEB), RAEB in transformation (RAEB-T) and chronic myelomonocytic leukemia (CMML). Some authors have suggested that CMML more likely belongs in the group of myeloproliferative disorders [10]. Patients with RA and RARS generally have a median survival of 2-4 years, a low incidence of evolution to AML, and often die of diseases unrelated to MDS [11-13]. In contrast, those patients with RAEB, RAEB-T and CMML have a very poor prognosis with median survival of 6-12 months, with approximately 50% of such patients evolving into AML. Recently a more refined prognostic scoring system has been developed which takes into consideration other biological considerations such as chromosome abnormalites and cytopenias in addition to the percentage of bone marrow blasts [14].

MDS is a disease most commonly seen in elderly patients with >70% of patients over the age of 60. Males and females are affected equally. The incidence of this disease has been estimated to be approximately 4 cases per 100,000 individuals. However, this incidence is increasing due to the advancing age of the population in the U.S. and Western Europe. The cause of this disorder is not known, however, it has been speculated that unrepaired damage to DNA may play an important role. Chromosomal abnormalities are common in MDS patients and are found in 40-70% of these individuals [15]. These abnormalities typically involve chromosomes 5, 7 or 8, with monosomy 5, 5q-, monosomy 7 and trisomy 8 being the most common findings. However, a variety of other chromosomal abnormalities have been found in these patients. Evidence of clonality has been demonstrated in MDS patients by X-linked genetic analysis including restriction fragment length polymorphism studies, as well as by cytogenetics and in-vitro culture [16].

Patients with MDS are often diagnosed following a routine blood test or one performed for non-specific complaints. Patients can present with isolated cytopenias or pancytopenia which typically prompts a bone marrow examination. This usually demonstrates a hypercellular bone marrow with evidence of dysplasia in at least two of the hematopoietic cell lines on the bone marrow aspirate. The clinical complications of MDS patients are typical of the patient's dominant cytopenia and include infections, bleeding and anemia. Red blood cell (RBC) transfusional needs are common, as well as antibiotic and platelet support in a lesser percentage of patients. In addition to the cytopenias, MDS patients often have abnormally functioning neutrophils, platelets and RBCs[17].

Therapy for MDS

Therapeutic options for patients with MDS are limited. The only curative approach has been allogeneic bone marrow transplantation in selected patients. In these studies approximately 40% of eligible patients enjoy long term control of their disease [18]. The advanced age of most patients with this disorder makes this impractical for many MDS patients. However, recent successes in transplanting older patients as well as the growth of the National Marrow Donor Program (NMDP) has increased options for MDS patients[19]. Cytotoxic chemotherapy has been employed for patients who show signs of evolution to AML, but with generally poor results. Newer topoisomerase-1 interacting drugs such as topotecan have resulted in clinical responses in some patients [20]. Various agents such as pyridoxine, androgens, danazol and corticosteroids have been used with limited benefit in a small proportion of patients [21,22]. Low-dose cytarabine and retinoids have been widely studied, but have not been shown to improve survival in clinical trials, including several randomized studies [23-25]. The standard approach for the treatment of MDS patients has been supportive.

Rationale for the Use of CSFs in MDS

The chronic cytopenias which characterize this disorder have led to the consideration of CSFs for the treatment of MDS. The major questions include not only whether patients will respond to these agents with an improvement in blood counts, but more importantly, will patients derive clinical benefit with a decreased need for transfusions and risk of infection. Central to the use of CSFs in MDS is concern whether such treatment alters the pace of disease progression towards AML.

Hematologic effects of G-CSF treatment of MDS patients.

G-CSF has been administered by both intravenous (IV) infusion and subcutaneous (SC) injection. We have utilized E. coli derived (non-glycosylated) G-CSF employing the SC route to treat patients with primary MDS since chronic administration of the drug is likely to be required for this disease. In the initial phase I/II dose-escalation study, the G-CSF was administered by daily SC injection at dosage levels between 0.1-3.0 µg/kg/d until a neutrophil response was demonstrated [26]. In this study of 18 patients, sixteen had a rise in WBC (two to 10-fold) and absolute neutrophil count (ANC; five to 40-fold). This was noted even among the eleven patients who were severely neutropenic (ANC <500/mm^3). In most patients, responses were seen at dosage levels between 0.3-1.0 µg/kg/d. Upon discontinuation of the G-CSF injections, blood counts returned to pre-treatment baseline values in all patients after a two to four week period.

A longer term study was performed to determine whether these responses could be sustained[27]. Eleven patients were treated with the dose of G-CSF required to maintain an ANC>1,800/mm^3 for six monthly periods. Following the initial dose-escalation trial, the blood counts returned to their pre-treatment levels. The G-CSF was re-started, again by daily SC injection, resulting in a rapid rise in WBC count and ANC. After six months, the G-CSF was discontinued and again the blood counts returned to their pre-treatment values, yet could be improved again by re-treatment.

Ten of the 11 patients enrolled in the maintenance phase study responded to the G-CSF with a normalization of the ANC. These effects could be maintained for prolonged periods up to several years. In six patients, the G-CSF was stopped after six months of treatment and in all patients the blood counts returned to pre-treatment levels. Red blood cell responses were also noted in four of the 10 anemic patients where two non-transfusion dependent patients had a greater than 20% rise in hematocrit and two more severely anemic, RBC transfusion dependent patients had a decrease in RBC requirements. Only a single patient had a sustained rise in platelet count. Other groups have also utilized G-CSF to treat patients with MDS. In an initial report of five patients treated with IV G-CSF, all patients had a short-term rise in ANC[28]. A second report of 41 patients, demonstrated that most responded with a rise in ANC following the IV administration of G-CSF[29]. In these studies, the G-CSF was derived from Chinese hamster ovary (CHO) cells and was glycosylated. The dose required for a response was generally between 2-5 μ/kg/d. Patients were treated for 14 days and no patient converted to AML over this short treatment period. In these studies, the response was limited to elevations of the WBC and primarily neutrophils. Several of the patients had resolution of active infections during treatment.

G-CSF has been extremely well tolerated even when administered chronically over long periods of time. The major toxicity associated with treatment with G-CSF has been bone pain. The SC injection of G-CSF has been self-administered in an outpatient setting. Several thrombocytopenic patients developed mild and tolerable ecchymoses at the injection sites. One patient with a history of psoriasis developed a flare of her skin disease while receiving G-CSF who had an elevated WBC count. This was severe enough to require discontinuation of the G-CSF, whereupon the psoriasis resolved [26]. Serum samples have indicated that no patient developed antibodies to G-CSF, including those individuals who transformed to AML.

To more definitively evaluate the in vivo effects of G-CSF a multi-center randomized Phase III clinical trial was performed. Patients with high risk MDS (RAEB and RAEBT) were randomly assigned to receive either G-CSF or to be observed. The dose of G-CSF was adjusted to maintain a normal ANC and the drug was administered by a daily SC injection. No crossover was allowed in this study. 102 patients were randomized, 70 with RAEB and 32 with RAEBT. The median ANC prior to treatment was <0.8 X 10^9/L in both groups. ANC responses were noted in all patients who received G-CSF wihin 2-3 weeks and the median ANC was >4 X 10^9/L. There was no change in the observation arm. Importantly, there were no significant differences in transformation to AML in either group and overall survival in the RAEBT patients was not different [30]. In the RAEB patients there was worse survival in the G-CSF treated group with an increase in non-leukemic disease-related deaths. In retrospect, this increased mortality was likely due to a higher proportion of high-risk RAEB patients in the treatment arm [30]. These results, although disappointing, demonstrate the safety of administering G-CSF to MDS patients with respect to the risk of transformation and underscore the need to perform randomized clinical trials to assess efficacy in this often variable and challenging disease. The use of G-CSF to treat those patients with MDS who develop an infection has not been extensively studied.

Hematologic effects of GM-CSF in MDS patients

GM-CSF has also been widely studied in MDS patients and a number of trials have been reported[31-35]. In the initial study of eight patients a dose range of 30-500 µg/m2/d was utilized by continuous intravenous infusion. A marked increase in peripheral blood leucocytes, particularly granulocytes of 5 to 373 fold was noted [32]. Three of the patients also had a rise in platelets which has not been reproduceably observed in other studies. The effects lasted for as long as the growth factor was administered. In a subsequent report a patient with therapy-related MDS who was transfusion dependent and thrombocytopenic had a complete remission following the treatment with GM-CSF including normalization of a cytogenetic abnormality [36]. These types of responses are unusual and the majority of patients who are treated with CSFs maintain the cytogenetic abnormalities and evidence for clonal hematopoiesis following therapy.

A number of other phase I/II trials have confirmed and extended these initial results. The majority of patients do have a hematologic response to GM-CSF therapy at surprisingly low doses of CSF. Both intravenous and subcutaneous dosing is effective with the later slightly better due to the longer bioavailibility of the growth factor following injection [37]. A study randomized between two different dosage levels from the EORTC Leukemia Cooperative Group found an identical response rate between a dosage of 108 vs 216 µg/kg/d over an eight week period [38].

A phase III randomized study with GM-CSF has been performed and reported in abstract form. In this study a cross-over design was utilized making it impossible to evaluate the effect of GM-CSF therapy on overall survival and progression of disease. This study was limited to patients who had <15% BM blasts and were therefore, at a relatively low risk of transformation to acute leukemia. Most patients who received GM-CSF had a rise in their neutrophil counts and a decreased incidence of infections were noted [39]. Because of the somewhat disappointing results from the randomized trials with both G-CSF and GM-CSF further testing of these agents in this disease has not been aggressively pursued. A critical question is whether those patients with MDS who develop infections would benefit from growth factor therapy has not been addressed.

Interleukin-3

Interleukin-3 (IL-3) has also been used to treat MDS patients in a limited number of patients over short treatment periods. Modest improvements in neutrophils were noted. A small number of patients also appeared to have transient increases in RBCs and platelets [40, 41]. These studies suggested that IL-3 may have biological activity in patients with MDS. However, the neutrophil responses were not as dramatic as observed with G-CSF or GM-CSF and effects on other cell lineages were modest.

Interleukin-6

Interleukin-6 (IL-6) was evaluated in one study of patients with MDS who had relatively low platelet counts (<100,000/µ?L) aqnd <5% BM blasts. Dosing was between 1-5 µg/kg/d given by subcutaneous injection. The maximally tolerated dose was found to be 3.75 µg/kg/d and all patients developed at least grade II fever. Eight patients (36%) had at least a transient improvement in platelet counts, however, toxicity has precluded further evaluation [42].

Erythropoietin

A large number of studies have been reported evaluating the effects of erythropoietin (EPO) on the ineffective RBC production which is characteristic of MDS patients. A variety of doses and schedules have been employed with generally disappointing results. To further evaluate the role of EPO therapy in MDS patients a meta-analysis has been performed of 17 studies which included 205 patients [43]. In this analysis 33 (16%) of patients were found to respond to EPO therapy. Those patients with RARS were less likely to respond as were patients with transfusional needs. The serum EPO level was also found to be significantly lower in responding patients but this alone could not be used to predict which patients who were most likely to respond. However, in patients with RARS who had a serum EPO level >200 U/L there were no responses. In another study, serum tumor necrosis factor levels were found to be predictive of those patients who were more likely to respond to EPO therapy [44].

Combination therapy of MDS patients

In vitro erythroid clonal growth in MDS demonstrated suboptimal responses of MDS erythroid precursors to EPO [5]. Analysis of the relationship between EPO levels in MDS and patients' erythroid progenitors suggested that the anemia was not due to an abnormality in the capacity of EPO to induce generation of CFU-E but was more likely influenced by the size of the BFU-E population [45]. These findings, which were consistent with the above discussed clinical studies, suggested that treatment of MDS patients with EPO alone was unlikely to have clinical benefit. We have demonstrated that G-CSF augments the in vitro EPO responsiveness of BFU-E in MDS [46]. Due to this synergy a phase II clinical trial was initiated using both G-CSF and EPO to treat MDS patients and 55 patients were treated [47]. Fifty three patients (96%) had a neutrophil response. Forty four patients were evaluable for an erythroid response and 21 (48%) responded with either an increase in hemoglobin level or a decrease in transfusion requirements. Erythroid responses were significantly more likely to occur in patients with relatively low serum erythropoietin levels[48]. To determine whether true in vivo synergy occurs between these two growth factors 17 patients who had responded for at least an 8 week maintenance phase had the G-CSF discontinued. All patients lost their neutrophil response, however, eight continued to have an erythroid response to erythropoietin alone [47]. In 7/9 of the remaining patients resumption of G-CSF was required for recurrent erythroid responses. A representative response to combination therapy is shown in Figure 1.

A similar study was performed by Hellstrom and colleagues who treated an additional 21 patients in whom 38% had an erythroid response [49]. The data from these two studies were analyzed together in an effort to determine which patients were most likely to respond to combined therapy with G-CSF and EPO. These results indicated that those patients with low serum epo levels (<100 U/L) and low RBC transfusion requirements (<2 units/month) had a 74% response rate to the combined therapy [50]. In contrast, those patients who had high serum epo levels (>500 U/L) and high RBC transfusion requirements (>2 units/month) had only a 10% chance of responding to combination therapy. The responses were quite durable in some patients [47, 51]. These data suggest that combination therapy with G-CSF + EPO may improve not only the neutropenia but also the anemia associated with this disorder in some MDS patients.

GM-CSF has also been combined with EPO with a similar response rate of 46% noted. Some of these responders also required both growth factors for maintaining a response suggesting a synergism between these two drugs [52]. The beneficial effects of combined therapy have been questioned however, in a small study of 10 patients where only two responded to these two drugs [53].

Aplastic Anemia (AA)

Patients with AA are at a dramatically increased risk of infection and bleeding. There are many causes of this disorder ranging from exposure to chemicals or drugs to infectious agents, however, the majority of patients present with idopathic disease. The appoach to the patient with AA is beyond the scope of this review, however, bone marrow transplantation has been extremely effective for those young patients who have HLA-matched sibling donors [54]. Other therapeutic approachs include the use of immunosuppressive drugs in the form of anti-thymocyte globulin (ATG) with cyclosporine-A and corticosteroids. Growth factor therapy has also been pursued for patients with AA especially for those with more moderate forms of the disease.

GM-CSF and G-CSF

The first patients with AA were treated with GM-CSF over a decade ago. In the initial study of 10 patients with moderate to severe disease a rise in WBC (1.6 to 10 fold) was noted in all of the patients [55]. In these patients the increase in WBC was mainly due to an increase in neutrophils and eosinophils. Similar results were reported for an additional 6 of 8 patients and no changes in RBC transfusional needs nor platelet counts were noted [35]. Early on it was noted that those patients who were more likely to respond were those with less severe disease [56, 57]. Similar responses were noted in children with AA [58, 59]. In one study very high doses of G-CSF of between 400 to 2,000 $\mu g/m^2/d$ were utilized for 4 weeks. Six of 10 patients had from a 10 to 60 fold increase in neutrophil counts with evidence for clinical efficacy as judged by the resolution of bacterial or fungal infections which were present prior to growth factor therapy [60]. Despite these responses most were in patients with mild to moderate disease and responses were only durable for the duration of CSF therapy. Because of this the role of CSF therapy in patients with moderate to severe AA was questioned [61], and it was recommended that CSF therapy be used only in conjunction with immunosuppressive therapy or for support while searching for a BMT donor.

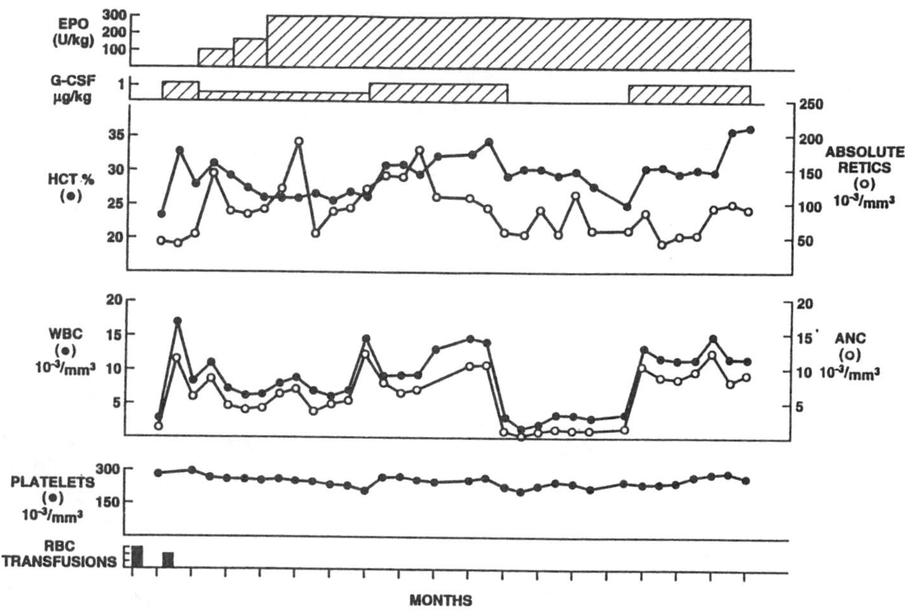

Figure 1. Clinical course of a patient treated with G-CSF/EPO combination therapy demonstrating that both drugs are required for a sustained red blood cell response. (Reprinted with permission from ref. #47)

Interleukin-3

IL-3 has also been explored in patients with AA. The hypothesis is that this CSF has broader biological activity and may help ameliorate the other cytopenias that these patients experience. In this first report nine patients with AA were treated with IL-3 between the dosages of 250-500 $\mu g/m^2$ administered as a subcutaneous injection daily for 15 days. Only one patient had a sustained increase in platelet count and four patients had an increase in reticulocyte counts [62]. The effects were again transient and mild side effects were observed. An addtional study of patients with AA were treated with escalating doses of IL-3 of between 0.5-10 $\mu g/kg/d$. A planned 21 day cycle was administered however, two patients could not complete this amount of therapy due to intolerable side effects. Multilineage effects were noted in only 5 or 20 evaluable patients [63]. Another study of 15 patients with refractory AA were treated with IL-3. Increases in neutrophil counts were noted in 9 of 16 patients treated at doses of between 4-16 $\mu g/kg/d$, however, these were not sustained and were associated with significant toxicity [64].

Interleukin-6

IL-6 has also been utilized in small numbers of patients with AA. In one study of 10 patients with AA whom had failed immunosuppressive therapy and were not candidates for BMT IL-6 was given as a subcutaneous injection for 28 days at doses ranging from 0.5 to 5 μg/kg. Only a single patient had a sustained increase in platelet count and therapy was associated with significant toxicity which required early discontinuation of the study [65]. IL-6 has not been pursued further in this disorder.

Combination Therapy of G-CSF with EPO in AA

Since only rare patients experienced multilineage effects with G-CSF alone studies have been performed using G-CSF in combination with EPO in an effort to stimulate multilineage hematopoiesis. A randomized study was performed which enrolled 131 patients who were treated with G-CSF either alone or in combination with two dosages of EPO. Fourteen of 38 (36.8%) patients treated with G-CSF and the higher dose of EPO (400 IU/kg for 12 weeks) as compared to <15% for the other two groups (p<0.05). The significant effects of EPO administration were primarily observed in those patients with non-severe AA [66].

Combination of CSFs with Immunosuppressive Therapy in Patients with AA

Due to the relatively modest effects of CSFs on their own a number of investigators have explored the role of CSFs as supportive therapy in those patients who are undergoing treatment with immunosuppression. The rationale for this approach is the risk of infectious complications that patients with severe AA exerience when undergoing therapy with immunosuppressive drugs. In one study of 40 patients with newly diagnosed untreated severe AA (ANC<0.5 X 10 ^{9}/L) G-CSF at a dose of 5 μg/kg/d was added to standard therapy with horse ALG, cyclosporine, and prednisone. The G-CSF was continued for 90 days. In this study 33 (82%) of patients had trilineage hematopoietic reconstitution and there were only three early deaths due to infection [67]. The G-CSF was well tolerated. A similar approach was employed in the treatment of seven children with newly diagnosed severe AA using GM-CSF at a dose of 5 μg/kg/d. All patients responded within 3.5 months of diagnosis and treatment was well tolerated [68]. IL-3 has been used in a similar fashion with good results when utilized at a dosage of 250 μg/m2/d [69]. These studies have demonstrated that growth factor therapy is likely a useful adjunct to immunosuppressive therapy especially in those patients with severe AA who are at significant risk of infection.

Toxicity of CSF Therapy

Both G-CSF and GM-CSF have been reported to cause bone pain in patients with AA as well as low grade fever mainly in the patients who were treated with GM-CSF. In addition, some unusual side effects have also been observed. These include the report of an adult patient and a child who developed Sweet's Syndrome (febrile neutrophilic dermatosis) while being treated with G-CSF [70, 71]. In addition, AML has developed in a case of aplastic anemia following G-CSF therapy, however, it is often difficult to be certain that this patient didn't have hypoplastic MDS [72].

Other Bone Marrow Failure States

CSFs have also been evaluated in patients with other forms of bone marrow failure. Fanconi's anemia is a congenital disorder characterized by multiple physical anomalies, progressive bone marrow failure and a predilection for developing acute leukemia. Both G-CSF and GM-CSF have been utilized in the treatment of this disorder. In these relatively small studies increases in neutrophils were noted in the majority of patients who were treated [73-75]. These studies suggested that these agents were safe to use and potentially effective in the treatment of neutropenia in patients with this disorder, however, the benefits were limited to the time when the drug was administered.

Patients with Diamond-Blackfan anemia (DBA) have also been treated with CSFs. In the initial small study of six transfusion-dependent, steroid-unresponsive patients with this disorder three patients had an increase in reticulocyte counts following the administration of GM-CSF but only one had a reduction in transfusion requirement. These same six patients were then treated with IL-3 and three had an increase in reticulocyte count two of whom had a reduction in transfusion requirements. One of these two patients remained transfusion independent for over a year since the completion of IL-3 therapy [76]. These data suggested that IL-3 may have a role in the treatment of patients with DBA and further investigation was pursued. In a larger study of 18 patients with DBA four patients experienced a clinically significant erythroid response following IL-3 therapy which was dose-escalated from 0.5-10 ?g/kg/d. Two patients had prolonged responses to the IL-3 therapy [77]. A large multicenter European study reported on the treatment of 40 DBA patients with IL-3. The IL-3 was begun at 2.5 µg/kg/d and dose-escalated every 21 days to 5 and then 10 µg/kg/d for a total duration of 12 weeks. Five patients had significant response (2 adults and 3 children), however, the responses in the adults was transient and not well tolerated [78]. Responses were noted in those patients who achieved some prior response to steroids suggesting a possible role for IL-3 treatment in this disorder.

A number of other isolated instances of BM failure following drug treatment have been treated with CSFs. These case reports include patients treated with methimazole, gold and ticlopidine who developed severe aplastic anemia and then responded to CSF therapy in the form of G-CSF or GM-CSF [79-81].

Conclusions

CSFs have dramatic effects on hematopoiesis in a variety of clinical settings. In patients with MDS and BM failure states responses have been noted some of which are multilineage and dramatic. Despite these responses there is little evidence that CSF therapy has a major impact on the clinical course of these diverse and often refractory disorders. In addition, the lessions learned from larger randomized clinical trials are extremely important where clear hematopoietic responses were noted in the majority of patients, however, were not associated with demonstrable clinical benefits. Newer

CSFs such as kit-ligand or stem cell factor, flt-3 ligand and thrombopoietin will be of interest in these disorders either as single agents or in combination with other CSFs.

References

1. Rajapaksa R, Ginzton N, Rott LS, Greenberg PL. Altered oncogene expression and apoptosis in myelodysplastic syndrome marrow cells. Blood 88:4275-4287, 1996.
2. Miyauchi J, Kelleher CA, Yang YC, et al. The effects of the three recombinant growth factors, IL3, GM-CSF and G-CSF on the blast cells of acute myeloblastic leukemia maintained in short-term suspension culture. Blood 76:657-663, 1987.
3. Metcalf D. The molecular biology and functions of the granulocyte-macrophage colony-stimulating factors. Blood 67:257-267, 1986.
4. Vellenga E, Young DC, Wagner K, et al. The effects of GM-CSF and G-CSF in promoting growth of clonogenic cells in acute myelogenous leukemia. Blood 69:1771-1776, 1987.
5. Greenberg PL. In vitro culture studies in myelodysplastic syndromes. Semin Oncol 19:34-46, 1992.
6. Greenberg PL. The smoldering myeloid leukemic states: clinical and biological features. Blood 61:1035-1044, 1983.
7. Block M, Jacobson LO, Bethard WF. Preleukemic acute leukemia. JAMA 152:1018-1021, 1953.
8. Linman JW, Bagby GCJ. The preleukemic syndrome (hematopoietic dysplasia). Cancer 1978 42:854-864.
9. Bennett JM, Catovsky D, Daniel MT, et al. Proposals for the classification of the myelodysplastic syndromes. Br J Haematol 51:189-199, 1982.
10. Gosquen JE, Bennett JM. Classification and morphologic features of the myelodysplastic syndromes. Sem Oncol 19:4-13, 1992.
11. Mufti GJ, Stevens JR, Oscier DG, et al. Myelodysplastic syndromes: a scoring system with prognostic significance. Br J Haematol 59:425-433, 1985.
12. Kerhofs N, Hermans J, Haak HL, et al. Utility of the FAB classification for myelodysplastic syndromes: investigation of prognostic factors in 237 cases. Br J Haematol 65:73-81, 1987.
13. Foucar K, Langdon RM, Armitage JO, et al. Myelodysplastic syndromes: A clinical and pathological analysis of 109 cases. Cancer 56:553-561, 1985.
14. Greenberg P, Cox L, LeBeau MM, et al. International scoring system for evaluating prognosis in myelodysplastic syndromes. Blood 89:2079-2088, 1997
15. Nowell PC. Chromosome abnormalities in myelodysplastic syndromes. Sem Oncol 19:25-33, 1992.
16. Greenberg PL. In vitro culture techniques defining the biologic abnormalities in the myelodysplastic syndromes and myeloproliferative disoreders. Clinics in Haematol 15:973-993, 1986.
17. Boogaerts MA, Nelissen V, Roeland C, Goossens W. Blood neutrophil function in primary myelodysplastic syndromes. Br J Haematol 55:217-227, 1983.
18. Anderson JE, Appelbaum FR, Fisher LD, et al. Allogeneic bone marrow transplantation for 93 patients with myelodysplastic syndrome. Blood 82:677-681, 1993.
19. Anderson JE, Anasetti C, Appelbaum FR, et al. Unrelated donor marrow transplantation for myelodysplasia (MDS) and MDS-related acute myeloid leukaemia. Br J Haematol 93:59-67, 1996.
20. Beran M, Kantarjian H, O'Brien S, et al. Topotecan, a topoisomerase I inhibitor, is active in the treatment of myelodysplastic syndrome and chronic myelomonocytic leukemia. Blood 88:2473-2479, 1996.
21. Cines DB, Cassileth PA, Kiss JE. Danazol therapy in myelodysplasia. Ann Intern Med 103:58-60, 1985.
22. Bagby GGJ, Gabourel JD, Linman JW. Glucocorticoid therapy in the preleukemic syndrome (hemopoietic dysplasia): identification of responsive patients using in-vitro techniques. Ann Int Med 92:55-58, 1980.
23. Cheson BD, Jasperse DM, Simon R, Freidman MA. A critical appraisal of low-dose cytosine arabinoside in patients with acute non-lymphocytic leukemia and myelodysplastic syndromes. J Clin Oncol 4:1857-1864, 1986.
24. Griffin JD, Spriggs D, Wisch JS, D.W. K. Treatment of preleukemic syndromes with continuous intravenous infusion of low-dose cytosine arabinoside. J Clin Oncol 3:982-991, 1985.
25. Tricot G, DeBock R, Dekker AW, et al. Low dose arabinoside (Ara-C) in myelodysplastic syndromes.

Br J Haematol 58:231-240, 1984.

26. Negrin RS, Haeuber DH, Nagler A, et al. Treatment of myelodysplastic syndromes with recombinant human granulocyte colony-stimulating factor. A phase I-II trial. Ann Int Med 110:976-984, 1989.

27. Negrin RS, Haeuber DH, Nagler A, et al. Maintenance treatment of patients with myelodysplastic syndromes using recombinant human granulocyte colony-stimulating factor. Blood 76:36-43, 1990.

28. Kobayashi Y, Okabe T, Ozawa K, et al. Treatment of myelodysplastic syndromes with recombinant human granulocyte colony-stimulating factor: A preliminary report. Am J Med 86:178-182, 1989.

29. Yoshida Y, Hirashima K, Asano S, Takaku F. A phase II trial of recombinant human granulocyte colony-stimulating factor in the myelodysplastic syndromes. Br J Haematol 78:378-384, 1991.

30. Greenberg P, Taylor K, Larson R, et al. Phase III randomized multicenter trial of G-CSF vs observation for myelodysplastic syndromes (MDS). Blood 82 suppl 1:196a., 1993

31. Thompson JA, Lee DJ, Kidd P, et al. Subcutaneous granulocyte-macrophage colony-stmulating factor in patients with myelodysplastic syndrome: Toxicity, pharmacokinetics and hematological effects. J Clin Oncol 7:629-637, 1989.

32. Vadhan-Raj S, Keating M, LeMaistre A, et al. Effects of recombinant human granulocyte-macrophage colony-stimulating factor in patients with myelodysplastic syndromes. N Engl J Med 317:1545-1552, 1987.

33. Herrmann F, Lindemann A, Klein H, et al. Effect of recombinant granulocyte-macrophage colony-stimulating factor in patients with myelodysplastic syndrome with excess blasts. Leukemia 3:335-338, 1989.

34. Ganser A, Volkers B, Greher J, et al. Recombinant human granulocyte-macrophage colony-stimulating factor in patients with myelodysplastic syndromes. Blood 73:31-37, 1989.

35. Antin JH, Smith BR, Holmes W, et al. Phase I/II study of recombinant granulocyte-macrohage colony-stimulating factor in aplastic anemia and myelodysplastic syndrome. Blood 72:705-713, 1988.

36. Vadhan-Raj S, Broxmeyer HE, Spitzer G, et al. Stimulation of nonclonal hematopoiesis and suppression of the neoplastic clone after treatment with recombinant human granulocyte-macrophage colony-stimulating factor in a patient with therapy-related myelodysplastic syndrome. Blood 74:1491-1498, 1989.

37. Rosenfeld CS, Sulecki M, Evans C, Shadduck RK. Comparison of intravenous versus subcutaneouus recombinant human granulocyte-macrophage colony-stimulating factor in patients with primary myelodysplasia. Exp Hematol 19:272-277, 1991.

38. Willemze R, van der Lely N, Zwierzina H, et al. A randomized phase-I/II multicenter study of recombinant human granulocyte-macrophage colony-stimulating factor (GM-CSF) therapy for patients with myelodysplastic syndromes and a relatively low risk of acute leukemia. EORTC Leukemia Cooperative Group. Ann Hematol 64:173-180, 1992.

39. Schuster MW, Thompson JA, Larson RA, et al. Randomized trial of subcutaneous granulocyte-macrophage colony-stimulating factor in patients with myelodysplastic syndrome or aplastic anemia. Proc Am Soc Clin Oncol A793, 1990.

40. Kuzrock R, Talpaz M, Estrov Z, et al. Phase I study of recombinant human interleukin-3 in patients with bone marrow failure. J Clin Oncol 9:1241-1250, 1991.

41. Ganser A, Seipelt G, Lindemann A, et al. Effects of recombinant human interleukin-3 in patients with myelodysplastic syndromes. Blood 76:455-462, 1990.

42. Gordon MS, Nemunaitis J, Hoffman R, et al. A phase I trial of recombinant human interleukin-6 in patients with myelodysplastic syndromes and thrombocytopenia. Blood 85:3066-3076, 1995.

43. Hellstrom-Lindberg E. Efficacy of erythropoietin in the myelodysplastic syndromes: a meta-analysis of 205 patients from 17 studies. Br J Haematol 89:67-71, 1995.

44. Stasi R, Brunetti M, Bussa S, et al. Serum levels of tumour necrosis factor-alpha predict response to recombinant human erythropoietin in patients with myelodysplastic syndrome. Clin Lab Haematol 19:197-201, 1997.

45. Merchav S, Nielson OJ, Rosenbaum H, et al. In vitro studies of erythropoietin-dependent regulation of erythropoiesis in myelodysplastic syndromes. Leukemia 4:771-774, 1990.

46. Greenberg PL, Negrin RS, Ginzton NL. G-CSF synergizes with erythropoietin for enhancing erythroid colony-formation in myelodysplastic syndromes. Blood 78(suppl1):38a, 1991.

47. Negrin RS, Stein R, Doherty K, et al. Maintenance treatment of the anemia of myelodysplastic syndromes with recombinant human granulocyte colony-stimulating factor and erythropoietin: evidence for in vivo synergy. Blood 87:4076-4081, 1996.

48. Negrin RS, Stein R, Vardiman J, et al. Treatment of the anemia of myelodysplastic syndromes using recombinant human granulocyte colony-stimulating factor in combination with erythropoietin. Blood

82:737-743, 1993.

49. Hellstrom-Lindberg E, Birgegard G, Carlsson M, et al. A combination of granulocyte colony-stimulating factor and erythropoietin may synergistically improve the anaemia in patients with myelodysplastic syndromes. Leuk Lymphoma 11:221-228, 1993.

50. Hellstrom-Lindberg E, Negrin RS, Stein R, et al. Erythroid response to treatment with G-CSF plus erythropoietin for the anaemia of patients with myelodysplastic syndromes: proposal for a predictive model. Br J Haematol 99:344-351, 1997.

51. Hellstrom-Lindberg E, Ahlgren T, Beguin Y, et al. Treatment of anemia in myelodysplastic syndromes with granulocyte colony-stimulating factor plus erythropoietin: results from a randomized phase II study and long-term follow-up of 71 patients. Blood 92:68-75, 1998.

52. Bernell P, Stenke L, Wallvik J, Hippe E, Hast R. A sequential erythropoietin and GM-CSF schedule offers clinical benefits in the treatment of anaemia in myelodysplastic syndromes. Leuk Res 20:693-699, 1996.

53. Runde V, Aul C, Ebert A, Grabenhorst U, Schneider W. Sequential administration of recombinant human granulocyte-macrophage colony-stimulating factor and human erythropoietin for treatment of myelodysplastic syndromes. Eur J Haematol 54:39-45, 1995.

54. Storb R, Leisenring W, Anasetti C, et al. Long-term follow-up of allogeneic marrow transplants in patients with aplastic anemia conditioned by cyclophosphamide combined with antithymocyte globulin. Blood 89:3890-3891, 1997.

55. Vadhan-Raj S, Buescher S, Broxmeyer HE, et al. Stimulation of myelopoiesis in patients with aplastic anemia by recombinant human granulocyte-macrophage colony-stimulating factor. N Engl J Med 319:1628-1634, 1988.

56. Nissen C, Tichelli A, Gratwohl A, et al. Failure of recombinant human granulocyte-macrophage colony-stimulating factor therapy in aplastic anemia patients with very severe neutropenia. Blood 72:2045-2047, 1988.

57. Champlin RE, Nimer SD, Ireland P, Oette DH, Golde DW. Treatment of refractory aplastic anemia with recombinant human granulocyte-macrophage colony-stimulating factor. Blood 73:694-699, 1989.

58. Kojima S, Fukuda M, Miyajima Y, Matsuyama T, Horibe K. Treatment of aplastic anemia in children with recombinant human granulocyte colony-stimulating factor. Blood 77:937-941, 1991.

59. Guinan EC, Sieff CA, Oette DH, Nathan DG. A phase I/II trial of recombinant granulocyte-macrophage colony-stimulating factor for children with aplastic anemia. Blood 76:1077-1082, 1990.

60. Kojima S, Matsuyama T. Stimulation of granulopoiesis by high-dose recombinant human granulocyte colony-stimulating factor in children with aplastic anemia and very severe neutrophenia. Blood 83:1474-1478, 1994.

61. Marsh JC, Socie G, Schrezenmeier H, et al. Haemopoietic growth factors in aplastic anaemia: a cautionary note. European Bone Marrow Transplant Working Party for Severe Aplastic Anaemia. Lancet 344:172-173, 1994.

62. Ganser A, Lindemann A, Seipelt G, et al. Effects of recombinant human interleukin-3 in aplastic anemia. Blood 76:1287-1292, 1990.

63. Nimer SD, Pacquette RL, Ireland P, Resta D, Young D, Golde DW. A phase I/II study of interleukin-3 in patients with aplastic anemia and myelodysplasia. Exp Hematol 22:875-880, 1994.

64. Bargetzi MJ, Gluckman E, Tichelli A, et al. Recombinant human interleukin-3 in refractory severe aplastic anaemia: a phase I/II trial. Br J Haematol 91:306-312, 1995.

65. Schrezenmeier H, Marsh JC, Stromeyer P, et al. A phase I/II trial of recombinant human interleukin-6 in patients with aplastic anemia. Br J Haematol 90:283-292, 1995.

66. Bessho M, Hirashima K, Asano S, et al. Treatment of the anemia of aplastic anemia patients with recombinant erythropoietin in combination with granulocyte colony-stimulating factor: a multicenter randomized controlled trial. Multicenter Study Group. Eur J Haematol 58:265-272, 1997.

67. Bacigalupo A, Broccia G, Corda G, et al. Antilymphocyte globulin, cyclosporine, and granulocyte colony-stimulating factor in patients with acquired severe aplastic anemia (SAA): a pilot study of the EBMT SAA Working Party. Blood 85:1348-1353, 1995.

68. Hord JD, Gay JC, Whitlock JA, et al. Long-term granulocyte-macrophage colony-stimulating factor and immunosuppression in the treatment of acquired severe aplastic anemia. J Pediatr Hematol Oncol 17:140-144, 1995.

69. Raghavachar A, Ganser A, Freund M, Heimpel H, Herrmann F, Schrezenmeier H. Long-term interleukin-3 and intensive immunosuppression in the treatment of aplastic anemia. Cytokines Mol Ther 2:215-223, 1996.

70. Shimizu T, Yoshida I, Eguchi H, Takahashi K, Inada H, Kato H. Sweet syndrome in a child with aplastic anemia receiving recombinant granulocyte colony-stimulating factor. J Pediatr Hematol Oncol 18:282-284, 1996.
71. Fukutoku M, Shimizu S, Ogawa Y, et al. Sweet's syndrome during therapy with granulocyte colony-stimulating factor in a patient with aplastic anaemia. Br J Haematol 86:645-648, 1994.
72. Izumi T, Muroi K, Takatoku M, Imagawa S, Hatake K, Miura Y. Development of acute myeloblastic leukaemia in a case of aplastic anaemia treated with granulocyte colony-stimulating factor. Br J Haematol 87:666-668, 1994.
73. Kemahli S, Canatan D, Uysal Z, Akar N, Cin S, Arcasoy A. GM-CSF in the treatment of Fanconi's anaemia. Br J Haematol 87:871-872, 1994.
74. Rackoff WR, Orazi A, Robinson CA, et al. Prolonged administration of granulocyte colony-stimulating factor (filgrastim) to patients with Fanconi anemia: a pilot study. Blood 88:1588-1593, 1996.
75. Guinan EC, Lopez KD, Huhn RD, Felser JM, Nathan DG. Evaluation of granulocyte-macrophage colony-stimulating factor for treatment of panyctopenia in children with fanconi anemia. J Pediatr 124:144-150, 1994.
76. Dunbar CE, Smith DA, Kimball J, Garrison L, Nienhuis AW, Young NS. Treatment of Diamond-Blackfan anaemia with hematopoietic growth factors, granulocyte-macrophage colony stimulating factor and interleukin-3: sustained remissions following IL-3. Br J Haematol 79:316-321, 1991.
77. Gillio AP, Faulkner LB, Alter BP, et al. Treatment of Diamond-Blackfan anemia with recombinant human interleukin-3. Blood 82:744-751, 1993.
78. Ball SE, Tchernia G, Wranne L, et al. Is there a role for interleukin-3 in Diamond-Blackfan anaemia? Results of a European multicentre study. Br J Haematol 91:313-318, 1995.
79. Arribalzaga K, Garcia-Suarez J, Lopez-Rubio M, Krsnik I, Calero MA, Del Campo JF. Sustained granulocyte recovery after G-CSF in a patient with ticlopidine-induced severe aplastic anemia. Am J Hematol 50:313, 1995.
80. Chasen MR, Sarembock B, Meyers OL. Successful treatment of gold-induced aplastic anaemia with granulocyte macrophage colony stimulating factor. Br J Rheumatol 31:428-429, 1992.
81. Lopez-Karpovitch X, Ulloa-Aquirre A, von Eiff C, Hurtado-Monroy R, Alanis A. Treatment of methimazole-induced severe aplastic anemia with recombinant human granuloctye-monocyte colony-stimulating factor and corticosteroids. Acta Haematol 87:148-150, 1992.

VII

The Use of Cytokines in Blood and Marrow Transplantation

19. Stem Cell Collection for Hematopoietic Transplantation: Stem Cell Sources, Mobilization Strategies, and Factors that Influence Yield

John R. Wingard, Frederick M. Weeks

Introduction

Over the past decade, it has become clear that the make-up of the stem cell product used in hematopoietic transplantation is one of the most important determinants of transplant outcome. The number of hematopoietic progenitor cells (HPC) is the major determinant of the speed of hematopoietic reconstitution and thereby a strong influence on the length of transplant hospitalization, the amount of resources needed to provide supportive care for the period of iatrogenic marrow failure, and the risk of treatment-related mortality. Both numbers and types of immune cells in the stem cell product also influence the speed and potency of immune reconstitution and the ability of the patient to withstand assault from opportunistic pathogens. In the case of an autologous hematopoietic transplant, contamination by tumor cells admixed with hematopoietic progenitors is strongly associated with the risk for recurrence of the disease for which the transplant is used. In the case of allogeneic hematopoietic transplantation, the presence of large numbers of T lymphocytes influences the risk for graft-versus-host disease (GVHD). With these observations in mind, a number of investigators have evaluated methods to enumerate HPCs, quantify and characterize immune cells, identify presence and number of contaminating tumor cells, and characterize what factors influence the yield of hematopoietic progenitors in the stem cell product.

The number of hematopoietic progenitors in the stem cell product is influenced by patient factors, disease characteristics, and the type and duration of prior treatment. Similarly, the source of stem cells, bone marrow or peripheral blood, influences the progenitor content as well as the types of progenitor cells present. In the case of peripheral blood as the source of stem cells, there are a variety of maneuvers that can be used to mobilize the HPC and these also are important determinants of stem cell yield. The mechanisms of growth factor mobilization are discussed in Section 7, Chapter 2. The data addressing various growth factor mobilizing regimens to enhance collection of stem cells is discussed in Section 7, Chapter 4. In this chapter, stem cell sources, mobilization strategies, and patient, disease, and treatment influences on stem cell collection will be discussed.

Myeloablative Treatment followed by Hematopoietic Reconstitution

During the 1950's, experiments in mice exposed to myeloablative doses of radiation indicated that shielding of the spleen could provide radioprotection. Subsequently, infusions of marrow cells from donors from a different strain had similar hematopoietic restorative properties. These observations were duplicated in other animal species. These experiments provided a basis for transplantation as a treatment for aplastic anemia and other marrow failure diseases. Such findings in animals also led to a consideration of whether very intensive chemoradiotherapy could be of help to individuals with hematologic malignancies by increasing the capacity to give intensive chemotherapy doses and improving the prospects for control of the neoplastic disease. In the late 1950's, patients with leukemia were given myeloablative doses of radiation followed by infusions of marrow cells from healthy donors. Restoration of hematopoietic function was noted two to four weeks later. During the ensuing decades, intensive study has led to refinements of supportive care of patients with marrow failure during the interval between myeloablation and hematopoietic restoration; introduction of tissue typing to permit matching between donor and recipient in the allogeneic transplant setting, development of effective immunosuppressive regimens to prevent both graft rejection and graft-versus-host disease (GVHD), development of techniques for cryopreservation of HPCs in the autologous transplant setting, and refinement of the conditioning regimens used to suppress host immunity and, in the case of neoplasia, provide effective antineoplastic control.

These advances now permit robust restoration of hematopoietic function in patients with marrow failure states or immunodeficiency syndromes (by allogeneic transplantation). The treatment of neoplastic diseases is facilitated by the ability to use dose intensive chemoradiotherapy (by either allogeneic or autologous transplantation) and obviating the threat of life threatening infection or hemorrhage during prolonged marrow failure.

The number of hematopoietic cells required for hematopoietic reconstitution after myeloablative treatment has been clarified in animal experiments. The HPC dose required for engraftment is similar in different animal species. Doses of autologous marrow cells of 10^7 to 10^8 nucleated cells/kg are uniformly effective in restoring hematopoietic function in animals exposed to myeloablative doses after whole body irradiation while higher doses of allogeneic marrow cells (10^8 to 10^9 cells/kg) are required for hematopoietic restoration. In general, there is a factor of 5-15 between the doses of autologous and allogeneic donor cells required for hematopoietic restoration[1].

For many years, bone marrow was the source of HPC used in human transplantation. Although initially there was concern as to the capacity of peripheral blood to provide durable engraftment after myeloablation, experiments in animals and observations in humans indicate robust and enduring hematopoietic reconstitution using blood-derived HPCs. Interest in collection of HPCs from blood has grown since it provides an option for individuals being considered for autologous transplantation where collection of HPCs from the bone marrow is not an option because of marrow fibrosis or tumor involvement. Multiple studies indicate quantitatively fewer tumor cells in peripheral blood than in bone marrow [2].

Enumeration of Hematopoietic Progenitor Cell Content

Several parameters have been used over the years to quantify the HPC content of the stem cell product. The mononuclear or nucleated cell count has been (and continues to be) routinely used for harvesting bone marrow. This parameter is quickly available to the clinician harvesting the stem cells during the procedure and allows the harvester to standardize the product obtained. Typically, the product is characterized as the number of mononuclear cells (MNC) obtained per kilogram of body weight of the recipient. Early studies demonstrated a correlation between rapidity of engraftment with the number of mononuclear cells. An optimal stem cell product consists of a minimum of 3 x 10^8 MNC/kg of recipient body weight in the allogeneic transplant setting (Table 1).

Table 1. Threshold numbers of hematopoietic cells needed for engraftment after transplantation

Allogeneic
Bone marrow   > 3.0 x 10^8 MNC/kg

Peripheral blood   > 3.0 x 10^6 CD34$^+$ cells/kg *

Autologous
Bone marrow   > 1.0 x 10^8 MNC/kg

Peripheral blood   > 2.5 x 10^6 CD34$^+$ cells/kg **

* Currently under study
** A cell dose of > 2.5 x 10^6 CD34$^+$ cells/kg ensures myeloid engraftment but a higher dose of > 5.0 x 10^6 CD34$^+$ cells/kg ensures platelet engraftment

---

Later, similar parameters were developed for autologous bone marrow harvesting. In the absence of an allogeneic barrier, animal transplant experiments demonstrated that fewer MNC were required to rescue animals after lethal irradiation. Similarly, in humans, lower numbers of MNC were found to be required for engraftment in the autologous setting (a minimum of 1 x 10^8 MNC/kg).

With recognition of the tremendous heterogeneity of mononuclear cell populations, more precise estimates of the repopulating potential of mononuclear cells were sought. The ability to grow hematopoietic colony-forming units (CFU) in soft agar led to the development of a wide variety of assays of hematopoietic progenitors. The most commonly used assays to estimate hematopoietic potential have been colony-forming units-granulocyte macrophage (CFU-GM) and burst forming units-erythroid (BFU-E). These assays are not gauges of the true pluripotent stem cell content, but rather measures of differentiated cells. Nevertheless, they have been used widely as measures of progenitor cell content and numerous studies have shown excellent correlation with engraftment in the transplant setting. A threshold dose of >2x10^5 CFU-GM/kg is associated with a high likelihood of engraftment [3-8]. Although, colony growth assays are an improvement over the less precise MNC counts, they have the disadvantage of requiring approximately two weeks for the result of the hematopoietic potential of the stem cell product. Accordingly, the search continued for better techniques to provide answers more quickly.

With the recognition and characterization of immunophenotypic charactistics of HPCs, the advent of monoclonal antibody technology, and the introduction of flow cytometry immunophenotypic assays to enumerate HPCs have been developed. The most commonly used antigen expressed by immature HPCs is the CD34 antigen, present not only on pluripotent stem cells but also on more committed, but still quite immature, HPCs. The CD34[+] cell content correlates well with engraftment[19-23] . Numerous studies have demonstrated a high degree of correlation between CD34[+] cell content and CFU-GM content [19] and both correlate with hematopoietic recovery after myeloablative therapy in the transplant setting. The CD34 assay provides a quantification of HPC content much more rapidly than colony-forming assays, but unfortunately still generally takes several hours for its performance. Accordingly, CD34[+] cell determination is at present not a substitute for MNC assessment for bone marrow harvesting where there is a need to minimize anesthesia time to optimize donor safety. But it is quite satisfactory in peripheral blood progenitors cell (PBPC) collection where the measurement of one day's apheresis yield can be used to determine the need for the subsequent collection the next day. A value of between 2.0 and 2.5×10^6 CD34[+] cells/kg of patient body weight is generally regarded as a threshold dose sufficient to reliably achieve neutrophil engraftment. This number, however, is not sufficient to provide for optimal platelet recovery levels, where up to 5.0×10^6 CD34 cells/kg may be necessary for prompt platelet recovery [13,21-23]. Finally, even in obese patients, ideal body weight appears to be the superior predictor of engraftment of both granulocytes and platelets when compared to actual body weight.

Although the enumeration of HPCs by CD34[+] cell count has become widely used, it is clear that there are methodologic problems with both colony assays and CD34[+] cell counting. Several studies have indicated wide variability in the enumeration by both CD34 [24-29] and CFU-GM [30,31] assays by different laboratories. Efforts are underway to standardize procedures such that results of studies from one center to another can be compared with greater reliability. Further, even among CD34[+] cells which represent only 1-4% of the nucleated cells in the bone marrow, there is tremendous heterogeneity as assessed by other immunophenotypic markers and growth in long-term colony assays. Some studies, but not others, suggest certain CD34[+] subsets, such as CD34[+]/CD33[+] [19] or CD34[+]/CD71[-] [32] cells are better predictors of engraftment than the total CD34[+] cell count. Such observations serve as a reminder that there is much yet to learn and undoubtably more refined assays will be developed in the future to guide optimization of hematopoietic cell content.

Studies using measures of more primitive HPCs have been limited by technologic hurdles. Long-term culture initiating cells (LTC-ICs) are primitive HPCs able to produce clonogenic progenitors of multiple lineages after 5 weeks of culture in the presence of irradiated stroma. LTC-ICs are more primitive than CFU colony assays and copurify with long-term in vivo repopulating cells. They circulate in blood infrequently, but increase after chemotherapy followed by growth factors due to a rebound of CD34[+] cells and CFU-GM coincident with leukocyte recovery. However, the numbers of LTC-ICs do not correlate well with numbers of CFU-GM or CD34[+] cells (or with the speed of engraftment) [33]. Moreover, there is considerable interpatient variability (more than 2 logs) and substantially fewer LTC-ICs are mobilized than CD34[+] cells and CFU-GM[33] . Further, the proliferative potential of the LTC-ICs collected during mobilization seems to be significantly lower than that of either normal donor blood or bone marrow at steady state [33]. In one study [34], LTC-ICs appeared to peak 1-2 days earlier than CD34 cells after G-CSF administration. Using immunophenotypic analyses, CD34[+] Th1+ cells (a population of very primitive CD34 cells) appear earlier in the peripheral blood than Thy 1- cells (more differentiated and less primitive cells) after mobilization [35]. The clinical significance of these observations are not as yet known.

The number and type of HPCs vary according to the source of stem cells. The number of CD34[+] cells in peripheral blood is typically quite low [36-39] and much less frequent than in the bone marrow. The CD34[+] cell content in peripheral blood increases 1-2 logs with recovery from chemotherapy-induced marrow suppression and this is augmented by administration of exogenous hematopoietic growth factors as discussed below. The potential for multiple phereses on consecutive days with monitoring of CD34[+] cell content each day provides the clinician much better control over obtaining the number of cells desired. For that reason, in the autologous BMT setting, peripheral blood as the source of stem cells has largely replaced bone marrow.

In the allogeneic setting, however, bone marrow still remains the source of stem cells in most patients because of concerns as to the safety of delivering large numbers of T lymphocytes when peripheral blood is used. Randomized trials comparing bone marrow and peripheral blood in the allogeneic transplant setting are underway. Preliminary data suggest that even though the number of T lymphocytes given to an allogeneic recipient with a peripheral blood stem product is 10 times or greater than a bone marrow product, the risk for acute GVHD does not appear to be increased [40,41]. Animal experiments suggest possible reasons for this counter-intuitive finding. The immunophenotype of T lymphocytes collected from blood of a donor after G-CSF administration demonstrates a shift from a Th1 to Th2 immunophenotype was comapred to non-G-CSF stimulated bone marrow [42,43]. The Th2 phenotype is characterized by increased synthesis of IL-4 and IL-10, and in animals, Th2 lymphocytes appear to suppress acute GVHD. However, the Th2 immunophenotype may also contribute to a greater risk for chronic GVHD. Preliminary reports in human trials likewise suggest a higher rate of chronic GVHD. Similar studies have also demonstrated that after G-CSF administration there is comobilization of CD4[-] CD8[-] T cells along with CD34[+] cells in the blood of normal donors[43,44]. Investigations in animals and humans indicate that CD4[-] CD8[-] T cells suppress the mixed leukocyte reaction and in animals such T cell populations suppress lethal GVHD [45]. Thus, whether the more rapid engraftment and lower treatment-related mortality seen with allogeneic peripheral blood compared to bone marrow offset the potentially greater morbidity from chronic GVHD remains to be seen with longer follow-up.

Preliminary reports from randomized studies have demonstrated that in the autologous setting peripheral blood compared to bone marrow results in more rapid hematopoietic recovery, shorter hospital stays, fewer infectious complications, and lower costs [46,47]. The question of whether these benefits are ascribable to the source (peripheral blood) or the prior treatment of hematopoietic growth factors has been raised. Accordingly, several studies have examined administration of hematopoietic growth factors to the donor prior to harvesting bone marrow [48,49]. In these studies, recipients of G-CSF primed bone marrow appeared to have the same rapid engraftment as recipients of G-CSF primed peripheral blood. The prior "priming" of the HPCs with growth factors rather the source of HPCs appears to be the key explanation for more robust hematopoietic reconstitution with PBPC.

The make-up of CD34[+] subpopulations in peripheral blood differs from bone marrow [50]. For example, expression of c-kit on CD34[+] cells from mobilized blood is much lower than on CD34[+] cells from steady state blood or bone marrow [40,51]. Measures of the cell cycle status of very primitive HPCs (CD34[+] Th1+) indicate that such primitive populations from bone marrow are much more likely to be in G0/G1 than similar cell populations from mobilized peripheral blood[52]. There is considerable interpatient variability in the cobblestone area forming cell (CAFC) content (another measure of primitive HPC) mobilized in PBPC and steady state bone marrow. Although the CAFC in PBPC products is lower than in bone marrow specimens, the ability of CAFC to generate CFC in long-term tissue culture is substantially greater [53]. PBPC-derived HPCs are less likely to be inhibited by stromal interactions in producing neutrophil progenitors in contrast to bone marow-derived HPC [54]. Whether such CD34 subgroup and colony growth differences are clinically important is not clear at this time.

The numbers of immune cells in a peripheral blood stem cell product are substantally greater than a bone marrow product. It has been speculated that this results in more rapid immune recovery and greater antitumor effects, but to date this subject has been poorly studied. Several reports in small numbers of patients suggest that immune response against opportunistic infectious pathogens may be more rapid but further study with larger numbers of patients and control of confounding factors are needed.

In the case of cord blood, the content of HPCs per cc, as measured by CFU-GM, is much greater than steady state adult blood (or bone marrow) [50,55-58]. CD34[+] cells in cord blood display similar phenotypic profiles and clonicity to G-CSF mobilized peripheral blood, and both differ from bone marrow [59]. The correlation of cell numbers in cord blood products with engraftment has been low in several studies [60,61], but in one study the nucleated cell dose correlated marginally with neutrophil engraftment and overall survival [62]. Clearly, the engraftment potential of cord blood is considerable. Much work remains to optimally charactize the hematopoietic potential of cord blood cells.

In the ensuing sections in this chapter, we will emphasize the use of peripheral blood stem cells rather than bone marrow because hematopoietic growth factors are not generally required for collection of bone marrow stem cells and because of the general replacement of bone marrow by peripheral blood as a source of stem cells in autologous transplantation and it is increasingly used in the allogeneic transplant setting as well.

Techniques to Mobilize and Collect HPC from Peripheral Blood

As noted, the number of HPCs circulating in the blood is ordinarily quite low [36-39], one to two logs less frequent than in bone marrow [63]. However, early studies demonstrated that by repeated aphereses, sufficient numbers of HPCs could be obtained from steady state blood to perform transplants [64,65]. Unfortunately, 6-12 phereses were typically required to obtain adequate numbers of HPCs. However, other studies demonstrated that the HPC frequency increased (by 1-2 logs compared to baseline) in the post-chemotherapy setting at the time of leukocyte recovery, with a rebound in the number of HPC and release into circulation [66,67]. Similarly, after administration of G-CSF or GM-CSF, [19,67-69] or the combination of chemotherapy followed by G-CSF or GM-CSF, enhancement of the yield of HPC occurs [19,67-70]. Mobilization by growth factors or the combination of chemotherapy followed by growth factors allows for a reduction in the number of apheresis procedures needed to collect target doses of HPCs and lead to substantially higher yields. These have in turn resulted in shorter times to engraftment in the transplant setting.

The yield of HPCs after the combination of chemotherapy plus growth factors is greater than the yield after growth factor administration alone [11]. Monotherapy using cyclophosphamide is one of the most commonly used regimens, given in doses between 1.5 g/m^2 to 7 g/m^2. Both dose of chemotherapy[71] and schedule of growth factor following the chemotherapy [72,73] appear to influence the HPC yield. In general, the higher the dose of cychophosphamide the greater the yield, but some studies have shown that lower doses with optimization of the schedule of growth factors produce excellent yields with less morbidity to the patient. Other single chemotherapy agents, including paclitaxel, carboplatin, and etoposide, have also been found to be effective mobilizers. Combination chemotherapy regimens have also been evaluated and multiple regimens are quite suitable for mobilizing HPC.

Different guidelines have been developed to time the start of apheresis after mobilization. In general, the collection of stem cells is begun during leukocyte recovery. Some investigators standardize collection to start on a given day after the chemotherapy regimen, while others use the achievement of a given level of neutrophil or leukocyte count. Still others use measurements of certain parameters such as $CD34^+$ cell count in the peripheral blood to determine when to begin stem cell collection. The data to support these indicators are discussed below. The maximal concentration of HPC circulating in peripheral blood after chemotherapy varies from patient to patient (and differs according to dose of chemotherapy and which drug regimen is used). This poses difficulties in planning the start of apheresis and requires flexibility of the apheresis and cell processing staff schedules. Moreover, the chemotherapy mobilizing regimens frequently result in neutropenia, hospitalization and the use of antibiotics, with attendant morbidity and expense. For these reasons, many clinicians prefer to use hematopoietic growth factor mobilization alone.

With the use of G-CSF or GM-CSF, yields are frequently satisfactory even though they may not be a large as after chemotherapy. Augmentation of the circulating pool of HPC typically peaks during the fifth to the eighth day after start of growth factor injections and apheresis can be timed to begin on the fifth day after start of growth factors. Dose and dose schedule of growth factor administration for HPC mobilization is discussed below in Section 7, Chapter 4.

The technique of apheresis also can influence HPC yield. Several reports have indicated that the volume of blood that is pheresed correlates highly with the number of stem cells. The larger the volume the more cells collected [8,74-77]. In some studies, the numbers of cells collected during the first 5-10 liters processed are lower than the numbers collected during the subsequent 5-10 liters. The reason for increasing efficiency of mobilization as the apheresis proceeds is not clear.

Patient Factors

There is considerable interpatient variability in the yield of HPCs after G-CSF mobilization [78-82]. Healthy donors are the best group of subjects to evaluate factors not explained by disease or prior treatment. Up to 20% healthy individuals are poor mobilizers of HPC after hematopoietic growth factors [82,83], with the target number of CD34$^+$ cells not being achieved in one or two aphereses.

Several factors have been identified as associated with lower HPC yield (Table 2). Several studies have identified older age as being associated with decreased HPC yield[83-87], while other studies, in contrast, have not [11,12].

Table 2. Factors associated with best hematopoietic progenitor cell yields in mobilized peripheral blood.

Category	Parameters
Patient	Younger age Male gender Obesity
Disease	Disease other than Hodgkin's Disease Disease other than Acute Myelogenous Leukemia
Prior Treatment	Fewer numbers of chemotherapy cycles Shorter duration of prior chemotherapy Avoidance of large field radiotherapy Avoidance of stem cell toxins Avoidance of dose dense chemotherapy regimens
Source of Stem Cells	Cord blood > PBPC > Bone marrow
Mobilization Strategy	Chemotherapy plus growth factors > growth factors > steady state
Collection Strategy	Large-volume leukapheresis
Cell Processing	Avoidance of ex vivo tumor purging procedures

Some studies have also suggested an association with gender: HPC yield in men being greater[81,88]. Body weight has also been evaluated: obese individuals having greater HPC yields in some studies, perhaps explained by larger doses of growth factors [81,83]. Several other studies have not found correlations with such patient variables [12,78,79].

The explanation for the individual variability in the efficiency of HPC mobilization remains poorly understood.

Disease and Treatment Factors

Several studies have noted different HPC yields in patients with different diseases (Table 2). Patients with Hodgkin's disease have lower HPC yields than patients with non-Hodgkin's lymphoma [12]. Other studies have noted greater HPC yields in patients with breast cancer compared to those with lymphoma [89]. For example, in our experience, 96% of breast cancer patients are successfully mobilized with growth factors alone, but only 60% of lymphoma patients achieved target cell yields [89]. Yields from patients with acute myelogenous leukemia have been noted by several investigators to be lower than patients with other diseases [5,87]. The impact of marrow tumor involvement has been less certain with contradictory findings [3,4,12]. A number of studies have pointed to the importance of prior therapy, both type and duration, in influencing the yield of HPCs. The number of previous cycles of chemotherapy are inversely correlated with the HPC yield [3-6,9-14,90-95]. Generally speaking, treatment less than 1 year is associated with higher HPC yields than treatment lasting more than 1 year. In addition, certain chemotherapeutic agents are associated with poor stem cell yields. Nitrosoureas, bleomycin, carboplatin, melphalan, and nitrogen mustard all have been associated with poor cell yields [5,13,14,94]. Dose-dense regimens may also deplete marrow HPC reserves and interfere with HPC yields [96]. In addition, the use of large field radiotherapy has also been associated with poor stem cell yields [5,11,12,15]. The depth of neutropenia observed with conventional dose chemotherapy during treatment prior to the mobilization has been inversely correlated with HPC yields [97]. Probably this is a reflection of bone marrow reserve: with a given dose of chemotherapy, patients with poor reserve would experience greater leukopenia than those with better marrow reserves.

Ex vivo manipulations of HPCs can also affect their engraftment potential. Pharmacologic agents or monoclonal antibodies used to purge the stem cell product from contaminating tumor lead to loss of HPC content [7,98-101] and a resultant prolonged pancytopenia. In contrast, procedures to select $CD34^+$ cells appear not to compromise myeloid engraftment potential but may impede platelet engraftment slightly [102,103].

Laboratory Tests Useful in Predicting Stem Cell Yields

Because of the inter-individual variability in stem cell yield, a number of studies have been conducted to evaluate the utility of various clinical laboratory parameters to assist in evaluating the suitability of a patient or donor for stem cell mobilization and to time start of apheresis after mobilization.

Tests to Assess Suitability for Mobilization. A bone marrow biopsy is frequently performed to assess cellularity and search for the presence of tumor cells (Table 3). In one study [97], reduced baseline bone marrow cellularity was associated with poor platelet engraftment. Of note, individuals with decreased cellularity had also experienced significant myelosuppression from conventional dose chemotherapy as a reflection of this poor bone marrow reserve. The CD34 percentage [20], $CD34^+/CD71^-$ count [32], and CFU-GM content [4] in the bone marrow prior to mobilization have all been shown to correlate with HPC yield [4]. Of interest, bone marrow $CD34^+$ subsets which are markers of proliferation and maturation capacity have largely not been shown to be predictive of CD34$^+$ mobilization [104].

Table 3. Parameters used to assess suitability for mobilization.

Marrow cellularity
Percentage of CD34$^+$ cells in bone marrow
Counts of CD34$^+$ cells, CD34$^+$/CD71$^-$ cells, CFU-GM colonies in bone marrow
Counts of CD34$^+$ cells in blood

Similarly, the CD34$^+$ cell count in the peripheral blood at steady state before mobilization has been shown to correlate very highly with the HPC yield during apheresis [104]. For example, a CD34$^+$ cell concentration of 0.4 cells x 10^6/liter in steady state peripheral blood has been shown to predict successful HPC collection [104], with a greater degree of correlation than steady state bone marrow CD34$^+$ cell count or CFU content.

<u>Tests to Optimize Timing of HPC Collection</u>. After initiation of the mobilization procedures, guidelines have been developed in different centers as to when to initiate HPC collection to optimize yield. If growth factors alone are the mobilizing strategy, the peak concentration of HPCs in the blood occurs between Day 4 and 7. The most common practice is to start apheresis on the fifth day of hematopoietic growth factor. Collections are continued until the target yield is achieved by consecutive aphereses on each subsequent day with monitoring of CD34$^+$ cell counts after each apheresis.

There is greater variability in the peak appearance of HPCs in the circulation after the combination of chemotherapy and hematopoietic growth factors as the mobilizing strategy. The leukocyte nadir and HPC rebound vary considerably between different chemotherapy regimens, different doses of a given chemotherapy, and the schedule and dose of growth factors. Accordingly, the initiation of apheresis must be individualized to the regimen (Table 4). In some studies, a given day after the start of the chemotherapy mobilization was chosen for HPC collection and reliable HPC yields were achieved. Because of interpatient variability of leukocyte recovery, other centers have chosen to choose a specific leukocyte count, such as 1.0, 5.0, or 8.0 x 10^9 leukocytes/L. Both a rapid increase [3,16] and the achievement of such leukocyte levels are successful guides for effective HPC collection [12,14,16,72,105] (Table 3). The platelet count on the day of pheresis has also been noted to correspond with engraftment in general, and platelet engraftment in particular [20]. Likewise, CD34$^+$ cell count [12,18,20], CD34$^+$ cell percentage [20], CFU-GM [104], number of circulating immature cells [106], and blast cell counts [107] in peripheral blood prior to apheresis all correlate highly with HPC yield during apheresis. For example, a CD34$^+$ cell count >50 x 10^6/L is highly predictive of achieving a target yield of 4 x 10^6 CD34 cells/kg in 1-2 leukophereses, while a level of <20 x 10^6/L is generally associated with failure to achieve this target yield [18]. With these observations, some centers use one or more of these laboratory parameters as guides in patients in which the combination of chemotherapy and hematopoietic growth factors are used to time start of collection of stem cells by apheresis.

Table 4. **Parameters used to optimize timing of collection of hematopoietic progenitor cells on the day of apheresis.**

Leukocytes >1.5, >5.0, or >8.0 x 10^9 cells/L
Rapidity of climb of leukocyte count
Platelet count
C34$^+$ cell count, CD34$^+$ cell percentage, number of CFU-GM colonies, number
   of circulating immature cells, number of blast cells in peripheral blood

---

The clinician is occasionally faced with a dilemma as to what to do in a patient with an inadequate HPC yield [89,108]. Options include proceeding to a bone marrow harvest, the administration of combination of chemotherapy plus growth factors if growth factor alone was the mobilization strategy in the first attempt, or use of higher doses of growth factors. Unfortunately, all of these strategies are suboptimal, none is superior to the others, and they are quite costly [109]. Further study is needed to identify such patients in advance and develop improved strategies for "hard to mobilize" patients.

Conclusion

The observations that hematopoietic growth factors cause a shift of HPCs from bone marrow to peripheral blood and the development of apheresis techniques to collect HPCs from blood has revolutionized the field of BMT. PBPC has replaced bone marrow as the source of stem cells for most autologous BMTs and is currently in study for allogeneic BMT as well. Preliminary studies suggest allogeneic PBPCs provide more rapid engraftment, a reduction in treatment-related morbidity and mortality without an increase in acute GVHD compared to bone marrow. Randomized studies are underway.

There is considerable interpatient variability in the concentration of HPCs in blood and variability in the timing of the appearance and peak concentration of HPCs in blood after mobilization. Improved understanding of the factors that underlie this is needed. In some patients, poor HPC yields are obtained, no matter which mobilization strategy is used, and this phenomenon seems to be indicative of poor bone marrow HPC results. Certain patient disease and treatment variables have been found to be associated with impaired HPC yields. Future study is needed to more precisely identify such individuals either before mobilization or prior to the start of apheresis so that alternative strategies can be tested.

References

1.	van Bekkum DW, De Vries MJ: Radiation Chimaeras. Logos Press Ltd London 1967.
2.	Sharp JG, Armitage J, Crouse D, et al: Are occult tumor cells present in peripheral stem cell harvests of candidates for autologous transplantation? In: Autologous bone marrow transplantation: Proceedings of the Fourth International Symposium. Dicke KA, Spitzer G, Jagannath S, Evinger-Hodges MJ, eds. 693, 1989

3.	To LB, Shepperd M, Haylock DN, et al: Single high doses of cyclophosphamide enable the collection of high numbers of hematopoietic stem cells from the peripheral blood. Exp Hematol 18: 442, 1990.

4.	Kotasek D, Shepherd KM, Sage RE, et al: Factors affecting blood stem cell collections following high-dose cyclophosphamide mobilization in lymphoma, myeloma and solid tumors. Bone Marrow Transplant 9: 11, 1992.

5.	Dreger P, Kloss M, Petersen B, et al: Autologous pregenitor cell transplantation: Prior exposure to stem cell toxic drugs determines yield and engraftment of peripheral blood progenitor cell but not of bone marrow grafts. Blood 86: 3970, 1995.

6.	Reiffers J, Faberes C, Boiron JM, et al: Peripheral blood progenitor cell transplantation in 118 patients with hematological malignancies: Analysis of factors affecting the rate of engraftment. J Hematother 3: 185, 1994.

7.	Rowley S, Zuehldsorf M, Braine HG, et al: CFU-GM content of bone marrow graft correlates with time to hematologic reconstitution following autologous bone marrow transplantation with 4-Hydroperoxycyclophosphamide-purged bone marrow. Blood 70: 271, 1987.

8.	Douay L, Gorin NC, Mary JY, et al: Recovery of CFU-GM from cryopreserved marrow and in vivo evaluation after autologous bone marrow transplantation are predictive of engraftment. Exp Hematol 14: 358, 1986.

9.	Shea TC, Mason JR, Breslin M, et al: Reinfusion and serial measurements of carboplatin-mobilized peripheral blood progenitor cells in patients receiving multiple cycles of high-dose chemotherapy. J Clin Oncol 12: 1012, 1994.

10.	Nademanee A, Sniecinski I, Schmidt GM, et al: High-dose therapy followed by autologous peripheral blood stem cell transplantation for patients with Hodgkin's disease and non-Hodgkin's lymphoma using unprimed and granulocyte colony-stimulating factor mobilized peripheral blood stem cells. J Clin Oncol 12: 2176, 1994.

11.	Bensinger W, Appelbaum FR, Rowley S, et al: Factors that influence collection and engraftment of autologous peripheral blood stem cells. J Clin Oncol 13: 2547, 1995.

12.	Haas R, Mohle R, Fruhauf S, et al: Patient characteristics associated with successful mobilizing and autografting of peripheral blood progenitor cells in malignant lymphoma. Blood 83: 3787, 1994.

13.	Tricot G, Jagannath S, Vesole D, et al: Peripheral blood stem cell transplants for multiple myeloma: Indentification of Favorable variables for rapid engraftment in 225 patients. Blood 85: 588, 1995.

14.	Watts MJ, Sullivan AM, Jamieson E, et al: Progenitor cell mobilization after low dose cyclophosphamide and granulocyte colony-stimulatieng factor: An analysis of progenitor cell quantity and quality and factors predicting for these parameters in 101 pretreated patients with malignant lymphoma. J Clin Oncol 15: 535, 1997.

15.	Bolwell BJ, Fishleder A, Andresen SW, et al: G-CSF primed peripheral blood progenitor cells in autologous bone marrow transplantation: parameters affecting bone marrow engraftment. Bone Marrow Transplant 12: 609, 1993.

16.	Pettengell R, Morgenstern GR, Woll PJ, et al: Peripheral blood progenitor cell transplantation in lymphoma and leukemia using a single apheresis. Blood 82: 3771, 1993.

17.	Zimmerman TM, Lee WJ, Bender JG, et al: Quantitative CD34 analysis may be used to guide peripheral blood stem cell harvests. Bone Marrow Transplant 9: 439, 1995.

18.	Remes K, Matinlauri I, Grenman S, et al: Daily measurements of blood $CD34^+$ cells after stem cell mobilization predict stem cell yield and post-transplant hematopoietic recovery. J Hematother 6: 13, 1997.

19.	Siena S, Bregni M, Brando B, et al: Flow cytometry for clinical estimation of circulating hematopoietic progenitors for autologous transplantation in cancer patients. Blood 77: 400, 1991.

20.	Passos-Coelho JL, Braine HG, Davis JM, et al: Predictive factors for peripheral blood progenitor cell collections using a single large-volume leukapheresis after cyclophosphamide and granulocyte-macrophage colony-stimulating factor mobilization. J Clin Oncol 13: 705, 1995.

21.	Bensinger WI, Longin K, Appelbaum FR, et al: Peripheral blood stem cells (PBSCs) collected after recombinant granulocyte colony stimulating factor (rhG-CSF): An analysis of factors correlating with the tempo of engraftment after transplantation. Br J Haematol 87: 825, 1994.

22.	Bensinger WI, Appelbaum FR, Rowley S, et al: Factors that influence collection and engraftment of autologous peripheral-blood stem cells. J Clin Oncol 13: 2547, 1995.

23.	Weaver CH, Hazelton B, Birch R, et al: An analysis of engraftment kinetics as a function of the CD34 content of peripheral blood progenitor cell collections in 692 patients after the administration of myeloablative chemotherapy. Blood 86: 3961, 1996.

24. Haas R, Mohle R, Murea S, et al: Characterization of peripheral blood progenitor cells mobilized by cytotoxic chemotherapy and recombinant human granulocyte colony-stimulating factor. J Hematother 3: 323, 1994.

25. Lumley MS, McDonald DF, Czarnecka HM, et al: Quality assurance of CD34[+] cell estimation in leucapheresis products. Bone Marrow Transplant 18: 791, 1996.

26. Holm M, Hokland P: A convergence fo methods for a worldwide standard for CD34[+] cell enumeration. J Hematother 7: 105, 1998.

27. Sutherland D: Assessment of pripheral blood stem cell grafts by CD34[+] cell enumeration: Toward a standardized flow cytometric approach. J Hematother 5: 209, 1996.

28. Knape CC: Standardization of absolute CD34 cell enumeration. J Hematother 5: 211, 1996.

29. Brecher ME, Sims L, Schmitz J, et al: North American multicenter study on flow cytometric enumeration of CD34[+] hematopietic stem cells. J Hematother 5: 227, 1996.

30. Rich IN: Standardization of the CFU-GM assay using hematopoietic growth factors. J Hematother 6: 191, 1997.

31. Lewis ID, Rawling T, Dyson PG, et al: Standardization of the CFU-GM assay using hematopoietic growth factors. J Hematother 6: 625, 1996.

32. Osma MM, Ortuna F, de Arriba F, et al: Bone marrow steady-state CD34[+]/CD71- cell content is a predictive value of rG-CSF-mobilized CD34[+] cells. Bone Marrow Transplant 21: 983, 1998.

33. Sutherland HJ, Eaves CJ, Lansdorp PM, et al: Kinetics of committed and primitive blood progenitor mobilization after chemotherapy and growth factor treatment and their use in autotransplants. Blood 83: 3808, 1994.

34. Suzuki T, Muroi K, Amemiya Y, et al: Analysis of peripheral blood CD34[+] cells mobilized with granulocyte colony-stimulating factor (G-CSF) using a long-term culture system. Bone Marrow Transplant 21: 751, 1998.

35. Murray L, Chen B, Galy A, et al: Enrichment of human hematopoietic stem cell activity in the CD34[+] and CD34 Thy1[+] Lin-subpopulation from mobilized peripheral blood. Blood 85: 368, 1995.

36. McKredie KB, Hersh EM, Freireich EJ: Cells capable of colony formation in the peripheral blood of man. Science 171: 293, 1971.

37. Epstein RB, Sarpel SC: Processing of peripheral blood cells of canines and man. Exp Hematol 3: 109, 1975.

38. Ogawa M, Brush OC, O'dell RF, et al: Circulating erythropoietic precursors assessed in culture: Characterization in normal men and patients with hemaglobinopathies. Blood 50: 1081, 1977.

39. Goodman JW, Hodgson GS: Evidence for stem cells in the peripheral blood of mice. Blood 19: 702, 1962.

40. Schmitz N, Bacigalupo A, Hasenclever D, et al: Allogeneic bone marrow transplantation vs filgrastim-mobilized peripheral blood progenitor cell transplantation in patients with early leukaemia: first results of a randomized multicentre trial on the European Group for Blood and Marrow Transplantation. Bone Marrow Transplant 21: 995, 1998.

41. Korbling M, Przepiorka D, Huh YO, et al: Allogeneic blood stem cell transplantation for refractory leukemia and lymphoma: Potential advantage of blood over marrow allografts. Blood 85: 1659, 1995.

42. LoVelle B: Fungicidal activation of murine macrophages by recombinant gamma interferon. Infect Immun 55: 2951, 1987.

43. Zeng D, Dejbakhsh-Jones S, Strober S: Granulocyte colony-stimulating factor reduces the capacity of blood mononuclear cells to induce graft-versus-host disease: Impact on blood progenitor cell transplantation. Blood 90: 453, 1997.

44. Chao NJ: Graft-versus-host disease: The viewpoint from the donor T cell. Biol Blood Marrow Transplant 3: 1, 1997.

45. Kusnierz-Glaz CR, Still BJ, Amano M, et al: Granulocyte colony-stimulating factor-induced comobilization of CD4[-]CD8[-]T cells and hematopoietic progenitor cells (CD34[+]) in the blood of normal donors. Blood 89: 2586, 1997.

46. Schmitz N, Linch DC, Dreger P, et al: Randomized trial of filgrastim-mobilised peripheral blood progenitor cell transplantation versus autologous bone marrow transplantation in lymphoma patients. The Lancet 347: 353, 1996.

47. Beyer J, Schwella N, Zingsem J, et al: Hematopoietic rescue after high-dose chemotherapy using autologous peripheral blood progenitor cells on bone marrow: A randomized comparison. J Clin Oncol 13: 1328, 1995.

48. Damiani D, Fanin R, Silvestri F, et al: Randomized trial of autologous filgrastim-primed bone marrow transplantation versus filgrastim-mobilized peripheral blood stem cell transplantation with lymphoma patients. Blood 90: 36, 1997.

49. Janssen WE, Smilee RC, Elfenbein GJ: A prospective randomized trial comparing blood- and marrow-derived stem cells for hematopoietic replacement following high-dose chemotherapy. J Hematotherapy 4: 139, 1995.

50. Knudtzon S: In vitro growth of granulocytic colonies from circulating cells in human cord blood. Blood 43: 357, 1974.

51. Mohle R, Haas R, Hunstein W: Expression of adhesion molecules and c-kit on CD34[+] hematopoitic progenitor cells: Comparison of cytokine mobilized blood stem cells with normal bone marrow and peripheral blood. J Hematother 2: 483, 1993.

52. Uchida N, He D, Friera AM, et al: The unexpected G0/G1 cell cycle status of mobilized hematopoietic stem cells from peripheral blood. Blood 89: 465, 1997.

53. Breems DA, van Hennik PB, Kusadasi N, et al: Individual stem cell quality in leukapheresis products is related to the number of mobilized stem cells. Blood 87: 5370, 1996.

54. Scott MA, Apperley JF, Bloxham DM, et al: Biological properties of peripheral blood progenitor cells mobilized by cyclophosphamide and granulocyte colony-stimulating factor. Br J Haematol 97: 474, 1997.

55. Ueno Y, Koizumi S, Yamagami M, et al: Characterization of hematopietic stem cells (CFU-C) in cord blood. Exp Hematol 9: 716, 1981.

56. Broxmeyer HE, Hangoc G, Cooper S, et al: Growth characteristics and expansion of human umbilical cord blood and estimation of its potential for transplantation in adults. Proc Natl Acad Sci USA 89: 4109, 1992.

57. Wang JCY, Doedens M, Dick JE: Primitive human hematopoietic cells are enriched in cord blood compared with adult bone marrow or mobilized peripheral blood as measured by the quantitative in vivo SCID-repopulating cell assay. Blood 89: 3919, 1997.

58. Piacibello W, Sanavio F, Garetto L, et al: Extensive amplification and self-renewal of human primitive hematopoietic stem cells from cord blood. Blood 89: 2644, 1997.

59. Steen R, Tjonnfjord GE, Egeland T: Comparison of the phenotype and clonogenicity of normal CD34[+] cells from umbilical cord blood, granulocyte colony-stimulating factor-mobilized peripheral blood and adult human bone marrow. J Hematother 3: 253, 1994.

60. Wagner JE, Rosenthal J, Sweetman R, et al: Successful transplantation of HLA-matched and HLA-mismatched umbilical cord blood from unrelated donors: Analysis of engraftment and acute graft-versus-host disease. Blood 88: 795, 1996.

61. Cairo MS, Wagner JE: Placental and /or umbilical cord blood: An alternative source of hematopoietic stem cells for transplantation. Blood 90: 4665, 1997.

62. Gluckman E, Rocha V, Boyer-Chammard A, et al: Outcome of cord-blood transplantation from related and unrelated donors. N Eng J Med 337: 373, 1997.

63. McCarthy DM, Goldman JM: Transfusion of circulating stem cells. CRC Crit Rec Clin Lab Scvi 20: 1, 1984.

64. Kessinger A, Armitage JO, Smith DM, et al: High-dose therapy and autologous peripheral blood stem cell transplantation for patients with lymphoma. Blood 74: 1260, 1989.

65. Kessinger A, Armitage J, Landmark J, et al: Autologous peripheral hematopoietic stem cell transplantation restores hematopoietic function following marrow ablative therapy. Blood 71: 723, 1988.

66. Richman CM, Weiner RS, Yankee RA: Increase in circulating stem cells following chemotherapy in man. Blood 47: 1031, 1976.

67. Siena S, Bregni M, Brando M, et al: Circulation of CD34[+] hematopoietic stem cells in the peripheral blood of high-dose cyclophosphamide-treated patients: Enhancement by intravenous recombinant human granulocyte macrophage colony-stimulating factor. Blood 74: 1905, 1989.

68. Gianni AM, Siena S, Bregni M, et al: Granulocyte-macrophage colony-stimulating factor to harvest circulating hematopoietic stem cells for autotransplantation. Lancet 2: 580, 1989

69. Gianni AM, Tarella C, Siena S, et al: Durable and complete engraftment of rhGM-CSF exposed peripheral blood progenitor cells. Bone Marrow Transplant 6: 143, 1990

70. Socinski MA, Elias A, Schnipper L, et al: Granulocyte-macrophage colony stimulating factor expands the circulating haemopoietic progenitor cell compartment in man. Lancet 1: 1194, 1988.

71. Rowlings PA, Rawling CM, To LB, et al: A comparison of peripheral blood stem cell mobilisation after chemotherapy with cyclophosphamide as a single agent in doses of 4 g/m^2 or 7 g/m^2 in

patients with advanced cancer. Aust NZ J Med 22: 660, 1992.

72. Jones HM, Jones SA, Watts MJ, et al: Development of a simplified single-apheresis approach for peripheral blood progenitor cell transplantation in previously treated patients with lymphoma. J Clin Oncol 12: 1693, 1994.

73. Scwartzberg L, Heffernan M, Birch R, et al: Comparison of different G-CSF schedules in conjunction with cyclophosphamide, etoposide, and cisplatin for peripheral blood stem cell (PBSC) mobilization. Blood 82: 641-Abstract #2548, 1993.

74. Hillyer CD, Tiegerman KO, Berkman EM: Increase in circulating colony-forming units granulocyte-macrophage during large-volume leukapheresis: Evaluation of a new cell separator. Transfusion 31: 327, 1997.

75. Comenco RL, Malachowski ME, Miller KB, et al: Engraftment with peripheral blood stem cells collected by large-volume leukapheresis for patients with lymphoma. Transfusion 32: 729, 1992.

76. Malachowski ME, Comenzo RL, Hillyer CD, et al: Large-volume leukapheresis for peripheral blood stem cell collection in patients with hematologic malignancies. Transfusion 32: 732, 1992.

77. Passos-Coelho JL, Machado MA, Lucio P, et al: Large-volume leukaphereses may be more efficient than standard-volume leukaphereses for collection of peripheral blood progenitor cells. J Hematother 6: 465, 1997.

78. Grigg A, Roberts A, Raunow H, et al: Optimizing dose and scheduling of filgrastim (granulocyte colony-stimulating factor) for mobiliation and collection of peripheral blood progenitor cells in normal volunteers. Blood 1995 85: 4437

79. Tabilio A, Falzetti F, Giannoni C, et al: Stem cell mobilization in normal donors. J Hematother 6: 227, 1997

80. Hoglund M, Smedmyr B, Simonsson B, et al: Dose-dependent mobilization of hematopoietic progenitor cells in healthy volunteers receiving glycosylated rHuG-CSF. Bone Marrow Transplant 18: 19, 1996

81. Stroncek D, Clay M, Smith J, et al: Composition of peripheral blood progenitor cell components collected from healthy donors. Transfusion 37: 411, 1997

82. Holm M, Hokland P: Not all healthy donors mobilize hametopoietic progenitor cells sufficiently after G-CSF administration to allow for subsequent CD34 purification of the leukapheresis product. J Hematother 7: 111, 1998.

83. Anderlini P, Korbling M: The use of mobilized peripheral blood stem cells from normal donors for allografting. Stem Cells 15: 9, 1997

84. Dreger P, Haferlach T, Eckstein V, et al: G-CSF-mobilized peripheral blood progenitor cells for allogeneic transplantation: Safety, kinetics of mobilization, and composition of the graft. Br J Haematol 87: 609, 1994.

85. Chatta S, Price T, Allan R, et al: Effects of in vivo recombinant methionyl human granulocyte colony-stimulating factor on the neutrophil response and peripheral blood colony-forming cells in healthy young and elderly adult volunteers. Blood 84: 2923, 1994.

86. Welte K, Gabrilove J, Bronchud M, et al: Filgrastim (r-metHuG-CSF): The first 10 years. Blood 88: 1907, 1996

87. Rowley SD, Piantadosi S, Marcellus DC, et al: Analysis of factors predicting speed of hematologic recovery after transplantation with 4-hydroperoxycyclophosphamide-purged autologous bone marrow grafts. Bone Marrow Transplant 7: 183, 1991.

88. Miflin G, Charley C, Stainer C, et al: Stem cell mobilization in normal donors for allogeneic transplantation: Analysis of safety and factors affecting efficacy. Br J Haematol 95: 345, 1996.

89. Sugrue MW, Williams KD, Hutcheson CE, et al: Characterization of a patient population in whom an optimal autologous peripheral blood stem cell dose cannot be achieved. J Hematothera 7: 267-(Abstract P10), 1998.

90. Demirer T, Buckner CD, Storer B, et al: Effect of Different chemotherapy regimens on peripheral blood stem cell collections in patients with breast cancer receiving granulocyte colony-stimulating factor. J Clin Oncol 15: 684, 1997.

91. Jagannath S, Vesole DH, Glenn L, et al: Low-risk intensive therapy for multiple myeloma with combined autologous bone marrow and blood stem cell support. Blood 80: 1666, 1992.

92. Martinez C, Sureda A, Martino R, et al: Efficient peripheral blood stem cell mobilization with low-dose G-CSF (50 ug/m^2) after salvage chemotherapy for lymphoma. Bone Marrow Transplant 20: 855, 1997.

93. Aurlien E, Holte H, Pharo A, et al: Combination chemotherapy with mitoguazon, ifosfamide, MTX, etoposide (MIME) and G-CSF can efficiently mobilize PBPC in patients with Hodgkin's and

non-Hodgkin's lymphoma. Bone Marrow Transplant 21: 873, 1998.

94. Olivieri A, Offidani M, Ciniero L, et al: Optimization of the yield of PBSC for autotransplantation mobilized by high-dose chemotherapy and G-CSF: proposal for a mathematical model. Bone Marrow Transplant 14: 273, 1994.

95. Papadopoulos KP, Ayello J, Tugulea S: Harvest quality and factors affecting collection and engraftment of CD34[+] cells in patients with breast cancer scheduled for high-dose chemotherapy and peripheral blood progenitor cell support. J Hematother 6: 61, 1997.

96. Freedman A, Neuberg D, Mauch P, et al: Cyclophosphamide, doxorubicin, vincristine, prednisone dose intensification with granulocyte colony-stimulating factor markedly depletes stem cell reserve for autologous bone marrow transplantation. Blood 90: 4996, 1997.

97. Elias AD, Ayash L, Anderson KC, et al: Mobilization of peripheral blood progenitor cells by chemotherapy and granulocyte macrophage colony-stimulating factor for hematologic support after high-dose intensification for breast cancer. Blood 79: 3036, 1992

98. Spitzer G, Verma DS, Fisher R, et al: The myeloid progenitor cell - its value in predicting hematopoietic recivery after autologous bone marrow transplantation. Blood 55: 317, 1980

99. Ritz J, Bast RC, Clavell LA, et al: Autologous bone marrow transplantation in CALLA-positive acute lymphoblastic leukemia after in vitro treatment with J-r monoclonal antibody and complement. Lancet 2: 60, 1982

100. Kaizer H, Levy R, Cote JP, et al: Autologous bone marrow transplantation in lymphoblastic lymphoma and T-cell lymphoma. Blood 60: 169a, 1982

101. Seager RC, Siegal SE, Sidell H, et al: Neuroblastoma: Clinical respectives, monoclonal antibodies and retinoic acid. Ann Intern Med 97: 873, 1982

102. Schiller G, Stewart AK, Ballester O, et al: A Phase III study evaluating CD34[+] selected versus unselected autologous peripheral blood progenitor cell transplantation for patients with advanced multiple myeloma: Engraftment results. Blood 90: 218a-Abstract #960, 1997.

103. Shpall EJ, LemIstre CF, Holland K, et al: A prospective randomized trial of buffy coat versus CD34-selected autologous bone marrow support in high-risk breast cancer patients receiving high-dose chemotherapy. Blood 90: 4313-4320, 1997.

104. Fruhauf S, Haas R, Conradt C, et al: Peripheral blood progenitor cell (PBPC) counts during steady-state hematopoiesis allow to extimate the yield of mobilized PBPC after filgrastim (R-metHuG-CSF)-supported cytotoxic chemotherapy. Blood 85: 2619, 1995.

105. Webb IJ, Eickhoff CE, Elias AD, et al: Kinetics of peripheral blood mononuclear cell mobilization with chemotherapy and/or granulocyte-colony-stimulating factor: Implications for timing and yield of hematopoietic progenitor cell collections. Transfusion 36: 160, 1996.

106. Teshima T, Sunami K, Bessho A, et al: Circulating immature cell counts on the harvest predict the yields of CD34[+] cells collected after granulocyte colony-stimulating factor plus chemotherapy-induced mobilization of peripheral blood stem cell. Blood 89: 4660, 1997.

107. Mijovic A, Fishlock K, Pagliuca A, et al: Blast counts in blood progenitor cell (BPC) correlate with CD34[+] cells and CFU-GM and are a useful predictor of haemopoietic recovery after autologous BPC transplantation collections. Bone Marrow Transplant 21: 869, 1998.

108. Weaver CH, Tauer K, Zhen B, et al: Second attempts at mobilization of peripheral blood stem cells in patients with initial low CD34[+] cell yields. J Hematother 7: 241, 1998.

109. Stiff P, LeMaistre CF, Luger S, et al: Resource utilization following PBPC mobilization failure. Proc ASCO 17: 83a-Abstract #319, 1998.

20. Mechanisms of Growth Factor Mobilization of Hematopoietic Progenitors

Daniel C. Link

Introduction

The use of hematopoietic progenitor cells (HPC) to reconstitute hematopoiesis following myeloablative therapy has significantly improved the clinical outcome for patients with a variety of diseases. Recently, mobilized peripheral blood HPC instead of bone marrow-derived HPC have been used because of their reduced engraftment times, relative ease of collection, and possibly reduced risk of acute graft-versus-host disease. Although the great majority of HPC reside within the bone marrow, a small number of HPC also continuously circulate in the peripheral blood. This number can be dramatically increased, or mobilized, by a wide variety of stimuli including hematopoietic growth factors, chemotherapy, and certain chemokines. Mobilization regimens utilizing hematopoietic growth factors alone recently have become popular because they avoid exposure to cytotoxic chemotherapy. These regimens are generally well-tolerated but not universally effective and are often associated with co-mobilization of neoplastic cells. A better understanding of the mechanisms that regulate HPC mobilization may lead to the design of novel mobilization strategies that overcome these limitations.

The Bone Marrow Microenvironment.

In humans and mice the principal site of hematopoiesis is the bone marrow; the spleen is a secondary site in mice [1]. In the bone marrow, hematopoiesis is restricted to the extravascular space where dense cords of hematopoietic cells are interspersed among the venous sinuses. The hematopoietic cells are surrounded by stromal cells that include endothelial cells, macrophages, fibroblasts, and adipocytes. The only complete barrier to the intravascular space are the endothelial cells lining the venous sinuses. The migration of hematopoietic cells through the endothelium is thought to occur near inter-endothelial cell junctions and in regions where the endothelial cell basement membrane extracellular matrix (ECM) is thinned or absent [2]. In addition to providing signals through direct cell-cell interactions with hematopoietic cells, the stromal cells also produce the ECM. The bone marrow ECM is primarily comprised of collagens, glycoproteins, and glycosaminoglycans. The ECM is thought to regulate hematopoietic cell activity through interaction with specific cell surface receptors and by localizing and facilitating interactions with growth factors [3]. In addition to their role in regulating hematopoietic cell growth and differentiation, the ECM and stromal cells are likely to play a major role in regulating hematopoietic cell migration.

Homing of HPC to the Bone Marrow Microenvironment.

Critical to the understanding of the mechanisms of HPC mobilization is the identification of the adhesive interactions that mediate the binding of HPC to the bone marrow ECM. It is likely that these adhesive interactions also contribute to the homing of HPC to the bone marrow, therefore a review of the data in this field of study is warranted. Homing of HPC has been defined as the set of molecular interactions that mediate the localization of HPC to the bone marrow microenvironment following intravenous infusion [4]. Recent studies have identified some of the potential mechanisms involved in HPC homing. Surface membrane lectins on HPC with specificities for galactose and mannose appear to play a role in homing, since infusion of synthetic neoglycoproteins with these specificities inhibits the reconstitution of hematopoiesis in mice following bone marrow transplantation [5]. Although a putative lectin homing receptor has been identified on HPC, its functional role in vivo has not been determined [6].

A number of adhesion molecules are expressed on HPC including: the $\alpha_4 \beta_1$, $\alpha_4 \beta_1$, and $\alpha_L \beta_2$ integrins {very late antigen-4 (VLA-4), VLA-5, and leukocyte function associated antigen-1 (LFA-1), respectively}[7] CD44 [8], selectins [9,10], platelet/endothelial cell adhesion molecule (PECAM-1) [11], and HEMCAM [12]. Perhaps the best characterized adhesion molecule on HPC is VLA-4. VLA-4 is expressed on the majority of HPC in a low-affinity state; however, in response to cytokines such as granulocyte-macrophage colony-stimulating factor (GM-CSF), interleukin-3 (IL-3), and stem cell factor (SCF) its function can be rapidly and transiently activated to promote adhesion to fibronectin [13]. Antibodies directed against VLA-4 largely inhibit the adhesion of purified CD34+ cells to bone marrow stromal cells [14]. More importantly, antibodies directed against VLA-4 significantly inhibit the homing of murine HPC to the bone marrow of lethally irradiated recipients [15]. Interestingly, treatment of mice or primates with anti-VLA-4 antibody results in the mobilization of HPC to the peripheral circulation [15,16]. Consistent with these observations, a study of chimeric mice generated from β_1-integrin-deficient embryonic stem cells showed that β_1-integrin-deficient cells failed to contribute to fetal liver hematopoiesis despite evidence that these cells could differentiate into hematopoietic cells in vitro [17]. Collectively, these data establish VLA-4 as a key adhesion molecule on HPC and suggest an important role for VLA-4 in HPC homing and mobilization.

Recent data also have implicated CD44 in the adhesive interactions of HPC to the bone marrow. CD44 is a highly polymorphic transmembrane glycoprotein that is expressed on all hematopoietic cells including primitive progenitors [8]. Antibodies to CD44 inhibit myelopoiesis and lymphopoiesis in murine long term bone marrow cultures [18]. Further, an antibody to a particular isoform of CD44 can inhibit the homing of murine HPC to the bone marrow [19,20]. Finally, mice lacking CD44 have decreased numbers of splenic HPC and an impaired mobilization response to G-CSF[21].

Recent evidence suggests that the chemokine stromal cell-derived factor-1 (SDF-1) also may play a role in HPC homing. SDF-1 is a C-X-C chemokine isolated from bone marrow stromal cells [22]. In addition to being a potent chemoattractant for T lymphocytes, SDF-1 is the only known chemoattractant for HPC [22,23]. Mice carrying a homozygous null mutation of this gene die perinatally [24]. These mice have dramatically reduced numbers of myeloid progenitors in their bone marrow despite having normal numbers in fetal liver, suggesting that SDF-1 is necessary for the migration of HPC from the fetal liver to the bone marrow [24].

Diversity of mobilizing stimuli

A notable feature of HPC mobilization is the diversity of stimulating agents. Hematopoietic growth factors, cytotoxic agents, and certain chemokines {interleukin-8,[25] macrophage inflammatory protein-2 (MIP-2) [26], and BB-1001027 (a genetically engineered form of MIP-1α)} can induce HPC mobilization. A partial list of hematopoietic growth factors capable of mobilizing HPC is shown in Table 1. A striking feature of this group is the diversity of their target cell populations. For example, hematopoietic growth factors that predominantly effect myeloid cells {granulocyte colony-stimulating factor (G-CSF) and granulocyte-macrophage colony-stimulating factor (GM-CSF)}, T-lymphocytes (interleukin-7), and natural killer cells (interleukin-12) are all potent mobilizing stimuli. The mobilization of HPC by cytokines with distinct cellular targets and biological actions suggests a common mechanism of action. Indeed, several common features are observed during mobilization with these agents. First, the kinetics of HPC mobilization are similar, with peak levels of circulating HPC (increases of 5- to 500-fold over baseline) generally achieved after 7 to 10 days of cytokine treatment. Second, the increase in circulating HPC is associated with a decrease in bone marrow HPC; with the exception of stimulation by flt-3 ligand [35], no increase in total HPC is observed. Third, a broad spectrum of HPC are mobilized including primitive pluripotent as well as committed myeloid, megakaryocytic and erythroid progenitors [50-53]. Fourth, with the exception of IL-12 and thrombopoietin [37,46], neutrophils are co-mobilized with HPC into the peripheral circulation by these cytokines.

Mechanisms of HPC mobilization

Mobilization of HPC could potentially occur by three general mechanisms. The mobilizing stimulus (e.g., hematopoietic growth factors) could induce proliferation of hematopoietic cells in the bone marrow such that HPC are "crowded out" and forced into the peripheral circulation. It is also possible that a mobilizing stimulus could result in phenotypic changes in the HPC themselves, leading to enhanced migration into the intravascular space. Finally, the mobilizing stimulus could lead to changes in the bone marrow microenvironment that facilitate HPC release. With the possible exception of flt-3 ligand, it does not appear that the first model is true. During peak HPC mobilization by growth factors, the HPC content of bone marrow is usually reduced (see table 1). Furthermore, studies of mobilization in G-CSF receptor deficient mice (see detailed discussion below) clearly demonstrate that increases in bone marrow cellularity and HPC content are not sufficient to induce HPC mobilization.

The second model predicts that the phenotype of mobilized peripheral blood HPC versus HPC that reside in the bone marrow under steady-state conditions should be different. In fact, several studies have consistently detected differences between these

Table 1. Cytokine Mobilization of Murine hematopoietic Progenitors

Cytokine	Primary Cell target	Blood PMN (inc.)	Blood HPC (inc.)	Spleen HPC (inc.)	Bone Marrow HPC	Time to Peak Response	Ref.
G-CSF	Myeloid	20-fold	20-100 fold	20-fold	2-fold	7-14 days	[28-30]
GM-CSF	Myeloid	7-fold	45-fold	UK	UK	7 days	[31]
SCF (kit-ligand)	Pluripotent and mast cell	24-fold	20-fold	24-fold	1.5-fold dec.	1-10 days	[32-34]
Flt-3 ligand	Pluripoetne and dndritic cell	10-fold	500-fold	100-fold	2-fold	10 days	[35,36]
Thrombopoietin	Pluripotent & megakaryocytes	NC	10-fold	UK	UK	7 days	[31,37]
Interleukin-1	Pleiotropic	5-fold	30-fold	UK	UK	4-8 hs	[38]
Interleukin-3[1]	Pleiotropic	2-fold	5-fold	UK	UK	15 days	[39-41]
Interleukin-6[2]	Pleiotropic	2-fold	3-fold	3-fold	UK	UK	[42]
Interleukin-7	B- & T-lymphocytes	3-fold	50-fold	50-fold	20-fold	7 days	[43,44]
Interleukin-11	Pluripotent	NR	2-fold	4-fold	1.5-fold dec.	7 days	[45]
Interleukin-12	Natural Killer & T-lymphoctes	NC	50-fold	40-fold	5-fold	7 days	[46]
Interleukin-8	Neutrophils	3-fold	10-fold	10-fold	UK	15-30 minutes	[24,47]
CY	Chemotherapy	8-fold	62-fold	10-fold	NC	8 days	[48,49]

NR=Not reported; UK=unknown; NC=No change; inc.=increase; dec.=decrease
Studies of hematopoietic progenitor cell (HPC) mobilizaton in mice are shown to facilitate comparisons. HPC werre enumerated using various assays. Fold-increases represent approximate averages of data published in the indicated studies. It is difficult to directly compare mobilization potency since the dose, strain of mice, and assay for HPC varied considerably in these studies. The chemokine IL-8 and the chemotherapeutic agent cyclophosphamide (CY) are shown for comparison.
[1]No response seen in mice (data is shown for humans).
[2]There are no published reports of the mobilization response to IL-6 in mice (data shown is for humans).

two groups (Table 2). First, expression of the VLA-4 integrin is consistently lower on peripheral blood HPC [10,11,54,55], a potentially important finding given the recent reports that anti-VLA-4 antibodies can mobilize HPC in mice [15]. Second, relative to bone marrow HPC, a higher percentage of peripheral blood HPC appear to be in a quiescent stage of the cell cycle [56-59]. For example, in one study 7% of peripheral blood versus 47% of bone marrow progenitors were observed to be in S-phase [57]. Third, mobilized HPC have decreased c-kit expression [51,60], another potentially important finding given the recent reports that HPC mobilization by G-CSF [61] or anti-VCAM antibodies[62] is

Table 2.	Phenotype of mobilized HPC

Feature	Comparison
Pluripotent vs. lineage-committed	Similar to bone marrow HPC. Both pluripotent and lineage-committed HPC
Cell cycle	Quiescent, majority in G_0/G_1
c-kit expression	Decreased
VLA-4 expression	Decreased

impaired in W/W^v (c-kit deficient) mice. Whether any of these phenotypic differences is responsible for the release of HPC from the bone marrow is not yet clear.

Recent studies of IL-8 administration in mice suggest that changes in the bone marrow microenvironment can lead to HPC mobilization. IL-8 is a C-X-C chemokine that is produced by a wide variety of cell types including neutrophils, monocytes, fibroblasts, and endothelial cells [63]. IL-8 is a potent chemoattractant for neutrophils and T lymphocytes [64]. In addition, IL-8 leads to neutrophil activation, degranulation, and upregulation of the β_2 integrin, Mac-1 [65-67]. Recently, it has been shown that IL-8 induces a rapid increase in the level of circulating HPC that is detectable 5 minutes after parenteral administration, peaks at 15 to 30 minutes, and returns to baseline within 2 hours [25,47]. Similar to the effects of chemotherapy and growth factors, IL-8 mobilizes both primitive and committed HPC [25,47]. Several observations have led to the hypothesis that IL-8 activation of neutrophils may be critical for IL-8 induced HPC mobilization. First, the rapid kinetics of IL-8 induced mobilization suggests a direct mechanism for IL-8. Second, neutrophils are the major known target for IL-8 [63]. Third, in mice the receptor for IL-8 (CXCR-2) does not appear to be expressed on HPC[68]. In support of this hypothesis, pretreatment of rhesus monkeys with neutralizing antibodies against gelatinase-B (a metalloprotease that is released from neutrophils upon IL-8 stimulation) completely inhibited IL-8-induced mobilization of HPC [69]. It should be noted that, although controversial, receptors for IL-8 have been detected on endothelial cells raising the possibility that alterations in endothelial cell function also may be important for IL-8 induced mobilization [70,71].

Role of G-CSF receptor signals in HPC mobilization

Granulocyte colony-stimulating factor (G-CSF) is the most commonly used agent to mobilize HPC because of its potency and lack of serious toxicity. In addition, G-CSF recently has been shown to act synergistically with cytotoxic agents [48,72,73], stem cell factor [34,74,75], and flt-3 ligand[36,76,77] to induce HPC mobilization. To explore the mechanisms of G-CSF-induced mobilization, we examined HPC mobilization in mice genetically deficient for the G-CSF receptor (G-CSFR) in response to three major types of mobilizing stimuli: cytotoxic agents (cyclophosphamide), hematopoietic growth factors (G-CSF, flt-3 ligand, and IL-12), and chemokines (IL-8) [78]. G-CSFR-deficient mice have chronic neutropenia with a uniform decrease in myeloid cells in the bone marrow [79]. No accumulation of immature granulocytic cells is present in the bone marrow, suggesting that residual granulocytic precursors present in these mice are able to differentiate normally into mature neutrophils. In agreement with this conclusion, residual neutrophils present in G-CSFR-deficient mice appear phenotypically normal as assessed by morphology and expression of myeloperoxidase, Gr-1, and Mac-1 [79]. The defect in hematopoiesis appears to be limited to granulopoiesis since the number and cytokine-responsiveness of myeloid progenitors in the bone marrow and spleen of these mice are nearly normal [79]. Further, the number and function of primitive multipotent progenitors, as measured in day 12 colony-forming unit-spleen (CFU-S) assays [80], are normal. In sum, G-CSFR-deficient mice appear to have an isolated but severe defect in granulopoiesis.

<u>Hematopoietic progenitor mobilization by cyclophosphamide in G-CSFR-deficient mice</u>. Cyclophosphamide is a potent stimulus for HPC mobilization in mice [48,49]. To determine whether cyclophosphamide-induced mobilization requires the G-CSFR, we challenged G-CSFR-deficient mice with this agent [78]. In comparison with wild-type mice, neutrophil recovery was delayed and blunted in G-CSFR-deficient mice. Wild-type mice had the expected mobilization response, with a 40-fold increase in blood circulating colony-forming units (CFU-C) observed 8 days after cyclophosphamide treatment. In contrast, no increase in CFU-C was detected in the blood of G-CSFR-deficient mice at any time during this study. Likewise, a significant increase in circulating CD34+ lineage- HPC was detected in wild-type but not G-CSFR-deficient mice. To determine whether the defect in HPC mobilization in G-CSFR-deficient mice extended to more primitive HPC, we measured the level of CFU-S (d12) progenitors in peripheral blood on day 8 after cyclophosphamide administration. In contrast to wild-type mice, no increase in CFU-S (d12) was detected in the blood of G-CSFR-deficient mice. To exclude the possibility that the lack of an increase in peripheral HPC was due to an inability of G-CSFR-deficient mice to regenerate HPC following cyclophosphamide administration, we quantified CFU-C in the bone marrow, spleen, and blood of these mice (Table 3). A similar increase from baseline of total body CFU-C was observed in wild-type and G-CSFR-deficient mice. In fact, the absolute number of CFU-C present in the bone marrow of G-CSFR-deficient mice on day 8 after cyclophosphamide administration was significantly increased relative to wild-type mice. However, despite the increase in total body CFU-C, no redistribution of these cells from the bone marrow to peripheral blood or spleen was observed. Interestingly, mature neutrophils (PMN) showed a similar pattern; the number of PMN in the bone marrow was increased without a concomitant increase in circulating PMN (Table 3). Collectively, these results demonstrate that the G-CSFR is absolutely required for HPC mobilization in response to cyclophosphamide treatment in mice.

Table 3. **Mobilization in G-CSFR deficient mice.**

Stimulus	Tissue	CFU-C		PMN	
		Wild-type	G-CSFR (+/-)	Wild Type	G-CSFR (+/-)
CY	Blood	45.5	0.5	8.1	1.5
	Spleen	9.4	0.5	NE	NE
	BM	1.4	2.8	3.7	2.3
Flt-3 Ligand	Blood	213.5	160.3	9.0	14.3
	Spleen	42.5	21.4	NE	NE
	BM	2.6	1.6	1.6	1.6
IL-12	Blood	3.6	16.4	1.3	6.8
	Spleen	13.3	44.0	NE	NE
	BM	0.7	2.7	1.6	3.0

Fold-change from baseline in colony forming cells (CFU-C) or mature neutrophils (PMN) in peripheral blood, spleen, or bone marrow (BM). Analyses were performed at baseline, 8 days after a single intraperitoneal injection of cyclophosphamide (CY), [200 mg/kg], or after 10 days of either flt-3 lingand (10 ug/day) or IL-12 (1 ug/day) administration. 4-6 age and sex-matched mice were used to generate each data entry. NE refers to not evaluated.

HPC mobilization in G-CSFR-deficient mice in response to G-CSF, flt-3 ligand, and IL-12. These cytokines were chosen because of their strong mobilization responses and distinct biological activities (flt-3 ligand and IL-12 predominantly affect pluripotent/dendritic cells and T lymphocytes/natural killer cells, respectively). In addition, mobilization by flt-3 ligand or IL-12 is associated with characteristic features suggesting unique mechanisms of mobilization. Flt-3 ligand mobilizes with delayed kinetics and is associated with a significant increase in HPC in the bone marrow as well as the peripheral circulation [35]. Mobilization by IL-12, in contrast to mobilization by most other hematopoietic growth factors, is not associated with an increase in the level of circulating neutrophils [46]. The mobilization response in G-CSFR-deficient mice to flt-3 ligand or IL-12 is summarized in Table 3. As expected, G-CSF treatment had no effect on the level of circulating neutrophils or HPC in G-CSFR-deficient mice. Although reduced relative to wild-type mice, administration of flt-3 ligand for 10 days resulted in a significant expansion of total body CFU-C in G-CSFR-deficient mice. Further, in sharp contrast to cyclophosphamide treatment, treatment with flt-3 ligand clearly resulted in the redistribution of HPC from the bone marrow to the spleen and blood. Likewise, treatment of G-CSFR deficient mice with IL-12 resulted in a significant increase in blood and spleen HPC. Interestingly, both flt-3 ligand and IL-12 treatment resulted in the mobilization of PMN to the peripheral circulation in

G-CSFR-deficient mice. These data demonstrate that the G-CSFR is not required for flt-3 ligand- or IL-12-induced HPC mobilization, and are consistent with the observation that G-CSF can synergize with flt-3 ligand to mobilize HPC.

<u>HPC mobilization by IL-8 in G-CSFR-deficient mice</u>. To determine whether IL-8-induced mobilization requires the G-CSFR, we challenged G-CSFR-deficient mice with IL-8 [78]. Although both wild-type and G-CSFR-deficient mice had the expected transient neutropenia following IL-8 administration, only the wild-type mice had the expected rebound neutrophilia. As reported previously, IL-8 administration in wild-type mice induced a rapid (peak response at 15 minutes) fourfold increase in circulating CFU-C [25]. In contrast, no increase in circulating CFU-C was detected at any time after IL-8 administration in G-CSFR-deficient mice. These results indicate that the G-CSFR is required for IL-8-induced HPC mobilization in mice.

In summary, the G-CSFR is required for mobilization of HPC from the bone marrow by cyclophosphamide or IL-8, but not flt-3 ligand or IL-12. This suggests that the G-CSFR plays an important and previously unexpected role in HPC mobilization. The G-CSFR is expressed on mature hematopoietic cells, HPC, and endothelial cells[81]; therefore, the loss of G-CSFR signals in any (or all) of these cell types may contribute to the mobilization defect. The defect in mobilization does not appear to be due to neutropenia per se for two reasons. First, there are significant numbers of neutrophils in the bone marrow of G-CSFR-deficient mice. Second, in isolated cases, we have observed G-CSFR-deficient mice that have normal levels of circulating neutrophils, yet these mice still fail to mobilize HPC in response to IL-8. To define the cell type responsible for the mobilization defect in G-CSFR-deficient mice, a series of radiation chimeras were generated by bone marrow transplantation. Preliminary results suggest that the defect in mobilization is intrinsic to transplantable hematopoietic cells, indicating that a functional G-CSFR on bone marrow stromal cells is not required for the generation of the mobilization signal. Within the transplantable hematopoietic cell compartment, the G-CSFR is expressed on HPC, neutrophils, monocytes, and possibly natural killer (NK) cells and B-lymphocytes [82-84]. G-CSFR signals in any or all of these cell types could potentially be required for HPC mobilization. To determine whether a functional G-CSFR on HPC is required, a series of "mixed" chimeras were generated in which both wild-type and G-CSFR deficient hematopoietic cells contributed equally to hematopoiesis. If a functional G-CSFR on HPC is required, then CY-induced mobilization of these mixed chimeras would be predicted to mobilize only the wild-type (G-CSFR-positive) HPC. Surprisingly, preliminary results showed that similar numbers of wild-type and G-CSFR deficient HPC were mobilized after CY treatment, indicating that a functional G-CSFR on mature hematopoietic cells but not on HPC is required for CY-induced mobilization. Collectively, these studies suggest a model in which (G-CSFR-dependent) signals generated by hematopoietic cells after certain stimuli (such as cyclophosphamide) lead to changes in the bone marrow microenvironment that in turn lead to HPC mobilization. In this model, HPC play a more passive role; changes in the bone marrow microenvironment rather than in the phenotype of the HPC themselves are responsible for mobilization.

Summary

The mobilization of HPC from the bone marrow to the peripheral circulation is likely to be a complicated process that is regulated by multiple adhesive interactions between the HPC and the bone marrow ECM. Some of the molecules on HPC important for mobilization (or homing) have been identified and include VLA-4, SDF-1 receptor, and possibly c-kit. Studies of IL-8-induced mobilization and mobilization responses in G-CSF receptor deficient mice suggest a model in which changes in the bone marrow microenvironment rather than the HPC itself may be important for mobilization. This model is consistent with the observation that the phenotype of mobilized HPC is similar for mobilizing stimuli with distinct biological actions and target cell populations. The identification of the molecule(s) responsible for the microenvironment changes should provide exciting avenues of future research.

References

1. Yoder MC, Williams DA: Matrix molecule interactions with hematopoietic stem cells. Exp Hematol 23:961-967, 1995
2. Lichtman M, Packman C, Constine L: Molecular and cellular traffic across the marrow sinuses, vol. 87. Clifton, NJ, Humana Press, 1989
3. Adams J, Watt F: Regulation of development and differentiation by the extracellular matrix. Development 117:1183, 1993
4. Tavassoli M, Hardy CL: Molecular basis of homing of intravenously transplanted stem cells to the marrow. Blood 76:1059-1070, 1990
5. Aizawa S, Tavassoli M: Molecular basis of the recognition of intravenously transplantated hemopoietic cells by bone marrow. Proc Natl Acad Sci USA 85:3180, 1988
6. Matsuoka T, Tavassoli M: Purification and partial characterization of membrane-homing receptors in two cloned murine hemopoietic progenitor cell lines. J Biol Chem 264:20193-8, 1989
7. Coulombel L, Auffray I, Gaugler MH, Rosemblatt M: Expression and function of integrins on hematopoietic progenitor cells. Acta Haematologica 97:13-21, 1997
8. Lesley J, Hyman R, Kincade PW: CD44 and its interaction with extracellular matrix. Advances in Immunology 54:271-335, 1993
9. Spertini O, Cordey AS, Monai N, et al. P-selectin glycoprotein ligand 1 is a ligand for L-selectin on neutrophils, monocytes, and CD34+ hematopoietic progenitor cells. J Cell Biol 135:523-31, 1996
10. Dercksen MW, Gerritsen WR, Rodenhuis S, et al. Expression of adhesion molecules on CD34+ cells: CD34+ L-selectin+ cells predict a rapid platelet recovery after peripheral blood stem cell transplantation. Blood 85:3313-9, 1995
11. Leavesley DI, Oliver JM, Swart BW, et al. Signals from platelet/endothelial cell adhesion molecule enhance the adhesive activity of the very late antigen-4 integrin of human CD34+ hemopoietic progenitor cells. J Immunol 153:4673-83, 1994
12. Vainio O, Dunon D, Aissi F, et al. HEMCAM, an adhesion molecule expressed by c-kit+ hemopoietic progenitors. J Cell Biol 135:1655-68, 1996
13. Levesque J-P, Haylock DN, Simmons PJ: Cytokine regulation of proliferation and cell adhesion are correlated events in human CD34+ hemopoietic progenitors. Blood 88:1168-1176, 1996
14. Simmons PJ, Masinovsky B, Longenecker BM, et al. Vascular cell adhesion molecule-1 expressed by bone marrow stromal cells mediates the binding of hematopoietic progenitor cells. Blood 80:388-395, 1992
15. Papayannopoulou T, Craddock C, Nakamoto B, et al. The VLA4/VCAM-1 adhesion pathway defines contrasting mechanisms of lodgement of transplanted murine hemopoietic progenitors between bone marrow and spleen. Proc Natl Acad Sci USA 92:9647-9651, 1995
16. Papayannopoulou T, Nakamoto B: Peripheralization of hemopoietic progenitors in primates treated with anti-VLA4 intergrin. Proc Natl Acad Sci USA 90:9374-9378, 1993
17. Hirsch E, Iglesias A, Potocnik AJ, et al. Impaired migration but not differentiation of haematopoietic

stem cells in the absence of beta1 integrins. Nature 380:171-5, 1996

18. Miyake K, Medina KL, Hayashi S, et al. Monoclonal antibodies to Pgp-1/CD44 block lympho-hemopoiesis in long-term bone marrow cultures. J Exp Med 171:477-88, 1990

19. Khaldoyanidi S, Denzel A, Zoller M: Requirement for CD44 in proliferation and homing of hematopoietic precursor cells. J Leukocyte Biol 60:579-92, 1996

20. Khaldoyanidi S, Schnabel D, Fohr N, Zoller M: Functional activity of CD44 isoforms in haemopoiesis of the rat. Br J Haematol 96:31-45, 1997

21. Schmits R, Filmus J, Gerwin N, et al. CD44 regulates hematopoietic progenitor distribution, granuloma formation, and tumorigenicity. Blood 90:2217-33, 1997

22. Aiuti A, Webb IJ, Bleul C, et al. The chemokine SDF-1 is a chemoattractant for human CD34+ hematopoietic progenitor cells and provides a new mechanism to explain the mobilization of CD34+ progenitors to peripheral blood. J Exp Med 185:111-20, 1997

23. Kim CH, Broxmeyer HE: In vitro behavior of hematopoietic progenitor cells under the influence of chemoattractants: stromal cell-derived factor-1, steel factor, and the bone marrow environment. Blood 91:100-110, 1998

24. Nagasawa T, Hirota S, Tachibana K, et al. Defects of B-cell lymphopoiesis and bone-marrow myelopoiesis in mice lacking the CXC chemokine PBSF/SDF-1. Nature 382:635-638, 1996

25. Laterveer L, Lindley IJ, Hamilton MS, et al. Interleukin-8 induces rapid mobilization of hematopoietic stem cells with radioprotective capacity and long-term myelolymphoid repopulating ability. Blood 85:2269-75, 1995

26. Wang J, Mukaida N, Zhang Y, et al. Enhanced mobilization of hematopoietic progenitor cells by mouse MIP-2 and granulocyte colony-stimulating factor in mice. Journal of Leukocyte Biology 62:503-9, 1997

27. Lord BI, Woolford LB, Wood LM, et al. Mobilization of early hematopoietic progenitor cells with BB-10010: a genetically engineered variant of human macrophage inflammatory protein-1 alpha. Blood 85:3412-5, 1995

28. Molineux G, Pojda Z, Hampson IN, et al. Transplantation potential of peripheral blood stem cells induced by granulocyte colony-stimulating factor. Blood 76:2153-2158, 1990

29. Molineux G, Pojda Z, Dexter TM: A comparison of hematopoiesis in normal and splenectomized mice treated with granulocyte colony-stimulating factor. Blood 75:563-569, 1990

30. Haan Gd, Dontje B, Engel C, et al. The kinetics of murine hematopoietic stem cells in vivo in response to prolonged increased mature blood cell production induced by granulocyte colony-stimulating factor. Blood 86:2986-2992, 1995

31. Molineux G, Hartley C, McElroy P, et al. Megakaryocyte growth and development factor accelerates platelet recovery in peripheral blood progenitor cell transplant recipients. Blood 88:366-76, 1996

32. Bodine DM, Seidel NE, Zsebo KM, Orlic D: In vivo administration of stem cell factor to mice increases the absolute number of pluripotent hematopoietic stem cells. Blood 82:445-55, 1993

33. Fleming WH, Alpern EJ, Uchida N, et al. Steel factor influences the distribution and activity of murine hematopoietic stem cells in vivo. Proc Natl Acad Sci USA 90:3760-3764, 1993

34. Molineux G, Migdalska A, Szmitkowski M, et al. The effects on hematopoiesis of recombinant stem cell factor (ligand for c-kit) administered in vivo to mice either alone or in combination with granulocyte colony-stimulating factor. Blood 78:961-966, 1991

35. Brasel K, McKenna HJ, Morrissey PJ, et al. Hematologic effects of flt3 ligand in vivo in mice. Blood 88:2004-12, 1996

36. Molineux G, McCrea C, Yan XQ, et al. Flt-3 ligand synergizes with granulocyte colony-stimulating factor to increase neutrophil numbers and to mobilize peripheral blood stem cells with long-term repopulating potential. Blood 89:3998-4004, 1997

37. Vadhan-Raj S, Murray LJ, Bueso-Ramos C, et al. Stimulation of megakaryocyte and platelet production by a single dose of recombinant human thrombopoietin in patients with cancer. Ann Intern Med 126:673-81, 1997

38. Fibbe WE, Hamilton MS, Laterveer LL, et al. Sustained engraftment of mice transplanted with IL-1-primed blood-derived stem cells. J Immunol 148:417-21, 1992

39. Ohi S, Sakamaki S, Matsunaga T, et al. Co-administration of IL3 with G-CSF increases the CFU-S mobilization into peripheral blood [published erratum appears in Int J Hematol 1995 Dec;62(4):261]. Int J Hematol 62:75-82, 1995

40. Geissler K, Peschel C, Niederwieser D, et al. Effect of interleukin-3 pretreatment on granulocyte/macrophage colony-stimulating factor induced mobilization of circulating haemopoietic progenitor cells. Br J Haematol 91:299-305, 1995

41. Geissler K, Peschel C, Niederwieser D, et al. Potentiation of granulocyte colony-stimulating factor-induced mobilization of circulating progenitor cells by seven-day pretreatment with interleukin-3. Blood 87:2732-9, 1996

42. Pettengell R, Luft T, de Wynter E, et al. Effects of interleukin-6 on mobilization of primitive haemopoietic cells into the circulation. Br J Haematol 89:237-42, 1995

43. Grzegorzewski K, Komschlies KL, Mori M, et al. Administration of recombinant human interleukin-7 to mice induces the exportation of myeloid progenitor cells from the bone marrow to peripheral sites. Blood 83:377-85, 1994

44. Damia G, Komschlies KL, Faltynek CR, et al. Administration of recombinant human interleukin-7 alters the frequency and number of myeloid progenitor cells in the bone marrow and spleen of mice. Blood 79:1121-9, 1992

45. Mauch P, Lamont C, Neben TY, et al. Hematopoietic stem cells in the blood after stem cell factor and interleukin-11 administration: Evidence for different mechanisms of mobilization. Blood 86:4674-4680, 1995

46. Jackson JD, Yan Y, Brunda MJ, et al. Interleukin-12 enhances peripheral hematopoiesis in vivo. Blood 85:2371-6, 1995

47. Laterveer L, Lindley IJ, Heemskerk DP, et al. Rapid mobilization of hematopoietic progenitor cells in rhesus monkeys by a single intravenous injection of interleukin-8. Blood 87:781-8, 1996

48. Neben S, Marcus K, Mauch P: Mobilization of hematopoietic stem and progenitor cell subpopulations from the marrow to the blood of mice following cyclophosphamide and/or granulocyte colony-stimulating factor. Blood 81:1960-7, 1993

49. Craddock CF, Apperley JF, Wright EG, et al. Circulating stem cells in mice treated with cyclophosphamide. Blood 80:264-9, 1992

50. Ho AD, Young D, Maruyama M, et al. Pluripotent and lineage-committed CD34+ subsets in leukapheresis products mobilized by G-CSF, GM-CSF vs. a combination of both. Exp Hematol 24:1460-8, 1996

51. To LB, Haylock DN, Dowse T, et al. A comparative study of the phenotype and proliferative capacity of peripheral blood (PB) CD34+ cells mobilized by four different protocols and those of steady-phase PB and bone marrow CD34+ cells. Blood 84:2930-9, 1994

52. Prosper F, Vanoverbeke K, Stroncek D, et al. Primitive long-term culture initiating cells (LTC-ICs) in granulocyte colony-stimulating factor mobilized peripheral blood progenitor cells have similar potential for ex vivo expansion as primitive LTC-ICs in steady state bone marrow. Blood 89:3991-7, 1997

53. Varas F, Bernad A, Bueren JA: Granulocyte colony-stimulating factor mobilizes into peripheral blood the complete clonal repertoire of hematopoietic precursors residing in the bone marrow of mice. Blood 88:2495-501, 1996

54. Watanabe T, Dave B, Heimann DG, et al. GM-CSF-mobilized peripheral blood CD34+ cells differ from steady-state bone marrow CD34+ cells in adhesion molecule expression. Bone Marrow Transplant 19:1175-81, 1997

55. Mohle R, Murea S, Kirsch M, et al. Differential expression of L-selectin, VLA-4, and LFA-1 on CD34+ progenitor cells from bone marrow and peripheral blood during G-CSF-enhanced recovery. Exp Hematol 23:1535-42, 1995

56. Rumi C, Rutella S, Teofili L, et al. RhG-CSF-mobilized CD34+ peripheral blood progenitors are myeloperoxidase-negative and noncycling irrespective of CD33 or CD13 coexpression. Exp Hematol 25:246-51, 1997

57. Uchida N, He D, Friera AM, et al. The unexpected G0/G1 cell cycle status of mobilized hematopoietic stem cells from peripheral blood. Blood 89:465-72, 1997

58. Roberts A, Metcalf D: Noncycling state of peripheral blood progenitor cells mobilized by granulocyte colony-stimulating factor and other cytokines. Blood 86:1600-1605, 1995

59. Ponchio L, Conneally E, Eaves C: Quantitation of the quiescent fraction of long-term culture-initiating cells in normal human blood and marrow and the kinetics of their growth factor-stimulated entry into S-phase in vitro. Blood 86:3314-3321, 1995

60. Mohle R, Haas R, Hunstein W: Expression of adhesion molecules and c-kit on CD34+ hematopoietic progenitor cells: comparison of cytokine mobilized blood stem cells with normal bone marrow and peripheral blood. J Hematother 2:483, 1993

61. Roberts AW, Foote S, Alexander WS, et al. Genetic influences determining progenitor cell mobilization and leukocytosis induced by granulocyte colony-stimulating factor. Blood 89:2736-44, 1997

62. Papayannopoulou T, Priestley G, Nakamoto B: Anti-VLA-4/VCAM-1-induced mobilization requires cooperative signaling through the kit/mkit ligand pathway. Blood 91:2231-2239, 1998

63. Hoch RC, Schraufstatter IU, Cochrane CG: In vivo, in vitro, and molecular aspects of interleukin-8 and the interleukin-8 receptors. Journal of Laboratory & Clinical Medicine 128:134-45, 1996

64. Peveri P, Walz A, Dewald B, Baggiolini M: A novel neutrophil-activating factor produced by human mononuclear phagocytes. J Exp Med 167:1547-59, 1988

65. Thelen M, Peveri P, Kernen P, et al. Mechanism of neutrophil activation by NAF, a novel monocyte-derived peptide agonist. FASEB Journal 2:2702-6, 1988

66. Detmers PA, Powell DE, Walz A, et al. Differential effects of neutrophil-activating peptide 1/IL-8 and its homologues on leukocyte adhesion and phagocytosis. J Immunol 147:4211-7, 1991

67. Luscinskas FW, Kiely JM, Ding H, et al. In vitro inhibitory effect of IL-8 and other chemoattractants on neutrophil-endothelial adhesive interactions. J Immunol 149:2163-71, 1992

68. Wang J, Zhang Y, Kasahara T, et al. Detection of mouse IL-8 receptor homologue expression on peripheral blood leukocytes and mature myeloid lineage cells in bone marrow. J Leukocyte Biol 60:372-81, 1996

69. Pruijt J, Fibbe W, Laterveer L, et al. Prevention of interleukin-8-induced mobilization of hematopoietic progenitor cells in rhesus monkeys by antibodies to the metalloproteinase gelatinase-B. Blood 88:455a, 1996

70. Schonbeck U, Brandt E, Petersen F, et al. IL-8 specifically binds to endothelial but not to smooth muscle cells. J Immunol 154:2375-2383, 1995

71. Koch A, Polverini P, Kunkel S, et al. Interleukin-8 as a macrophage-derived mediator of angiogenesis. Science 258:1798-1801, 1995

72. Yan XQ, Briddell R, Hartley C, et al. Mobilization of long-term hematopoietic reconstituting cells in mice by the combination of stem cell factor plus granulocyte colony-stimulating factor. Blood 84:795-9, 1994

73. Morrison SJ, Wright DE, Weissman IL: Cyclophosphamide/granulocyte colony-stimulating factor induces hematopoietic stem cells to proliferate prior to mobilization. Proc Natl Acad Sci USA 94:1908-13, 1997

74. Yan XQ, Hartley C, McElroy P, et al. Peripheral blood progenitor cells mobilized by recombinant human granulocyte colony-stimulating factor plus recombinant rat stem cell factor contain long-term engrafting cells capable of cellular proliferation for more than two years as shown by serial transplantation in mice. Blood 85:2303-7, 1995

75. Bodine DM, Seidel NE, Orlic D: Bone marrow collected 14 days after in vivo administration of granulocyte colony-stimulating factor and stem cell factor to mice has 10-fold more repopulating ability than untreated bone marrow. Blood 88:89-97, 1996

76. Papayannopoulou T, Nakamoto B, Andrews RG, et al. In vivo effects of Flt3/Flk2 ligand on mobilization of hematopoietic progenitors in primates and potent synergistic enhancement with granulocyte colony-stimulating factor. Blood 90:620-9, 1997

77. Sudo Y, Shimazaki C, Ashihara E, et al. Synergistic effect of FLT-3 ligand on the granulocyte colony-stimulating factor-induced mobilization of hematopoietic stem cells and progenitor cells into blood in mice. Blood 89:3186-91, 1997

78. Liu F, Poursine-Laurent J, Link DC: The granulocyte colony-stimulating factor receptor is required for the mobilization of murine hematopoietic progenitors into peripheral blood by cyclophosphamide or interleukin-8 but not Flt-3 ligand. Blood 90:2522-2528, 1997

79. Liu F, Wu HY, Wesselschmidt R, et al. Impaired production and increased apoptosis of neutrophils in granulocyte colony-stimulating factor receptor deficient mice. Immun 5:491-501, 1996

80. Liu F, Poursine-Laurent J, Wu H, Link D: IL-6 and the G-CSF receptor are major independent regulators of granulopoiesis in vivo but are not required for lineage commitment or terminal differentiation. Blood 90:2583-2590, 1997

81. Demetri GD, Griffin JD: Granulocyte colony-stimulating factor and its receptor. Review. Blood 78:2791-808, 1991

82. Inukai T, Sugita K, Iijima K, et al. Expression of granulocyte colony-stimulating factor receptor on CD10-positive human B-cell precursors. Br J Haematol 89:623-6, 1995

83. Iszuka K, Kaneko H, Tamada T, et al. Host F1 mice pretreated with granulocyte colony-stimulating factor accept parental bone marrow grafts in hybrid resistance system. Blood 89:1446-1451, 1997

84. Nicola NA, Metcalf D: Binding of I125-labeled granulocyte colony-stimulating factor to normal murine hematopoietic cells. J. Cell Physiol 124:313, 1985

21. The Use of Cytokines to Enhance Collection of Stem Cells for Marrow and Blood Transplantation

Susan Roman-Unfer, Elizabeth J. Shpall

Introduction

High-dose therapy with hematopoietic cell support is effective treatment for selected high-risk patients with hematologic malignancies[1] or solid tumors[2] in whom standard-dose therapy has minimal benefit. Over the past decade, rapid and substantial advances have been made in the procurement and manipulation of hematopoietic progenitor cells for transplantation. The advances include the development and continued refinement of peripheral blood progenitor cell (PBPC) mobilization regimens using chemotherapy and/or growth factor(s), purging of malignant cells from marrow or blood, the isolation of purified hematopoietic cell subpopulations using flowcytometry, immunoadsorption or immunomagnetic techniques, and the ex vivo expansion of hematopoietic progenitors using static or continuously perfused liquid culture systems.

The major sources of human hematopoietic cells for clinical transplantation include bone marrow and peripheral blood. More recently, umbilical cord blood has been employed as an alternative source of hematopoietic cells. Allogeneic transplantation of marrow,[3] peripheral blood[4], and cord blood[5] has been performed with cells from both related and unrelated donors. Autologous transplants, where the patient serves as his/her own donor, are typically performed with either marrow and/or PBPCs [6].

When clinically indicated, patients receive a high-dose therapy regimen, followed by infusion of fresh (allogeneic marrow or PBPCs) or previously cryopreserved (autologous marrow and/or peripheral blood, allogeneic cord blood) hematopoietic cells. Within days of high-dose therapy administration, the patients develop profound myelosuppression which is ameliorated by the hematopoietic cell transplant. The time to hematopoietic reconstitution or "engraftment," which is commonly defined as a white blood cell (WBC) count of 500 cells x 10^9/L and a platelet count of 20 x 10^9/L, reflects the quality of the infused progenitors.

Quality Control of a Hematopoietic Graft

What constitutes an adequate hematopoietic product has not been universally defined. The reproducible murine hematopoietic stem cell assays, such as the colony forming unit-spleen (CFU-S)[7] and competitive repopulation studies in lethally irradiated recipients[8] do not exist for the human hematopoietic stem cell. The lack of information with any of the available in vitro or in vivo assays to detect and quantitate human hematopoietic cells with long-term, multilineage, in vivo repopulation capacity underscores the difficulty of assessing the reconstitution potential of hematopoietic grafts. Several different assays are currently employed to evaluate parameters which are felt to be surrogate markers of human hematopoietic cell repopulation potential. Flow cytometric analysis of CD34[+] cell content is commonly employed to assess hematopoietic grafts. Short-[9] and long-term[10] in vitro tissue culture assays, as well as in vivo severe combined immunodeficiency (SCID)-mouse repopulating assays[11] have also been used to quantitate the content of progenitors present in human hematopoietic cell fractions.

Short-Term Tissue Culture Assay. Short-term methylcellulose-based tissue culture assays are often used to quantitatively assess the content of committed colony forming cells in culture (CFC), which include colony forming units-granulocyte macrophage (CFU-GM)[9], consisting primarily of myeloid and burst forming units erythroid (BFU-E) progenitors in hematopoietic cell fractions. A fibrin clot assay[12], is less commonly employed to assess the megakaryocyte colony forming units (CFU-MK) of the progenitor cell fractions. The obligate 10-14 day period required before the cultures can be analyzed make the clinical use of these assays difficult, given the immediate decisions regarding hematopoietic graft quality often necessary for optimal patient care.

Long-Term Tissue Culture Assay. Sutherland et al., developed the long-term culture initiating cell (LTC-IC) assay which is being used with increasing frequency in research laboratories to assess a more primitive human hematopoietic progenitor than that represented by the CFC[10]. The assay measures cells that give rise to clonogenic progenitors detectable in methylcellulose after a minimum of five weeks of culture in the presence of preirradiated stroma. When compared directly in murine experiments, LTC-IC were shown to be more primitive than many CFU-S and to co-purify with long-term in vivo repopulating cells[10]. Although this assay may be useful in preclinical hematopoietic graft manipulation studies to determine the optimal procedures to be used clinically, the multi-week delay before it can be analyzed makes it impossible to use clinically for the analysis of specific grafts.

SCID-Mouse Assay. The SCID syndrome was first described in mice in 1991 by selectively breeding a colony of mice deficient in mature B and T lymphocytes[13]. Because of this immunodeficiency, the SCID mouse was noted to be permissive for the growth of human hematopoietic cells. Approximately 1% of the human bone marrow cells infused into irradiated SCID mice were still detectable several months following the infusion[14]. The administration of human growth factors to the SCID mice, following injection, significantly enhanced the level of human hematopoietic cell reconstitution to greater than 10% and resulted in the detection of multilineage engraftment. More recently, substantial reconstitution of SCID mice with human cord blood progenitors, which require no exogenous growth factor support, was reported with a very high fraction (70%) of human cells detected six months following transplant[15,16]. Reconstitution in SCID mice is an vivo assay of repopulating potential that will likely be of major importance in the research laboratories developing new hematopoietic graft manipulation(s) that will ultimately be used in the clinical setting. However, given the technical complexity of performing and several month delay in evaluating the assay, it is obviously not suitable for clinical use.

Future Directions. In clinical studies, time to hematopoietic reconstitution has been shown to correlate with the number of mononuclear cells (MNCs),[17] CFU-GM,[18] and

CD34[+] cells[19] contained in the hematopoietic products. As discussed above, the clinical use of short- and/or long-term tissue culture or SCID mice is generally not feasible given the time delays inherent in those assays. Because of the current lack of CD34[+] cell assay standardization among hematopoietic cell processing laboratories, the total cells (marrow) or MNCs (PBPCs, cord blood) is probably the most consistent, although not necessarily the most predictive, parameter currently in use. Studies have been initiated by the International Society of Hematotherapy and Graft Engineering (ISHAGE) to rapidly standardize the flow cytometric analysis of CD34[+] cells in North American hematopoietic cell processing laboratories. The number of CD34[+] cells which possess short- and/or long-term hematopoietic repopulation potential are likely a better measure of graft quality than the number of cells in the more heterogeneous MNC fraction. Once standardized, flow cytometric assessment of CD34[+] cell number will likely become the primary assay for evaluating hematopoietic graft quality in the next several years.

From the time bone marrow or peripheral blood is harvested until it is infused or cryopreserved, the viability of hematopoietic cells declines at a continual rate [20]. Thus, irrespective of quality control assays, it is generally accepted that, with respect to quality of the progenitors and the safety of the patients, the sooner a graft can be processed following harvest the better.

Bone Marrow

Bone marrow has been successfully used to support the myelosuppression produced by high-dose chemotherapy since 1957 [21]. The marrow is generally harvested from the posterior iliac crests of the donor or patient under general anesthesia [22], and then either infused or cryopreserved as described above. A final marrow volume of approximately 800-2000 ml is collected and infused fresh (allogeneic) or cryopreserved (autologous). Generally, transplant centers attempt to collect a total of 0.5 - 4.0 x 10^8 MNCs/kg patient weight, depending upon the additional manipulations which are planned.

Although reproducible hematopoietic reconstitution is achieved with bone marrow, which cells are actually responsible respectively for the short and long-term engraftment is unknown. In murine models, separable progenitor cell subpopulations with short- and long-term repopulating potential have been reported [23]. Baum et al. showed that the Thy1.1(lo) Lin(-) Sca-1(+) subpopulation of mouse bone marrow cells contained all cells capable of long-term repopulation in lethally irradiated mice [23]. More recently, their group compared the kinetics of reconstitution using purified Thy1.1(lo) Lin(-) Sca-1(+) cells, to that achieved with unfractionated marrow containing an equivalent number of the highly purified cells [24]. Surprisingly, they found that the short-term or early phase (day 7-21) and middle phase (day 21 to 35) of hematopoietic reconstitution in lethally irradiated mice could be achieved exclusively with the highly purified stem cell fraction. Furthermore, there was no significant difference in the rate of hematopoietic recovery after transplantation of the highly purified (although still heterogeneous) cells, when compared to recipients transplanted with whole marrow containing comparable numbers of the same. These data suggest that either this specific subpopulation contains cells with both short- and long-term repopulating potential, or alternatively, the subpopulation could be heterogeneous, containing cells with different repopulating potentials.

In humans, it is commonly believed that a subpopulation of CD34[+] pluripotent bone marrow cells are responsible for the long-term repopulation, and that a distinct CD34[+] subpopulation of more differentiated hematopoietic progenitors can produce an early phase of more rapid hematopoietic recovery; however, neither of these assumptions has been formally tested clinically. Whether a highly purified marrow subpopulation could produce both short- and long-term engraftment in patients is unknown. Whether there is a subpopulation with the ability to increase the rate of short-term engraftment is also unknown. Similarly, although current evidence suggests that all human long-term repopulating cells will be CD34[+], the possibility that some or even all such cells are CD34-negative (-), has also not yet been excluded. With the dramatic advances in hematopoietic graft engineering, the answers to these fundamental questions about human bone marrow transplantation should be forthcoming in the near future.

Peripheral Blood Progenitor Cells

PBPCs have replaced bone marrow as the major source of hematopoietic progenitor cell support in patients receiving high-dose chemotherapy. This trend is due, in part, to the perception that multiple leukapheresis procedures are less morbid than a marrow harvest. Additionally, several studies have demonstrated improvements in the rate of platelet recovery for patients who received PBPCs alone [25], or in combination with marrow [26,27] when compared to patients who received bone marrow alone or with posttransplant growth factor support. Initially, a major concern in the transplant community was whether PBPCs as sole hematopoietic support would produce durable long-term engraftment. Several studies with multi-year follow-up have confirmed the durability of hematopoietic reconstitution produced using PBPCs alone [1,28-30] which has led to the increasing use of this technology.

<u>Harvesting of PBPCs</u>. PBPCs are collected by an outpatient "leukapheresis" procedure using a continuous-flow blood cell separator such as the COBE-Spectra or the Fenwall CS-3000. Approximately 9-14 liters of patient blood is processed, which takes three to four hours. The vast majority of the processed blood is returned to the patient. A final PBPC volume of approximately 200 ml is collected and infused (allogeneic) or cryopreserved (autologous). Transplant centers usually attempt to collect a total of 4.0 - 6.0 x 10^8 MNCs per kilogram of patient weight [25]. The number of leukaphereses performed depends upon several factors, including the patient's disease, amount of prior myelotoxic therapy, extent of tumor involvement in the marrow and/or blood, whether the cells are collected from patients in a "steady state," or following mobilization from the marrow to the blood with chemotherapy and/or growth factors. In the steady state, six or more leukaphereses may be required to reach the target MNC number described above [1,31]. Because of delayed platelet recovery in patients transplanted with PBPCs collected in the steady state, such collections are now generally reserved for patients who are mobilization failures as a result of extensive prior therapy, substantial tumor contamination of the marrow, or rarely, no apparent reason. With mobilized PBPCs, one to five leukaphereses may be required, depending upon the mobilization regimen used. Whether tumor cells are also mobilized with chemotherapy and/or growth factors is unknown and requires investigation.

Mobilization Regimens

PBPCs can be mobilized with growth factors and/or chemotherapy. Granulocyte-colony stimulating factor (G-CSF, Filgrastim) and granulocyte-macrophage colony stimulating factor (GM-CSF, sargramostim) are the growth factors most commonly used. Newer growth factors such as stem cell factor (SCF), IL-3, and Flt-3 ligand however are currently being evaluated in combination with G-CSF and GM-CSF to determine if a better mobilization product can be obtained.

Chemotherapy and Growth Factors. Sutherland et al., reported that PBPCs mobilized with cyclophosphamide contained higher numbers of primitive hematopoietic precursors than PBPCs mobilized with cyclophosphamide plus GM-CSF [10]. Udomsakdi et al., demonstrated that the clonogenic progenitor-producing potential of LTC-IC present in PBPC harvests collected, following mobilization with cyclophosphamide and/or growth factors, was significantly lower than that of LTC-IC in normal bone marrow or peripheral blood samples [32].

Granulocyte-Colony Stimulating Factor (G-CSF, Filgrastim). Human G-CSF is a 204 amino acid protein of approximately 25 kDa [33,34]. The G-CSF receptor is found on neutrophilic progenitors, mature neutrophils, and various myeloid leukemia cells [35-37]. The use of autologous PBPCs collected, following mobilization with G-CSF, results in rapid engraftment with the time to reach an absolute neutrophil count (ANC) of $500/\mu l$ and $20,000/\mu l$ significantly reduced when compared to steady-state PBPCs [38-40].

It has not been definitely shown that raising the dose of G-CSF above 10 $\mu g/kg/day$ can also attain a higher degree of mobilization; however, there are several reports to suggest that the hypothesis should be tested. Animal data suggests that SCF will enhance the PBPC mobilization of a broad range of doses of G-CSF. For example, baboons treated with 10 or 250 $\mu g/kg/day$ G-CSF showed synergistic mobilization when SCF (25 $\mu g/kg/day$) was added to the mobilization regimen [41].

Weaver et al., reported the results of a randomized dose-finding study with Filgrastim in patients with stage IV breast cancer having received $\leq$ two prior chemotherapy regimens [42]. Four cohorts of 20 to 37 patients were evaluated in terms of mobilization of CD34$^+$ cells. While a Filgrastim dose response was observed, a plateau of mobilization effect was observed at the higher doses. This effect is somewhat contradicted by the findings of Sheridan et al., where equivalent effects of 12 and 24 $\mu g/kg/day$ of Filgrastim on mobilization were observed [43,44].

Granulocyte-Macrophage Stimulating Factor (GM-CSF), Sargramostim. Human GM-CSF is a 127 amino acid protein of approximately 23 kDa [45]. GM-CSF receptors are found on hematopoietic cells and non-hematopoietic cells such as trophoblasts, endothelial cells, oligodendrocytes, and on various malignant cells [46]. The use of GM-CSF mobilized PBPCs, following ablative chemotherapy, also results in rapid engraftment [47]. No large randomized trial has been performed comparing Filgrastim and GM-CSF-mobilized PBPCs, however both appear to be effective mobilizing agents. Filgrastim is more commonly used as a mobilizing agent, due to the increased side effects associated with GM-CSF. Bone pain, headaches, and fatigue tend to be more severe when associated with GM-CSF. Additionally, a flu-like syndrome could also be induced by GM-CSF that may cause a rash and elevated liver function tests. Capillary leak syndrome is a dose-limiting toxic effect [48].

Stem Cell Factor (SCF). More recently discovered, hematopoietic cytokines are currently under investigation for the mobilization of PBPCs. Human SCF is a glycoprotein that acts on hematopoietic blood cell progenitors [49]. While recombinant methionyl human SCF (r-metHuSCF) alone exerts little colony-stimulating activity on normal human bone marrow cells, the combination of r-metHuSCF with IL-3, Filgrastim, GM-CSF, or EPO results in a synergistic increase in the number of colonies[50]. The types of colonies produced are determined by the other hematopoietic growth factors used in conjunction with r-metHuSCF. The synergism between r-metHuSCF and other hematopoietic growth factors has also been demonstrated with bone marrow cells from patients with bone marrow failure diseases [48].

In rodents, dogs, and baboons the combination of low doses of species-specific recombinant SCF plus optimal doses of recombinant G-CSF caused a synergistic increase in PBPCs that were capable of rescuing animals from otherwise lethal irradiation [41,51,52]. In mice, PBPCs mobilized with the combination of PEGylated r-met-rat SCF (r-metRSCF) plus Filgrastim provided faster engraftment, and fewer cells were required to achieve engraftment, as compared with PBPCs mobilized by PEGylated r-metRSCF or Filgrastim alone [47]. These animal models demonstrated that low doses of recombinant SCF, which do not mobilize PBPCs, synergize with recombinant G-CSF to mobilize greater numbers of PBPCs than can be mobilized by G-CSF alone. The mobilized PBPCs established both short- and long-term engraftment, and hematologic recovery was more rapid than seen with PBPCs mobilized by G-CSF alone [53].

Toxicology studies have been performed in primates that received r-metHuSCF (100-6000 μg/kg/day) by intravenous or subcutaneous injection. At doses of up to approximately 300 times the anticipated human dosage, subcutaneous dosing for 21 days caused minimal toxicities and the expected biological effects. The expected dose-dependent increases in bone marrow and extramedullary hematopoiesis and in mast-cell numbers were observed in cynomolgus monkeys administered r-metHuSCF subcutaneously for 13 weeks at 100, 1000, and 6000 μg/kg/day. Pathogenic changes seen at 1000 and 6000 μg/kg/day included increased pigmentation of the skin, development of skin papules, and proliferation of mast cells in virtually all organs and tissues. The incidence and severity of the pharmacological and biological effects were greater in the higher dose groups, and these effects, for the most part, were reversible.

Several studies in nonhuman primates have demonstrated the potential for serious anaphylactoid reactions following rapid intravenous administration ("IV push") of r-metHuSCF. This effect was initially observed in cynomolgus monkeys after intravenous administration of very high levels of r-metHuSCF (6000 μg/kg). Subsequently, these reactions were observed in baboons at doses as low as 40 μg/kg r-metHuSCF administered by intravenous injection.

These reactions and the efficacy of premedications were evaluated in a randomized, blinded GLP study in baboons utilizing 80 μg/kg r-metHuSCF administered by intravenous injection. (Amgen data on file). Acute anaphylactoid reactions were observed in at least 60% of the baboons that were not premedicated. The reactions were characterized by more frequent and severe hypotension, bronchoconstriction, and markedly fewer cutaneous findings that were observed following administration of subcutaneous r-metHuSCF in clinical studies. Pathophysiology indicated that these reactions were mast cell-mediated, as are the systemic allergic-like reactions in man.

This study included evaluation of the protective effect of H_1 antihistamines (i.e., diphenhydramine, cetirizine), and H_2 antihistamine (ranitidine), an inhaled bronchodilator (albuterol), and a corticosteroid (methylprednisolone). In this baboon model of r-metHuSCF-induced anaphylactoid reactions, hypotension and bronchoconstriction were most effectively prevented by the three-drug combination of H_1 and H_2 antihistamines, plus either the inhaled bronchodilator or the corticosteroid, though the addition of corticosteroids appeared superior by some measures.

Phase I clinical non-PBPC trials have been performed in patients with advanced non-small cell lung cancer, as well as in patients with advanced breast cancer. In these studies, patients were given r-metHuSCF (5-50 μg/kg/day) either before and/or after conventional chemotherapy. The most common side effect observed was the development of dermatologic reactions at the injection site, with most patients developing a raised pruritic wheal with surrounding erythema. Mild urticaria at distant sites, with or without respiratory symptoms, were seen in some patients, but were reversible and transient [54,55]. All subsequent trials, including the use of r-metHuSCF, have included the use of a histamine (H_1- receptor antagonist) given concurrently with the r-metHuSCF.

SCF Plus Filgrastim. Several trials (phases I-III) are completed or in progress to assess the ability of r-metHuSCF in combination with Filgrastim to safely mobilize PBPCs in patients. The combination of r-metHuSCF plus Filgrastim at the doses studied to date, given with a premedication scheme, has been safe and well tolerated [54,56-60]. From these studies, there have been 16 systemic allergic-like reactions. Two reactions (3%) at 15 μg/kg/day r-metHuSCF, 13 reactions (4%) at 20 μg/kg/day, and one reaction (8%) at 30 μg/kg/day, in combination with Filgrastim have been reported. The safety experience of r-metHuSCF in PBPC trials appears superior to that observed in phase I non-PBPC trials [55,61].

Doses of r-metHuSCF from 5 to 30 μg/kg/day have been administered thus far in combination with 10 μ/kg/day Filgrastim. In a phase I/II study of patients with breast cancer, patients treated with the cytokine combination had increased WBCs, ANCs, MNCs, and CD34$^+$ cells in the peripheral blood, as compared to patients who received Filgrastim alone. Leukapheresis harvests obtained after mobilization with Filgrastim plus r-metHuSCF at $\geq$ 15 μg/kg/day yielded increased numbers of MNC, CD34$^+$ cells, CFU-GM, and BFU-E compared with harvests obtained after mobilization with Filgrastim alone. The median leukapheresis harvest of CD34$^+$ cells was approximately 3 x 10^6 cells/kg for patients mobilized with Filgrastim alone as compared with a median of approximately 8 x 10^6 cells/kg for patients who mobilized with Filgrastim plus r-metHuSCF (15 μg/kg/day) [62]. The mobilization data from this study indicated that 20 μg/kg/day is the most appropriate dose of r-metHuSCF for combination with 10 μg/kg/day Filgrastim for PBPC mobilization [62].

In a phase I/II study of 205 breast cancer patients randomized to receive either Filgrastim (10 μg/kg/day) or SCF (20 μg/kg/day) and Filgrastim (10 μg/kg/day), approximately 55% reached 5 x 10^6 CD34 cells by five pheresis procedures. This mobilization effect highlights the fact that some patients still require multiple apheresis procedures to achieve optimal transplant harvest. The development of a more efficient PBPC mobilization method that increases the harvest is an important clinical goal.

Recently, several randomized controlled studies have been performed comparing the addition of r-metHuSCF to Filgrastim vs Filgrastim alone. One study in high-risk breast cancer patients evaluated r-metHuSCF (20 μ/kg/day) plus Filgrastim (10 μg/kg/day) vs Filgrastim alone (10 μg/kg/day) [63]. There was a significant increase in CD34[+] cell yield on most days of apheresis associated with a statistically significant decrease in the number of aphereses required to reach a target yield between patients receiving r-metHuSCF plus Filgrastim and those receiving Filgrastim alone. The median number of aphereses to achieve the target was four days for the r-metHuSCF plus Filgrastim group, and for the Filgrastim alone group was $\geq$ 6 days (i.e., less than 50% of the patients reached the target in five apheresis collections). Similar phase III trials in patients with myeloma and lymphoma are currently underway [63].

Another randomized study in heavily pretreated non-Hodgkin's lymphoma and Hodgkin's lymphoma patients also evaluated SCF (20 μ/kg/day) plus Filgrastim (10 μg/kg/day) vs Filgrastim alone (10 μg/kg/day). Their results were similar with significant increases in the total number of CD34[+] cells collected (median 3.6 x 10^6/kg in SCF plus Filgrastim patients versus 2.4 x 10^6/kg in Filgrastim alone patients), the proportion of patients reaching > 5.0 x 10^6/kg and the number of aphereses to reach this target. The most common side effects were mild-to-moderate dermatologic changes at the injection site, most commonly involving erythema/ pruritus, occurring in 78% of the patients [64].

Finally, a third randomized study in 129 multiple myeloma patients evaluated SCF 20 μg/kg/day with Filgrastim 5 μg/kg/day and cyclophosphamide ($4g/m^2$) versus Filgrastim and cyclophosphamide alone. All patients receiving SCF were given prophylactic antihistamines. An interim analysis of 29 patients revealed similar results with a greater four-fold increase in the CD34[+] cell number in the first leukapheresis product in patients treated with the regimen containing SCF. The number of leukaphereses needed to reach 5 x 10^6 CD34[+] cells/kg was 1 for SCF and Filgrastim patients versus 2.5 for Filgrastim alone patients. Injection site reactions occurred in 46% of patients, and there were no systemic allergic-like reactions [65].

Clinical studies of PBPC transplantation have shown a general relationship between the quantity of PBPCs infused (as measured by either the number of CD34[+] cells or CFU-GM) and the rate of hematologic recovery, particularly for platelet recovery [66-68]. When high numbers of PBPCs were infused, hematologic recovery was almost invariably rapid [69]. When low numbers of PBPCs were infused, the rate of hematologic recovery was variable with a higher proportion of patients showing delays in platelet recovery. Therefore, there is a clinical benefit to increasing the mobilization and collection of CD34[+] cells.

In summary, the data in three animal models and from the clinical trials conducted to date indicate that administration of r-metHuSCF in combination with Filgrastim yields higher numbers of PBPCs and appears to be a superior mobilization method compared with Filgrastim alone.

Basser et al., reported on a study of stage II or III chemotherapy-naive breast cancer patients receiving three days of priming with r-metHuSCF 10 μg/kg/day before seven days of combination cytokine at 12 μg/kg/day Filgrastim and 10 μg/kg/day r-metHuSCF [70]. The median cumulative CD34[+] cell yield obtained was 24.5 x 10^6/kg compared to 11.4 x 10^6/kg CD34[+] cells in patients receiving Filgrastim alone (12 μg/kg/day) for seven days. A separate cohort receiving the seven-day combination of

10 μg/kg/day of r-metHuSCF and 12 μg/kg/day of Filgrastim had a median cumulative CD34$^+$ cell yield of 20.9 x 10^6 kg, suggesting that there might be a benefit with respect to PBPC yield in priming with r-metHuSCF, prior to administration of the cytokine combination (Amgen study report, SCF9216). The PBPC harvests, as measured by the number of CFU-GMs in the total leukapheresis yield, were higher in the 10-day r-metHuSCF cohort than the seven-day combination, or the Filgrastim alone cohort (1002, 675, and 392 x 10^6/kg respectively) [32].

The combination of H_1, H_2 antihistamines and albuterol has proven effective in preventing serious allergic-like reactions in prior r-metHuSCF clinical studies. Preclinical studies in primates indicated that prednisone is at least as effective as albuterol, in combination with H_1 and H_2 blockers in preventing hypotension and bronchoconstriction, the most serious mast cell-mediated adverse events observed. In the current clinical study, prednisone will replace albuterol in the premedication regimen.

Flt-3 Ligand. Multiple isoforms of human Flt-3 ligand have been identified [71-74]. The biological role of these different isoforms is currently unknown. The predominant isoform of human Flt-3 ligand is a transmembrane protein [71,72,74]. Flt -3 ligand receptor has not been found on mature hematopoietic cells however has been detected on the surface of stem and progenitor cells [75].

Data in both mice[76] and primates[77] suggest that Flt-3 ligand is capable of increasing the number of colony-forming cells in peripheral blood. The potential use of Flt-3 ligand in the mobilization of PBPCs in humans is promising and requires further study.

In summary, whether different mobilization regimens will produce PBPC harvests with different repopulating potentialities or unique potentialities for progenitor expansion ex vivo, requires further investigation and will be evaluated in current and future clinical studies.

References

1. Philip T, Armitage JO, Spitzer G, et al. High-dose therapy and autologous bone marrow transplantation after failure of conventional chemotherapy in adults with intermediate-grade or high-grade non-Hodgkin's lymphoma. N Engl J Med 316:1493-8, 1987.
2. Shpall EJ, Jones RB, Bearman SI. High-dose therapy with autologous bone marrow transplantation for the treatment of solid tumors. Curr Science 6:135-8, 1994.
3. Thomas ED, Buckner CD, Clift RA, et al. Marrow transplantation for acute nonlymphoblastic leukemia in first remission. N Engl J Med 301:597-9, 1979.
4. Anasetti C, Martin PJ, Storb R, and Hansen JA. Engraftment of allogeneic hematopoietic stem cells in patients conditioned only with anti-CD3 monoclonal antibody BC3 plus methylprednisolone. Blood 84:249a (980), 1994.
5. Broxmeyer HE, Kurtzberg J, Gluckman E, et al. Umbilical cord blood hematopoietic stem and repopulating cells in human clinical transplantation. Blood Cells 17:313, 1991.
6. Peters WP, Ross M, Vredenburgh JJ, et al. High-dose chemotherapy and autologous bone marrow support as consolidation after standard-dose adjuvant therapy for high-risk primary breast cancer. J Clin Oncol 11:1132-43, 1993.
7. McCullogh E and Till J. The radiation sensitivity of normal mouse bone marrow cells, determined by quantitative marrow transplantation into irradiated mice. Radiat Res 13:15-125, 1960.
8. Philips RA. Hematopoietic stem cells: Concepts, assays, and controversies. Sem Immunol 3:337-41, 1991.
9. Rowley S, Sharkis S, Hattenburg C, Sensenbrenner L. Culture from human bone marrow of blast progenitor cells with an extensive proliferative capacity. Blood 69:804-8, 1987.

10. Sutherland HJ, Lansdorp PM, Henkelmean DH, Eaves AC, Eaves CJ. Functional characterization of individual human hematopoietic stem cells cultured at limiting dilution on supportive marrow stromal layers. Proc Natl Acad Sci USA 87:3584-8, 1990.

11. Shpall EJ, Jones RB, Franklin W, et al. Transplantation of enriched CD34 positive ($^+$) autologous marrow into breast cancer patients following high-dose chemotherapy: Influence of CD34$^+$ peripheral blood progenitors and growth factors on engraftment. J Clin Oncol 12:28-36, 1994.

12. Briddell RA, Bruno E, Cooper RJ, et al. Plasma clot assay for the evaluation of megakaryocyte progenitor cells. Blood 78:2854-9, 1991.

13. Bosma MJ, Carroll AM. The SCID mouse mutant: Definition, characterization, and potential uses. Ann Rev Immunol 9:323-50, 1991.

14. Lapidot T, Pflumio F, Doedens M, Murdoch B, Williams DE, and Dick JE. Cytokine stimulation of multi lineage hematopoiesis from immature human cells engrafted in SCID mice. Science 255:1137, 1992.

15. Vormoor J, Lapidot T, Pflumio F, et al. Immature human cord blood progenitors engraft and proliferate to high levels in severe combined immunodeficient mice. Blood 83:2489-98, 1994.

16. Lowry PA, Schultz LD, Greinier D, et al. Human hematopoietic progenitor engraftment into NOD-SCID/SCID mice not require cytokine support. Exp Hematol 22:803, 1994.

17. Kessinger A, and Armitage JO. The evolving role of autologous peripheral stem cell transplantation following high-dose therapy for malignancies. Blood 77:211-13, 1991.

18. Douay L, Gorin N, Mary J, et al. Recovery of CFU-GM from cryopreserved marrow and in vivo evaluation after autologous bone marrow transplantation are predictive of engraftment. Exp Hematol 14:358-65, 1986.

19. Sienna S, Bregni M, Brando B, et al. Flow cytometry for clinical estimation of circulating hematopoietic progenitors for autologous transplantation in cancer patients. Blood 77:400-6, 1991.

20. Treleaven J. Bone marrow harvesting and reinfusion. In: Bone Marrow Processing and Purging, A Practical Guide. Ed: Gee A: CRC Press, Pp 31-8, 1991.

21. Storb R, Thomas ED. The scientific foundation of marrow transplantation based on animal studies. In: Bone Marrow Transplantation. Eds Forman S, Blume K, and Thomas ED. Blackwell Scientific Publications, Boston Part 1, Chapter 1, pp. 3-11, 1994.

22. Peggy D, Kemp N. Collection, storage, and administration of autologous bone marrow. Lancet 2:1426-8, 1960.

23. Baum CM, Weissman IL, Tsukamoto AS, et al. Isolation of a candidate human hematopoietic stem cell population. Proc Natl Acad Sci USA 89:2804-8, 1992.

24. Uchida N, Combs A, Conti S, et al. The in vivo hematopoietic population of a rhodamine 123 low population of human marrow. Exp Hematol 22:755, 1994.

25. Kessinger A, Armitage JO, Landmark JD, Smith DM, and Weisenburger D. Autologous peripheral hematopoietic stem cell transplantation restores hematopoietic function following marrow ablative therapy. Blood 71:723-7, 1988.

26. Sheridan W, Begley CG, Juttner CA, et al. Effect of peripheral blood progenitor cells mobilized by filgrastim (Filgrastim) on platelet recovery after high-dose chemotherapy. Lancet 640-4, 1992.

27. Peters WP, Davis R, Shpall EJ, et al. Adjuvant chemotherapy involving high-dose combination CPA/BCNU/cDDP with bone marrow support for stage II/III breast cancer involving ten or more lymph nodes (CALGB 8782): A preliminary report. Proc Amer Soc Clin Oncol 31:22, 1990.

28. Juttner CA, To LB, Roberts MM, et al. Comparison of hematologic recovery, toxicity, and supportive care of autologous PBSC, autologous BM, and allogeneic BM transplants. Int J Cell Cloning 10:160, 1992.

29. Reiffers J, Castaigne S, Tilly H, et al. Hematopoietic reconstitution after autologous blood stem cell transplantation. A report of 46 cases. Plasma Ther Transfus Technol 8:360-4, 1987.

30. Stiff PJ, Murgo AJ, Wittes RE, et al. Quantification of peripheral blood colony forming unit-culture rise following chemotherapy: Could leukocytaphereses replace bone marrow for autologous transplantation? Transfusion 23:500-3, 1983.

31. Williams SF, Bitran JD, Richards JM, et al. Peripheral blood-derived stem cell collections for use in autologous transplantation after high-dose chemotherapy: an alternative approach. Bone Marrow Transplant 5:129-33, 1990.

32. Udomsakdi C, Eaves CJ, Swolin B, et al. Rapid decline of chronic myeloid leukemic cells on long-term culture due to a defect at the leukemic stem cell level. Proc Natl Acad Sci USA 89:6192-6, 1992.

33. Nagata S, Tsuchiya M, Asano S, et al. Molecular cloning and expression of cDNA for human granulocyte colony-stimulating factor. Nature 319, 415-418, 1986.

34. Souza LM, Boone TC, Gabrilove J, et al. Recombinant human granulocyte colony-stimulating factor effects on normal and leukemic myeloid cells. Science 232, 61-65, 1986.

35. Nicola NA, Peterson L. Identification of distinct receptors for two hematopoietic growth factors (granulocyte colony-stimulating factor and multipotential colony-stimulating factor) by chemical cross linking. J Biol. Chem. 261, 12384-12389, 1986.

36. Park LS, Waldron PE, Friend D, et al. Interleukin-3, GM-CSF, and G-CSF receptor expression on cell lines and primary leukemia cells: receptor heterogeneity and relationship to growth factor responsiveness. Blood 74, 56-65, 1989.

37. Fukunaga R, Ishizaka-Ikeda E, Nagata S. Purification and characterization of the receptor for murine granulocyte colony-stimulating factor. J Biol. Chem. 265, 14008-14015, 1990.

38. Bensinger W, Singer J, Appelbaum F, et al. Autlogous transplantation with peripheral blood mononuclear cells collected after administration of recombinant granulocyte colony-stimulating factor. Blood 81:3158-63, 1993.

39. Sheridan WP, Begley CG, Juttner CA. Effect of peripheral-blood progenitor cells mobilized by filgrastim (G-CSF) on platelet recovery after high-dose chemotherapy. Lancet 339: 640-4, 1992.

40. Chao N, Long G, Negrin R, et al. G-CSF and peripheral blood progenitor cells (letter). Lancet 339: 1410, 1992.

41. Andrews RG, Briddell RA, Knitter GH, et al. In vivo synergy between recombinant human stem cell factor and recombinant human granulocyte colony-stimulating factor in baboons: enhanced circulation of granulocytic, erythrocytic, and megakaryocytic progenitor cells. Blood 84:800-10, 1994.

42. Weaver CH, Hazelton B, Palmer PA, et al. A randomized dose finding study of filgrastim for mobilization of peripheral blood progenitor cells (PBPCs). Proc Am Soc Clin Oncol 15:341, 1996.

43. Sheridan WP, Begley GC, To LB, et al. Phase II study of autologous Filgrastim (G-CSF) -mobilized peripheral blood progenitor cells to restore hematopoiesis after high-dose chemotherapy for lymphoid malignancies. Bone Marrow Transplant 14:105-11, 1994.

44. Sheridan WP, Begley CG, Juttner CA, et al. Effect of peripheral blood progenitor cells mobilized by filgrastim (G-CSF) on platelet recovery after high-dose chemotherapy. Lancet 339:640-4, 1992.

45. Rasko JEJ, Gough NM. Granulocyte-macrophage colony stimulating factor. In The Cytokine Handbook, 2nd edn. (Ed. A.W. Thomson), Academic Press, London, pp. 343-369, 1994.

46. Morrissey PJ, Bressler L, Park LS, Alpert A, and Gillis S. Granulocyte-macrophage colony-stimulating factor augments the primary antibody response by enhancing the function of antigen presenting cells. J. Immunol. 139: 1113-1119, 1987.

47. Haas R, Ho AD, Bredthauer U, et al. Successful autologous transplantation of blood stem cells mobilized with recombinant human granulocyte-macrophage colony-stimulating factor. Exp Hematol 18:94-8, 1990.

48. Krause DS, Mechanic SA, and Snyder E. Mobilization an Collection of Peripheral Blood Progenitor Cells. In Apheresis Principles and Practice (Ed. B. McLeod), AABB Press, Bethesda, Maryland, pp 436, 1996.

49. Bernstein ID, Andrews RG, Zsebo KM. Recombinant human stem cell factor enhances the formation of colonies by CD34$^+$ and CD34$^+$lin- cells, and the generation of colony-forming cell progeny from CD34$^+$lin- cells cultured with interleukin-3, granulocyte colony-stimulating factor, or granulocyte-macrophage colony-stimulating factor. Blood 77:2316-21, 1991.

50. McNiece IK, Langley KE, Zsebo KM. Recombinant human stem cell factor synergizes with GM-CSF, G-CSF, L-3 and Epo to stimulate human progenitor cells of the myeloid and erythroid lineages. Exp Hematol 19:226-31, 1991.

51. Briddell RA, Hartley CA, Smith KA, McNiece IK. Recombinant rat stem cell factor synergizes with recombinant human granulocyte colony-stimulating factor in vivo in mice to mobilize peripheral blood progenitor cells that have enhanced repopulating potential. Blood 82:1720-3, 1993.

52. de Revel T, Appelbaum FR, Storb R, et al. Effects of granulocyte colony-stimulating factor and stem cell factor, alone and in combination, on the mobilization of peripheral blood cells that engraft lethally irradiated dogs. Blood 83:3795-9, 1994.

53. Yan XQ, Briddell R, Hartley C, Stoney G, Samal B, McNiece I. Mobilization of long-term hematopoietic reconstituting cells in mice by the combination of stem cell factor plus granulocyte colony-stimulating factor. Blood 84:795-9, 1994.

54. Basser R, Begley CG, Maher D, et al. The use of peripheral blood progenitor cells (PBPC) mobilized by stem cell factor (SCl:) and filgrastim (G-CSF) to support multiple cycles of high-dose chemotherapy in untreated women with poor prognosis breast cancer. Brit J Haematol 87 (suppl 1):90(Abst.), 1994.

55. Demetri G, Costa J, Hayes D, et al. A phase I trial of recombinant methionyl human stem cell factor

(SCF) in patients with advanced breast carcinoma pre- and postchemotherapy (chemo) with cyclophosphamide (C) and doxorubicin (A). Proc Am Soc Clin Oncol 12:142(Abst.), 1993.

56. Glaspy J, McNiece I, LeMaistre F, et al. Effects of stem cell factor (rhSCF:) and filgrastim (rhG-CSF) on mobilization of peripheral blood progenitor cells (PBPC) and on hematological recovery posttransplant: early results from a phase VII study. Proc Am Soc Clin Oncol 13:68(Abst.), 1994.

57. McNiece I, Glaspy J, LeMaistre F, Briddell R, Menchaca D, Shpall EJ. Effects of recombinant methionyl human stem cell factor (rhSCE) and filgrastim (rhG-CSF) on mobilization of peripheral blood progenitor cells: preliminary laboratory results from a phase I/II study. Blood 82a(Abst.), 1993.

58. Briddell R, Glaspy I, Shpall EJ, LeMaistre F, Menchaca D, McNiece I. Mobilization of myeloid, erythroid, and megakaryocyte progenitors by recombinant human stem cell factor (rhSCE7) plus filgrastim (rhG-CSF) in patients with breast cancer. Proc Am Soc Clin Oncol 13:77(Abst.), 1994.

59. Glaspy I, McNiece I, LeMaistre F, et al. Effects of stem cell factor (rhSCE:) and filgrastim (rhG-CSF) on the mobilization of peripheral blood progenitor cells (PBPC) and hematological recovery post transplant: preliminary phase VII study results. Brit J Haematol 87(suppl 1):156(Abst.), 1994.

60. Briddell R, Glaspy J, Shpall EJ, LeMaistre F, Menchaca D, McNiece L. Recombinant human stem cell factor (rhSCE7) and filgrastim (rhG-CSF) synergize to mobilize myeloid erythroid and megakaryocyte progenitors in patients with breast cancer. Brit J Haematol 87(suppl 1):92(Abst.), 1994.

61. Crawford J, Lau D, Erwin R, Rich W, McGuire B, Meyers F. A phase I trial of recombinant methionyl human stem cell factor (SCI;) in patients (pts) with advanced non-small cell lung carcinoma (NSCLC). Proc Am Soc Clin Oncol 12:135(Abst.), 1993.

62. Glaspy J, McNiece IK, LeMaistre F, et al. Effects of stem cell factor (rhSCF) and filgastrim (rhG-CSF) an the mobilization of peripheral blood progenitor cells (PBPC) and hematological recovery post transplant: preliminary phase I/II sudy results [Abstract. Br. J Hematol 1994; 87:156a.

63. Shpall EJ, Wheeler CA, Turner SA, et al. A randomized Phase III study of PBPC mobilization by stem cell factor (SCF, STEMGEN®) and filgrastim in patients with high-risk breast cancer. Blood 90(10):591a, 1997.

64. Stiff P, Gingrich S, Luger S, et al. Emmanouilides. Improved PBPC collection using STEMGEN (stem cell factor, SCF) and Filgrastim (G-CSF) compared to G-CSF alone in heavily pretreated lymphoma (NHL) and Hodgkin's Disease patients (pts). Blood 90: 2628, 1998.

65. Facon T, Harousseau J, Maloisel F, et al. Stem Cell Factor (SCF, Stemgen) in combination with Filgrastim following chemotherapy improves peripheral blood progenitor cell (PBPC) yield in multiple myeloma patients. ASCO Proceedings, 17:299, 1998.

66. Bensinger WI, Appelbaum FR, Rowley SD, et al. Factors that influence collection and engraftment of autologous peripheral-blood stem cells. J Clin Oncol 12:2547-55, 1995.

67. Tricot G, Jagannath S, Vesole DH, et al. Peripheral blood stem cell transplants for multiple myeloma identification of favorable variables for rapid engraftment in 225 patients. Blood 85:558-96, 1995.

68. Weaver CH, Hazelton B, Birch R, et al. An analysis of engraftment kinetics as a function of the CD34 content of peripheral blood progenitor cell collections in 692 patients after the administration of myeloablative chemotherapy. Blood 86:3961-9, 1995.

69. McNiece I, Glaspy J, Shpall EJ, et al. CD34$^+$ cells in pheresis harvests from patients mobilized by growth factors predict engraftment post transplantation.. Blood 84(suppl 1):10(Abst.), 1994.

70. Basser R, Begley CG, Mansfield R, et al. Mobilization of PBPC by priming with stem cell factor (SCF) before filgrastim compared to concurrent administration. Blood 86:687(Abst.), 1995.

71. Lyman SD, James L, Vanden Bos T, et al. Molecular cloning of a ligand for the flt3/flk-2 tyrosine kinase receptor: a proliferative factor for primitive hematopoietic cells. Cell 75:1157-67, 1993.

72. Lyman SD, James L, Johnson L, et al. Cloning of the human homologue of the murine flt3 ligand: a growth factor for early hematopoietic progenitor cells. Blood 83:2795-801, 1994.

73. Lyman SD, James L, Escobar S, et al. Identification of soluble and membrane-bound isoforms of the murine flt3 ligand generated by alternative splicing of mRNAs. Oncogene 10:149-57, 1995.

74. Hannum C, Culpepper J, Cambell D, et al. Ligand for FLT3/FLK2 receptor tyrosine kinase regulates growth of hematopoietic stem cells and is encoded by variant RNAs. Nature 368:643-8, 1994.

75. Small D, Levenstein M, Kim E, et al. STK-1, the human homolog of Flk-2/Flt-3, is selectively expressed in CD34$^+$ human bone marrow cells and is involved in the proliferation of early progenitor/stem cells. Proc Natl Acad Sci USA 91:459-63, 1994.

76. Brasel K, McKenna HJ, Morrissey PJ, et al. Hematologic effects of flt-3 ligand in vivo in mice. Blood 88:2004-12, 1996.

77. Winton EF, Bucur SZ, Bond LD, et al. Recombinant human (rh) Flt3 ligand plus rhGM-CSF or rhG-CSF causes a marked CD34$^+$ cell mobilization to blood in rhesus monkeys. Blood 88(Suppl 1):642A, 1996.

22. The Use of Cytokines during Blood and Marrow Transplantation

John Nemunaitis

Introduction:

Worldwide three recombinant human colony-stimulating factors (rhCSFs) are available for clinical use in stem cell transplant patients. Granulocyte (G)-CSF and granulocyte macrophage (GM)-CSF are available worldwide, and macrophage (M)-CSF is only available in Japan. G-CSF is indicated therapy in the United States as prophylaxis following autologous bone marrow transplant (BMT), and for mobilization of peripheral blood hematopoietic progenitor cells (PBPC). GM-CSF is indicated therapy in neutropenic patients after autologous or allogeneic BMT following marrow graft failure, and for mobilization of autologous PBPC. M-CSF is an acceptable treatment in Japan for autologous BMT. In addition to FDA-approved indications, these molecules have also been utilized to enhance neutrophil and monocyte function in patient populations with infection or at high risk of developing infection.

G-CSF

<u>Myelosuppressive Chemotherapy</u>. G-CSF was initially approved following completion of a trial comparing the tolerability of cyclophosphamide, doxorubicin, and etoposide in 210 patients with small-cell lung cancer (NSCLC)[1]. G-CSF was administered subcutaneously at a dosage of 4-8µg/kg/day from Days 4 to 17 after completion of chemotherapy. The duration of neutropenia was reduced by 2 days over all cycles in patients receiving rhG-CSF. The incidence of neutropenic fever was also reduced from 76% in placebo-treated patients to 40% in G-CSF-treated patients. Furthermore, hospitalization was reduced from 69% in placebo-treated patients to 52% in G-CSF-treated patients. No significant adverse events, no alterations in survival, or tumor relapse were observed. Toxicity at doses between 4-8µg/kg/day include medullary pain in approximately 25% of patients, and skin rashes in 10-20% of patients. Less frequent adverse events included low grade fever, bone pain, and abdominal pain. Rarely, adverse reactions have included reversible elevations of uric acid, elevation of lactic dehydrogenase, elevation of alkaline phosphatase, seizures, anaphylactic reactions, and transient hypotension[1-30]. Given the good tolerability of G-CSF, consistent evidence of enhancement of neutrophil recovery, and reduction of febrile neutropenia episodes with the use of myelosuppressive chemotherapy, several studies were performed to explore the role of G-CSF in enabling a higher maximum tolerated dose of myelosuppressive agents [31-42]. Chemotherapy agents evaluated for dose escalation in combination with G-CSF and other cytotoxic agents include paclitaxel, epirubicin, mitomycin, ifosfamide, cyclophosphamide, doxorubicin, etoposide, carboplatin, navelbine, irinotecan, and cisplatin. The use of G-CSF appears to enable higher dose levels to be achieved, and these higher dose regimens occasionally result in higher response rates and rarely associated with prolonged survival duration

compared to historical survival with standard dose regimens. These data suggest potential benefit with further chemotherapy dose intensification through concurrent use of G-CSF in certain subsets of patients (e.g., lymphoma, responsive breast cancer).

Data from 35 dose intensive trials were recently reviewed[36]. Unfortunately, none of these studies evalualuated dose intensity in comparison to a <u>prospective</u> control group to explore survival differences. So no firm conclusions can be drawn regarding the use of G-CSF enabling greater dose intensification to improve survival.

Despite an FDA-approved indication for use of G-CSF as secondary prophylaxis in patients who initially developed neutropenic fever, many have also considered the use of G-CSF at the time of development of neutropenic fever as an adjunct to antimicrobial therapy. Results of such trials[43-45] suggest no real benefit to the initiation of G-CSF after the patient develops febrile neutropenia. The duration of neutropenia was shortened slightly, but no significant differences were observed with respect to fever duration, infection, IV antibiotics, hospitalization, or survival. Thus, the primary value of G-CSF appears to be with use as a prophylactic agent to reduce duration of severe neutropenia, thereby limiting febrile neutropenic episodes and duration of hospitalization. Regimens associated with a transient prolonged period of neutropenia (possibly between 7-14 days) are more likely to derive benefit with the administration of G-CSF following chemotherapy.

<u>Bone Marrow Transplantation (BMT)</u>. Several trials have been performed confirming that patients who receive G-CSF achieve an absolute neutrophil count (ANC) of $\geq$ 500 cells/mm^3 earlier than controls[45-63] following autologous or allogeneic BMT (see Table 1). Neutrophil recovery to 500 cells/mm^3 is generally 7 days earlier, platelet recovery is not affected, infection is either not affected or is less frequent, and hospital stay is generally not affected or is of shorter duration in G-CSF-treated patients. No adverse effects of G-CSF with graft-versus-host disease (GVHD), rate of relapse, survival, or the occurrence of graft failure or infection have been observed. A daily subcutaneous route of administration between 5 and 10µg/kg/day is well tolerated.

<u>Peripheral Blood Progenitor Cell Transplant (PBPCT)</u>. Both neutrophil and platelet recovery have been shown to be enhanced with the infusion of PBPC harvested after a short course of G-CSF (10µg/kg/day)[62-75]. The use of G-CSF mobilized PBPC following treatment with myeloablative regimens has been shown to have greater benefit when compared to infused marrow with respect to neutrophil recovery, platelet recovery, and duration of hospitalization, and no adverse effects (see Table 2). If one summarizes data provided in Table 2 in patients receiving the same chemotherapy regimen, the median time to achieve a neutrophil count of $\geq$ 500 cells/mm^3 was 19 days (10-21) in patients who received marrow, and 12 days (9-15) in patients who received PBPC. The duration of platelet recovery to $\geq$ 50,000/mm^3 was 17 days in patients receiving PB compared to 35 days in patients who received marrow. Hospital stay was 18 days in patients receiving PB compared to 27 days in marrow-treated patients.

Little has been done to confirm the use of G-CSF after transplant with PBPCs. Data suggest no real added improvement of neutrophil recovery with the use of G-CSF after infusion of G-CSF-mobilized PBPCs[63,64,70,7,73,75]. Data from most trials indicate that a 5 to 7-day course of G-CSF at a dose of 10µg/kg/day (subcutaneous injection) is required for adequate mobilization, and that the peak period for circulation of multipotent progenitors (at which time patients need to be harvested), occurs between days 4 and 6 [62]. The most common use of G-CSF mobilized stem cell support is in patients with breast cancer. Prospective controlled trials comparing the use of dose intensive therapy to standard dose therapy in breast cancer patients remain in progress. Until their completion, data from Phase II studies suggest good tolerability to the use of cytokine-mobilized PBPC following high dose chemotherapy. One study [76] recently summarized 5 years of investigation in which 67 breast cancer patients with Stage II or III disease involving $\geq$ 10 axilary nodes, who received sequential high dose therapy with cyclophosphamide, metothrexate, and melphalan. Sixty-three patients completed the program. One patient died of regimen-related toxicity. Median follow-up of the 67 patients was 48.5 months, and the relapse-free survival was 57% with an overall survival of 70%. Comparison was made to a similar historical control group of 58 patients who received standard dose treatment. Relapse-free survival was 41% in the standard dose treated patients. The median time of hospitalization associated with the high dose regimen was 32 days. In another recent Phase II study,[77] high dose cyclophosphamide, etoposide, and carboplatin was administered to breast cancer patients with Stage II (n=10), Stage IIIA (n=12), Stage IIIB (n=11), or Stage IV (n=37) disease. Following administration of chemotherapy, all patients received autologous hematopoietic stem cell rescue. Thirty-one of the 70 patients who underwent transplant had detectable disease at the time of transplant. Fifty-five percent of these patients achieved a partial or complete response following the chemotherapy regimen. The median follow-up of all patients was 545 days with a 2-year disease-free survival of 86% in patients with Stage II disease, 75% in patients with Stage IIIA disease, 42% in patients with Stage IIIB disease, and 13% in patients with Stage IV disease. Factors found to be independently predictive of longer progression-free survival by multivariate analysis included lower stage of disease, status of disease at transplant (if the patients was in complete remission or not), and positive estrogen receptor status. Factors predictive of more rapid neutrophil engraftment by multivariate analysis included post-transplant administration of hematopoietic growth factors, greater number of infused CFU-GM and mobilization with G-CSF. Toxicity associated with the high dose regimen was predominantly limited to hospitalization for management of febrile neutropenia. One patient died of regimen-related toxicity within 100 days after administration of chemotherapy. In a third trial involving breast cancer patients with 4-9 nodes, patients received high dose cyclophosphamide, cisplatin, and carmustine followed by mobilized PBPCs. Fifty-four patients were evaluable for relapse-free survival, and 43 patients remain alive without disease for a median of 947 days after transplant. Twenty-nine patients developed late pulmonary regimen-related toxicity, which resolved after a 10-week course of steroids in all but one patient, who did die of pulmonary toxicity. One patient also developed myelodysplastic syndrome 809 days after the start of chemotherapy. Four-year survival and disease-free survival from the start of treatment are 84 and 71%, respectively. Results of these trials suggest that high dose therapy is reasonably well tolerated and that a low mortality rate has been observed. However, survival assessment, despite appearing favorable in comparison to historical controls and previously published data, remains to be compared with randomized prospective control patients.

Table 1. Results of Controlled Trials with RhG-CSF in BMT

NUMBER OF PATIENTS		DAY ANC > 500/mm^3		DAY PLATELET-INDEPENDENT		% PATIENTS WITH INFECTION		DAY OF INITIAL DISCHARGE		REFERENCES
G-CSF	Control	G-CSF	Control	G-CSF	Control	G-CSF	Control	G-CSF	Control	
15	18	11	20	33	45	53	61	23	29	46
18	58	13	22	28	32	17	36	NR	NR	47
24	24	S	S	NS	NS	18	35	NR	NR	48,49
25[a]	NR	16	NR	NR	NR	NR	NR	NR	NR	50
96[b]	25	14	19	NR	NR	31	12	24	36	51

S = Values not given but reported as being significantly earlier in patients who received rhG-CSF

NS = Values not given but reported not significantly different

NR = Not reported

a   Patients who received Methotrexate and Cyclosporin for GVHD prophylaxis after sibling HLA-matched BMT.

b   Randomized trial in patients undergoing allogeneic or autologous BMT. Mortality in G-CSF arm 9% versus 0% in control.

Table 2. Results of G-CSF-mobilized Peripheral Blood Stem (Progenitor) Cell Infusion (PBSC) Following Myeloablative Chemotherapy

DISEASE	MOBILIZING REGIMEN	NO. PATIENTS	DAY ANC >500mm^3		DAY PLATELET COUNT >50,000/mm^3		DURATION OF HOSPITAL STAY (Days)		CYTOKINE POST-INFUSION		REF.
			BMT	PBSC	BMT	PBSC	BMT	PBSC	BMT	PBSC	
Breast	F, Ep, C/G-CSF	29		9					-	+	65
Breast, non-Hodgkin's Lymphoma	G-CSF	15[a]	19	13		35	27	18	+	+	62
	IL-3 → G-CSF	23[a]	19	12		25	27	19	+	+	62
Hodgkin's Disease, non-Hodgkin's Lymphoma	Chemo/G-CSF	10		15					-	-	70
Multiple Myeloma	C, P/G-CSF	37		12			27	18	-	+	66
Neuroblastoma (pediatric)	C, E/G-CSF	5	19	12					-	-	71
	G-CSF	6		14					-	-	71
Non-Hodgkin's Lymphoma	G-CSF	26		10					-	+	74
	G-CSF	27[b]	14						+	+	72
	CA, Mi/G-CSF	30		13					-	-	73
	G-CSF	39		10					-	+	74
	CE, Mi/G-CSF	20		12		16.5		21	-	-	75
	CA, Mi/G-CSF	20		10		14.5		21	-	+	75
	G-CSF	29		10		15		13	-	+	67
Non-Hodgkin's Lymphoma, Breast	G-CSF	49[a]	19	10			39	29	-	+	68
Various	CA, E/G-CSF	42[a]		13			29	19	-	-	63
	C/G-CSF	42		14		13		16	-	+	69
	G-CSF	12		13					-		64

a   Historical BMT controls (the prospective patients received the cytokine)

b   Prospective BMT controls.

Abbreviations: A = Doxorubicin (Adriamycin); ANC = Absolute Neutrophil Count; BMT = Bone Marrow Transplant; C = Cyclophosphamide; CA = Cytarabine; Chemo = Chemotherapy; E = Etoposide; Ep = Epirubicin; F = Fluorouracil; IL = Interleukin; Mi = Mitoxantrone; P = Prednisone; "-" = Cytokine Not Administered; "+" = Cytokine Administered

G-CSF mobilized progenitors have also been administered to patients undergoing allogeneic transplant. Results suggest more rapid neutrophil and platelet recovery with no adverse effects on acute GVHD, although chronic GVHD may be increased [79-83].

Conclusion. Efficacy of G-CSF is shown after myelosuppressive chemotherapy with prophylactic usage following the development of febrile neutropenia with a prior chemotherapy regimen. Neutrophil recovery is enhanced, and the incidence of febrile neutropenia is reduced, and with some regimens, reduced hospitalization duration was also observed. G-CSF also optimized mobilization of PBPC, thereby reducing both neutrophil and platelet recovery following reinfusion of the harvested mobilized product after myeloablative chemotherapy regimens in both allogeneic or autologous transplantation. Hospital duration appears to have been substantially shortened in patients receiving G-CSF mobilized PBPC suggesting a greater likelihood of benefit. No effect on incidence of documented infection was observed in most trials with comparing G-CSF, and conclusions regarding the potential use of G-CSF to improve survival can not be made.

The recommended dose of G-CSF ranges between 5 and 10μg/kg/day administered subcutaneously once a day with high doses potentially being of greater efficacy over a short duration to stimulate mobilization of multipotent progenitor cells and lower doses being administered for prophylactic treatment of induced febrile neutropenia by chemotherapy. It is also indicated that G-CSF should be administered until achieving a neutrophil level $\geq$ 10,000 cells/mm^3, however, no data is provided to support the necessity of achieving such a high neutrophil level prior to discontinuation of G-CSF. Most can safely administer G-CSF to achievement a neutrophil level >1,500 cells/mm^3. Occasionally, a reduction in neutrophil levels will occur following discontinuation of G-CSF in patients recovering from chemotherapy, although the reduction of neutrophil levels is generally transient, and will range from 20 to 50% of the neutrophil level at the time of discontinuation.

GM-CSF

Myelosuppressive Chemotherapy. GM-CSF has similar activity to G-CSF, but toxicity (low grade fevers, myalgias, bone pains, abdominal pains) may be slightly greater. Enhanced macrophage function is observed in patients receiving GM-CSF, potentially enabling greater effect on infection, thereby suggesting the use of GM-CSF in patient populations with more prolonged neutropenia and higher risk of infection.

Autologous Bone Marrow Transplant. The primary trial in autologous BMT which led to approval of GM-CSF involved the use of GM-CSF in patients with lymphoid malignancy undergoing autologous BMT [84]. In this trial, time to achieve an ANC of > 500 cells/mm^3 was 6 days less (18 vs. 24 days), time to reach an ANC > 1,000 cells/mm^3 was 8 days less (25 vs. 32 days), and the duration of hospitalization was 10 days less (21 vs. 31 days) in patients who received rhGM-CSF compared to placebo. The duration of infection and duration of antibacterial therapy were also significantly shorter in GM-CSF-treated patients. A summary of Phase I/II studies is shown in Table 3. Summarized Phase III studies are shown in Table 4 [84,92-95]. These results are consistent with the FDA approval trial.

A recent comparison[96] of GM-CSF to GM-CSF/IL-3 fusion molecule (PIXY) in

177 patients with lymphoid malignancy undergoing autologous BMT was recently completed. Data revealed that the time to achieve neutrophil recovery to 500 cells/mm^3 (17 days for PIXY and 19 days for GM-CSF), and time to platelet transfusion-independence (25 days for PIXY and 23 days for GM-CSF), was similar. Toxicity was slightly greater with PIXY, and there was no difference in survival.

Despite a perception of higher toxicity to GM-CSF in patients receiving this molecule following standard chemotherapy, no statistically significant difference in toxicity was observed with GM-CSF compared to placebo in the FDA-approved trial when used in patients undergoing autologous BMT [84]. The potential role of GM-CSF in infection has been further explored in one retrospective analysis in which infection complications of 106 consecutive historical patients who underwent autologous BMT for lymphoid malignancy were compared with those in 50 consecutive similarly treated patients who received prophylactic GM-CSF [97]. Forty percent of control patients developed infection compared to only 13% of the GM-CSF-treated patients. It was suggested that there was a benefit from GM-CSF during the period of severe neutropenia before differences in neutrophil levels between study groups were detectable. This leads to the conclusion that the functional enhancing effect of GM-CSF may be of benefit in BMT patients, thereby suggesting potential application in patients with prolonged graft delay or failure after transplant [98].

<u>Marrow Graft Failure</u>. Patients who fail to achieve adequate neutrophil recovery following autologous or allogeneic transplant have a poor survival. Without the use of GM-CSF, less than 20% of patients had an expected survival of 5 years [99,100]. Phase II trials investigating the use of GM-CSF in patients with graft failure revealed that GM-CSF was well tolerated and that neutrophil recovery occurred at a more rapid rate compared to matched historical controls [99,101.] Furthermore, infectious complications, survival and mortality related to infection was significantly reduced [99,101]. Survival of patients who underwent allogeneic transplant was improved from 35 days to 97 days with the administration of GM-CSF, and survival of patients with graft failure following autologous transplant was improved from 161 days to 474 days [99,101]. Multivariate analysis of possible factors which may have affected survival in both cohorts of patients, failed to identify differences in the populations other than administration of GM-CSF. Other trials have subsequently supported the initial observations [102-104]. Results of the use of GM-CSF in the population of patients who underwent allogeneic transplant also revealed no adverse effects on GVHD, thereby opening the door to initiate investigation of cytokines in allogeneic transplantation.

<u>Allogeneic Bone Marrow Transplant</u>. Trials investigating the use of GM-CSF in matched sibling and unrelated donor transplant reveal that neutrophil recovery is enhanced, infection rates are reduced in subsets of patients, and hospitalization duration is less. No differences in relapse or survival are observed[105-117] (see Table 5). As a result, FDA expanded the indication of GM-CSF to involve allogeneic transplantation. In the FDA approval trial[108] in which GM-CSF was compared to placebo, neutrophil recovery to a level of 500 cells/mm^3 was 4 days shorter in patients receiving GM-CSF (13 vs. 17 days), time to achieve an ANC $\geq$ 1,000 cells/mm^3 was 5 days shorter (14 vs. 19 days), and the number of patients with infection was less (30 vs. 42 patients). The number of patients with bacteremia was also less (9 vs. 19 patients), and significantly fewer days were spent in the hospital (24 vs. 25 days) in the

Table 3. Results of Phase I/II Trials with rhGM-CSF Following Autologous BMT Compared to Historical Control Patients

NUMBER OF PATIENTS		DAY ANC > 500/mm^3		PLATELET-INDEPENDENT (day)		INFECTION (% patients)		DURATION OF HOSPITALIZATION AFTER BMT (Days)		REF
GM-CSF	Control	GM-CSF	Control	GM-CSF	Control	GM-CSF	Control	GM-CSF	Control	
19	24	14	19	NS	NS	16	35	NR	NR	85
22	86	17	25	28	38	18	30	32	41	86,87
6	86	22	25	30	38	0	30	30	41	86,87
12	19	18	25	30	28	58	68	30	30	88
5	27	14	24	NR[a]	NR[a]	NR	52	36	47	89
15	27	18	24	NR[b]	NR[b]	NR	52	50	47	89
5	27	23	24	NR[b]	NR[b]	NR	52	43	47	89
6	NR	11	20	NR	NR	NR	NR	NR	NR	90
16	52	14	20	24	26	6	NR	NR	NR	91

a   Day of platelet transfusion independence was not reported, but the number of platelet units required were significantly less during the first 28 days (81 vs. 149 units compared to historical controls).

b   Number of platelet units infused from Day 0-28 of all patients who received ≤ 0.45 CFU-GM/kg (n=30) was 215 in the GM-CSF-treated patients and 149 in the control group.

Abbreviations: NS = Values not shown, but reported as not significantly different; NR = Not reported.

Table 4. Results of Phase III Trials with rhGM-CSF Following Autologous BMT

NO. PATIENTS		ANC > 500/mm^3 (day)		PLATELET-INDEPENDENCE (day)		INFECTION (% patients)		INITIAL DISCHARGE (days)		REF
GM-CSF	Placebo	GM-CSF	Placebo	GM-CSF	Placebo	GM-CSF	Placebo	GM-CSF	Placebo	
65	63	19	26	26	29	17	30	27	33	84
41	47	14	21	19	19	39	47	23	28	92
39	40	15	28	39	31	38	70	30	31	93
36	33	12	16	35	52	3	19	27	27	94
12	12	NR	NR	14	21	NS	NS	32	41	95

Day ANC > 1,000 x 10 ^{9}/µl was Day 16 in the GM-CSF group vs. Day 27 in the placebo group.
Abbreviations: NR = Not Reported; ND = Not Done

GM-CSF-treated group. The incidence of severe mucositis (Grade III/IV) was also significantly improved in the GM-CSF group (4 of 53 patients vs. 16 of 56 patients). Improvement of mucositis has not been shown in subsequent studies. The severity and duration of GVHD, relapse rate, and survival were not different between GM-CSF and placebo treated patients. Patients undergoing unrelated donor marrow transplant also showed earlier neutrophil recovery, but no other factors such as infection, hospital duration, or mucositis were improved [107,111,112,114]. On a previously mentioned trial, long-term follow-up of patients who underwent allogeneic transplant, in which 20 patients received placebo and 20 patients received GM-CSF for 14 days, revealed a comparable incidence of GVHD, transplant-related mortality, and relapse and survival[117]. Patients were followed for a median of 5.5 years, and no late complications such as chronic GVHD, graft failure, or myelodysplasia occurred in the GM-CSF-treated patients.

Peripheral Blood Stem Cell Transplant. Generally, the goal of mobilization is to induce sufficient circulation of multipotent progenitors for rapid and stable long-term hematopoietic cell recovery over a minimum time for harvesting. Ideally, 3×10^8 to 6×10^8 mononuclear cells/kg (with $> 2 \times 10^6$ CD34+ cells/kg) are necessary to enable sufficient neutrophil and platelet recovery following myeloablative chemo/radiotherapy [118]. Use of GM-CSF has been explored in combination with high dose cyclophosphamide to mobilize early progenitors [119-124]. GM-CSF reduced the duration of neutropenia, infection-related complications, and appeared to enhance mobilization of progenitors. However, substantial morbidity still resulted with cyclophosphamide despite the use of GM-CSF (see Table 6). Despite continued use of chemotherapy combined with cytokines for mobilization in Europe and occasionally in the United States, mobilization is sufficient for adequate long-term engraftment utilizing G-CSF or GM-CSF alone. Since G-CSF appears to induce a more rapid rate of increase in neutrophil levels as compared to GM-CSF, and is perceived as being less toxic, G-CSF has been much more commonly used for mobilization when administered alone. There is no significant evidence that tumor cells are mobilized into circulation during recovery after chemotherapy alone, after chemotherapy combined with growth factors, or after growth factors alone [125-128]. Contaminating tumor cells are less frequently identified in mobilized peripheral blood than in bone marrow. The rate of neutrophil recovery, and the frequency of clinical complications following the infusion of GM-CSF mobilized PBPCs are similar to those obtained with G-CSF[121,123,129-135,62-78]. Studies directly comparing PBPCT against autologous BMT in similar patient populations suggest that there is a marked advantage to the use of PBPCs after myeloablative regimens over BMT with or without prophylactic cytokines, particularly with respect to platelet recovery [62,123]. Other cytokines such as IL-3, when used in combination with G-CSF or GM-CSF, appear to be well tolerated, and there was some suggestion of earlier platelet recovery when combined with IL-3 for mobilization (see Table 7) [136].

Table 5. Granulocyte-macrophage Colony-stimulating Factor (GM-CSF) in Allogeneic Bone Marrow Transplant

CYTOKINE	TYPE OF BMT	NO. PATIENTS	GVHD PROPHYLAXIS	ANC > 500/mm^3 (day)	PLATELET-INDEPENDENT (day)	GVHD ≥ GRADE III[a] (% patients)	SURVIVAL (Y) (%)	REF
Placebo	Matched sibling	28	T-cell depletion	20	NR	6	2 (40)	105
GM-CSF	Matched sibling	29	T-cell depletion	15	NR	3	2 (58)	
Placebo	Matched sibling	20	CSP	16	NR	15	1 (20)	106,
GM-CSF	Matched sibling	20	CSP	13	NR	5	1 (42)	107
Placebo	Unrelated	63	CSP/MTX	22	NR	NR	1 (51)	107
GM-CSF	Unrelated	61	CSP/MTX	20	NR	NR	1 (39)	
Placebo	Matched sibling	56	CSP/P	17	24	12	1 (63)	108
GM-CSF	Matched sibling	53	CSP/P	13	20	15	1 (55)	
Placebo	Matched sibling	16	CSP/MTX	22	NR	NR	1 (56)	109
GM-CSF	Matched sibling	16	CSP/MTX	14	NR	NR	1 (48)	
Historical controls	Matched sibling	50	CSP/P	19	21	ND		110
GM-CSF	Matched sibling	28	CSP/P	14	23	14		
Historical controls	Matched sibling	43	CSP/MTX	24	20	ND		111, 112
GM-CSF	Matched sibling	19	CSP/MTX	20	23	6	2 (49)	
Historical controls	Unrelated	78	CSP/MTX	23	31	ND	2 (57)	
GM-CSF	Unrelated	103	CSP/MTX	21	23	25		
Historical controls	Matched sibling	40	CSP/MTX	18	23	ND		113
GM-CSF	Matched sibling	20	CSP/MTX	14	16	ND		
GM-CSF	Unrelated	9	CSP/P	16	NR	50		114
GM-CSF	Matched sibling	2	CSP/P	13	NR	50		115
GM-CSF	Matched sibling	6	CSP/P	12	14	0		116

a   Grade III or IV GVHD indicates that the condition is "very severe."

Abbreviations: ANC = Absolute Neutrophil Count; BMT = Bone Marrow Transplant; CSP - Cyclosporin; GVHD = Graft-versus-Host Disease; MTX = Methotrexate; ND = Not different from comparator group (specific percentages not reported); NR = Not Reported; P = Prednisone.

<u>Conclusion</u>.   Efficacy of GM-CSF is shown following myeloablative chemotherapy in patients undergoing autologous or allogeneic transplant. Mobilization of progenitors used to supplement dose intensive chemotherapy, and patients who develop graft delay or graft failure after autologous or allogeneic transplant also appear to derive benefit with the prophylactic use of GM-CSF. The primary advantage of GM-CSF appears to be to stimulate earlier neutrophil recovery enabling, in some trials, the reduction of infection and shorter hospital duration. In general, no effect was observed on the incidence or duration of acute GVHD, rate of relapse, or survival in patients receiving GM-CSF as compared to placebo after allogeneic or autologous transplantation. However, chronic GVHD in patients receiving GM-CSF-stimulated allogeneic PBSCs may be greater. Whether or not this would be of benefit or detriment with respect to a "graft-versus-tumor" effect remains to be studied in prospective controlled trials with longer follow-up.

M-CSF

M-CSF has been sparsely explored in the United States. It was initially explored as a highly purified product, and received approval in Japan to enhance neutrophil recovery following allogeneic transplant, dose intensive therapy for ovarian cancer, and after consolidation chemotherapy for AML [137-140]. In allogeneic transplant recipients, M-CSF was administered to 51 patients in one trial and the results were compared to concurrent nonrandomized controls [137-139]. Other than occasional low grade fever, no significant toxicity was described. The incidence and severity of GVHD, the rate of graft failure and the rate of recurrent disease and survival were not different. Patients received 10 daily doses of M-CSF and achieved an ANC of 500 and 1,000 cells/mm^3 4 and 8 days earlier than controls. Another randomized placebo-controlled trial was recently completed in which 88 patients received M-CSF following consolidation chemotherapy for AML. The results were compared to 94 placebo-treated patients.[140] The dose of M-CSF was 8 x 10^6 IU by 2-hour intravenous infusion for 14 days following consolidation chemotherapy. Patients receiving M-CSF achieved earlier neutrophil recovery, and the duration of neutropenic fever was 4 days less in M-CSF-treated patients.

Recombinant M-CSF was investigated in the United States in patients who underwent autologous or allogeneic transplant, which was complicated by fungal infection. In an initial Phase I trial, M-CSF was administered concomitantly with Amphothericin-B to 24 patients who developed invasive fungal infection in association with BMT [141]. Other than transient thrombocytopenia, no significant toxicity was observed. GVHD was not adversely affected, however, neutrophil, monocyte, and lymphocyte recovery was not altered. Six of these patients achieved complete histologic and radiologic resolution of fungal infection during the study period. Ten of the 24 patients (42%) survived 100 days after the initiation of therapy. No patients developed recurrent disease while receiving M-CSF. After completion of this Phase I trial, 22 additional patients received M-CSF at the maximum tolerated dose of 2,000µg/m^2/day by intravenous infusion [142,98]. Analysis of all 46 patients compared to historical controls revealed that those patients with a Karnofsky Score > 20% at the time of entry into trial, who received M-CSF, and had invasive *Candida* infection had

Table 6. Morbidity Related to Mobilization with Cyclophosphamide

References	Kotasek [119]		To [120]		Jagannath [121]		Boiron [122]		Rosenfeld [123]		Sureda [124]	
Dose of Cyclophosphamide	$7\ g/m^2$	$4\ g/m^2$	$7\ g/m^2$	$4\ g/m^2$	$6\ g/m^2$	$6\ g/m^2$ + GM-CSF	$7\ g/m^2$	$7\ g/m^2$ + GM-CSF	$4\ g/m^2$	$4\ g/m^2$ + GM-CSF	$4\ g/m^2$	$4\ g/m^2$ + GM-CSF
Number of cycles	23	52	23	37	36	39	21	10	10	10	12	15
Day ANC $<1,000/<500/mm^3$	10/NR	7/NR	NR/NR	NR/NR	NR/18	NR/15	NR/20	NR/14	15/NR	12/NR	NR/10	NR/7
Day platelet count $<50,000/mm^3$	7	1	NR	NR	18	15	15	13	NR	NR	NR	NR
Percentage of patients with febrile neutropenia	100	21	100	44	57[a]	57[a]	NR	NR	50	0	92	73
Percentage of sepsis	39	10	NR	NR	23[a]	23[a]	5	20	NR	NR	42	26
Duration of hospital stay (days)	NR	NR	NR	NR	NR	NR	23	22	NR	NR	NR	NR

a   57% of patients developed febrile neutropenia and 23% documented infections in both groups. GM-CSF was described as not making a difference in infection morbidity, but data were not shown.

Abbreviations: ANC = Absolute Neutrophil Count; GM-CSF = Granulocyte-Macrophage Colony-Stimulating Factor; NR = Not Reported.

Table 7. Cytokine-mobilized Peripheral Blood Stem Cell Transplant Versus Historical Bone Marrow Transplant with and Without Cytokines [136]

	ARM 1[a]	ARM 2[b]	ARM 3[c]	HISTORICAL PLACEBO	HISTORICAL GM-CSF
Mononuclear cell count/kg/apheresis	2.5	-1.3	1.3		
Day ANC:					
> 100/mm^3	12	16	11	14	13
> 500/mm^3	14	24	13	26	19
> 1,000/mm^3	16	23	15	33	26
Day platelet count > 20,000/mm^3	15	28	10	29	26
Duration of hospital stay (days)	19	27	18	33	27

a = rhIL-3 5µg/kg/day prior to rhG-CSF 5µg/kg/day; b = rhIL-3 5µg/kg/day prior to rhGM-CSF 5µg/kg/day; c = rhIL-3 25µg/kg/day combined with rhG-CSF 5µg/kg/day.

Abbreviations: rhIL-3 = recombinant human Interleukin-3

Table 8. Survival of Patients Who Received RhM-CSF Compared to Historical Controls [142]

GROUP	> 20% KARN/*CANDIDA*	> 20% KARN/*ASPERGILLUS*	≤ 20% KARN/*CANDIDA*	≤ 20% KARN/*ASPERGILLUS*	TOTAL
rhM-CSF	50% (n=20)[b]	20% (n=10)	0% (n=11)	0% (n=5)	27% (n=46)
Control	15% (n=33)[b]	0% (n=5)	9% (n=11)	0% (n=9)	5% (n=58)
p Value[a]	0.004	0.675	0.565	0.228	0.027

a = Mantel-Cox analysis.

b = Includes one patient with mucormycosis who did not survive as a result of progressive infection.

Abbreviations: Karn = Karnofsky performance score.

better survival compared to historical controls (see Table 8). No adverse effect on engraftment or GVHD were observed.

Conclusions

Few conclusions can be made with respect to the use of M-CSF in transplant patients. The purified product used in Japan has a similar effect as recombinant G-CSF or GM-CSF after autologous transplant. It may also have a similar or, possibly, greater effect than GM-CSF on enhancing macrophage function with potential application in patients with infection. Further clinical investigation is needed.

Acknowledgment:

The author wishes to thank Ana Petrovich for excellent manuscript preparation.

References:

1. Crawford J, Ozer H, Stoller R, et al.: Reduction of granulocyte colony-stimulating factor of fever and neutropenia induced by chemotherapy in patients with small-cell lung cancer. N Engl J Med 325:164-170, 1991.
2. Gabrilove JL, Jakibowski A, Scher H, et al.: Effect of granulocyte colony-stimulating factor on neutropenia and associated morbidity due to chemotherapy for transitional cell carcinoma of the urothelium. N Engl J Med 318(22):1414-1422, 1988.
3. Neidhart J, Mangalik A, Kohler W, et al.: Granulocyte colony-stimulating factor stimulates recovery of granulocytes in patients receiving dose intensive chemotherapy without bone marrow transplantation. J Clin Oncol 7(1):1685-1692, 1989.
4. Kotaket T, Miki T, Akaza H, et al.: Effect of recombinant granulocyte colony stimulating factor (rG-CSF) on chemotherapy-induced neutropenia in patients with urogenital cancer. Cancer Chemother Pharmacol 27(4):253-257, 1991.
5. Chung YS, Sowa M, Kato Y, et al.: A clinical study on the effect of recombinant human G-CSF in gastric cancer patients with neutropenia induced by chemotherapy (EAP). J Jpn Soc Cancer Ther 26:802-807, 1991.
6. Trillet-Lenoir V, Green J, Manegold C, et al.: Recombinant granulocyte colony stimulating factor reduces the infectious complications of cytotoxic chemotherapy. Eur J Cancer 29A:319-324, 1993.
7. Pettengell R, Gurney G, Randford J, et al.: Granulocyte colony stimulating factor to prevent dose limiting neutropenia in non-Hodgkin's lymphoma: A randomized controlled trial. Blood 80(6):1430-1436, 1992.
8. Penella J, Hodgetts J, Lomax L, et al.: Can cytotoxic dose-intensive be increased by using granulocyte colony-stimulating factor? A randomized controlled trial of lenograstim in small-cell lung cancer. J Clin Oncol 13(3):652-659, 1995.
9. Chevallier B, Chollet P, Merrouche Y, et al.: Lenograstim prevents morbidity from intensive induction chemotherapy in the treatment of inflammatory breast cancer. J Clin Oncol 13(7):1564-1571, 1995.
10. Nguyen B, Chevallier B, Chevreau C, et al.: Efficacy of Lenograstim on hematologic tolerance to MAID chemotherapy in patients with advanced soft tissue sarcoma and consequences on treatment dose-intensity. J Clin Oncol 13(10):2629-2636, 1995.
11. Fukuoka M, Masuda N, Takada M, et al.: Dose-intensive chemotherapy in extensive-stage small cell lung cancer. Semin Oncol 21(1 suppl):43-47, 1994.
12. Ochiai K, Terashima Y: Chemotherapy and granulocyte colony-stimulating factor in ovarian cancer. Sem Oncol 21(1 suppl):23-28, 1994.
13. Fischer JR, Manegold C, Bulzebruck H, et al.: Induction chemotherapy with and without recombinant human granulocyte colony-stimulating factor support in locally advanced Stage IIIA/B

non-small cell lung cancer. Semin Oncol 21(3 suppl):20-27, 1994.

14. Mori K, Saitoh Y, Tominage K: Recombinant human granulocyte colony-stimulating factor in patients receiving intensive chemotherapy for non-small cell lung cancer. Eur J Cancer 29A(5):677-680, 1993.

15. Avilés A, Diaz-Maqueo JC, Talavera A, et al.: Effect of granulocyte colony-stimulating factor in patients with diffuse large cell lymphoma treated with intensive chemotherapy. Leukemia and Lymphoma 15:153-157, 1994.

16. Vokes EE, Haraf DJ, Mick R, et al.: Intensified concomitant chemo/radiotherapy with and without Filgrastim for poor-prognosis head and neck cancer. J Clin Oncol 12(11):2351-2359, 1994.

17. Bertini M, Freiline R, Vitolo U, et al.: P-VEBEC: A new 8-weekly schedule with or without rG-CSF for elderly patients with aggressive non-Hodgkin's lymphoma (NHL). Ann Oncol 5:895-900, 1994.

18. Gebbia V, Valenza R, Testa A, et al.: Escalating doses of Mitoxantrone with granulocyte colony-stimulating factor (G-CSF) rescue plus 5-Fluorouracil and high-dose levofolinic acid in metastatic breast cancer. Eur J Cancer 30A:1734-1736, 1994.

19. Christman K, Saltz L, Schwartz G, et al.: Granulocyte colony-stimulating factor: Effective in ameliorating Fluorouracil-based myelosuppression? J Nat Cancer Inst 85(10):826-827, 1993.

20. Bronchud MH, Scarffe JH, Thatcher N, et al.: Phase I/II study of recombinant human granulocyte colony-stimulating factor in patients receiving intensive chemotherapy for small cell lung cancer. Br J Cancer 56(6):809-813, 1987.

21. Eguchi K, Sasaki S, Tamura T, et al.: Dose escalation study of recombinant human granulocyte-colony stimulating factor (KRN8601) in patients with advanced malignancy. Cancer Res 49(18):5221-5224, 1989.

22. Eguchi K, Shinkai T, Sasaki Y, et al.: Subcutaneous administration of recombinant human granulocyte colony-stimulating factor (KRN8601) in intensive chemotherapy for patients with advanced lung cancer. Jpn J Cancer Res 81(11):1168-1174, 1990.

23. Ota K, Ariyoshi Y, Fukuoka M, et al.: Clinical effect of recombinant human G-CSF on neutropenia induced by chemotherapy for lung cancer. rG-CSF Cooperation Study Group. Gan To Kagaku Ryoho 17(1):65-71, 1990.

24. Tsukimoto I, Hanawa Y, Takaku F, et al.: Clinical evaluation of recombinant human G-CSF in children with cancer. Rinsho Ketsueki 31(10):1647-1655, 1990.

25. Kosaka T, Suzaki Y, Kinoshita K, et al.: Effect of rhG-CSF on the neutropenia induced by chemotherapy for relapsed gastric carcinoma. J Jpn Soc Cancer Ther 26:51-55, 1991.

26. Kudoh S, Fukuoka M, Negoro S, et al.: Weekly dose intensive chemotherapy in patients with small cell lung cancer: A pilot study. Am J Clin Oncol 15:29-34, 1992.

27. Oyama A, Ota K, Asano S, et al.: Clinical effect of recombinant human G-CSF on neutropenia induced by chemotherapy for non-Hodgkin's lymphoma. Nippon Gan Chiryo Gakkai Shi 25(8):1619-1634, 1990.

28. Yoshida T, Nakamura S, Ohtake S, et al.: Effect of granulocyte colony stimulating factor on neutropenia due to chemotherapy for non-Hodgkin's lymphoma. Cancer 66(9):1904-1909, 1990.

29. Oyama A, Ota K, Asano S, et al.: A double blind crossover clinical induced by chemotherapy for non-Hodgkin's lymphoma. Nippon Gan Chiryo Gakkai Shi 25(10):2533-2548, 1990.

30. Ogawa M, Masaoka T, Mizoguchi H, et al.: A phase III study of KRN8601 (rhG-CSF) on neutropenia induced by chemotherapy for malignant lymphoma - a multi-institutional placebo controlled double blind comparative study. Gan To Kagaku Ryoho 17(3):365-373, 1990.

31. Niitsu N, Umeda M: Biweekly COP-BLAM (Cyclophosphamide, vincristine, prednisone, Bleomycin, doxorubicin and procarbazine) regimen combined with granulocyte colony-stimulating factor (G-CSF) for intermediate-grade non-Hodgkin's lymphoma. Eur J Haematol 56:163-167, 1996.

32. Bronchud MH, Howell A, Crowther D, et al: The use of granulocyte colony-stimulating factor to increase the intensity of treatment with doxorubicin in patients with advanced breast and ovarian cancer. Br J Cancer 60:121-125, 1989.

33. SarosY G, Kohn E, Stone DA, et al.: Phase I study of Taxol and granulocyte colony-stimulating factor in patients with refractory ovarian cancer. J Clin Oncol 10:1165-1170, 1992.

34. Noda K, Eguchi K, Nakasa K, et al.: Dose escalation study of VM-26 with CDDP and rhG-CSF in patients with small cell lung cancer (SCLC). Proc Am Soc Clin Oncol 10:263 (abstr), 1991.

35. Demetri GD, Younger J, Shapiro C, et al.: A Phase I study of dose-intensified CAF chemotherapy with adjunctive r-metHuG-CSF (G-CSF) in patients with advanced breast cancer. Proc Am Soc Clin Oncol 11:108 (abstr), 1992.

36. Nemunaitis J: A comparative review of colony-stimulated factors. Drugs 54(5):709-729, 1997.

37. Calvert AH, Lind MJ, Shazal-Asward S, et al.: Carboplatin and granulocyte colony-stimulating factor as first-line treatment for epithelial ovarian cancer: A Phase I dose-intensity escalation study. Semin Oncol 21(5):1-6, 1994.

38. Crowford J, O'Rourke MA: Vinorelbine (Navelbine)/Carboplatin combination therapy: Dose intensification with granulocyte colony-stimulating factor. Semin Oncol 21(5):73-78, 1994.

39. O'Reily SM, Smithe DB, Newlands ES, et al.: Dose intensification in the treatment of patients with testicular germ cell tumors abstract. Eur J Cancer 30A(5):723, 1994.

40. Frasci G, Comella G, Comella P, et al.: Mitoxantrone plus Vinorelbine with granulocyte colony-stimulating factor (G-CSF) support in advanced breast cancer patients: A dose and schedule finding study. Br Cancer Res Treat 35:147-156, 1995.

41. Miles DW, Foggarty CM, Ash RM, et al.: Received dose-intensity: A randomized trial of weekly chemotherapy with and without granulocyte colony-stimulating factor in small-cell lung cancer. J Clin Oncol 12(1):77-82, 1994.

42. Masuda N, Fukouka M, Kidoh S, et al.: Phase I study of Irinotecan and Cisplatin with granulocyte colony-stimulating factor support for advanced non-small cell lung cancer. J Clin Oncol 12(1):90-96, 1994.

43. Maher DW, Lieschke GJ, Green M, et al.: Filgrastim in patients with chemotherapy-induced febrile neutropenia. Ann Intern Med 121:492-501, 1994.

44. Mayordomo JI, Reivera F, Diaz-Puente T, et al.: Improving treatment of chemotherapy-induced neutropenia fever by administration of colony-stimulated factors. J Natl Cancer Inst 87(11):803-808, 1995.

45. Mayordomo JI, Reivera F, Diaz-Puente T, et al.: Improving treatment of chemotherapy-induced neutropenic fever by administration of colony-stimulating factors. J Natl Cancer Inst 87(11):803-808, 1995.

46. Sheridan WP, Morstyn G, Wolf M, et al.: Granulocyte colony-stimulating factor and neutrophil recovery after high-dose chemotherapy and autologous bone marrow transplantation. Lancet 2:891-895, 1989.

47. Taylor KM, Jagannath S, Spitzer G, et al.: Recombinant human granulocyte colony-stimulating factor hastens granulocyte recovery after high-dose chemotherapy and autologous bone marrow transplantation in Hodgkin's disease. J Clin Oncol 7:1791-1799, 1989.

48. Peters WP: The effect of recombinant human colony-stimulating factors on hematopoietic reconstitution following autologous bone marrow transplantation. Semin Hematol 26(2):18-23, 1989.

49. Auer I, Ribas A, Gale RP: What is the role of recombinant colony-stimulating factors in bone marrow transplantation. Bone Mar Transpl 6:79-87, 1990.

50. Masaoka T, Takaku F, Kato S, et al.: Recombinant human granulocyte colony-stimulating factor in allogeneic bone marrow transplantation. Exp Hematol 17:1047-1050, 1989.

51. Gisselbrecht C, Prentice HG, Bacigalupo A, et al.: Placebo-controlled Phase III trial of Lenograstim on bone marrow transplantation. Lancet 343:696-698, 1994.

52. Kennedy MJ, Davis J, Passos-Coelho J, et al.: Administration of human recombinant granulocyte colony-stimulating factor (Filgrastim) accelerates granulocyte recovery following high-dose chemotherapy and autologous marrow transplantation with 4-hydroperoxycyclophosphamide-purged marrow in women with metastatic breast cancer. Cancer Res 53:5424-5428, 1993.

53. Schriber JR, Chao NJ, Long GD, et al.: Granulocyte colony-stimulating factor after allogeneic bone marrow transplantation. Blood 84(5):1680-1684, 1994.

54. Vey N, Molnar S, Faucher C, et al.: Delayed administration of granulocyte colony-stimulating factor after autologous bone marrow transplantation: Effect on granulocyte recovery. Bone Mar Transpl 14:779-782, 1994.

55. Clark RE, Shlebak AA, Greagh MD: Delayed commencement of granulocyte colony-stimulating factor following autologous bone marrow transplantation accelerates neutrophil recovery and is cost-effective. Leuk Lymph 16:141-146, 1994.

56. Khwaja A, Mills W, Leveridge K, et al.: Efficacy of delayed granulocyte colony stimulating factor after autologous BMT. Bone Mar Transpl 11:479-482, 1993.

57. Madero L, Muñoz A, Diaz de Heredia A, et al.: G-CSF after autologous bone marrow transplantation for malignant diseases in children. Bone Mar Transpl 15:349-351, 1995.

58. Gomez AT, Jimenez MA, Alvarez MA, et al.: Optimal timing of granulocyte colony-stimulating factor (G-CSF) administration after bone marrow transplantation. A prospective randomized study.

Ann Hematol 71:65-70, 1995.

59. Schmitz N, Linch DC, Dreger P, et al.: Randomized trial of Filgrastim-mobilized peripheral blood progenitor cell transplantation versus autologous bone marrow transplantation in lymphoma patients. Lancet 347:353-357, 1996.

60. Locatelli F, Zecca M, Ponchio L, et al.: Pilot trial of combined administration of erythropoietin and granulocyte colony stimulating factor to children undergoing allogeneic bone marrow transplantation. Bone Mar Transpl 14:929-935, 1994.

61. Takahashi S, Okamoto SI, Shirafuji N, et al.: Recombinant human glycosylated granulocyte colony-stimulating factor (rhG-CSF)-combined regimen for allogeneic bone marrow transplantation in refractory acute myeloid leukemia. Bone Mar Transpl 13:239-245, 1994.

62. Nemunaitis J: Cytokine-mobilized peripheral blood progenitor cells. Semin Oncol 23(4):9-14, 1996.

63. Pigaditou A, Marini G, Johnson PWM et al.: Myeloablative therapy with peripheral blood progenitor cell (PBSC) support in patients with haematological malignancy. Ann Oncol 6:53-58, 1995.

64. Kessinger A, Armitage JO: The evolving role of autologous peripheral stem cell transplantation following high-dose therapy for malignancies. Blood 77:211-213, 1991.

65. van der Wall E, Nooijen WJ, Baars JW, et al.: High-dose carboplatin, thiotepa and Cyclophosphamide (CTC) with peripheral blood stem cell support in the adjuvant therapy of high-risk breast cancer: A practical approach. Br J Cancer 71:857-862, 1995.

66. Schiller G, Vescio R, Freytes C, et al.: Transplantation of CD34+ peripheral blood progenitor cells after high dose chemotherapy for patients with advanced multiple myeloma. Blood 86(1):390-397, 1995.

67. Sheridan WP, Begley CG, To OP, et al.: Phase II study of autologous Filgrastim (G-CSF)-mobilized peripheral blood progenitor cells to restore hematopoiesis after high dose chemotherapy for lymphoid malignancies. Bone Marrow Transplant 14:105-111, 1994.

68. Bolwell BJ, Fishleder A, Andersen SW, et al.: G-CSF primed peripheral blood progenitor cells in autologous bone marrow transplantation: Parameters affecting bone marrow engraftment. Bone Marrow Transplant 12:609-614, 1993.

69. Haynes A, Hunter A, McQuaker G, et al.: Engraftment characteristics of peripheral blood stem cells mobilized with Cyclophosphamide and the delayed addition of G-CSF. Bone Marrow Transplant 16:359-363, 1995.

70. Hohaus S, Goldschmidt H, Ehrhardt R, et al.: Successful autografting following myeloablative conditioning therapy with blood stem cells mobilized by chemotherapy plus rhG-CSF. Exper Hematol 21:508-14, 1993.

71. Kanold J, Rapatel C, Berger M, et al.: Use of G-CSF alone to mobilize peripheral blood stem cells for collection from children. Br J Haematol 88:633-635, 1994.

72. Schmitz N, Dreger P, Zander AR, et al.: Results of a randomized controlled, multicenter study of recombinant human granulocyte colony-stimulating factor (Filgrastim) in patients with Hodgkin's disease and non-Hodgkin's lymphoma undergoing autologous bone marrow transplantation. Bone Marrow Transplant 15:261-266, 1995.

73. Haas R, Moos M, Karcher A, et al.: Sequential high-dose therapy with peripheral blood progenitor cell support in low grade non-Hodgkin's lymphoma. J Clin Oncol 12(8):1685-1692, 1994.

74. Nademanee A, Sniecinski I, Schmidt GM, et al.: High dose therapy followed by autologous peripheral blood stem cell transplantation for patients with Hodgkin's disease and non-Hodgkin's lymphoma using unprimed and granulocyte colony-stimulating factor mobilized peripheral blood stem cells. J Clin Oncol 12(10):2176-2186, 1994.

75. Cartelazzo S, Viero P, Bellavita P, et al.: Granulocyte colony stimulating factor following peripheral blood progenitor cell transplant in non-Hodgkin's lymphoma. J Clin Oncol 13(4):935-941, 1995.

76. Gianni AM, Siena S, Bregni M, et al.: Efficacy, toxicity, and applicability of high-dose sequential chemotherapy as adjuvant treatment in operable breast cancer with 10 or more involved axillary nodes: Five-year results. J Clin Oncol 15(6):2312-2321, 1997.

77. Klumpp TR, Goldberg SL, Magdalinski AJ, et al.: Phase II study of high-dose Cyclophosphamide, Etoposide, and carboplatin (CEC) followed by autologous hematopoietic stem cell rescue in women with metastatic or high-risk non-metastatic breast cancer: Multivariate analysis of factors affecting survival and engraftment. Bone Marrow Transplant 20(4):273-281, 1997.

78. Bearman SI, Overmoyer BA, Bolwell BJ, et al.: High-dose chemotherapy with autologous peripheral blood progenitor cell support for primary beast cancer in patients with 4-9 involved axillary lymph nodes. Bone Marrow Transplant 20(11):931-937, 1997.

79. Rosenfeld C, Collins R, Pineiro L, et al.: Allogeneic blood cell transplantation without post-transplant colony stimulating factors in patients with hematopoietic neoplasm: A Phase II study. J Clin Oncol 14(4):1314-1319, 1996.

80. Schmitz N, Dreger P, Suttopr M, et al.: Primary transplantation of allogeneic peripheral blood progenitor cells mobilized by Filgrastim (granulocyte colony-stimulating factor). Blood 85(15):1666-1672, 1995.

81. Nemunaitis J, Rosenfeld C, Collins R, et al.: Allogeneic transplant combining mobilized blood and bone marrow in patients with refractory hematologic malignancies. Transfusion 35:666-73, 1995.

82. Korbling M, Przepiorka D, Huh TO, et al.: Allogeneic blood stem cell transplantation for refractory leukemia and lymphoma: Potential advantage of blood over marrow allografts. Blood 85:1659-1665, 1995.

83. Bensinger WI, Weaver CH, Appelbaum FR, et al.: Transplantation of allogeneic peripheral blood stem cells mobilized by recombinant human granulocyte colony stimulating factor. Blood 85:1655-1658, 1995.

84. Nemunaitis J, Rabinowe SN, Singer JW, et al.: Recombinant granulocyte macrophage colony stimulating factor after autologous bone marrow transplantation for lymphoid cancer. N Engl J Med 324:1773-1778, 1991.

85. Brandt SJ, Peters WP, Atwater SK, et al.: Effect of recombinant human granulocyte macrophage colony stimulating factor on hematopoietic reconstitution after high dose chemotherapy and autologous bone marrow transplantation. N Engl J Med 318:869-876, 1988.

86. Nemunaitis J, Singer JW, Buckner CD, et al.: Use of recombinant granulocyte/macrophage colony stimulating factors in autologous bone marrow transplant for lymphoid malignancies. Blood 72:834-836, 1988.

87. Nemunaitis J, Singer JW, Buckner CD, et al.: Use of Recombinant Human Granulocyte Macrophage Colony Stimulating Factor rhGM-CSF in Autologous Marrow Transplantation for Lymphoid Malignancies. In: Dicke KA (ed.) Autologous bone marrow transplantation: Proceedings of the third international symposium. Houston: University of Texas pp:631-636, 1989.

88. Devereaux S, Linch DC, Gribben JG, et al.: GM-CSF accelerates neutrophil recovery after autologous bone marrow transplantation for Hodgkin's disease. Bone Mar Transpl 4:49-54, 1989.

89. Blazar BR, Kersey JH, McGlave PB, et al.: In vivo administration of recombinant human granulocyte macrophage colony stimulating factor in acute lymphoblastic leukemia patients receiving purged autografts. Blood 73:849-857, 1989.

90. Link H, Freund M, Kirchner H, et al.: Recombinant human granulocyte macrophage colony stimulating factor (rhGM-CSF) after bone marrow transplantation. Behring Inst Mitt 83:313-319, 1988.

91. Lazarus HM, Coiffer B, Hyatt M, et al.: Recombinant granulocyte macrophage colony stimulating factor after autologous bone marrow transplantation for relapsed non-Hodgkin's lymphoma: Blood and bone marrow progenitor growth studies. A Phase II Eastern cooperative Oncology Group Trial. Blood 78:830-837, 1991.

92. Rabinowe SN, Nemunaitis J, Armitage J, et al.: The impact of myeloid growth factors on engraftment following autologous bone marrow transplantation for malignant lymphoma. Semin Hematol 28(suppl 2):6-16, 1991.

93. Gorin NC, Coiffier B, Hayat M, et al.: rhuGM-CSF shortens aplasia duration after ABMT in non-Hodgkin's lymphoma: A randomized placebo-controlled double blind study. Bone Mar Transpl 7(suppl 2):82, 1991.

94. Advani R, Chao NJ, Horning SJ, et al.: Granulocyte macrophage colony stimulating factor (GM-CSF) as an adjunct to autologous hematopoietic stem cell transplantation for lymphoma. Ann Intern Med 116:183-189, 1992.

95. Gulati SC, Bennett CL: Granulocyte macrophage colony stimulating factor (GM-CSF) as adjunct therapy in relapsed Hodgkin's disease. Ann Intern Med 116:177-182, 1992.

96. Vose JM, Pandite AN, Beveridge RA, et al.: Granulocyte-macrophage colony-stimulating factor/IL-3 infusion protein versus granulocyte-macrophage colony-stimulating factor after autologous bone marrow transplantation for non-Hodgkin's lymphoma: Results of a randomized double-blind trial. J Clin Oncol 15(4):1617-1623, 1997.

97. Nemunaitis J, Buckner CD, Dorsey KS, et al.: Retrospective analysis of infectious disease in patients who receive rhGM-CSF versus patients not receiving a cytokine who underwent autologous bone marrow transplant for treatment of lymphoid cancer. Am J Clin Oncol (in press).

98. Nemunaitis J: Macrophage function activating cytokines: Potential clinical application. Crit Rev

Oncol/Hematol 14:153-171, 1993.

99. Nemunaitis J, Singer JW, Buckner CD, et al.: Use of recombinant granulocyte macrophage colony stimulating factor in graft failure after bone marrow transplantation. Blood 76:245-253, 1990.

100. Bolger GB, Sullivan KM, Storb R, et al.: Second marrow infusion for poor graft function after allogeneic marrow transplantation. Bone Marrow Transplant 1:21-30, 1986.

101. Bierman P, Appelbaum F, Oette D, et al.: Granulocyte macrophage colony stimulating factor for engraftment failure following autologous or allogeneic bone marrow transplantation [abstract. Blood 80(1):269a, 1992.

102. Nemunaitis J: The role of GM-CSF and G-CSF in stem cell transplantation. Oncology 7(12):27-32, 1993.

103. Klingermann HG, Eaves AC, Barnett MJ, et al.: Recombinant GM-CSF in patients with poor graft function after bone marrow transplantation. Clin Invest Med 13:77-81, 1990.

104. Vose JM, Bierman PJ, Dessinger A, et al.: The use of recombinant human granulocyte macrophage colony stimulating factor for the treatment of delayed engraftment following high dose therapy and autologous hematopoietic stem cell transplantation for lymphoid malignancies. Bone Marrow Transplant 7:139-143, 1991.

105. Dewitte T, Gratwohl A, Vanderley N, et al.: Recombinant human granulocyte macrophage colony stimulating factor (rhGM-CSF) reduced infection-related mortality after allogeneic T-cell depleted bone marrow transplantation. Bone Marrow Transplant 2(7 suppl.):83, 1991.

106. Powels R, Smith C, Mulan S, et al.: Human recombinant GM-CSF in allogeneic bone marrow transplantation for leukemia: A double-blind placebo controlled trial. Lancet 336:1417-1420, 1990.

107. Anasetti C, Anderson G, Appelbaum FR, et al.: Phase III study of rhGM-CSF in allogeneic marrow transplantation from unrelated donors [abstract]. Blood 82:454a, 1993.

108. Nemunaitis J, Rosenfeld C, Ash R, et al.: Phase III randomized double-blind placebo controlled trial of rhGM-CSF following allogeneic bone marrow transplant. Bone Marrow Transplant 15:949-954, 1995.

109. Hiraoka A, Massaoka T, Moriyama A, et al.: A double-blind placebo controlled test of recombinant human nonglycosylated GM-CSF for allogeneic bone marrow transplantation. Bone Marrow Transplantation (in press).

110. Nemunaitis J, Buckner CD, Appelbaum FR, et al.: Phase I/II trial of recombinant human granulocyte macrophage colony stimulating factor following allogeneic bone marrow transplantation. Blood 77:2065-2071, 1991.

111. Nemunaitis J, Anasetti C, Buckner CD, et al.: Long-term follow-up of 103 patients who received rhGM-CSF after unrelated donor bone marrow transplant (BMT). Blood 81(3):865, 1993.

112. Nemunaitis J, Anasetti C, Storb R, et al.: Phase II trial of recombinant human granulocyte macrophage colony stimulating factor (rhGM-CSF) in patients undergoing allogeneic bone marrow transplantation from unrelated donors. Blood 79(10):2572, 1992.

113. Naparstek E, Hardogen Y, Ben-Shahar A, et al.: Enhanced marrow recovery by short preincubation B of marrow allografts with human recombinant Interleukin-3 and granulocyte macrophage colony stimulating factor. Blood 80:1673-1678, 1992.

114. Nemunaitis J, Anasetti C, Bianco J, et al.: rhGM-CSF after allogeneic bone marrow transplant from unrelated donors: A pilot study of cyclosporine and prednisone as graft-versus-host disease prophylaxis. Leuk Lymph 10:177, 1993.

115. Chap L, Schiller G, Nimer SD: The use of recombinant GM-CSF following allogeneic bone marrow transplantation for aplastic anemia. Bone Mar Transpl (in press).

116. Nemunaitis J, Rosenfeld C, Collins R, et al.: Allogeneic transplantation combining mobilized blood and bone marrow in patients with refractory hematologic malignancies. Transfusion 35:666-673, 1995.

117. Singhal S, Powels R, Treleaven J, et al.: Long-term safety of GM-CSF (molgramostim) administration after allogeneic bone marrow transplantation for hematologic malignancies: Five-year follow-up of a double-blind randomized placebo-controlled study. Leuk Lymphoma 23(3-4):301-307, 1997.

118. Lowry PA, Tabbara IA: Peripheral hematopoietic stem cell transplantation: Current concepts. Exp Hematol 20:937-942, 1992.

119. Kotasek D, Shephers KM, Sage RE, et al.: Factors affecting blood stem cell collections following high dose Cyclophosphamide mobilization in lymphoma, myeloma and solid tumors. Bone Mar Transpl 9:11-17, 1992.

120. To LB, Roberts MM, Haylock DN, et al.: comparison of hematological recovery times and

supportive care requirements of autologous recovery phase peripheral blood stem cell transplant autologous bone marrow transplant and allogeneic bone marrow transplants. Bone Marrow Transplant 9(4):277-284, 1992.

121. Jagannath S, Vesole DH, Glenn L, et al.: Low risk intensive therapy for multiple myeloma with combined autologous bone marrow and blood stem cell support. Blood 80(7):1666-1672, 1992.

122. Boiron JM, Marit G, Faberes C, et al.: Collection of peripheral blood stem cells in multiple myeloma following single high dose Cyclophosphamide with and without recombinant human granulocyte macrophage colony stimulating factor (rhGM-CSF). BMT 12:49-55, 1993.

123. Rosenfeld CS, Gremba C, Shadduck RK, et al.: Engraftment with peripheral blood stem cells using non-controlled rate cryopreservation: Comparison with autologous marrow transplantation. Exp Hematol 22:290-294, 1994.

124. Sureda A, Brunet S, Martinez E, et al.: A randomized study comparing Cyclophosphamide vs Cyclophosphamide + granulocyte macrophage colony stimulating factor as mobilization therapy for multiple myeloma patients. Bone Mar Transpl 15(suppl 3):74-77, 1995.

125. Ross AA, Copper BW, Lazarus HM, et al.: Detection and viability of tumor cells in peripheral blood stem cell collections from breast cancer patients using immunocytochemical and clonogenic assay techniques. Blood 82(9):2605-2610, 1993.

126. Kessinger A, Armitage JO, Smith DM: High dose therapy and autologous peripheral blood stem cell transplantation for patients with lymphoma. Blood 74:1260, 1989.

127. Moss TJ, Sanders DG, Lasky LC, et al.: Contamination of peripheral blood stem cell harvests by circulating neuroblastoma cell. Blood 76:1879, 1990.

128. Vose JM, Bierman PJ, Anderson JR, et al.: High dose chemotherapy with hematopoietic stem cell rescue for non-Hodgkin's lymphoma: Evaluation of event-free survival bases on histologic subtype and rescue product. Proc Am Soc Clin Oncol 11:318, 1992.

129. Tepler I, Cannistra SA, Frei E: Use of peripheral blood progenitor cells abrogates the myelotoxicity of repetitive outpatients high dose carboplatin and Cyclophosphamide chemotherapy. J Clin Oncol 11(8):1583-1591, 1993.

130. Haas R, Hohaus S, Egerer G, et al.: Recombinant human granulocyte macrophage colony stimulating factor (rhGM-CSF) subsequent to chemotherapy improves collection of blood stem cells for autografting in patients not eligible for bone marrow harvest. Bone Mar Transpl 9:459-465, 1992.

131. Ho AD, Gluck S, Germond C, et al.: Optimal timing for collections of blood progenitor cells following induction chemotherapy and granulocyte macrophage colony stimulating factor for autologous transplantation in advanced breast cancer. Bone Mar Transpl 6:269-275, 1992.

132. Shea TC, Mason JR, Storniolo AM, et al.: Sequential cycles of high dose carboplatin administered with recombinant human granulocyte macrophage colony stimulating factor and repeated infusions of autologous peripheral blood progenitor cells: A novel and effective method for delivering multiple courses of dose intensive therapy. J Clin Oncol 10:464-473, 1992.

133. Kritz A, Crown JP, Motzer RJ, et al.: Beneficial impact of peripheral blood progenitor cells in patients with metastatic breast cancer treated with high dose chemotherapy plus granulocyte macrophage colony stimulating factor: A randomized trial. Cancer 71(8):2515-2521, 1993.

134. Ho AD, Haas R, Korbbling M, et al.: Utilization of recombinant human GM-CSF to enhance peripheral progenitor cell yield for autologous transplantation. Bone Marrow Transplant 7:13-17, 1991.

135. Peters WP, Rosner G, Ross M, et al.: Comparative effects of granulocyte macrophage colony stimulating factor (GM-CSF) and granulocyte colony stimulating factor (G-CSF) on priming peripheral blood progenitor cells for use with autologous bone marrow after high dose chemotherapy. Blood 81(7):1709-1719, 1993.

136. Rosenfeld C, Bolwell B, LeFever A, et al.: Comparison of four cytokine regimens for mobilization of peripheral blood stem cells: IL-3 alone and combined with GM-CSF or G-CSF. Bone Marrow Transplant 17(2):179-183, 1996.

137. Motoyoshi T, Takaku F: Human monocyte colony stimulating factor (hM-CSF), Phase I/II clinical studies. In: Mertelsmann R, Hermann F (eds.) Hematolpoietic growth factors in clinical applications. New York: Marcel Dekker pp:161-175, 1990.

138. Masaoka T, Motohoshi K, Takaku F, et al.: Administration of human urinary colony stimulating factor after bone marrow transplantation. Bone Marrow Transplant 3:121-127, 1988.

139. Masaoka T, Shibata H, Ohno R, et al.: Double blind test of human urinary macrophage colony stimulating factor for allogeneic and syngeneic bone marrow transplantation: Effectiveness of

treatment and 2-year follow-up for relapse of leukemia. Br J Haematol 76:501-505, 1990.

140. Ohno R, Miyawaki S, Hatake K, et al.: Macrophage colony stimulating factor (M-CSF) reduces the incidence and duration of febrile neutropenia and shortens the period required to finish three courses of intensive consolidation therapy in acute myeloid leukemia (AML): A double-blind controlled study [abstract]. Blood 86(10):266, 1995.

141. Nemunaitis J, Meyers D, Buckner CD, et al.: Phase I trial of recombinant human macrophage colony stimulating factor in patients with invasive fungal infections. Blood 78(4):907-913, 1991.

142. Nemunaitis J, Dorsy KS, Appelbaum FR, et al.: Long-term follow-up of patients with invasive fungal disease who received adjunctive therapy with recombinant human macrophage colony stimulating factor. Blood 82(5):1422-1427, 1993.

Index

Acquired immunodeficiency syndrome (AIDS): 128, 209
Acute respiratory distress syndrome (ARDS): 128
Adherence: 63, 64, 122, 124, 180, 227, 358, 365
Adhesion molecules: 65, 358
Alkylating agents: 139
Anemia: 143, 187, 188
    associated with cancer: 187, 188, 192, 193, 198, 201, 202, 205, 208, 320
    associated with chronic disease (ACD): 187, 191, 194, 195
    associated with end stage renal disease: 199, 207, 209
    associated with iron deficiency: 187, 192, 195, 248
Antibody-dependent cellular cytotoxicity (ADCC): 126, 180, 346-348, 350
Apheresis: 179, 181, 182, 270, 347, 348, 350, 372, 375
Aplastic anemia (AA): 37, 253, 326, 332-335, 342
Apoptosis: 9, 13, 66, 127

Bacteremia: 171
Basophils: 27
Bioreactor: 63
Bone marrow harvesting: 371
Bone marrow reserve: 349
Breast cancer: 144, 145, 240, 242, 245, 247, 249, 282, 286, 289, 301, 349, 373, 375, 382, 383, 385
Burst forming units-erythroid (BFU-E): 20, 66, 189, 331, 343, 370
Burst forming units-megakaryocyte (BFU-MK): 220

C-kit: 21, 245, 346, 361
C-kit receptor: 246
C-mpl: 27, 224, 225
C-mpl ligand: 224, 231, 269, 271

Carboplatin: 273
Carmustine: 203
CD3-CD4-CD8- cells: 75
CD4+ cells: 77
CD4-CD8- cells: 345
CD8+ cells: 77
CD14: 127
CD16: 77
CD34: 66, 344
CD34+ cells: 59, 66, 121, 344, 348, 350, 358, 370, 371, 376
CD34- cells: 372
CD34+ CD33-: 362
CD34+ Th1+: 344, 346
CD34+CD71-: 349
CD34+CD38- cells: 59, 60, 61, 67, 220
CD34+CD38+ cells: 67
CD40 Ligand: 32
CD44: 358
CD45RA: 79
CD45RO: 79
CD56: 77
CD64: 124
Cell adhesion molecule (CAM): 56, 64
Chemokines: 251, 358, 362
    receptors: 11
Chemotherapy:
    dose dense: 145, 349
    dose escalation: 145, 381, 383
    dose intensity: 139, 140, 145, 168, 279, 280-289, 291, 294, 317 , 382
    high-dose sequential: 303
    resistance: 281
    with stem cell support: 288, 300-302
Chimeric molecule: 105
Cisplatin: 188, 202
Clonogenic assays: 57
Cobblestone area forming cell (CAFC): 345
Colon cancer: 144
Colony-forming units (CFU): 343,

circulating colony-forming units (CFU-C): 362-364
colony-forming units-granulocyte-macrophage (CFU-GM): 20, 58, 66, 343, 346, 349, 370, 376
colony-forming unit granulocyte erythrocyte macrophage (CFU-GEMM): 20, 66
colony-forming unit-MK (CFU-MK): 20, 220, 242, 370
colony-forming unit-spleen (CFU-S): 37, 362, 369, 370
colony stimulating factors (CSF): 137, 139, 145, 279, 326, 328, 334, 381
Cord blood: 62, 346, 369
Cost: 138, 139, 147, 150, 151, 210, 211, 254
analysis: 151, 152
effectiveness: 151, 155, 169
Cyclins: 229, 230
Cytarabine: 328

Daniplestim: 92, 95, 96, 250
Delta (pre-CFU): 58
Dendritic cells: 58
Diamond-Blackfan anemia (DBA): 326, 335
Donation
autologous blood: 206
platelets: 253, 270

Economic analyses: 156
Endotoxin: 25
Engraftment: 349, 369-371, 373, 376, 382, 383, 387, 388, 390
Eosinophils: 26
Erythropoiesis: 13, 19, 189, 190, 194, 195, 202
Erythropoietin (EPO): 2, 3, 13, 20, 27, 102, 103, 137, 141, 143, 146, 187, 188, 191, 193, 198-201, 203, 206, 209-211, 218, 292, 320, 326, 331, 374
dose schedule: 203, 207
level: 192, 199, 201-203, 321
receptors: 13, 21

response: 208
Ex vivo manipulations: 56, 57, 349, 370
Ex vivo expanded cells: 56, 58, 63, 82, 109, 120
Extracellular matrix: 218, 227, 357

Fanconi anemia: 37, 326, 335
Fas: 13, 17, 18
Ferritin: 208
Fibronectin: 65, 66, 228, 358
Filgrastim (G-CSF): 97, 140, 142, 272, 274, 373, 375-377
Flt-3 ligand (FL): 6, 22, 36, 37, 59, 68, 82, 251, 359-364, 373, 377
levels: 37

Germ cell tumors: 282, 288, 289
Granulocyte colony-forming stimulating factor (G-CSF): 3, 22, 25, 98-101, 118, 119, 120, 122, 125, 137, 142, 143, 166, 168, 170, 179, 181, 283, 285, 287, 289, 294, 313, 315, 316, 319, 326, 328, 332, 333, 335, 347, 358-363, 373, 381, 383-386, 394
levels: 121
G-CSF R: 25, 120, 361-364
Granulocyte-macrophage colony-forming stimulating factor (GM-CSF): 2, 3, 22, 25, 118, 119, 120, 122, 125, 137, 142, 143, 168, 171, 173, 174, 179, 181, 243, 244, 249, 279, 292, 293, 313, 314, 318, 326, 330, 332, 335, 347, 358-360, 373, 381, 386-392
GM-CSF R: 22
Graft engineering: 371
Graft failure: 387
Graft-vs-host disease (GVHD): 79, 81, 345, 387, 390, 392
Granulocyte transfusions: 178, 179
Granulopoiesis: 22, 23

Hematopoietic growth factors (HGF): 9, 56, 90, 179, 316
receptors: 12, 64, 65
chemokines: 11

receptors with cytoplasmic tyrosine kinase domains: 11, 15, 82
    Type I: 9, 10
    Type II: 11, 16
    TNF-R: 11
Hematopoietic progenitor cells (HPC): 56, 341-345, 347-349, 358, 361, 364, 365
Hematopoietic reconstitution:
Hemorrhage: 138, 327
High proliferative potential (HPP) colonies: 57, 220
Hodgkin's disease: 81, 154, 282, 349, 376, 385
4-hydroperoxycyclophosphamide (4HC): 62
Hypoxia: 188, 193, 199

Infection: 121, 138, 143, 159, 161, 170, 178, 180, 314, 317, 327, 329, 346 387-389, 393, 394
Insulin-like growth factor-1 (IGF-1): 3, 21, 22
Integrins: 65, 124, 358
Interferons : 77, 191, 224
    interferon-α: 81, 251, 252
    interferon-γ: 80, 81
Interleukins:
    IL-1: 7, 22, 25, 38, 39, 80, 81, 191, 224, 250, 360
    IL-2: 5, 30, 32, 77, 79, 80
    IL-3: 6, 22, 27, 36, 91, 93, 95, 96, 118, 122, 189, 218, 223, 242-244, 320, 330, 333, 335, 358, 360, 373, 390, 394
    IL-3 receptor agonist: 105
    IL-4: 5, 33, 34, 77, 79
    IL-5: 4, 26, 79
    IL-6: 7, 27, 29, 38, 109, 110, 218, 224, 243, 244, 247, 254, 320, 330, 360
    IL-7: 5, 30, 75, 78, 359, 360
    IL-8: 8, 359-362, 364
    IL-9: 7, 37
    IL-10: 5, 30, 33
    IL-11: 4, 22, 27, 28, 29, 146, 218, 224, 238, 240, 241, 242, 254, 320, 360
    IL-11Rα: 240
    IL-12: 6, 33, 34, 79, 359, 360, 362-364
    IL-13: 6, 34
    IL-14: 6, 35
    IL-15: 5, 32, 79
    IL-16: 6, 35
    IL-17: 8, 39, 40
    IL-18: 8, 40
Iron: 187, 190, 191, 196, 208

Jak/stat: 13

Lenograstim: 97
Leukemia: 138, 140, 146, 165, 205, 313
    acute leukemia: 166, 253
    acute lymphoblastic leukemia (ALL): 171, 253, 316
    acute myelogenous leukemia (AML): 153, 253, 303, 314-316, 318-320, 326, 327, 349, 392
    chronic myelogenous leukemia (CML): 81
Leukemia inhibitory factor (LIF): 27, 223, 250
Lipopolysaccharide: 127
Long-term culture initiating cells (LTC-IC): 37, 62, 82, 344, 370, 373
Lung cancer: 188, 271, 282, 284, 286, 288, 289, 375, 381
Lymphocytes:
    B cells: 32
    T cells: 32, 74, 76, 78-81, 341
Lymphoma, non-Hodgkin's (NHL): 140, 153, 170, 243, 247, 273, 282, 288, 294, 301, 303-308, 349, 376, 382, 385, 387
Lymphopoiesis: 30, 31

Macrophage: 25, 191

Macrophage inflammatory protein (MIP): 359

Megakaryoblast: 222

Megakaryocyte growth and development factor (MGDF): 60, 100, 269, 270-275, 320

Megakaryocytes: 28, 60, 221, 222, 237

Megakaryocytopoiesis: 27, 218-221, 223, 229, 251

Melphalan: 349

Mobilization: 180, 181, 341, 346
    CD34 cells: 180, 247, 274, 346-351, 358-365, 369, 372-377, 383, 385, 390, 392-394
    neutrophils: 180-183, 359, 363

Monocyte-macrophage colony-stimulating factor (M-CSF): 2, 4, 22, 25, 118, 122
381, 392, 394, 395

M-CSF R: 26

Monocyte function: 25, 124, 191, 314

Myelodysplasia: 140, 249, 253, 320, 326-332

Mucositis: 390

Multiple myeloma: 81, 140, 294, 376, 385

Myelopoietins: 105, 107, 108, 250

Myelosuppression: 37, 138, 141, 290, 317, 326, 327, 383, 386

Nartograstim: 96

Natural killer cells (NK): 32, 74, 77, 82

Neuroblastoma: 385

Neutropenia: 138, 151, 159, 161, 162, 170, 178, 180, 314, 315, 349

Neutropenic fever: 138, 142, 146, 153, 159-168, 171, 172, 173, 175, 279, 381, 383, 393

Neutrophils: 22, 118, 119, 361
    apoptosis: 127
    chemokinesis: 123
    engraftment:
    function: 123, 180
    margination:
    priming: 126, 181

Opreleukin: 254

Oncostatin-M: 250

Ovarian cancer: 284, 392

Pancytopenia:

Pegylation: 97, 98

Peripheral blood progenitor cells (PBPC): 154, 181, 351, 357, 369, 372,
373, 381, 382, 385, 390

Phagocytosis: 24, 124, 180

Pixykine (PIXIE321): 104, 106, 244, 245, 386

Platelets: 27, 28, 222, 350
    collection: 270, 271
    function: 273, 274
    mass: 225
    recovery: 272

Platelet factor 4 (PF4): 224, 251

Pneumonia: 171

Pre-CFCs: 20

Promegakaryoblasts (ProMKBs): 221

Promegapoietin: 251

Prophylaxis (of neutropenic infection): 141, 144, 152
    primary: 142, 144, 174, 279
    secondary: 142, 144, 279, 382

Protein engineering: 91

Public policy: 155

Quality of life: 143, 146, 150, 151, 188, 200, 209, 211, 320

Radiotherapy: 349

Recruitment: 57, 67

Retinoids: 328

Sarcoma: 245

Sargramostim (GM-CSF): 143, 314, 373

Severe combined immunodeficiency (SCID): 78
    mouse: 370

Selectins: 124, 358
    L-selectin: 122
    P-selectin: 66, 273

Sialomucins: 66, 67
Solid tumors : 138, 139, 144, 166, 168, 205, 244, 253, 282, 284, 369
Steel factor (SF): 3, 20, 22, 27
Stem cell factor (SCF): 68, 189, 218, 224, 245, 358, 360, 361, 373, 374
Stromal cell microenvironment: 56, 62, 191, 225, 364
Stromal cells: 218, 227, 357, 358
Stromal cell derived factor-1: 358
Supportive care: 341, 342
Synergy: 57, 59, 118, 223, 240, 243, 251, 361, 374

T cell receptors: 75
TGF-β: 20, 224, 251
Th1 response:
Th2 response:
Thrombocytopenia: 138, 224, 225, 249, 253, 272, 273, 320
Thrombocytosis: 248
Thrombopoiesis: 239
Thrombopoietin (TPO): 4, 27, 28, 29, 60, 68, 218, 224, 226, 231, 237, 240, 254, 269, 274, 320, 359, 360
   levels: 27, 225
   TPO-R: 27, 225, 226
Thrombospondin: 228
Thymus: 74
Tumor necrosis factor (TNF):
   TNF-α: 7, 25, 39, 80, 191
Topotecan: 328
Toxicities:
   EPO: 204, 205
   G-CSF: 140, 289, 290, 321, 329, 334, 381
   GM-CSF: 140, 249, 292, 315, 321, 334, 373
   IL-3: 243
   IL-6: 248, 249, 254
   IL-11: 241
   MGDF: 275
   PIXIE321: 245, 387
   SCF: 247, 374-376
   TPO: 275
Transferrin: 191, 194, 195

Transfusion: 198
   platelets: 241, 252, 253, 254
   red cells: 206, 208, 210
Transplantation: 139
   allogeneic: 327, 341, 343, 369, 382, 387, 391
   autologous: 154, 343
   bone marrow (ABMT): 143, 155, 242, 273, 282, 305, 343, 345, 382, 386, 388, 389
   stem cell (ASCT): 155, 253, 273, 282, 343, 345, 382

VCAM-1: 65
VLA-4: 65, 66, 358, 359, 361
   antibody: 360
VLA-5: 65, 66, 358